Dr Agarwals' Textbook on
CORNEAL TOPOGRAPHY
Including Pentacam and Anterior Segment OCT

Dr Agarwals' Textbook on
CORNEAL TOPOGRAPHY
Including Pentacam and Anterior Segment OCT

THIRD EDITION

Editor
Amar Agarwal
MS FRCS FRCOphth
Chairman and Managing Director
Dr Agarwal's Group of Eye Hospitals
and Eye Research Center
Chennai, Tamil Nadu, India

Foreword
Bonnie An Henderson

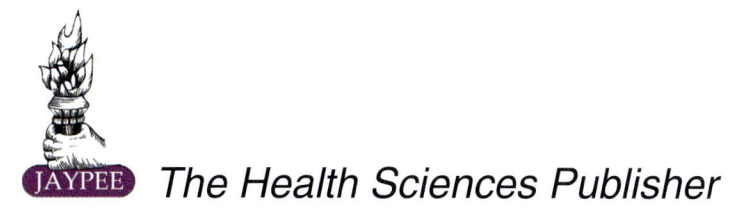

JAYPEE The Health Sciences Publisher

New Delhi | London | Philadelphia | Panama

Jaypee Brothers Medical Publishers (P) Ltd.

Headquarters
Jaypee Brothers Medical Publishers (P) Ltd.
4838/24, Ansari Road, Daryaganj
New Delhi 110 002, India
Phone: +91-11-43574357
Fax: +91-11-43574314
E-mail: jaypee@jaypeebrothers.com

Overseas Offices

J.P. Medical Ltd.
83, Victoria Street, London
SW1H 0HW (UK)
Phone: +44 20 3170 8910
Fax: +44 (0)20 3008 6180
E-mail: info@jpmedpub.com

Jaypee-Highlights Medical Publishers Inc.
City of Knowledge, Bld. 237, Clayton
Panama City, Panama
Phone: +1 507-301-0496
Fax: +1 507-301-0499
E-mail: cservice@jphmedical.com

Jaypee Medical Inc.
The Bourse
111, South Independence Mall East
Suite 835, Philadelphia, PA 19106, USA
Phone: +1 267-519-9789
E-mail: jpmed.us@gmail.com

Jaypee Brothers Medical Publishers (P) Ltd.
17/1-B, Babar Road, Block-B
Shaymali, Mohammadpur
Dhaka-1207, Bangladesh
Mobile: +08801912003485
E-mail: jaypeedhaka@gmail.com

Jaypee Brothers Medical Publishers (P) Ltd.
Bhotahity, Kathmandu, Nepal
Phone: +977-9741283608
E-mail: kathmandu@jaypeebrothers.com

Website: www.jaypeebrothers.com
Website: www.jaypeedigital.com

© 2015, Jaypee Brothers Medical Publishers

The views and opinions expressed in this book are solely those of the original contributor(s)/author(s) and do not necessarily represent those of editor(s) of the book.

All rights reserved. No part of this publication may be reproduced, stored or transmitted in any form or by any means, electronic, mechanical, photocopying, recording or otherwise, without the prior permission in writing of the publishers.

All brand names and product names used in this book are trade names, service marks, trademarks or registered trademarks of their respective owners. The publisher is not associated with any product or vendor mentioned in this book.

Medical knowledge and practice change constantly. This book is designed to provide accurate, authoritative information about the subject matter in question. However, readers are advised to check the most current information available on procedures included and check information from the manufacturer of each product to be administered, to verify the recommended dose, formula, method and duration of administration, adverse effects and contraindications. It is the responsibility of the practitioner to take all appropriate safety precautions. Neither the publisher nor the author(s)/editor(s) assume any liability for any injury and/or damage to persons or property arising from or related to use of material in this book.

This book is sold on the understanding that the publisher is not engaged in providing professional medical services. If such advice or services are required, the services of a competent medical professional should be sought.

Every effort has been made where necessary to contact holders of copyright to obtain permission to reproduce copyright material. If any have been inadvertently overlooked, the publisher will be pleased to make the necessary arrangements at the first opportunity.

Inquiries for bulk sales may be solicited at: jaypee@jaypeebrothers.com

Dr Agarwals' Textbook on Corneal Topography Including Pentacam and Anterior Segment OCT

First Edition: **2006**

Second Edition: **2010**

Third Edition: **2015**

ISBN: 978-93-5152-785-5

Printed at Replika Press Pvt. Ltd.

Dedicated to

Sonia Yoo
a wonderful Surgeon
and human being

CONTRIBUTORS

Ahmad MM Shalaby MD
Instituto Oftalmologico De Alicante
Alicante, Spain

Amar Agarwal MS FRCS FRCOphth
Chairman and Managing Director
Dr Agarwal's Group of Eye Hospitals
and Eye Research Center,
Chennai, Tamil Nadu, India

Amin Ashrafzadeh MD
Northern California Eye Physicians
Modesto and Turlock, CA
Assistant Clinical Professor of
Ophthalmology
University of California
Davis, USA

Arun C Gulani MD MS
Director
Gulani Vision Institute
Jacksonville, Florida, USA

Athiya Agarwal MD FRSH DO
Dr Agarwal's Group of Eye Hospitals
and Eye Research Center
Chennai, Tamil Nadu
India

Cristina Simón-Castellvi MD
Simon Eye Clinic
Barcelona, Spain

David P Piñero PhD
Instituto Oftalmologico De Alicante
Alicante, Spain

Dhivya Ashok Kumar MD
Dr Agarwal's Group of Eye Hospitals
and Eye Research Center
Chennai, Tamil Nadu, India

Erik L Mertens MD FEBO
Medical Director
Antwerp Eye Center
Belgium

Francisco Sánchez León MD
Instituto NovaVision
Medical Director
Cornea, Refractive and Anterior
Segment Clinic
Cd de México, Acapulco
Mexico

Gemma Walsh B Optom
New Vision Clinics
Melbourne, Australia

Gregg Feinerman MD FACS
Feinerman Vision Center
Newport Beach
California
Associate Professor
University of California, Irvine
California, USA

Guillermo L Simón-Castellvi MD
Chief Anterior Segment Surgeon
Refractive Surgery Unit
Simon Eye Clinic
Barcelona, Spain

Helen Boerman OD
Wang Vision Institute
Nashville, TN, USA

Hoo Yeun Kim
Feinerman Vision Center
Newport Beach
California, USA

Jairo E Hoyos MD PhD
Chairman of Ophthalmology of the
Instituto Oftalmológico Hoyos
KM Study Group
President Sabadell
Barcelona, Spain

Jairo Hoyos-Chacón MD
Ophthalmologist of the
Instituto Oftalmológico Hoyos
Sabadell, Barcelona, Spain

Jorge L Alió MD PhD
Instituto Oftalmologico De Alicante
Alicante, Spain

José I Belda Sanchis MD PhD
Instituto Oftalmologico De Alicante
Alicante, Spain

José Maria Simón-Castellvi MD
Chairman
Simon Eye Clinic
Barcelona, Spain

Karolinne Maia Rocha MD PhD
Cleveland Clinic Foundation
Cole Eye Institute, USA

Laurent Laroche
Center Hospitalier National
d'Ophtalmologie des XV-XX, Pierre and
Marie Curie University
Paris 06, Research Team 968, Institut de la
Vision, Paris, France

Marcus Solorzano
USA

Masanao Fujieda MA
Nidek Ltd, Co, Japan

Melania Cigales MD
Ophthalmologist of the Instituto
Oftalmológico Hoyos
Sabadell
Barcelona, Spain

Ming Wang MD PhD
Wang Vision Institute
Nashville, TN, USA

Mohamad Rosman MD FRCS(Ed) FAMS
Instituto Oftalmologico De Alicante
Alicante, Spain

Mohamed Alaa El-Danasoury MD
Magrabi Eye Hospital Jeddah
Saudi Arabia

Mukesh Jain PhD
Nidek Ltd, Co, Australia

N Timothy Peters MD
Clear Advantage Vision Correction Center
Portsmouth, New Hampshire, USA

Noel A Alpins MD FRACO FRCOphth FACS
University of Melbourne
Australia

Otman Sandali
Center Hospitalier National
d'Ophtalmologie des XV-XX, Pierre and
Marie Curie University
Paris 06, Research Team 968
Institut de la Vision
Paris, France

Paul Karpecki OD FARO
Director (Research)
Moyes Eye Center
Kansas City
USA

Roger F Steinert MD
Professor of Ophthalmology
Professor of Biomedical Engineering
Vice Chair of Clinical Ophthalmology
Director of Cornea, Refractive,
and Cataract Surgery
University of California
Irvine, California
USA

Ronald R Krueger MD MSE
Cleveland Clinic Foundation
Cole Eye Institute, USA

Sarabel Simón-Castellvi MD
Simon Eye Clinic
Barcelona, Spain

Shiela Scott MD
USA

Soosan Jacob MS FRCS DNB MNAMS
Dr Agarwal's Group of Eye Hospitals
and Eye Research Center
Chennai, Tamil Nadu
India

Tracy Schroeder Swartz OD MS FAAO
Wang Vision Institute
Nashville, TN, USA

Vincent Borderie
Center Hospitalier National
d'Ophtalmologie des XV-XX, Pierre and
Marie Curie University
Paris 06, Research Team 968
Institut de la Vision
Paris, France

FOREWORD

Being a surgeon is a humbling experience. While most surgeons are competent in their field, every surgeon will experience a horrible case or two. After suffering through a particularly difficult case, where my surgical performance was less than ideal (to put it kindly), I was in full self-flagellation mode. As I was sullenly licking my wounds, I happened to attend my first Dr Amar Agarwal lecture. If you have not heard Dr Agarwal lecture, you are in for a treat. It is a cross between a heart stopping thriller, a Cirque du Soleil performance of exceptional surgical skill, and a slap-stick comedy. Amar delivered a memorable lecture of surgical acrobatics complete with self-effacing and good-humored criticism.

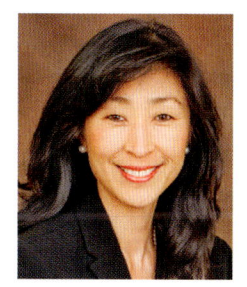

Amar Agarwal approaches life in this same manner. Always gracious and humble, he is the hardest working and most productive person that I know. He replies to emails almost instantaneously, at any hour of the day or night. I tried to test the hypothesis that he does not sleep by sending random emails at all hours. Without fail, he replies within minutes—even at 2 am in his native time zone. While traveling, I will often work-off my jet lag in the hotel fitness center in the off hours. The treadmill somehow seems more inviting when you cannot sleep in the middle of the night. Much to my delight, I often find Dr Agarwal as my sole workout partner.

When Amar asked me to write a foreword for the 3rd edition of *Textbook on Corneal Topography*, my first thought was "you are writing another book!". This will be his 60th textbook on ophthalmology. The book is a comprehensive reference tool for anterior segment surgeons. It helps readers to understand the currently available machine capabilities, differences, and highlights special uses. With the merging of the fields of cataract and refractive surgeries, anterior segment surgeons must be well-versed in understanding diagnostic technologies. The cornea, which by all accounts should be a simple tissue, is a difficult organ to understand and evaluate. Corneal topographies have been the gold standard to evaluate the anterior surface but new machines have been developed not only to evaluate this surface in more detail but also to evaluate the posterior and inner portions of the cornea. Using these technologies help determine the health of the cornea and thereby assess any surgical risk. These technologies assist in both the preoperative evaluation and the postoperative diagnosis of corneal abnormalities.

In the same fashion as his previous textbooks, Amar Agarwal delivers another complete but yet entertaining educational resource for ophthalmologists worldwide. Most people have a goal to have published the same number of articles as their age. Amar has raised that goal to another level and will have published not just articles but more full textbooks than his age. By the time you read this book, Dr Amar Agarwal will probably have written another 5 books.

Bonnie An Henderson MD
Ophthalmic Consultant
Boston, USA

PREFACE TO THE THIRD EDITION

To recapitulate the considerations that have led to the publication of the 3rd edition of *Textbook on Corneal Topography Including Pentacam and Anterior Segment OCT* are that the manual is prepared with the idea that revisions must be made periodically in order to have an available text that represents the status and details of corneal topography. The book provides a detailed text to assist with the interpretation and diagnosis of corneal surface disorders and also provides an up-to-date reference book for all the ophthalmologists. The editor hopes that this judicious compilation of work from various authors across the globe that highlights the fundamentals and the advanced stage disorders of cornea by topography analysis are well appreciated.

Amar Agarwal

PREFACE TO THE FIRST EDITION

Medical frontiers are never ending, there can be no end to division, the more you go deeper and deeper into any subject, the more we understand how little we know of it. "Multiplication ruins everything", says Lao-Tsu the author of Tao Te Ching.

However, we still need to understand the lakes, mountains and valleys of the corneal surface, for us to be able to understand how to modify the surface to suit the patients' refractive needs. Just as we understand the geography of the land by seeing from far its topography, so to the corneal surface.

Today, we not only use the topographical analysis for our LASIK cases, with our knowledge on relaxing incisions, we have stretched the doors to include cataract cases where incisions can be made to decrease the preoperative astigmatism. Wavefront technology heralds yet another dimension when the topography is fed into the LASIK machine to give us a customized ablation.

Aberrations have long played havoc with vision, and doctors world over have only now really understood where the problem really lies. The understanding has brought in better modalities of its treatment, we not only have LASIK treating aberrations, we have customized intraocular lenses taking the aberrations into consideration.

The same concept is also being used for the making of lens power to be fitted to spectacles where not only the spherical and cylindrical diopters are fed into lens power-cutting machines, they are surface modified to fit the aberration as well; thus, we come into an era of customized fittings of eyeglass power.

Authors from all over the world give you a taste of their facts and figures with their cohesive findings for topographical documentation and assessment. To grasp a meaning into this world of multicolored charts, we bring the textbook on corneal topography to keep on your desk, to enable you to read a picture effortlessly.

Sunita Agarwal
Athiya Agarwal
Amar Agarwal

CONTENTS

SECTION I: Introduction to Corneal Topography and Orbscan

1. Fundamentals on Corneal Topography 3
*Guillermo L Simón-Castellvi (Spain), Sarabel Simón-Castellvi (Spain),
José Maria Simón-Castellvi (Spain), Cristina Simón-Castellvi (Spain)*

Human Optics and the Normal Cornea *3* • Instruments to Measure
the Corneal Surface *4* • Topography Maps of the Normal Cornea *14*

2. Topographic Machines 22
*Guillermo L Simón-Castellvi (Spain), Sarabel Simón-Castellvi (Spain),
José Maria Simón-Castellvi (Spain), Cristina Simón-Castellvi (Spain)*

Zeiss Humphrey Systems® Atlas™ Corneal Topography System Models 993 and
Eclipse 995 *22* • Technomed® Color Ellipsoid Topometer *23* • Dicon® CT200 *23*
• Eyesys® 2000 *26* • KERATRON™ Corneal Topographer (Optikon 2000® SpA,
Italy-Europe) *26* • ET-800 Corneal Topography System *27* • Eye Map EH-290
Alcon® Corneal Topography System *27* • Tomey® Autotopographer *28*
• Oculus® Keratograph™ and Haag-Streit® Keratograph Ctk 922 *28*
• Orbscan IIz™ -Bausch And Lomb® Surgical, Inc. (USA) *30*

3. Corneal Topography and the Orbscan 33
Amar Agarwal (India), Athiya Agarwal (India)

Paraxial Optics *33* • Raytrace or Geometric Optics *33* • Elevation *33* • Orbscan I and II *34*
• Specular vs Back-Scattered Reflection *34* • Imaging in the Orbscan *35* • Map Colors Conventions *35*
• Analysis of the Normal Eye by the Orbscan Map *35* • Clinical Applications *37*

4. The Orbscan IIz Diagnostic System and Zywave Wavefront Analysis 40
*Gregg Feinerman (USA), N Timothy Peters (USA), Hoo Yeun Kim (USA),
Marcus Solorzano (USA), Shiela Scott (USA)*

Orbscan *40* • Quad Map *40* • Power Maps *42* • Pachymetry Map *42*
• Reading Corneal Elevation Maps *42* • Posterior Corneal Elevation Maps *43*
• Three Step Rule *44* • Preoperative Lasik Screening *46* • Middle Box *47*
• Orbscan Risk of Ectasia Indices *47* • Clinical Examples *49* • Zyoptix *57*

SECTION II: Orbscan and Refractive Surgery

5. Orbscan Corneal Mapping in Refractive Surgery 61
Francisco Sánchez León (Mexico)

Orbscan Corneal Mapping for Refractive Surgery Diagnostics *61* • Selection Criteria *66*

6. Anterior Keratoconus 71
Amar Agarwal (India), Athiya Agarwal (India)

Orbscan *71* • Technique *71* • Anterior Keratoconus *71* • Discussion *71*

7. **Posterior Corneal Changes in Refractive Surgery** — 76
   Amar Agarwal (India), Soosan Jacob (India), Athiya Agarwal (India)
   Topography 76 • Orbscan 76 • Primary Posterior Corneal Elevation 76 • Iatrogenic Keratectasia 80
   • Effect of Posterior Corneal Change on Intraocular Lens Calculation 82

8. **Corneal Ectasia Post-LASIK: The Orbscan Advantages** — 83
   Erik L Mertens (Belgium), Arun C Gulani (USA), Paul Karpecki (USA)
   Corneal Ectasia 83 • Selection Criteria 83 • Composite/Integrated Information 85
   • Future Thoughts 91

SECTION III: Pentacam and Anterior Segment Optical Coherence Tomography

9. **Pentacam** — 95
   Tracy Schroeder Swartz (USA)

10. **Evaluation of Patients for Refractive Surgery with Visante Anterior Segment OCT and the Combined Data Link with ATLAS Corneal Topographer** — 111
    Amin Ashrafzadeh (USA), Roger F Steinert (USA)
    Visante Anterior Segment Optical Coherence Tomography 111 • Atlas Corneal Topographer and the Visante 3.0 software 112 • LASIK Patients 112 • Phakic Intraocular Lenses 124

11. **Corneal Inflammation and Optical Coherence Tomography** — 130
    Dhivya Ashok Kumar (India), Amar Agarwal (India)
    Normal Corneal Texture 130 • Pathology In Corneal Inflammation 130
    • Role of OCT in Keratitis 130 • Advantage of OCT in Corneal Infiltration 132
    • As OCT for Prognosis 132 • As OCT Assessment for Surgery Plan 133

12. **Optical Coherence Tomography in Corneal Ectasia** — 135
    Otman Sandali (France), Vincent Borderie (France), Laurent Laroche (France)
    Keratoconus 135 • OCT in keratoconus screening 135 • OCT in Keratoconus Evaluation 135
    • OCT in the Follow-up of Keratoconus Treatments 137 • Intracorneal Rings Implantation 138
    • Corneal Keratoplasty 139 • Other corneal Ectatic Disorders 140 • Keratoglobus 142

13. **Spectral-domain Anterior Segment Optical Coherence Tomography in Refractive Surgery** — 143
    Karolinne Maia Rocha (USA), Ronald R Krueger (USA)
    Refractive Surgery Screening and Corneal Ectasia Risk Scoring System 143 • Epithelial Thickness Remodeling in Refractive Surgery 144 • LASIK Flap Mapping by Spectral-domain Optical Coherence Tomography 146 • Advances in Anterior Segment Biometry and Intraocular Lens Calculation 147
    • Advanced Spectral-domain Optical Coherence Tomography Imaging—Case Report 148

SECTION IV: Aberropia, Aberrations and Topography

14. **Corneal Topographers and Wavefront Aberrometers: Complementary Tools** — 155
    Tracy Schroeder Swartz (USA), Ming Wang (USA), Arun C Gulani (USA)
    Keratometers 155 • Corneal Topography 155 • Elevation Based Topography 156
    • Wavefront: Another View of Corneal Optics 156 • Cases 160

15. Aberrometry and Topography in the Vector Analysis of Refractive Laser Surgery — 168
Noel A Alpins (Australia), Gemma Walsh (Australia)

Measurement of Astigmatism *168* • Surgical Planning—Refraction, Topography, or Both? *168* • Vector Analysis by the Alpins Method *169* • Aberrometry and Wavefront Guided Treatment *169* • Treatment of Irregular Astigmatism *172*

16. Aberropia: A New Refractive Entity — 175
Amar Agarwal (India), Athiya Agarwal (India)

Materials and Methods *175* • Discussion *176*

17. Differences Between Various Aberrometer Systems — 184
Ronald R Krueger (USA)

Mapping a Profile of the Whole Eye *184* • Different Methods Available *184* • Wavefront Analysis in Conjunction with Corneal Topography *186* • Personalized LASIK Nomograms *186*

18. Corneal Wavefront Guided Excimer Laser Surgery for the Correction of Eye Aberrations — 187
Jorge L Alió (Spain), David P Piñero (Spain), Mohamad Rosman (Spain)

Impact of Higher-Order Aberrations *187* • Wavefront Guided Refractive Surgery *189* • Corneal Wavefront Guided Refractive Surgery *190* • Results of Corneal Wavefront Guided Refractive Surgery *191* • Methods *191* • Results *193* • Discussion *193* • Methods *193* • Results *194* • Discussion *195* • Methods *195* • Results *196* • Discussion *197* • Limitations of Corneal Wavefront Guided Refractive Surgery *197*

19. Ocular Higher Order Aberration Induced Decrease in Vision (Aberropia): Characteristics and Classification — 200
Amar Agarwal (India), Soosan Jacob (India), Dhivya Ashok Kumar (India), Athiya Agarwal (India)

Aberropia *200* • Case Report *200* • Discussion *203*

20. Topographic and Aberrometer Guided Laser — 209
Amar Agarwal (India), Athiya Agarwal (India)

Aberrations *209* • Zyoptix Laser *209* • Orbscan *209* • Aberrometer *209* • Zylink *210* • Results *210* • Discussion *211*

21. NAVWave: Nidek Technique for Customized Ablation — 214
Masanao Fujieda (Japan), Mukesh Jain (Australia)

OPD-Scan *214* • Topography and Wavefront Analyzer *214* • OPD Power Map *215* • OPD Power Map and Wavefront Map *216* • OPD Map and Corneal Topography Map *216* • Aligning Topography Data with OPD Data *217* • Measurement of Pupillary Diameter *217* • Final Fit Software: Outline and Features *217*

SECTION V: Refractive Procedures and Conditions

22. Post-LASIK Iatrogenic Ectasia — 223
Melania Cigales (Spain), Jairo Hoyos-Chacón (Spain), Jairo E Hoyos (Spain)

Subclinical Keratoconus *223* • Corneal Thickness Limits *229* • Keratectasia Treatments *232*

23. Decentered Ablations — 238
Helen Boerman (USA), Ming Wang (USA), Tracy Schroeder Swartz (USA)
Clinical Definition 238 • Topographic Decentration 238 • Wavefront Aberrations 238

24. Irregular Astigmatism: LASIK as a Correcting Tool — 251
Jorge L Alió (Spain), José I Belda Sanchis (Spain), Ahmad MM Shalaby (Spain)
Etiology of Irregular Astigmatism 251 • Diagnosis of Irregular Astigmatism 252 • Clinical Classification of Irregular Astigmatism Following Corneal Refractive Surgery 252 • Corneal Topography Patterns of Irregular Astigmatism 252 • Evaluation of Irregular Astigmatism 252 • Treatment of Irregular Astigmatism 255 • Surgical Techniques with Excimer Laser 255 • Selective Zonal Ablation (SELZA) 256 • Excimer Laser Assisted by Sodium Hyaluronate (ELASHY) 257 • Topographic Linked Excimer Laser Ablation (Topolink) 260 • The Future 261 • Other Procedures 262

25. Posterior Chamber ICL and Toric ICL — 264
Mohamed Alaa El-Danasoury (Saudi Arabia)
Evolution 264 • Indications of ICL and T-ICL 266 • Selection Criteria and Preoperative Assessment 266 • Surgical Techniques 269 • Postoperative Care 271 • Clinical Results 271 • Complications 277

26. Nidek OPD Scan in Clinical Practice — 283
Gregg Feinerman (USA), N Timothy Peters (USA), Hoo Yeun Kim (USA), Marcus Solorzano (USA), Shiela Scott (USA)
Nidek OPD Scan 283 • Clinical Examples 285

SECTION VI: Cataract

27. Corneal Topography in Cataract Surgery — 291
Athiya Agarwal (India), Amar Agarwal (India)
Cornea 291 • Keratometry 291 • Keratoscopy 292 • Computerized Videokeratography 292 • Orbscan 292 • Normal Cornea 292 • Cataract Surgery 293 • Extracapsular Cataract Extraction 294 • Nonfoldable IOL 294 • Foldable IOL 294 • Astigmatism Increased 294 • Basic Rule 296 • Unique Case 296 • Phakonit 296

28. Corneal Topography in Phakonit with a 5 mm Optic Rollable Intraocular Lens — 299
Amar Agarwal (India), Athiya Agarwal (India)
Rollable Intraocular Lens 299 • Surgical Technique 299 • Topographic Analysis and Astigmatism 300 • Microphakonit (Cataract Surgery through a 0.7 mm Tip) 300 • Discussion 302

29. Glued IOL Position: An OCT Assessment — 305
Dhivya Ashok Kumar (India), Amar Agarwal (India)
Background 305 • Technique 305 • Anterior Segment Optical Coherence Tomography 305 • IOL Tilt Estimation in OCT 306 • IOL Optic Position in Glued IOL 306 • Ocular Residual Astigmatism 306 • Scleral Apposition with Glue 307 • Glued Ion in Various Indications 307 • Comparison with Microscopic Tilt in Ultrasound Biomicroscopy 308 • Glued IOL Versus Sutured Scleral Fixated IOL 310

Index — 313

Section 1

Introduction to Corneal Topography and Orbscan

CHAPTERS

1. **Fundamentals on Corneal Topography**
2. **Topographic Machines**
3. **Corneal Topography and the Orbscan**
4. **The Orbscan IIz Diagnostic System and Zywave Wavefront Analysis**

Chapter 1

Fundamentals on Corneal Topography

Guillermo L Simón-Castellvi (Spain), Sarabel Simón-Castellvi (Spain)
José Maria Simón-Castellvi (Spain), Cristina Simón-Castellvi (Spain)

HUMAN OPTICS AND THE NORMAL CORNEA

The cornea is the highest diopter of human eye, accounting alone for about 43–44 diopters at corneal apex (about two thirds of the total dioptric power of the eye). It has an average radius of curvature of 7.8 mm. A healthy cornea is not absolutely transparent: It scatters almost 10% of the incident light, primarily due to the scattering at the stroma.

The corneal geography can be divided into four geographical zones from apex to limbus, which can be easily differentiated in color corneal videokeratoscopy:

1. *The central zone (4 central millimeters):* It overlies the pupil and is responsible for the high definition vision. The central part is almost spherical and called apex.
2. *The paracentral zone:* Where the cornea begins to flatten
3. The peripheral zone
4. The limbal zone.

Refractive surgery refers to a surgical or laser procedure performed on the cornea, to alter its refractive power. The major refractive component of the cornea being its front surface, it is not difficult to understand that most refractive techniques have involved this frontal surface (PRK, radial keratotomies, ...). Nevertheless, posterior surface of the cornea also accounts, and that is the reason why a "posterior surface corneal topographer" like the Orbscan™ - Bausch and Lomb® was developed by Orbtek®, in the race for a more precise refractive surgery.

The cornea of an eagle is almost as transparent as glass: There is almost no scattering of incident light. That alone explains the resolution of an eagle eye being much better than ours. As we are never satisfied, we are now developing new tools and extremely promising laser surgical techniques that have proven to increase human being visual acuity by reducing corneal aberrations: we reduce diopters and also improve visual acuity. The new dream is "supervision". Topographic and aberrometer-linked LASIK are on the way to achieve this goal of better-than-normal vision. Bausch and Lomb®'s *Zywave*™ combines topography and wavefront measurements to achieve customized computer controlled flying spot excimer laser ablation, which appears to be fundamental in treating irregular astigmatisms or retreating unsatisfied LASIK patients to regularize the corneal shape. Regularizing the corneal shape has the theoretical advantage of improving the quality of vision by means of reduction of halos, glare and any other optical aberrations. We are on the way to achieve an aberration-free visual system, though the influence of all other dioptric surfaces (vitreous, lens, ...) and interfaces still has to be ascertained **(Table 1.1)**.

In this chapter, we will try to introduce the novice to this interesting new world of instruments recently developed due to the advent of refractive corneal surgery. We have tried to show different maps from different systems, trying to make an interesting basic atlas of corneal topography. Corneal maps of rare cases and complications can be found in the different chapters of this book. Please refer to them for better knowledge. There is no perfect system to assess true corneal surface shape, but we still have to rely on the instruments we have, waiting for new instruments and methods being developed for better accuracy. With that goal in mind BioShape AG® has developed the *EyeShape*™ system, based on a principle called fringe projection. Patterns of parallel lines are first imaged onto a

Table 1.1 Indications and uses of corneal topographers

The use of computerized corneal topography is indicated in the following conditions:

1. Preoperative and postoperative assessment of the refractive patient
2. Preoperative and postoperative assessment of penetrating keratoplasty
3. Irregular astigmatism
4. Corneal dystrophies, bullous keratopathy
5. Keratoconus (diagnostic and follow-up)
6. Follow-up of corneal ulceration or abscess **(Figure 1.3)**
7. Post-traumatic corneal scarring
8. Contact lens fitting
9. Evaluation of tear film quality
10. Reference instrument for IOL-implants to see the corneal difference before and after surgery
11. To study unexplained low visual acuity after any surgical procedure (trabeculectomy, extracapsular lens extraction, ...).
12. Preoperative and postoperative assessment of Intacs™ corneal rings (intrastromal corneal rings)

reference and then onto the surface to be measured. Detection of the lines with a digital camera under a tilted angle yields distorted line patterns. The deviation of the detected lines from the original lines together with the tilt make it possible to calculate the absolute height at any point on the surface of the cornea (or not).

INSTRUMENTS TO MEASURE THE CORNEAL SURFACE

The normal corneal surface is smooth: A healthy tear film neutralizes corneal irregularities. The cornea, acting as a convex "almost transparent" mirror, reflects part of the incident light. Different instruments have been developed to assess and measure this corneal reflex. These noncontact instruments use a light target (lamp, mires, Placido discs, etc.) and a microscope or another optic system to measure corneal reflex of these light targets **(Tables 1.2 and 1.3)**.

Keratometry

A keratometer quantitatively measures the radius of curvature of different corneal zones of 3 mm (diameter). The present day keratometer allows the operator to precisely measure the size of the reflected image, converting the image size to corneal radius using a mathematical relation r = 2 a Y/y, where,

Table 1.2 Advantages and disadvantages of projection-based systems over reflection-based ones

Advantages
Measurement of direct corneal height
Ability to measure:
Irregular corneal surfaces
Nonreflective surfaces
Higher resolution (theoretical)
Uniform accuracy across the whole cornea
Less operator dependent
Do not suffer from spherical bias
Disadvantages
Not standard instruments (most are still prototypes):
Complex to use
Need clinical experience validation
Nonstandard presentation maps (more difficult to learn)
Longer examination time:
Longer image acquisition time
Longer image analysis
Fluorescein instillation needed (in some, like the Euclid Systems Corporation® ET-800™)

Table 1.3 Different methods of measuring corneal surface used by modern corneal topographers

Placido systems (small cone or large disc) are the most popular
Placido cone with arc-step mapping (Keratron™ from Optikon 2000®)
Placido's disc with arc-step mapping (Zeiss Humphrey® Atlas™)
Slit-lamp topo-pachymetry (Orbscan™ - Bausch and Lomb®)
Fourier profilometry (Euclid Systems Corporation® ET-800™)
Fringe projection or Moiré interference fringes (EyeShape® from BioShape AG™)
Triangulation ellipsoid topometry (Technomed™ color ellipsoid topometer)
Laser interferometry (experimental method, it records the interference pattern generated on the corneal surface by the interference of two lasers or coherent wave fronts)

 r : anterior corneal radius
 a : distance from mire to cornea (75 mm in kerotometer)
 Y : *image size*
 y : *mire size (64 mm in keratometer)*

The keratometer can convert from corneal radius r (measured in meters) into refracting power RP (in Diopters) using the relationship:

$$RP = 337.5/r$$

Modern—automated or not-keratometers also known as ophthalmometers directly convert from radius to diopters and inversely. They are mainly used to calculate the power of intraocular lenses through different formulas (Hoffer, SRK-T, SRK-II, Holladay, Enrique del Rio and S Simón, ...). Although the theory of measuring corneal reflex may appear to be simple, it is not, since eye movement, decentration or any tear film deficiency may make it difficult to measure accurately, thus creating errors. Modern video methods (topographers) can freeze the reflected cornea image, and perform the measurements once the image is captured on the video or computer screen, allowing greater precision. Notice that most traditional keratometers perform measurements of the central 3 mm, while computerized topographers can cover almost the whole corneal surface.

Keratoscopy or Photokeratoscopy

It is a method to evaluate qualitatively the reflected light on the corneal surface. The projected light may be a simple flash lamp or a Placido's disc target, which is a series of concentric rings (10 or 12 rings) or a tube (cone) with illuminated rings lining the inside surface. When we look at the keratoscope, an elliptical distortion of mires suggest astigmatism, and small, narrow and closely spaced mires suggest corneas that have high power (steep regions or short radius of curvature) **(Figure 1.1)**.

The use of keratoscopes is being abandoned in favor of computerized modern topographers which allow qualitative

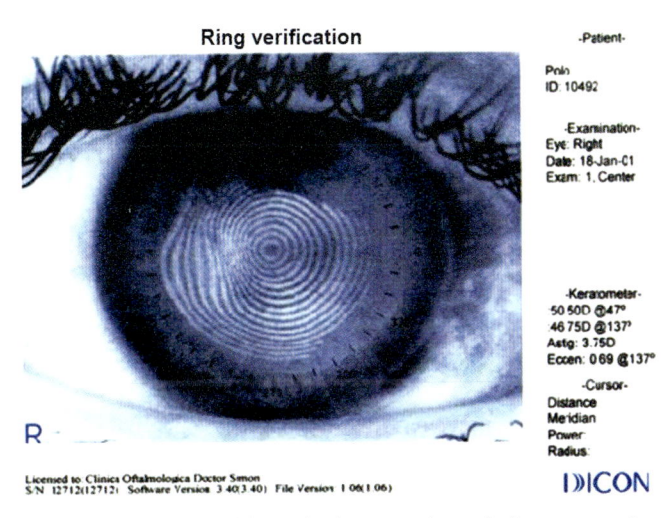

Figure 1.1 The "ring verification display" in modern videokeratoscopes is a static picture of what the explorer viewed at the keratoscope. Looking at the keratoscope, the explorer is able to evaluate qualitatively the corneal surface. In this case, notice the huge distortion of the mires on the temporal side of a right eye of a patient who underwent a keratoplasty for a keratoconus, and is wearing a soft plano-T therapeutic contact lens. The distortion of the mires is due to an irregularity at contact lens surface: air is in between the cornea and the lens

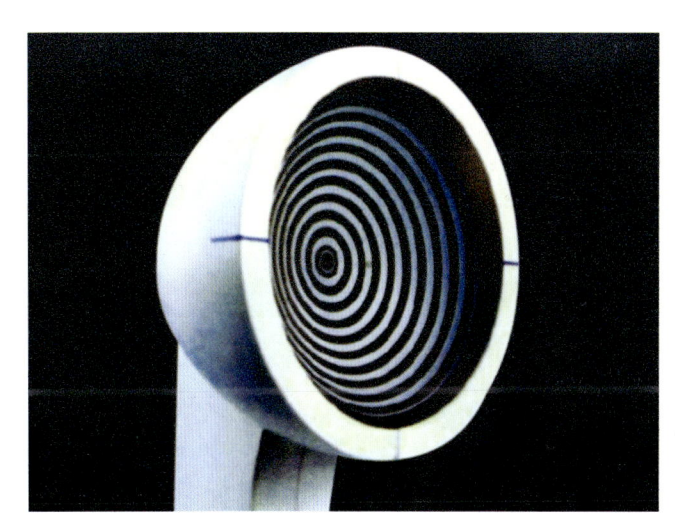

Figure 1.2 The Placido cone consists of a series of concentric dark and light rings in the configuration of a cone of different sizes depending on the number of rings and the manufacturer. Usually, it is better to have a large number of rings, since more corneal radius values can be measured. Notice that while describing the technical characteristics of videokeratographers some manufactures count both clear and dark rings, while others only count light ones. The mires of most systems exclude the very central cornea (where the video camera or CCD is located) and the paralimbal area. Picture shows a large cone of the Haag-Streit® Keratograph CTK 922™ with 22 rings (dark and light rings). (Published with permission from Haag-Streit® AG International)

and quantitative measurements of the corneal surface, with higher definition and accuracy (more than 20 rings), and more sensitivity in the peripheral cornea.

Some of the known deficiencies of the Placido's method are:
- It requires assumptions about the corneal shape
- It misses data on the central cornea (not all topographers)
- It is only able to acquire limited data points
- It measures slope not height.

Some more subjective complaints include:
- It is difficult to focus and align
- In most topographers, the patient is exposed to highlight.

Large Placido's disc systems work far away from the eye, while small Placido cones get much closer to the eye. While Placido's disc systems easily create shadows caused by the nose and brow blocking the light of the rings, small cone systems fit under the brow and beside the nose, avoiding shadows, but can get in contact with large noses and make the patient blink and be afraid. Most small cones have a reputation for difficult focusing: Some manufacturers—like Optikon 2000®—have worked out worthwhile automatic capture devices for improved accuracy, precision, and repeatability of measurements.

Computerized Videokeratoscopy: Modern Corneal Topographers

Corneal topography has gained wide acceptance as a clinical examination procedure with the advent of modern laser refractive surgery. It has many advantages over traditional keratometers or keratoscopes: They measure a greater area of the cornea with a much higher number of points and produce permanent records that can be used for follow-up.

Basically, a projection corneal topographer consists of a Placido's disc or cone (large or small) that illuminates the cornea by sending a mire of concentric rings, a video camera that captures the corneal reflex from the tear layer and a computer and software that perform the analysis of the data through different computer algorithms. The computer evaluates the distance between a series of concentric rings of light and darkness in a variable number of points. The shorter the distance, the higher the corneal power, and inversely. Final results can be printed in colors or black-and-white.

The Placido's disc **(Figure 1.2)** consists of a series of concentric dark and light rings in the configuration of a disk or a cone, of different sizes, depending on the number of rings and the manufacturer. Usually, it is better to have a large number of rings, since more corneal radius values can be measured. The mires of most systems exclude the very central cornea and the paralimbal area.

The reproducibility of videokeratography measurements is mainly dependent on the accuracy of manual adjustment in the focal plane. Videokeratoscopes having small Placido cones show a considerable amount of error when the required working distance between cornea and keratoscope is not maintained. The advantages of small cones (optimal illumination and the reduction of anatomically caused shadows) are in no proportion to the disadvantage—poor depth of focus, resulting in poor reproducibility. Which one should you choose, a small Placido cone or large Placido's disc? Not

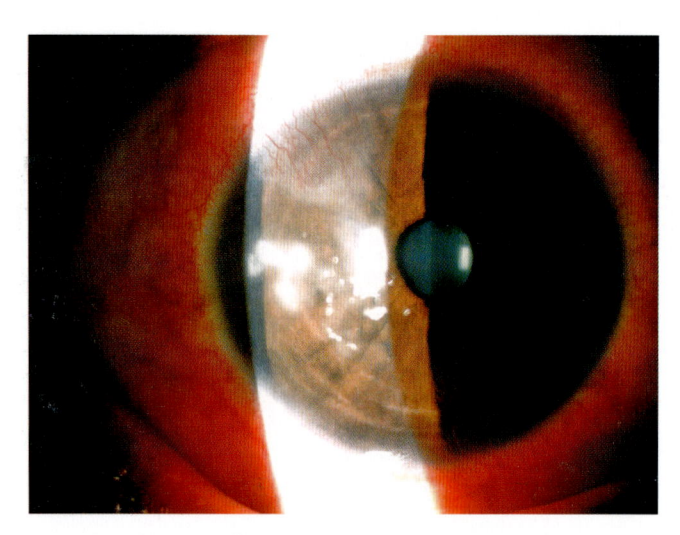

Figure 1.3 There are different methods of following the clinical course of a corneal ulceration or corneal abscess. While daily slit-lamp examination and daily photographs are invaluable, corneal topographic maps, being less "explorer dependant", can also be very useful in the follow-up. (*Courtesy: Dr Agarwal's Eye Hospital*)

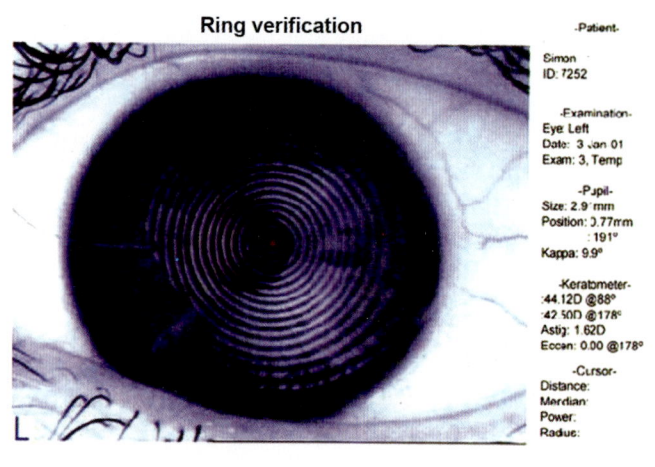

Figure 1.4 With large Placido's disc topographers, large eyelashes project shadows on the superior cornea: The topographer will be unable to accurately perform the map of that zone. Danger is that extrapolation performed by some systems distorts the true map of the paracentral cornea. Trichiatic cilia projects a shadow that may interfere with the mapping. This situation should be addressed prior to corneal topography

easy to answer: Each family of topographers has advantages and disadvantages. Being no ideal instrument, topographer potential buyers will have to decide upon other important factors, like software ability to exactly reproduce real corneal height, number of rings, price, ...

There are two main groups of corneal topographers: Those which use the principle of reflection (most), and those which use the principle of projection.

Let's notice that the image captured by most topographers is produced by the thin tear layer covering the cornea that almost reproduces the shape or contour of the corneal surface. Most instruments perform indirect measurements of the corneal surface (*reflection technique*) and extrapolate to know the height of each point of the cornea. Reflection techniques amplify the corneal topographic distortions **(Figure 1.3)**.

Euclid Systems Corporation® ET-800 uses a completely different method of topography called Fourier profilometry using filtered blue light that induces fluorescence of a liquid that has been applied to the tear film before the examination. This *projection technique* visualizes the surface directly while a reflection technique amplifies the corneal topographic distortions.

Causes of Artefacts of the Corneal Topography Map

- Shadows on the cornea from large eyelashes *or* trichiasis **(Figure 1.4)**
- Ptosis or nonsufficient eye opening **(Figure 1.5)**
- Irregularities of the tear film layer (dry eye, mucinous film, greasy film) **(Figure 1.6)**
- Too short working distance of the small Placido disc cone
- Incomplete or distorted image (corneal pathology) **(Figures 1.7A and B)**.

Understanding and Reading Corneal Topography

The meaningful interpretation of topographic maps requires the examiner to have detailed knowledge and clinical experience on the patterns detailed in them. At first, one must understand how to read the color scales. The untrained eye may find some confusion and sometimes misinterpretation in evaluating corneal maps. Modern topographers (videokeratographers) use the Louisiana State University Color-Coded Map to display corneal superficial powers. The power values (measured in diopters) are preferred by clinicians over the radius values (measured in millimeters), although all topographers can map the corneas using both values.

Projection-based topography systems, adopted a similar color scale to represent their height maps. High areas are depicted by warm colors, while low areas are depicted by cool colors.

The Louisiana State University Color—Coded Map

Colors correspond to the following:

Cool colors (violets and blues): Low powers. They correspond to flat curvatures (low diopter)

Greens and yellows: Colors found in the normal corneas

Warm or hot colors (oranges and reds): Higher powers. They correspond to steep curvatures (high diopter).

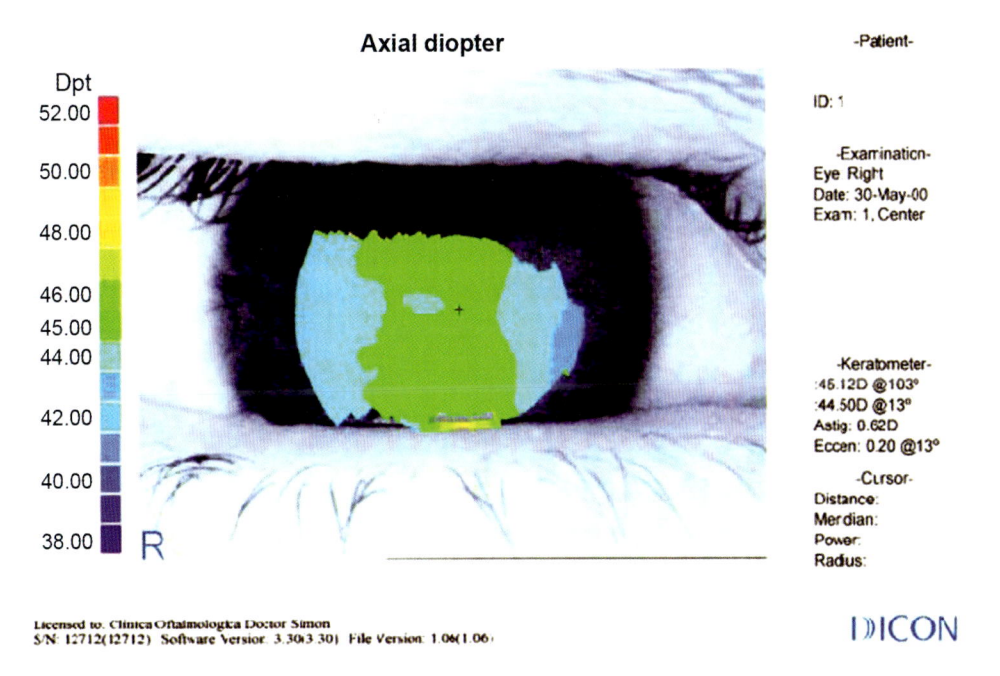

Chapter 1: Fundamentals on Corneal Topography 7

Figure 1.5 Ptosis or nonsufficient eye opening because of induced photophobia or patient anxiety limits and distorts the mapping of the cornea. Notice that the map is not round but oval

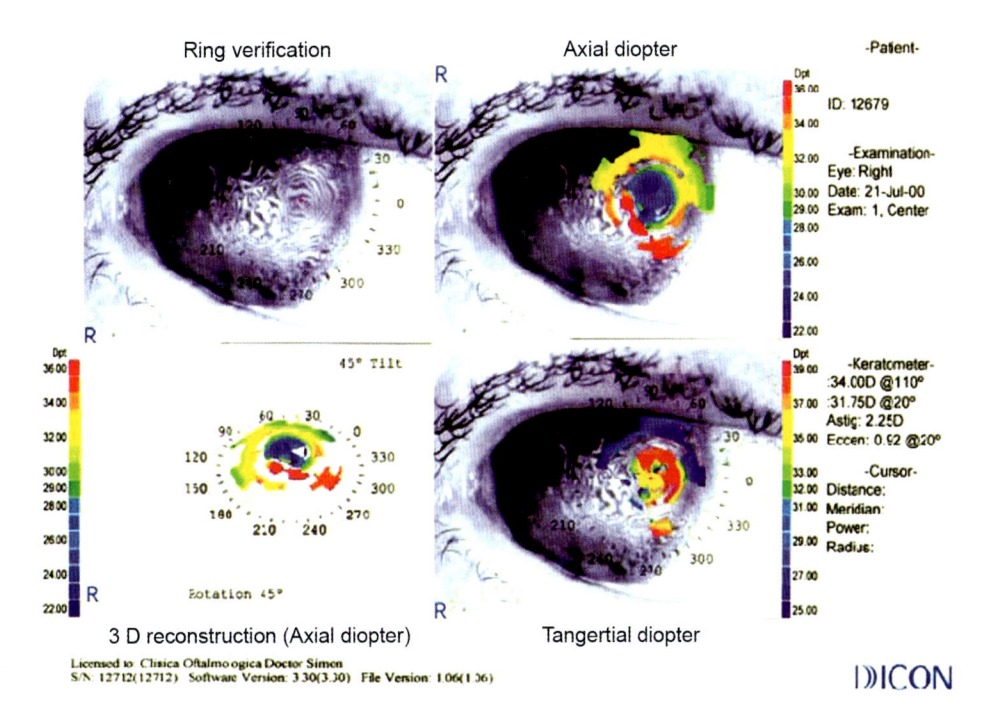

Figure 1.6 An advanced corneal herpetic keratopathy produces an irregular completely distorted corneal map in which no regular pattern can be identified. Notice that the low-vision patient is unable fixate the fixation light

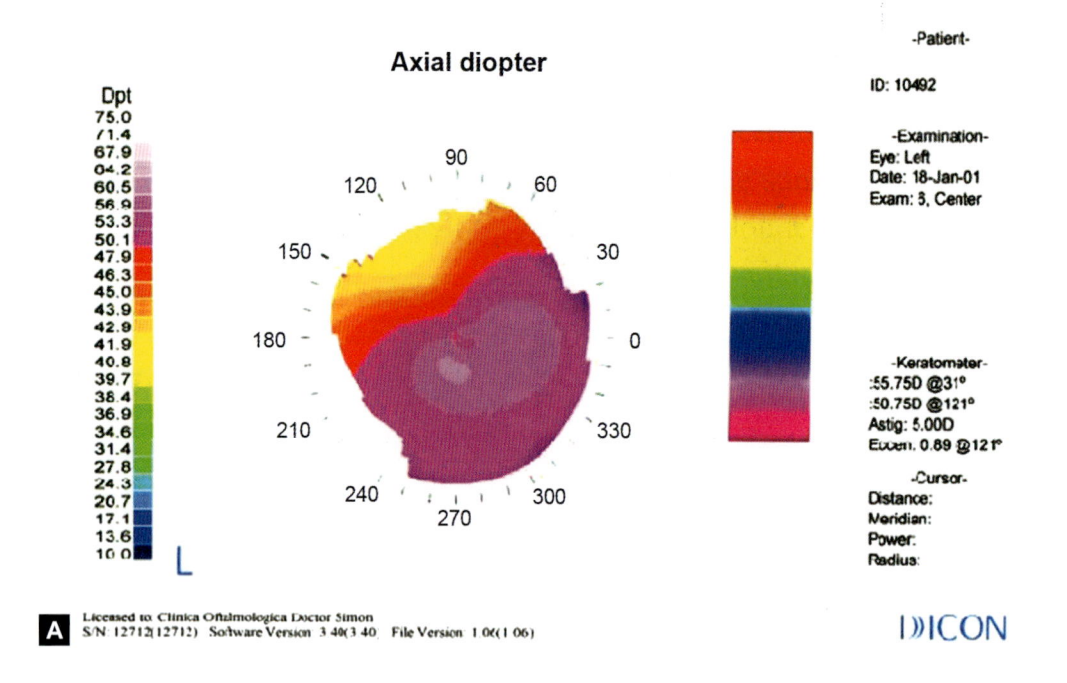

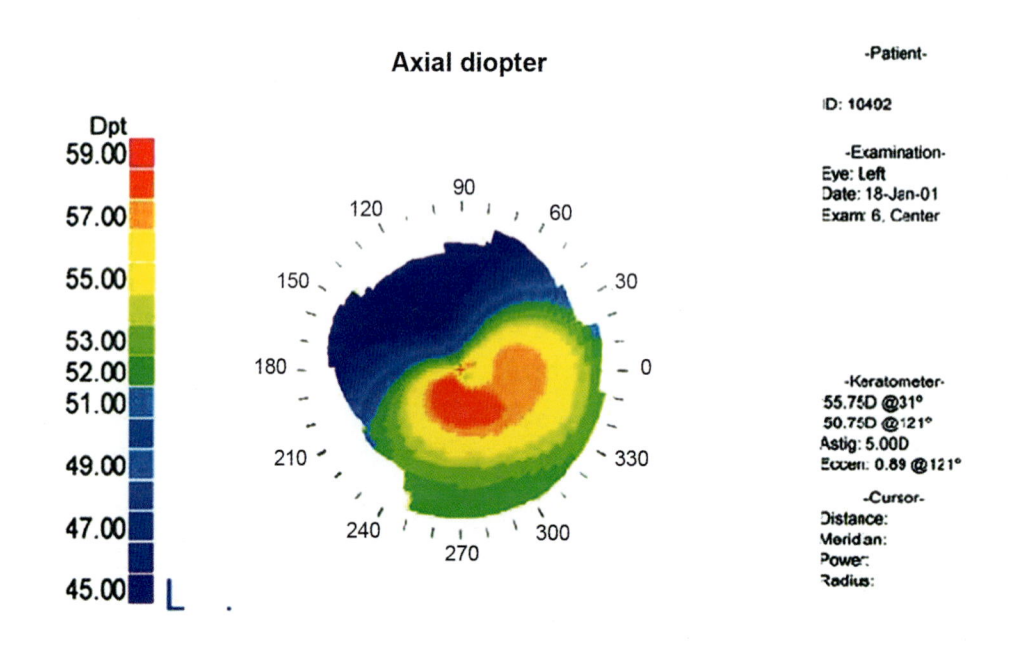

Figures 1.7A and B These two maps may look different but are the same axial diopter map of the left eye of the same patient (keratoconus) measured in different scales, absolute on the left and relative on the right. Notice very high diopter values under corneal vertex, where corneal surface is most elevated

Facing a corneal topography, care has to be taken to interpret colored maps, since scales (and sometimes color coding) can be modified in most topographers' software. For patient examination manufacturer sets default values which are operator adjustable (diopter interval, radius interval). When operator adjusts the values to new parameters, color scales are modified.

Rare are the topographers that directly measure the corneal elevation: Most act by extrapolation from corneal curvature and power at each measured point. The Optikon 2000® Keratron™ is one of those systems that accurately maps aspheric surfaces by means of its own method of arc-step mapping.

The range of powers found in the normal cornea range from 39 D found at peripheral cornea, close to the limbus, to 48 D found at corneal apex.

The colors do not always represent an elevation map, they correspond to curvature values. Therefore, the cornea is most curved towards the center (green) and flattens out towards the periphery (blue). The nasal side becomes blue more quickly, indicating that the nasal cornea is flatter than the temporal. Some advanced instruments like the Optikon 2000® Keratron™, are able to directly represent a colored elevation map.

Apart from color maps, most topographers also display values of simulated keratometry, that should be equivalent to those obtained by a keratometer. Simulated keratometry values are obtained from the radius values at the corneal position (3 central millimeters) where the reflection from the keratometer mires would take place.

Topographic Scales

Two basic scales are commonly used: Absolute and relative.

Absolute, Standardized or International Standard Scale

Same scale for every map produced. Good for direct comparisons between different maps, for screening and for gross pathologies. It was designed to make only clinically relevant information obvious, by setting the interval between the contours of the power plot (i.e. in practice, the contours of colors) at 1.5 diopters (which means it has low resolution).

Relative, Normalized or Adaptative Color Scale

Different scale for each map. The computer determines maximum and minimum curvatures for the map and automatically distributes the range of colors. The computer contracts or expands its color range according to the range of colors present in a given cornea. It is best suited for looking at variations for a particular cornea. It has the advantage of offering great topographic detail since incremental steps are smaller (around 0.8 diopters) giving high resolution, but suffers from some inconveniences: the meanings of colors are lost (explorer and clinician have to carefully check the meaning of the colors, according to the new scale), a normal cornea may look abnormal while abnormal corneas may appear closer to normal. With this scale, subtle features are made apparent, being good for detail.

Computer Displays: Presentation of Topographic Information

When confronted to a topography display, either a printed report or on screen, one should study it in a structured way to avoid mistakes in interpretation, and get the most of it. Proceed as follows:

- Check the name of the patient, date of exam and examined eye.
- Check the scale:
  — Type of measurement (height in microns, curvature in mm, power in diopters)
  — Step interval
- Study the map (type of map, form of abnormalities, ...)
- Evaluate statistical information (cursor box, statistical indices when given ...)
- Compare with topography of the other eye (always perform bilateral exams, when possible)
- Compare with the previous maps first verifying they are in the same scale)
- Apply statistical analysis or other needed software application (contact lens fit, surgical modules, 3-D color maps, neural networks, ...)
- Explain the exam's results to the patient

To present a corneal topography, each software application (i.e. each instrument) has a large number of computer displays. Most are produced from data of a single application, and are software dependent. Most instruments are able to show: A ring verification, a numerical display, a large number of corneal maps, a simulated keratometry, a meridional plot, and some can display a 3-D reconstruction of the corneal surface.

- *Ring verification (keratoscopic raw image) (Figure 1.1):* Displays a keratoscopic image of the Placido rings reflex on the examined cornea. It is a raw image, that allows qualitative evaluation of the image taken (irregularity of tear film layer, lids aperture, ...), helping the examiner to either accept or reject the taken image. It is very useful when there is a question regarding the accuracy of the displayed data.
- *Numeric display* of a number of corneal power values along several meridians shown in a radial display. Helpful to make the data amenable to statistical methods **(Figures 1.8A and B)**.
  - *Corneal maps:* Details of the most common (axial, tangential, 3-D, ...) will be discussed later in this chapter. Each topographer offers different maps or ways of presenting the results. Please refer to your topographer's manual for more details.

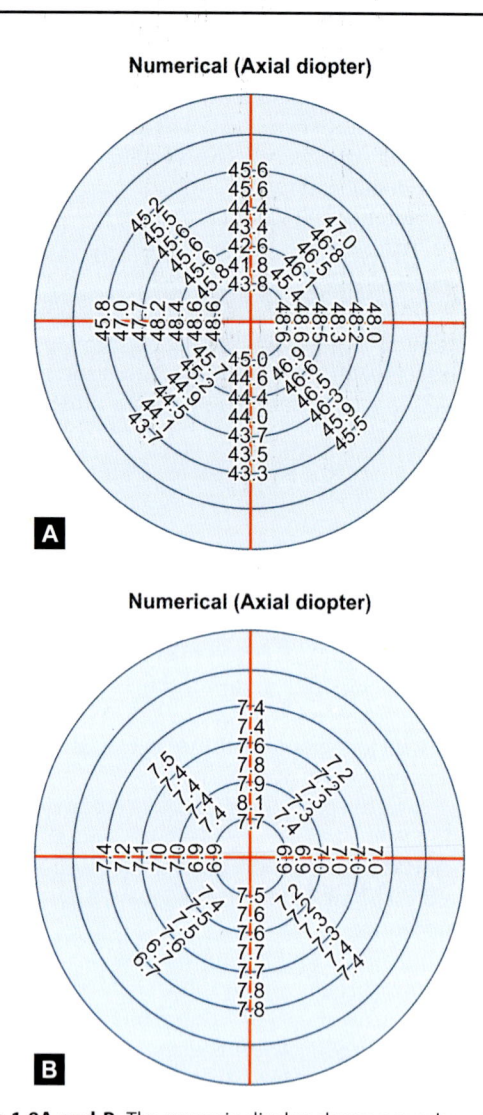

Figures 1.8A and B The numeric display shows a number of corneal power values along several meridians in a radial display. It is a very helpful presentation to make the data amenable to statistical methods. Notice that picture on the left (axial diopter) displays corneal powers in diopters and that on the right (axial radius) shows the same values in millimeters (corneal radius). Most topographers allow you to choose the way you want the results to be shown

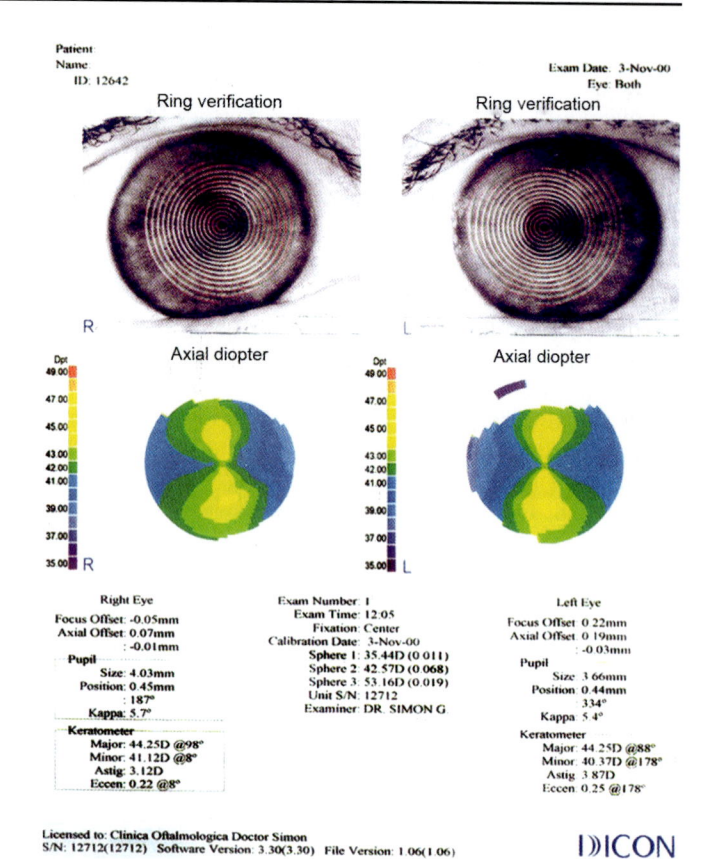

Figure 1.9 Axial diopter displays are showed for both right and left eyes. The patient suffered from regular astigmatism (with-the-rule), that gives an oval corneal map, being the most common deviation from optically perfect spherical (round) cornea. The long axis is near the vertical meridian. The shape and colors of the bow tie are influenced by the rate of peripheral corneal flattening: notice the nasal peripheral flattening in left eye (purple color). This binocular report from Dicon's CT-200 topographer shows pupil size and simulated keratometry of both eyes. RE size pupil is 4.03 mm, and astigmatism 3.12 D at 8°. Notice that the two eyes present a mirror image of each other: This phenomenon is called enantiomorphism

- *Simulated keratometry readings (SimK):* Obtained from the radius values at the corneal position (3 millimeters central zone) where, the reflection from the keratometer mires would take place. The major axis is that with the greatest power, and the minor axis is at 90° to it (perpendicular axis). The cylinder is the difference between the major and minor axis. The meridian with the lowest mean power can also be displayed.
- *Meridional plot:* Shows the minimum and the maximum corneal power values, displaying a cross-sectional profile of the cornea along the chosen meridian. It is used to show the general shape of the cornea to the patient, and assessing the toricity for contact lens adaptation. The helps identifying the ablation zone limits following LASIK or PRK.

Common Corneal Maps

1. *Axial map:* It is the original and most commonly used map. It provides measurements based on the keratometer formula. It is helpful is evaluating the overall characteristics of the cornea and classify the corneal map (normal or abnormal). It can differentiate between spherical, astigmatic or irregular corneas. It is the most stable type of map, but may confuse the explorer when evaluating the peripheral cornea **(Figure 1.9)**.
2. *Height map:* True height data (in microns) is immediately available from systems using the principle of projection,

although a reflection system like the Optikon 2000® Keratron™ does a good job with its own arc-step method of representing corneal height. Very useful in numeric or cross-sectional format to quantify the elevation or the depth of a corneal defect (ulceration, laser ablation zone, keratoconus, ...). Some topographers display the spherical height map relative to a reference spherical surface, by comparing to a best fit calculated reference sphere.

3. *Tangential map* **(Figures 1.10 and 1.11)***:* This very useful display provides a measurement of corneal power over a large portion of the cornea, based on a mathematical radius formula. It is more accurate than axial map in the corneal periphery, but is subject to greater variation when comparing several exams that are repeated. It may help detecting mild corneal changes that might not be detected by standard axial map. It is used for locating corneal distances on the map, and to locate a cone or peak position in keratoconus, as well as to locate the ablation diameter and position after laser refractive surgical ablation.

4. *Refractive map:* It is a map based on an axial map, using Snell's law to calculate the refractive power of the cornea. It is mainly used in pre- and postcorneal surgery.

5. *Elliptical elevation map:* It represents the height of the cornea in microns, at different corneal positions, relative to a reference elliptical surface. It is useful to visualize corneal shape. In contrast to the spherical height map—which uses a simple spherical reference—the elliptical elevation map matches better to the inherently elliptical shape of the healthy cornea.

6. 3-D reconstruction map is used to visualize the overall shape of the cornea in a more realistic way. Understandable for the patient, it can be rotated and tilted as desired. Some instruments like Oculus® Keratograph and Haag-Streit® Keratograph CTK 922 offer excellent comprehensive kinetic three-dimensional (3-D) analysis of corneal topography for simple explanation to the patient **(Figures 1.12A and B)**.

7. *Irregularity map:* It calculates a best sphere/cylinder correction for the cornea, subtracting the correction from either axial or tangential data and presents the remaining irregularities. Used after refractive surgery to detect irregularities that may explain a low visual acuity. It reports an index that measures eccentricity (a measure of asphericity) and the amount of astigmatism that has been subtracted from the original corneal data.

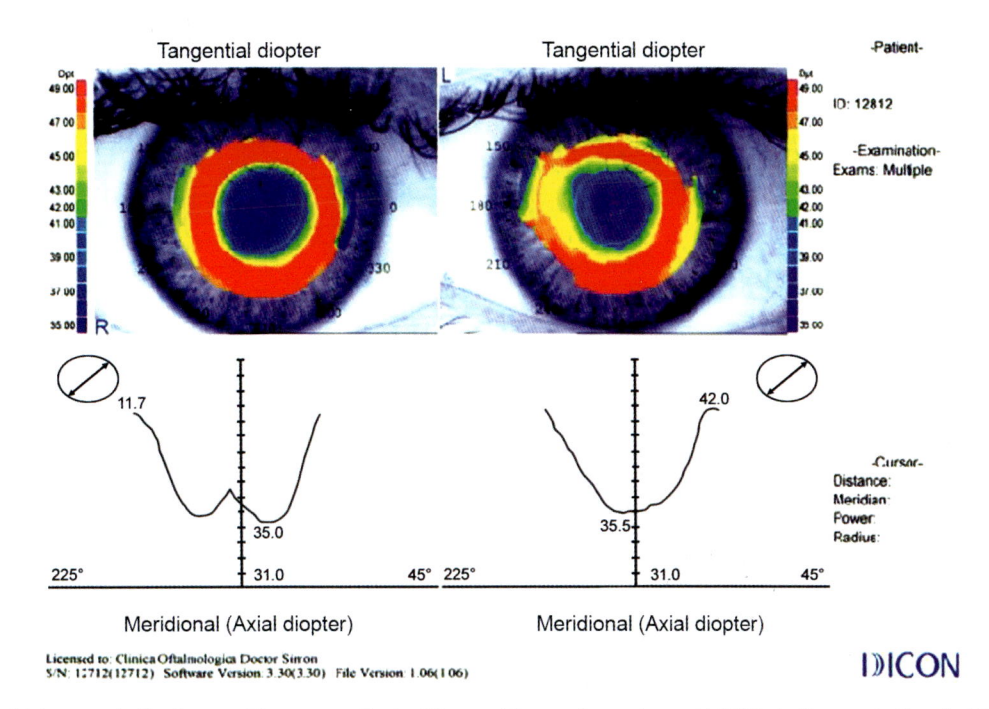

Figure 1.10 A "multiple exams" of both eyes of the same patient, a 38-year-old man who underwent LASIK in both eyes at a time for high myopia. Corneal map is overlaid upon the keratoscope eye image to aid interpretation. The overlay shows the spatial relationship between the pupil, the ablation zone and the cornea. Notice that immediately after surgery (the day after), ablation zones differ from each other: it is due to the fact that a different excimer laser was used for each eye. Schwind® Keratom™ was used on right eye, while left eye was operated using the Bausch and Lomb®-Chiron Technolas 217™. Although ablation zone seems more perfect and regular on right eye (tangential diopter map), this does not mean that visual result is better. The meridional plots shown under tangential diopter maps help the surgeon to evaluate the effectiveness and ablation pattern of the excimer laser he or she uses

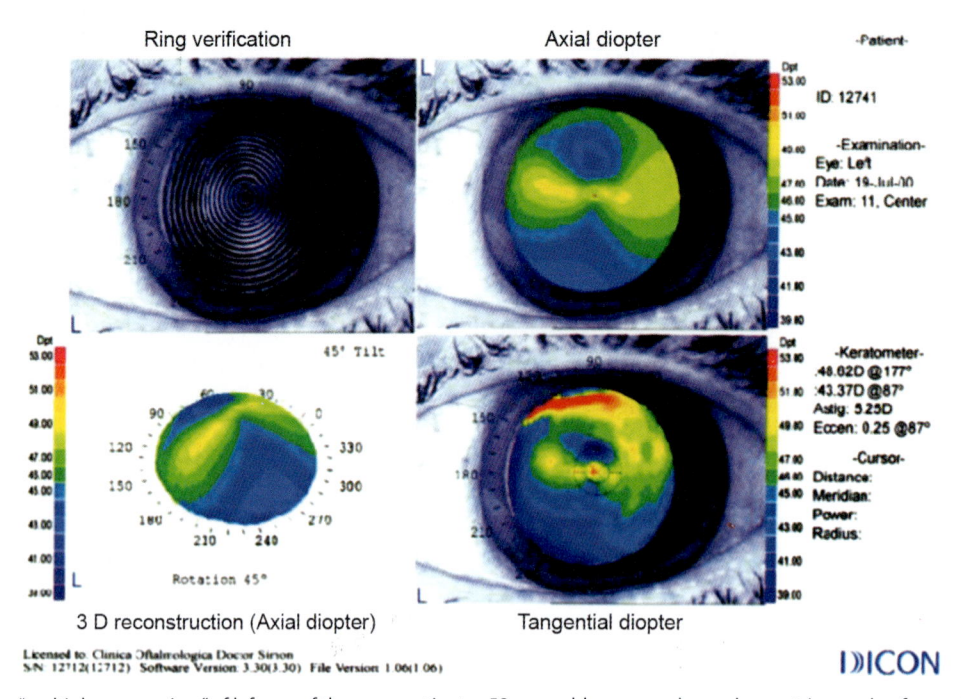

Figure 1.11 Shows a "multiple exams view" of left eye of the same patient, a 58-year-old woman who underwent (a couple of years before consultation) complicated phacoemulsification converted to extracapsular surgery. In the hurry, surgeon sutured the cornea too loose, thus creating a peripheral superior corneal wound defect. High against-the-rule astigmatism is well represented by the axial diopter display (superior right), and well measured by the keratometer display (5.25 D at 87°). But only tangential diopter map (down-right) accurately represented the corneal wound suture defect: notice the red superior area where the sutures used to be

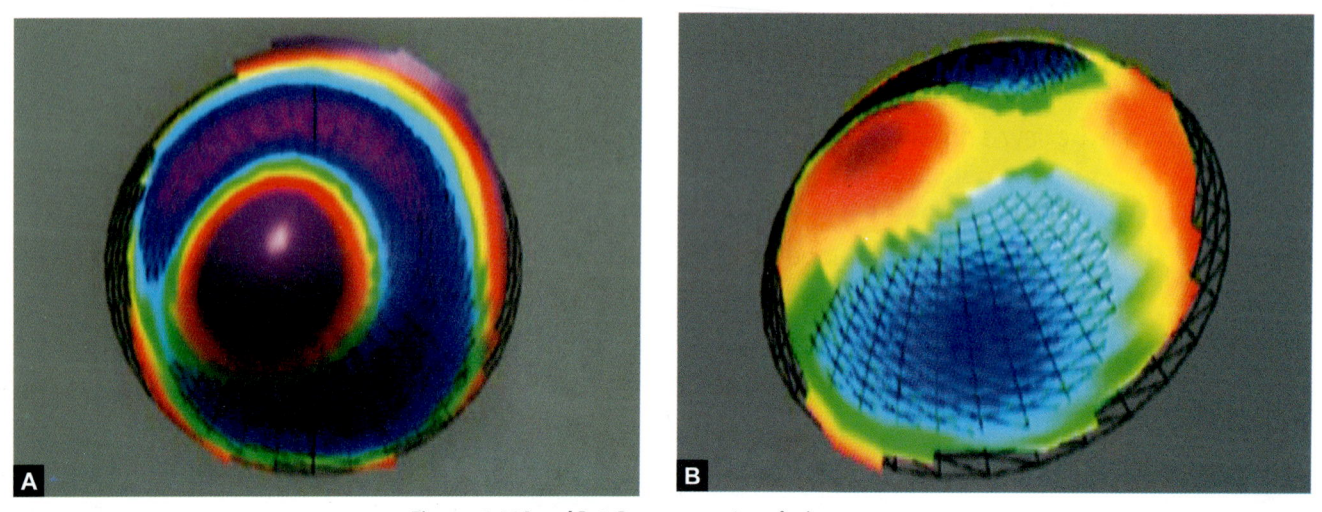

Figures 1.12A and B 3-D reconstruction of orbscan map
(Courtesy: Dr Agarwal's Eye Hospital)

Special Software Applications and Displays

Each available instrument is sold with standard software package and most offer optional packages at additional price. The most common are:

Multiple display option: A customisable multiple display allows simultaneous screen display for rapid analysis and ease of use. Depending on the software of your topographer, you can simultaneously view either one, two or four maps. Extremely practice in daily use to ease work and interpretation.

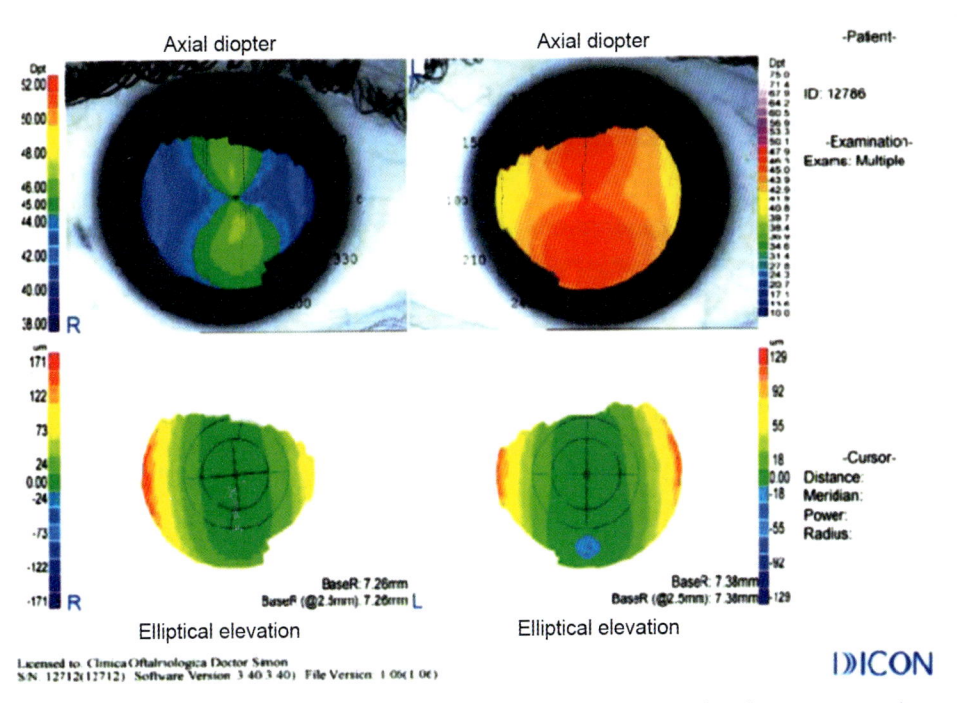

Chapter 1: Fundamentals on Corneal Topography 13

Figure 1.13 Shows a "multiple exams view" of both eyes of the same patient, a young man referred for refractive surgery who—to our surprise—was never diagnosed astigmatic. Axial diopter maps are displayed, in normalized (right eye) and absolute scales (left eye). Elliptical elevation with keratometer overlay maps help better assess true corneal shape and direction or axis of astigmatism. Radius of the reference ellipse are displayed and can be modified by operator: BaseR refers to central radius value, and BaseR (2.5 mm) refers to the radius value at 2.5 mm

Table 1.4 Common overlays that can be added to a topography map to help interpretation

Pupil margin: Displays the visually important region. Helps evaluating photopic pupillary size, and the centration or refractive surgery.

Grids square: Helps defining size and location of abnormalities.

Circular: Helps defining size and location of abnormalities.

Polar: Helps defining axis of abnormalities and the assessment of radial keratotomies.

Optical zone: Useful in refractive surgery for planning procedures or assessing results.

Angular scale: Useful in refractive surgery of astigmatism for planning procedures or assessing results. It is similar in use to polar grid **(Figure 1.13)**.

Eye image: More realistic than a simple map, it eases patient's interpretation of the map.

Keratoconus: A peak or keratoconus overlay can be applied by Dicon's CT-200. It is called Bull's Eye target. If one peak area exists with an index of 10 or greater, the system automatically marks it with a target, indicating the location of this elevation to some but not all maps **(see Figures 1.14 and 1.15)**.

Keratometer mires: It is a graphic reference showing a 3 mm circle with both major and minor meridians, representing the calculated keratometry readings, 90 degrees apart (perpendicular). It also shows a 5 mm with the steepest and flattest meridians **(see Figure 1.13)**.

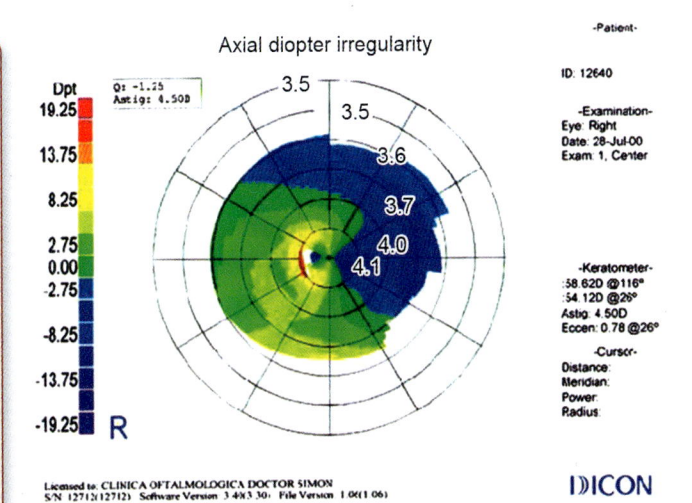

Figure 1.14 An "axial irregularity map" in diopters of the right eye of a 55-year-old man suffering from a paracentral progressive corneal ectasia (central keratoconus). Notice the Q index with a value of −1,25 (measuring eccentricity) and an astigmatism of 4.5 D, resulting from the subtraction of the original corneal data and the best sphere/cylinder for that cornea. An overlay option adds an irregularity index to the map for increasing circles of 1 mm radius, best visualized thanks to the overlay circular grid option. Normal values would be 0.2 or 0.4, but this exceptional case shows 3.5 and 4.0 zonal indices

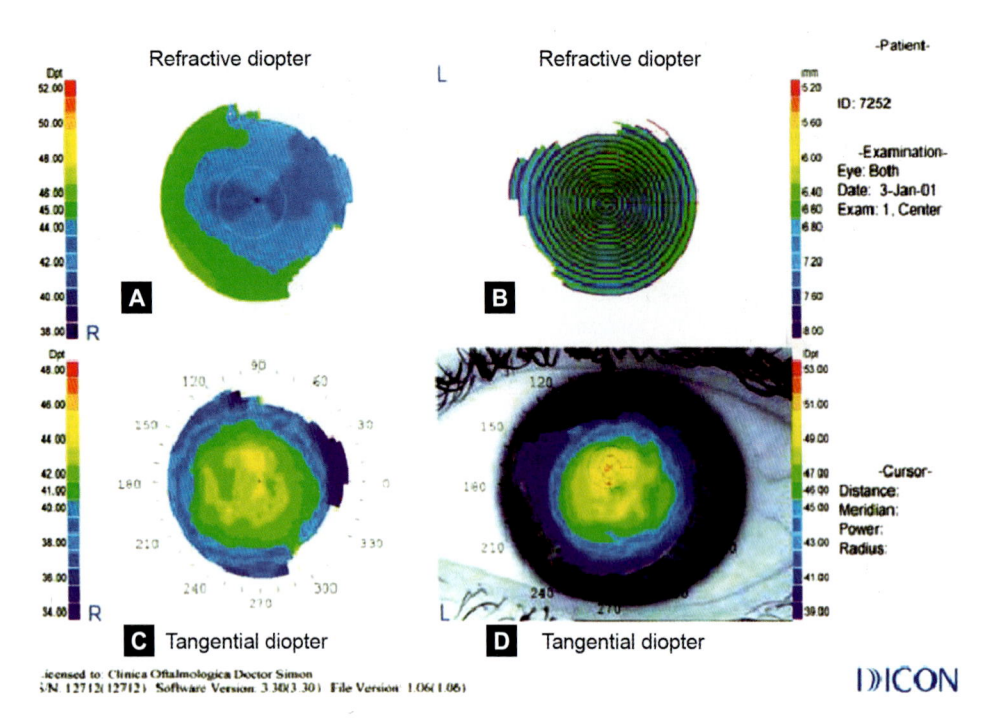

Figures 1.15A to D Different overlays can be added to a topography to help interpretation. The Figure shows a quadruple view of an almost normal cornea of a young contact lens user with mild corneal warpage only diagnosed by means of the tangential maps (C and D). Notice that (B) is displayed in radius (mm) while the rest of maps are displayed in diopters (see the color scale). Map (A) displays a center overlay (small red cross) that indicates where the true center of the cornea is, and a pupil outline overlay that reproduces pupil margin, the visually important region. Map (B) shows a "verify rings" overlay, to better asses the quality of the taken image. Red and green concentric rings should alternate and not cross. The red rings should be located on the outer edge of the white rings, and the green rings should be located on the outer edge of the black rings. Map (C) shows an angular scale that helps to locate the axis of astigmatism. Map (D) shows "eye image" overlay, the image of the patient's eye is displayed to ease patient's interpretation of the map. Notice that a paracentral target marks an elevation zone that has to be carefully inspected. Angular scale is also displayed in map **(Table 1.4)**

Surgical applications: Used to predict the results of refractive surgery, and for postoperative evaluation. Some but not all allow refractive surgery simulations and topography linked laser refractive surgery with special excimer laser brand names **(Figures 1.16A and B)**.

Contact lens fitting application: They are used for contact lens fitting, and help choosing the best suggested lens for each case, by simulating the fluorescein pattern and contact lens position of rigid contacts. Not all topographers offer this feature. In some cases this software module is sold as an option. For instance, Dicon's CT-200™ offers as standard the Mandell Contact Lens Module "Easy-Fit™", and as an option the Mandell Contact Lens Module "Advanced-Fit"™ for toric, bi-toric, keratoconic fitting and postsurgical fitting with Labtalk™. Contact your dealer for more precise information.

The simulated fluorescein feature is intended to reduce fitting time by viewing the effect of changing lens parameters on a personalized basis, depending on the patient's corneal exam. Let's notice that the true "*in vivo*" result of any computerized fluorescein test may vary due to differences caused by lid action on the lens (aperture and weight).

Ask the manufacturer of your topographer for special software applications, and for the possibility to link your topographer and your excimer laser for better results.

TOPOGRAPHY MAPS OF THE NORMAL CORNEA

When considering the topography of a normal cornea, we feel the need to remember that there is a wide spectrum of normality. No human cornea demonstrates the kind of regularity found in the calibration spheres of a topographer. The eye is not moulded glass-made. Normal corneal topography can take on many topographic patterns (*see* **Table 1.5** and **Figure 1.17**):

Regular astigmatism (with-the-rule) gives an oval axial corneal map, being the most common deviation from optically perfect spherical (round) cornea. If the bow tie is vertical (the long axis is near the vertical meridian) in an axial map, it represents a cornea having with-the-rule-astigmatism.

If the bow tie is horizontal, it represents an "against-the-rule" astigmatism, ninety degrees rotated when compared to a with-the-rule astigmatism.

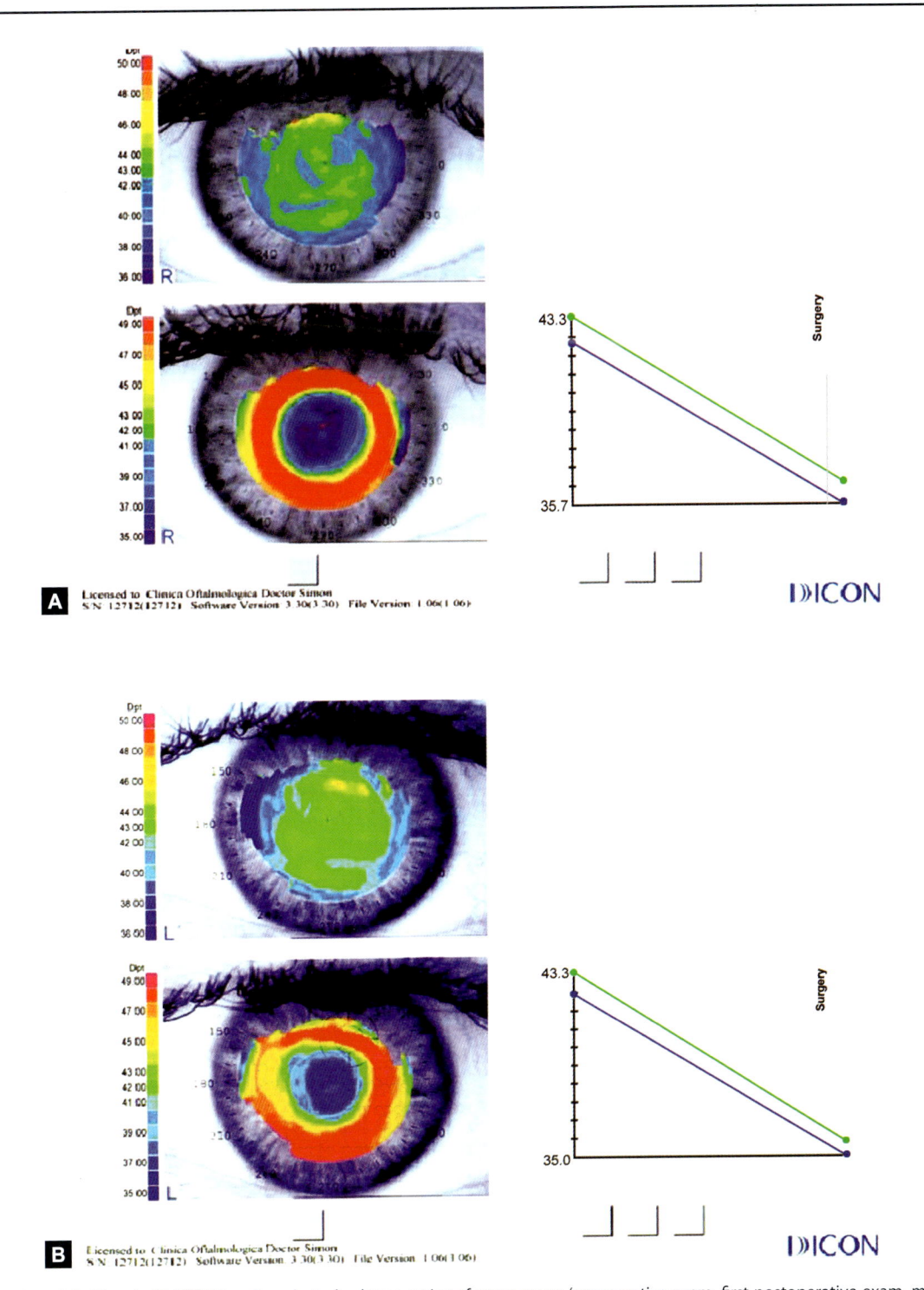

Chapter 1: Fundamentals on Corneal Topography 15

Figures 1.16A and B Dicon's CT-200™ trend analysis displays a series of exam maps (preoperative exam, first postoperative exam, most recent exam and a choice of a K-trend graph, a pre/postoperative difference map or a post-last difference map. Shown are trend analysis of both eyes of a patient who underwent myopic LASIK with two different excimer lasers. Shown are axial diopter preoperative, tangential diopter immediate postoperative and K-trend graph. Notice that immediately after surgery (the day after), ablation zones differ from each other: It is due to the fact that a different excimer laser was used for each eye. Schwind® Keratom™ was used on right eye, while left eye was operated using the Bausch and Lomb®-Chiron Technolas 217™. K-trend graph shows the major (green) and minor (blue) K values for all exams in the series. The Y axis is power in diopters, and the X axis is the exams' number spaced out over time. The vertical line marks the date of surgery. Trend analysis eases a rapid overview of healing trend over time

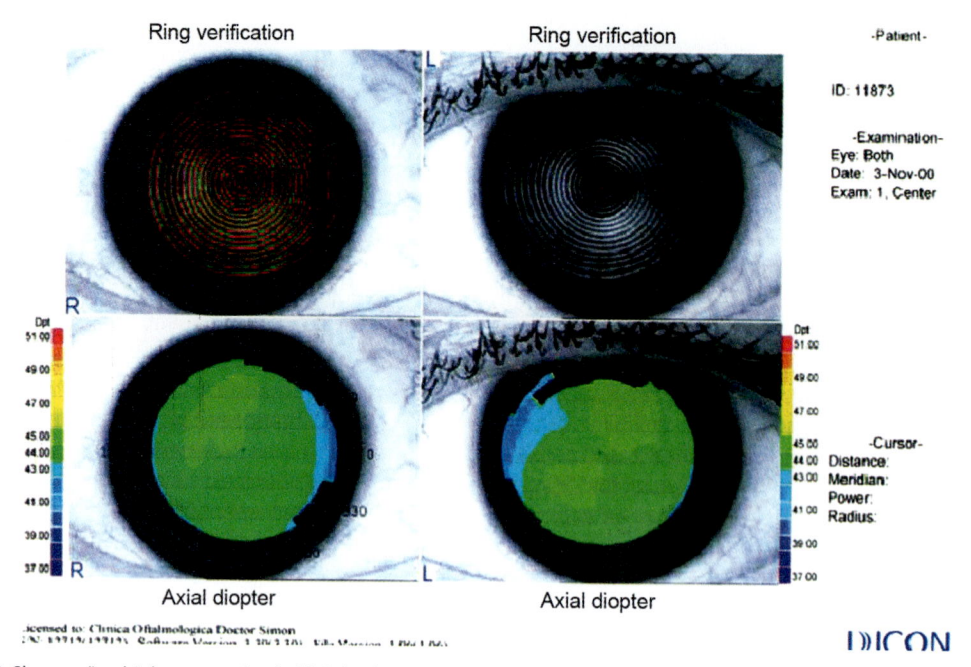

Figure 1.17 Shows a "multiple exams view" of left both eyes of the same patient, a 38-year-old woman prior to LASIK surgery. Corneal topography remains a routine exam for preoperative and postoperative assessment of the refractive patient. This report shows normal, spherical (round), corneas in both eyes (44 D at vertex, and mostly green color in the map). The color zones are approximately circular in shape. Notice that lid aperture is not the same in both eyes, thus making it more difficult to map superior corneal periphery in left eye

Table 1.5 Normal topographic patterns

Spherical	(Round) **(Figure 1.18)**	20%
With-the-rule	(Oval) **(Figure 1.19)**	20%
With-the-rule	(Symmetric bow tie)	17%
With-the-rule	(Asymmetric bow tie)	30%
Against-the-rule		
Displaced apex:	Inferiorly	
	Nasally	
Irregular		7%
Causes of irregularity:	Dry eye	
	Corneal scar or ulceration	
	Trauma	
	Corneal degeneration	
	Corneal edema	
	Pterygium	
	Contact lens overuse (corneal warpage)	
	Surgery (cataract, keratoplasty, . . .)	

When the bow tie is diagonal, it represents a cornea having an oblique astigmatism. The shape and colors of the bow tie are influenced by the rate of peripheral corneal flattening, and the appearance is influenced by the scale interval chosen by the explorer. The bow tie may be symmetrical or asymmetrical along the perpendicular meridian. One-half of the bow tie is significantly larger than the other, the corneal apex being located in the direction of the larger bow half, slightly decentered from the visual axis.

In the normal eye, nasal cornea is flatter than temporal. The nasal side of a healthy corneal map becomes blue more quickly, indicating that the nasal cornea is flatter than the temporal. There is a physiological astigmatism of around 0.75 diopter. Physiologically, the axis may not be the same superiorly than inferiorly. In an axial map, the rate of flattening is greater when the color scale interval is larger, and there are many color zones. A focal steepening inferiorly may exist due to the lower tear meniscus.

Generally, the two eyes of the same subject are very similar, and present a mirror image of each other **(Figures 1.9 and 1.18)**. This phenomenon is called enantiomorphism. The knowledge of this fact is useful to decide whether a cornea is normal or not, by comparing to the map of contralateral eye. Small changes in corneal shape do occur throughout life:
- In infancy the cornea is fairly spherical

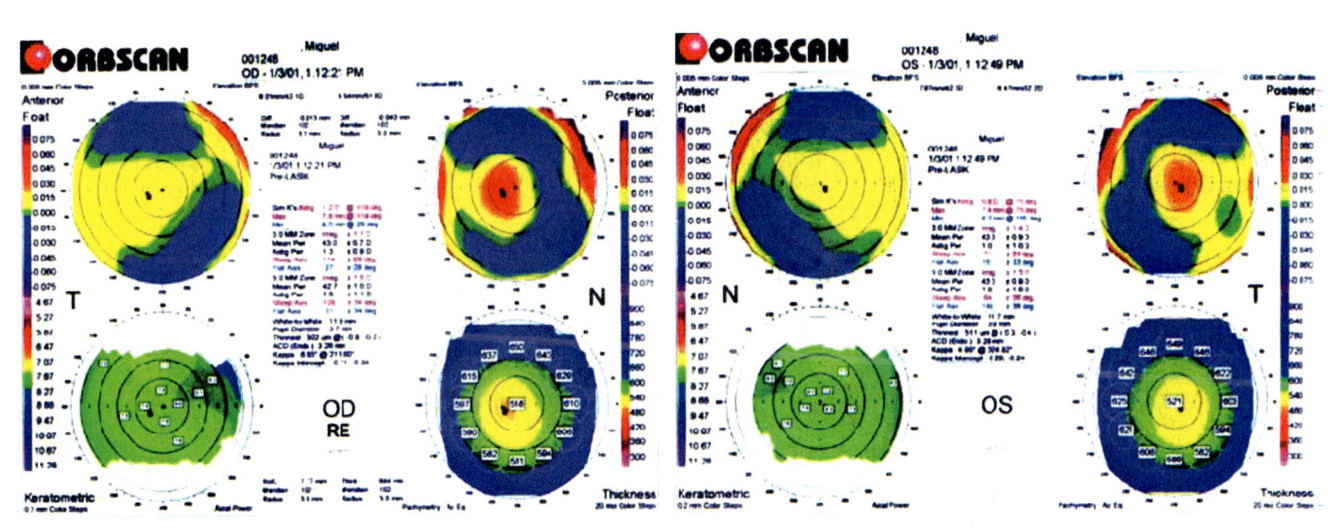

Figure 1.18 Enantiomorphism is the phenomenon wherein an individual's topographies are nonsuperimposable almost mirror images of each-other. The knowledge of this fact is useful to decide whether a cornea is normal or not, by comparing to the map of contralateral eye. Notice that even pachimetry maps reflect this phenomenon (Corneal thickness was mapped with Bausch and Lomb® Orbscan™ topo-pachimeter)

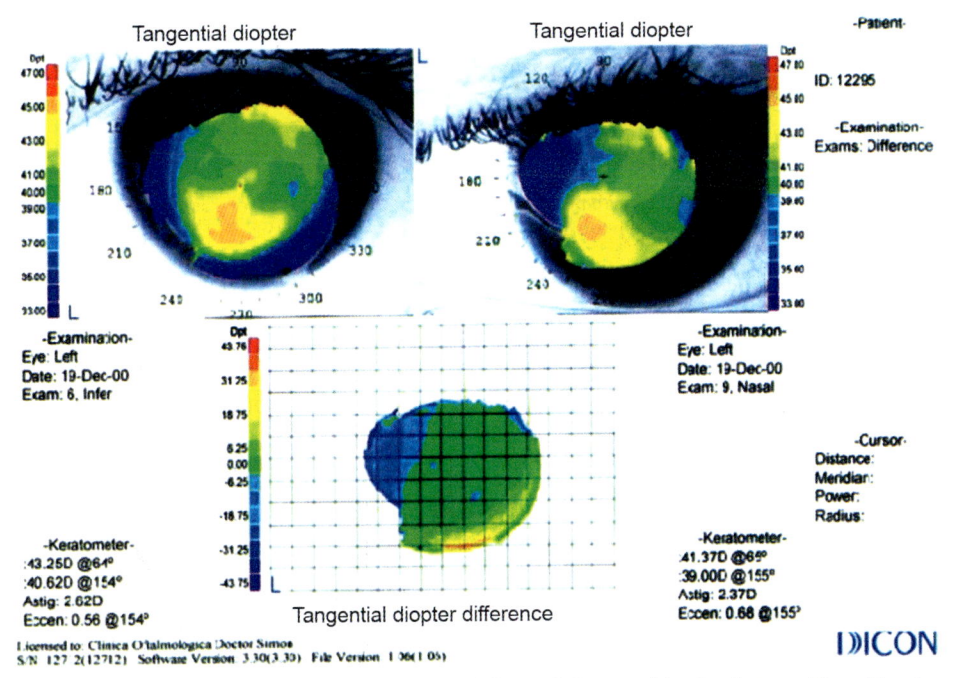

Figure 1.19 A tangential diopter difference map to the left eye of a 21-year-old patient is shown. The subtraction has been performed between two different eye fixations to determine the existence of any irregularity in the ablation zone. The patient underwent a successful bilateral LASIK surgery to correct a high myopic astigmatism in both eyes a year before

- In childhood and adolescence, probably due to eyelid pressure on a young tissue, cornea becomes slightly astigmatic with-the-rule
- In the middle age, cornea tends to recover its sphericity
- Late in life, against-the-rule astigmatism tends to develop.

Short-term fluctuation and diurnal variations are not rare, and usually remain unnoticed by individuals with normal corneas. Some conditions like corneal dystrophies, ocular

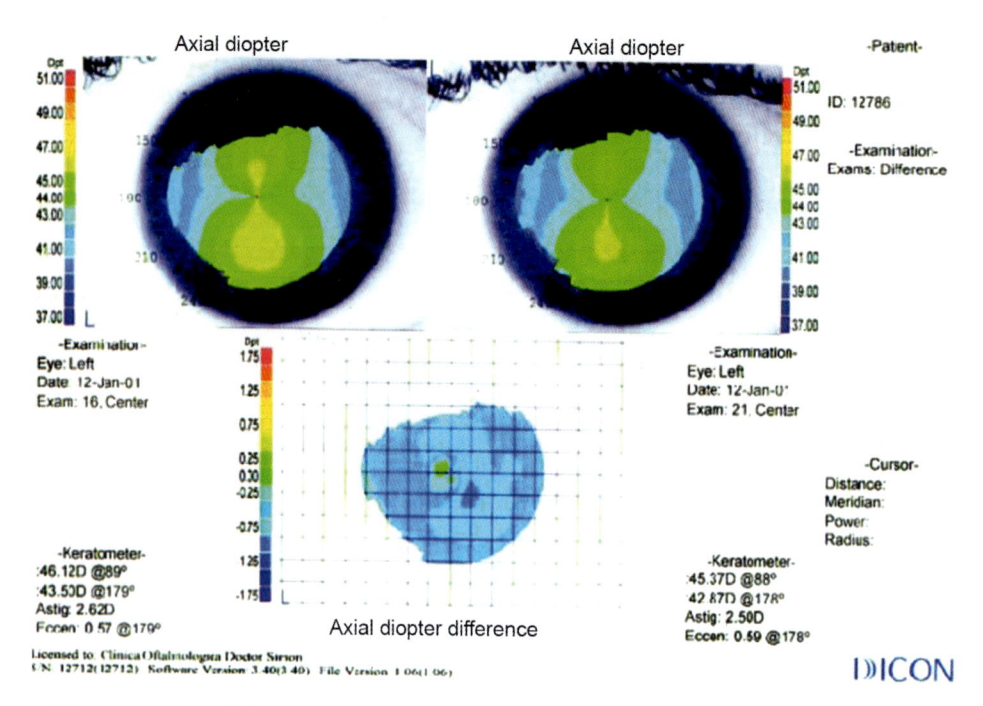

Figure 1.20 A diopter difference map is useful to assess the validity of the different exams with the same fixation performed in the same session. Low differences due to tear film irregularities, lid aperture and blinking is acceptable. In case of difference between maps taken at the same moment, they need to be repeated, after a few blinks from the patient. If significant difference persists, try instilling a tear substitute in both eyes and wait a few minutes. Should differences persist, repeat the exams in a few days. Image shows a left eye with regular (with-the-rule) high astigmatism. Both axial diopter maps were taken in the same session. Differences exist between the exams. Eye fixation is the same (center). Differences are attributable to different lid aperture and form blinking. Axial diopter difference (down, with a square grid overlay) shows that differences are almost nonsignificant (around 0.25–0.50 diopters), but exist. Such differences are physiological. Difference maps allow validation of various exams taken in a same session

hypotony, radial keratotomies or contact lens use can make them apparent (**Table 1.6**).

Comparing Displays

Maps can be compared directly only on the same scale, when taken with the same instrument, and preferably by the same explorer. It is not a good idea to compare maps taken with different instruments. Every instrument uses a different measuring algorithm that may confuse you, specially when comparing subtle details.

Most software applications allow the comparison of different maps (**Table 1.7**) over time, and even subtract values from two different exams (substraction or difference maps) (**Figure 1.19**). They are invaluable to the refractive surgeon.

Table 1.6 Factors that slightly affect the normal curvature of the cornea

Lid closure during sleep time
Tear film quality
Lid pressure on the cornea (weight, exophthalmos)
Intraocular pressure
Menstruation
Pregnancy

Table 1.7 Uses of substraction or difference maps

Validation of various exams taken in a same session (**Figure 1.20**)
Ascertain the existence of progressive corneal astigmatism (**Figure 1.21**)
Comparison of preoperative and postoperative corneal maps (LASIK and PRK)
Follow-up of myopic regression (LASIK and PRK)
Establishing ablation zone centration (LASIK and PRK)
Assessing resolution of corneal warpage in rigid contact lens users
Assessing evolution of a corneal ulcer or abscess

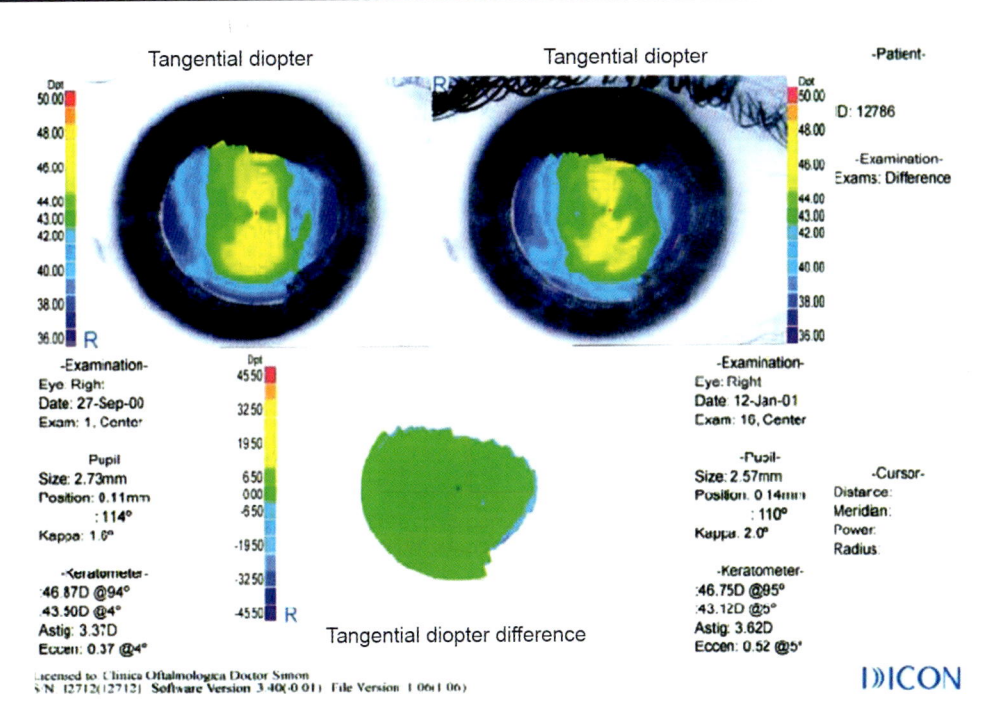

Figure 1.21 Difference maps ease the astigmatism progression follow-up. Tangential diopter displays show right eye maps of a 22-year-old myopic patient referred for refractive surgery. To our surprise, neither glasses nor contacts had astigmatism. The existence of astigmatism was ascertained with the keratometer, subjective refraction and skiascopy. Corneal topography was performed and helped the demonstration of its existence. Figure shows a difference map between two exams taken with a 3 months delay (see the dates of the exams). Tangential diopter difference is 0 (green), meaning that no changes have occurred in that period of time. The first impression is that the guy never had good refraction, but new topographic exams will be performed 6 months and one year later, before refractive surgery is decided, so as to make sure that no keratoconic formation is on the way

BIBLIOGRAPHY

1. Applegate RA, Nunez R, Buettner J, et al. How accurately can videokeratographic systems measure surface elevation? Optom Vis Sci. 1995;72:785-92.
2. Arffa RC, Warnicki JW, Rehkopf PG. Corneal topography using rasterstereography. Refract Corneal Surg. 1989;5:414-17.
3. Belin MW, Litoff FK, Strods SJ, et al. The PAR technology corneal topography system. Refract Corneal Surg. 1992;8:88-96.
4. Belin MW, Ratliff CD. Evaluating data acquisition and smoothing functions of currently available videokeratoscopes. J Cataract Refract Surg. 1996;22:421-6.
5. Belin MW, Zloty P. Accuracy of the PAR corneal topography system with spatial misalignment. CLAO J. 1993;19:64-68.
6. Borderie VM, Laroche L. Measurement of irregular astigmatism using semimeridian data from videokeratographs. J Refract Surg. 1996;12:595-600.
7. Brancato R, Carones F. Topografia corneale computerizzata. Milano, Italy: Fogliazza, ed. 1994.
8. Cantera E, Carones F, Brancato R, et al. Evaluation of a new autofocus device for computer-assisted corneal topography. Invest Ophthalmol Vis Sci. 1994;35(Suppl):2063.
9. Chan WK, Carones F, Maloney RK. Corneal topographic maps: a clinical comparison. International Society of Refractive Keratoplasty 1994—Abstract book.
10. Cohen KL, Tripoli NK, Holmgren DE, et al. Assessment of the height of radial aspheres reported by a computer-assisted keratoscope. Invest Ophthalmol and Vis Sci. 1993;34 (Suppl): 1217.
11. Cohen KL, Tripoli NK, Holmgren DE, et al. JM. Assessment of the power and height of radial aspheres reported by a computer-assisted keratoscope. Am J Ophthalmol. 1995;ll9:723-32.
12. Corbett MC, O'Brart DPS, Stultiens Bath, et al. Corneal topography using a new moiré image-based system. Eur J Implant Ref Surg. 1995;7:353-70.
13. Corbett MC, Rosen ES, O'Brart DPS. Corneal topography: Principles and applications. BMJ books, Great Britain; 1999.
14. Dekking HM. Zur Photographie der Hornhautoberfl-Eche. Graefes Arch Ophtalmol. 1930;124:708-30.
15. Dingeldein SA, Klyce SD, Wilson SE. Quantitative descriptors of corneal shape derived from the computer-assisted analysis of photokeratographs. Refract Corneal Surg. 1989;5:372-8.
16. Doss JD, Hutson RL, Rowsey JJ, et al. Method for calculation of corneal profile and power distribution. Arch Ophthalmol. 1981; 99:1261-5.
17. Duke Elder S. System of Ophthalmology, St Louis, Mo: CV Mosby Co, 1970, V, 96-101.
18. Ediger MN, Pettit GH, Weiblinger RP. Noninvasive monitoring of excimer laser ablation by time-resolved reflectometry. Refract Corneal Surg. 1993;9:268-75.
19. Eghbali F, Yeung KK, Maloney RK. Topographic determination of corneal asphericity and its lack of effect on the outcome of radial keratotomy. Am J Ophthalmol. 1995;119:275-80.

20. el-Hage SG. Suggested new methods for photokeratoscopy: A comparison of their validities. I. Am J Optom Arch Am Acad Optom. 1971;48:897-912.
21. el-Hage SG. The computerized corneal topographer EH-270. In: Shanzlin DJ, Robin JB, eds. Corneal topography: measuring and modifying the cornea. New York: Springer-Verlag 1991;l:1-24.
22. Fleming JF. Should refractive surgeons worry about corneal asphericity? Refract Corneal Surg. 1990;6:455-57.
23. Friedman NE, Zadnik K, Mutti DO, et al. Quantifying corneal toricity from videokeratography with fourier analysis. J Refract Surg. 1996;12:108-13.
24. Gardner BP, Klyce SD, Thompson HW, et al. Centration of photorefractive keratectomy: topographic assessment. Invest Ophthalmol Vis Sci; 1993. pp. 35, 803.
25. Greivenkamp JE, Mellinger MD, Snyder RW, Schwiegerling JT, Lowman AE, Miller JM. Comparison of three videokeratoscopes in measurement of toric test surfaces. J Refract Surg. 1996;12: 229-39.
26. Grimm BB. Communicating with keratography. J Refract Surg 1996;12:156-9.
27. Hannush SB, Crawford SL, Waring GO III, Gemmill MC, Lynn MJ, Nizam A. Accuracy and precision of keratometry, photokeratoscopy and corneal modeling on calibrated steel balls. Arch Ophtalmol. 1989;107:1235-9.
28. Holladay J, Warring GO. Optics and topography in radial keratotomy. In: Warring GO, ed. Refractive keratectomy for myopia and Astigmatism. Mosby-Year book, Inc; 1992. pp. 37-144.
29. Holladay JT, Cravy TV, Koch DD. Calculation of surgically induced refractive change following ocular surgery. J Cat Refract Surg 1992;18:429-43.
30. Holladay JT. Corneal topography using the Holladay diagnostic summary. J Cat Refract Surg. 1997;23:209-21.
31. Holladay JT. The Holladay diagnostic summary. In: Corneal topography: the state of art, James P. Gills editor, Slack Inc. 1995; 309-23.
32. Huber C, Huber A, Gruber H. Three-dimensional representations of corneal deformations from kerato-topographic data. J Cat Refract Surg. 1997;23:202-8.
33. Johnson DA, Haight DH, Kelly SE, et al. Reproducibility of videokeratographic digital subtraction maps after excimer laser photorefractive keratectomy. Ophthalmology. 1996;103: 1392-8.
34. Jongsma FHM, Laan FC, Stultiens BATh. A moiré based corneal topographer suitable for discrete Fourier analysis, Proc Ophthal Tech. 1994;2126:185-92.
35. Kawara T. Corneal topography using moiré contour fringes. Appl Optics. 1979;18:3675-8.
36. Kelman SE. Introduction of neural networks with applications to ophthalmology. In: Masters BR (ed) Non-invasive diagnostic techniques in ophthalmology. Springer-Verlag, New York. 1990.
37. Klein SA, Mandell RB. Axial and instantaneous power conversion in corneal topography. Invest Ophthalmol Vis Sci. 1995;36:2155-9.
38. Klein SA. A corneal topography algorithm that produces continuous curvature. Optom Vis Sci. 1992;69:829-34.
39. Klyce SD, Dingeldein SA. Corneal topography. In: Masters BR, ed. Noninvasive diagnostic techniques in ophthalmology. New York: Springer-Verlag; 1990. pp. 78-91.
40. Klyce SD, Wang JY. Considerations in corneal surface reconstruction from keratoscope images. In: Masters BR, ed. Noninvasive diagnostic techniques in ophthalmology. New York: Springer-Verlag, New York; 1990. p. 76.
41. Klyce SD. Computer-assisted corneal topography: High resolution graphic presentation and analysis of keratoscopy. Invest Ophthalmol Vis Sci. 1984;25:1426-35.
42. Koch DD, Foulks GN, Moran CT, et al. The corneal EyeSys System: Accuracy analysis and reproducibility of first-generation prototype. J Refract Corneal Surg. 1989;5:424-29.
43. Le Geais JM, Ren Q, Simon G. Computer-assisted corneal topography: Accuracy and reproducibility of the topographic modeling system. Refract Corneal Surgery. 1993;9:347-57.
44. Leroux Les Jardins, Pasquier N, Bertrand I. Modification de la chirurgie de l'astigmatisme en fonction des résultats de la topographie cornéenne computérisée. Bull Soc Opht. France, 1991, 12, XCLS, 1097-1104.
45. Leroux Les Jardins, Pasquier N, Bertrand I. Topographie cornéenne computérisée: Résultats apres kératotomie Radiaire et « T-Cuts ». Bull Soc Opht. France, 1991, 8-9, XCL, 729-34.
46. Lundergan MK. The Orbscan corneal topography system: Verification of accuracy. International Society of Refractive Keratoplasty 1994—Abstract book.
47. Maeda M, Klyce SD, Smolek MK. Neural network classification of corneal topography. Invest Ophthalmol Vis Sci. 1995;36:1327-35.
48. Maeda N, Klyce SD, Smolek MK, et al. Automated keratoconus screening with corneal topography analysis. Invest Ophthalmol Vis Sci. 1994;35:2749-57.
49. Maguire LJ, Singer DE, Klyce SD. Graphic presentation of computer analysed keratoscope photographs. Arch Ophthalmol. 1987;105:223-30.
50. Maguire LJ, Wilson SE, Camp JJ, et al. Evaluating the reproducibility of topography systems on spherical surfaces. Arch Ophthalmol. 1993;111:259-62.
51. Maloney RK, Bogan SJ, Waring GO III. Determination of corneal image-forming properties from corneal topography. Am J Ophthalmol. 1993;l15:31-41.
52. Mandell RB, Horner D. Alignment of videokeratoscopes. In: Sanders DR, Koch DD, (Eds). An Atlas of Corneal Topography. Thorofare NJ: Slack. 1993. pp. 197-206.
53. Mandell RB. Contact lens practice, 4th ed. Springfield, IL: Charles C.Thomas. 1988. pp. 107-35.
54. Mandell RB. Keratometry and contact lens practice. Optometric. 1965. pp. 69-75.
55. Mattioli R, Carones F, Cantera E. New algorithms to improve the reconstruction of corneal geometry on the Keratron™ videokeratographer. Invest Ophthalmol Vis Sci. 1995;36:s302.
56. Mattioli R, Carones F. How accurately can corneal profiles heights be measured by Placido-based videokeratography? Invest Ophthalmol Vis Sci. 1996;37:s932.
57. Mattioli R, Tripoli NA. Corneal geometry reconstruction with the Keratron Videokeratographer. Optom Vis Sci. 1997;74:881-94.
58. Merlin U. I cheratoscopi: Caratteristiche e attendibilita. In: Buratto L, Cantera E, Dal Fiume E, Genisi C, Merlin U, (Eds). Topografia Corneale. Milano Italy: CAMO. 1995. pp. 43-56.
59. Mishima S. Some physiological aspects of the precorneal tearfilm. Arch Ophthalmol. 1965;73:233.
60. Munger R, Priest D, Jackson WB, et al. Reliability of corneal surface maps using the PAR CTS. Invest Ophthalmol Vis Sci. 1996;37: s562.
61. Naufal SC, Hess JS, Friedlander MH, et al. Rasterstereography-based classification of normal corneas. J Cat Refract Surg. 1997;23: 222-30.
62. O'Bart DPS, Corbett MC, Rosen ES. The topography of corneal disease. Eur J Implant Ref Surg. 1995;7:173-83.

63. Olsen T, Dam-Johansen M, Beke T, et al. Evaluating surgically induced astigmatism by Fourier analysis of corneal topography data. J Cat Refract Surg. 1996;22:318-23.
64. Parker PJ, Klyce SD, Ryan BL, et al. Central topographic islands following photorefractive keratectomy. Invest Ophthalmol Vis Sci. 1993;34:803.
65. Prydal JI, Campbell FW. Study of precorneal tear film thickness and structure by interferometry and confocal microscopy. Invest Ophthalmol Vis Sci. 1992;33:1996-2005.
66. Rabinowitz YS, Garbus JJ, Garbus C, et al. Contact lens selection for keratoconus using a computer-assisted videokeratoscope. CLAO J. 1991;17:88-93.
67. Rabinowitz YS, McDonnell PJ. Computer-assisted corneal topography in keratoconus. Refract Corneal Surg. 1989;5:400-08.
68. Roberts C. Characterization of the inherent error in a spherically-biased corneal topography system in mapping a radially aspheric surface. J Refract Corneal Surg. 1994;10:103-16.
69. Roberts C. The Accuracy of power maps to display curvature data in corneal topography systems. Invest Ophthalmol Vis Sci. 1994; 35:3524-32.
70. Rowsey JJ, Reynolds AE, Brown DR. Corneal topography. Corneascope. Arch Ophthalmol. 1981;99:1093-100.
71. Ruiz-Montenegro J, Mafra CH, Wilson SE, et al. Corneal topography alterations in normal contact lens wearers. Ophthalmology. 1993;100:128-34.
72. Salabert D, Cochener B, Mage F, et al. Kératocone et anomalies topographiques cornéennes familiales. J Fr Ophtalmol. 1994;17:lI, 646-56.
73. Sanders RD, Gills JP, Martin RG. When keratometric measurements do not accurately reflect corneal topography. J Cat Refract Surg. 1993;19 (Suppl):131-5.
74. Seiler T, Reckmann W, Maloney RK. Effective spherical aberration of the cornea as a quantitative descriptor in corneal topography. J Cat Refract Surg. 1993;19 (Suppl):155-65.
75. Takeda M, Ina H, Kobayashi S. Fourier-transform method of fringe-pattern analysis for computer-based topography and interferometry. J Optical Soc Am. 1982;72:156-60.
76. Taylor CT, Sutphin JE. Accuracy and precision of the Orbscan topography unit in measuring standardized radially aspheric surfaces. Invest Ophthalmol Vis Sci. 1996;37:s561.
77. Thall EH, Lange SR. Preliminary results of a new intraoperative corneal topography technique. J Cat Refract Surg. 1993;19 (Suppl): 193-7.
78. Tripoli NK, Cohen KL, Holmgren DE, et al. Assessment of radial aspheres by the arc-step algorithm as implemented by the Keratron keratoscope. Am J Ophthalmol. 1995;120:658-64.
79. Tripoli NK, Cohen KL, Obla P, et al. Height measurement of astigmatic test surfaces by a keratoscope that uses plane geometry reconstruction, Am J Ophthalmol. 1996;121:668-76.
80. Vass C, Menapace R, Amon M, et al. Batch-by-batch analysis of topographic changes induced by sutured and sutureless clear corneal incisions. J Cat Refract Surg. 1996;22:324-30.
81. Vass C, Menapace R, Rainer G, et al. Improved algorithm for statistical batch-by-batch analysis of corneal topographic data. J Cat Refract Surg. 1997;23:903-12.
82. Vass C, Menapace R. Computerised statistical analysis of corneal topography for the evaluation of changes in corneal shape after surgery. Am J Ophthalmol. 1994;118:177-84.
83. Wang J, Rice DA, Klyce SD. A new reconstruction algorithm for improvement of corneal topographical analysis. J Refract Corneal Surg. 1989;5:379-87.
84. Warnicki JW, Rehkopf PG, Arrra RC, et al. Corneal topography using a projected grid. In: Schanzlin DJ, Robin JB (Eds). Corneal topography. Measuring and modifying the cornea. Springer-Verlag, New York, 1992.
85. Warnicki JW, Rehkopf PG, Curtin DY, et al. Corneal topography using computer analyzed rasterstereographic images. Appl Optics. 1988;27:1135-40.
86. Warning GO, Hannush SB, Bogan SJ, et al. Classification of corneal topography with videotopography. In: Shanzlin DJ, Robin JB, eds. Corneal topography: measuring and modifying the cornea. New York, NY, Springer-Verlag; 1992. pp. 47-73.
87. Wilson SE, Klyce SD, Husseini ZM. Standardized color-coded maps for corneal topography. Ophthalmology. 1993;100:1723-27.
88. Wilson SE, Klyce SD. Quantitative descriptors of corneal topography. A clinical study. Arch Ophthalmol. 1991;109: 349-53.
89. Wilson SE, Verity SM, Conger DL. Accuracy and precision of the corneal analysis system and the topographic modeling system. Cornea. 1992;11:28-35.
90. Wilson SE, Wang JY, Klyce SD. Quantification and mathematical analysis of photokeratoscopic images. In: Shanzlin DJ, Robin JB eds. Corneal topography: Measuring and modifying the cornea. New York, Springer-Verlag; 1991. pp. 1-81.
91. Young JA, Siegel IM. Isomorphic corneal topography: A clinical approach to 3-D representation of the corneal surface. Refract Corneal Surg. 1993;9:74-8.
92. Young JA, Siegel IM. Three-dimensional digital subtraction modeling of corneal topography. J Refract Surg. 1995;11: 188-93.

Chapter 2

Topographic Machines

Guillermo L Simón-Castellvi (Spain), Sarabel Simón-Castellvi (Spain)
José Maria Simón-Castellvi (Spain), Cristina Simón-Castellvi (Spain)

ZEISS HUMPHREY SYSTEMS® ATLAS™ CORNEAL TOPOGRAPHY SYSTEM MODELS 993 AND ECLIPSE 995

Zeiss Humphrey Systems® ATLAS™ Corneal Topography System Models 993 and Eclipse 995 **(Figure 2.1)** are best sellers in the USA. They measure true elevation data **(Figure 2.2)** through an advanced arc-step algorithm (similar to Optikon 2000® Keratron™), by means of 20–22 ring conical Placido's disk. The Atlas Eclipse 995 offers ultra-low illumination and increased peripheral coverage (limbus to limbus). They also offer automatic pupil measurement. Software displays are viewed in a 10.4″ TFT 640 × 480 pixel resolution in 18 bit color; they include: Photokeratoscope view, axial map, tangential map, numeric view, and profile view. Very interesting optional software packages are available at a price: MasterFit™ contact lens module, corneal elevation map, corneal irregularity map, refractive power map, keratoconus detection map, VisioPro™ ablation planing software and Healing Trend/STARS™ display.

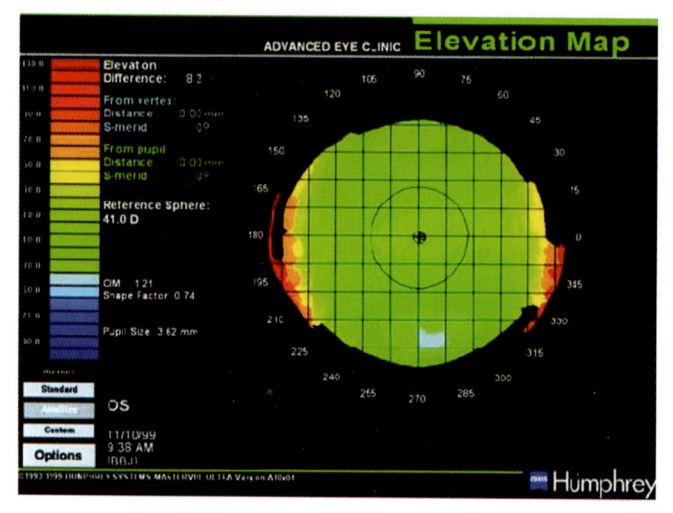

Figure 2.2 Elevation data as seen on Humphrey elevation map

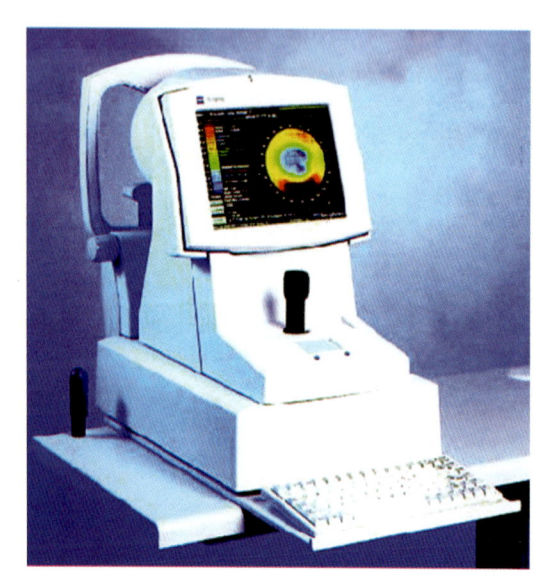

Figure 2.1 Zeiss Humphrey Systems® ATLAS™ Corneal Topography System Models 993 and Eclipse 995

Zeiss Humphrey Systems® ATLAS™ Corneal Topography System
Models 993 and Eclipse 995
Technical Specifications

	ATLAS 993	ATLAS ECLIPSE 995
Working distance	70 mm	70 mm
Field of view	11.4 mm	12.5 mm
Number of rings	20	22 (18 superiorly)
Dioptric range	9 to 108 D	9 to 108 D
Optics	High-res CCD camera	High-res CCD camera
Repeatability (test object)	+ 0.1 D	+ 0.1 D
Repeatability (normal corneas)	+ 0.25 D	+ 0.25 D
Luminosity	Visible light	Infrared (very low-light)
Voltage	100/120/220/240 V AC	100/120/220/240 V AC
Size (Width × Depth × Height) mm	313 × 466 × 457 mm	313 × 466 × 457 mm
Weight	17 kg	20 kg

Hardware: Configuration may vary (450 MHz microprocessor, 64 MB RAM memory, 20 GB hard disk drive, 3.5″ floppy disk drive, USB and Ethernet sockets, 10.4″ TFT flat panel monitor display, one button joystick control, compact keyboard, Glidepoint™ touchpad. Model 955 incorporates infrared chin rest sensors in the patented chin rest design.

TECHNOMED® COLOR ELLIPSOID TOPOMETER

The reproducibility of videokeratography measurements is mainly dependent on the accuracy of manual adjustment in the focal plane. Videokeratoscopes having small Placido cones show a considerable amount of error when the required working distance between cornea and keratoscope is not maintained. The advantages of small cones (optimal illumination and the reduction of anatomically caused shadows) are in no proportion to the disadvantage, poor depth of focus, resulting in poor reproducibility.

The Color Ellipsoid Topometer compensates defocusing errors with the use of software and hardware, by means of triangulation measurement, enhancing precision and theoretically avoiding measuring artefacts. It is the only Placido (30 ring) system with color coded rings (three colored rings). By means of a laser, it measures 10800 points, providing real height values and has ray tracing software. A new module enables topography-driven laser ablation. This unit is specially useful in diagnosing postoperative problems in a refractive practice, specially in those cases with a loss of vision that cannot be explained. The Color Ellipsoid Topometer can predict the quality of vision based on the shape of the cornea and pupil.

DICON® CT200

The reproducibility of videokeratography measurements is mainly dependent on the accuracy of manual adjustment in the focal plane. The Dicon® CT-200 **(Figure 2.3)** is a cheap easy to use instrument with autofocus and autoalignment that eliminate joystick and explorer subjectivity, thus improving repeatability. The big Placido's disk cone is managed from the computer by means of the mouse. Final alignment (up and down) and focusing (forwards and backwards) are automatically performed by the motorized instrument head.

It can explore the whole cornea (apex and limbus to limbus) thanks to an offset-fixation. The patient can fixate different green lights, to allow complete cornea coverage. Offset-fixation mapping allows for more precise mapping of the central 3 mm of the cornea. More true data points from the apex and true limbus-to-limbus measurements over a large corneal area provide for better coverage without extrapolation **(Figure 2.4)**.

Nevertheless, we miss a different chin rest to allow faster examination by eliminating the need for patient's head re-centration from one eye to the other.

The system generates maps in seconds and detailed customized reports can be printed in less than a minute with any color printer running under MS Windows '95™ operating system.

A very interesting feature of this instrument is the Bull's Eye Targetting™: The system automatically targets the apex position of a cone (keratoconus or other), providing a numerical index for that cone. An autoalarm is activated so that any suspicious case of keratoconus (or excessive corneal elevation with an index higher than 10) is automatically detected and acoustically signalled and a peak detection warning window appears in the display after the image capture is complete. New users will appreciate this feature: A low index is not uncommon, and does not always mean that we face a pathologic cornea. High indices in a tangential map almost always mean that we face a keratoconus or another kind of corneal ectasia **(Figure 2.5)**.

Peak detection can be triggered by any suspect peak, including mucous in the tear film, or localized areas of film break-up. In one such case, always have the patient close the eyes for a while and blink a few extra times before retaking the Figure. In case of doubt, it is advisable to retake the figure again. The determination of the condition producing the corneal elevation needs to be confirmed by other clinical tests, like slit lamp examination or others.

The Dicon® CT-200™ software includes an optional refractive module that allows single analysis, trend analysis of multiple displays and a special package called VISX® STAR S2™ Ablation Planner **(Figures 2.6A to D)**.

The VISX® STAR S2™ Ablation Planner is offered as an option and is intended to learn the control system for the VISX® laser. It offers a custom display of the CT 200 Elliptical Elevation Map, and access to the VISX® STAR S2™ control panel. It allows a simulated (not real) image of the before/after laser ablation for better comprehension of the procedure.

Developed by Dr Robert B. Mandell is a simplified contact lens fitting software, with fluorescein simulation. You can design unique lenses for each cornea (personalized designs) and send the data directly to the manufacturer (via modem) or print the ordersheet for faxing or mailing.

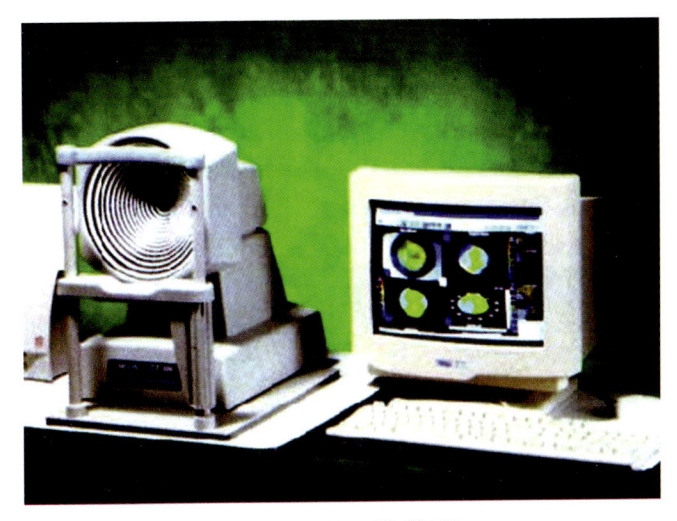

Figure 2.3 Dicon's® CT 200

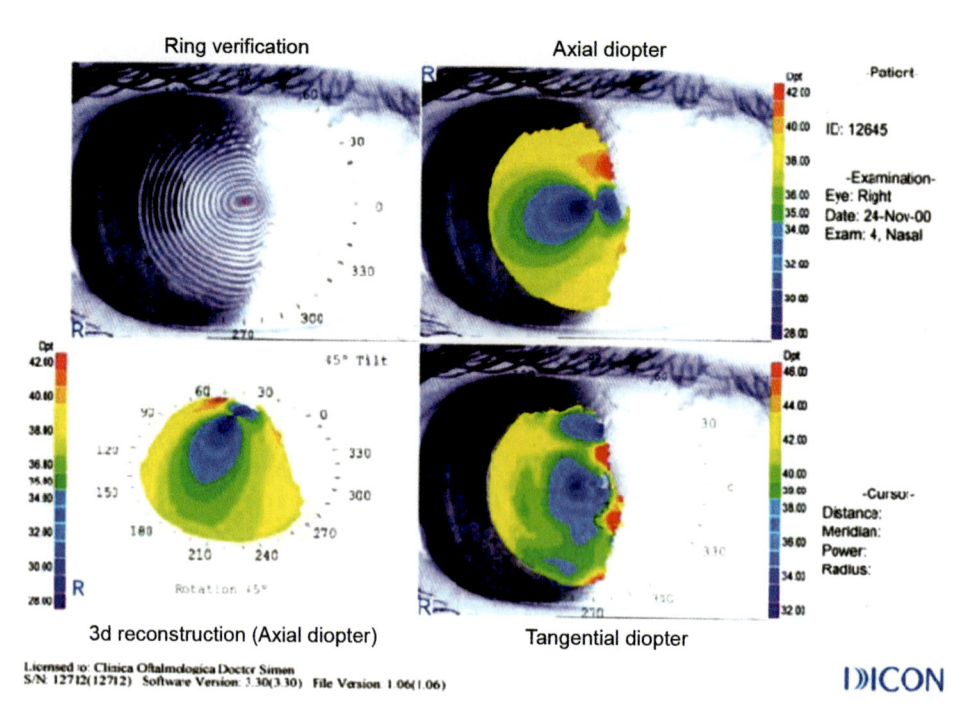

24 Section I: Introduction to Corneal Topography and Orbscan

Figure 2.4 Dicon's CT-200™ can explore the whole cornea (apex, and limbus-to-limbus) thanks to an offset-fixation. Patient fixates different green lights: shown is a quadruple view of right eye, corneal maps, display a nasal fixation, including 3-D reconstruction with a 45° tilt (left and down). Optional software (Multiview™) provides total cornea coverage using the mentioned multiple fixation targets. Limbal measurements are not always reliable, being subject to many artefacts

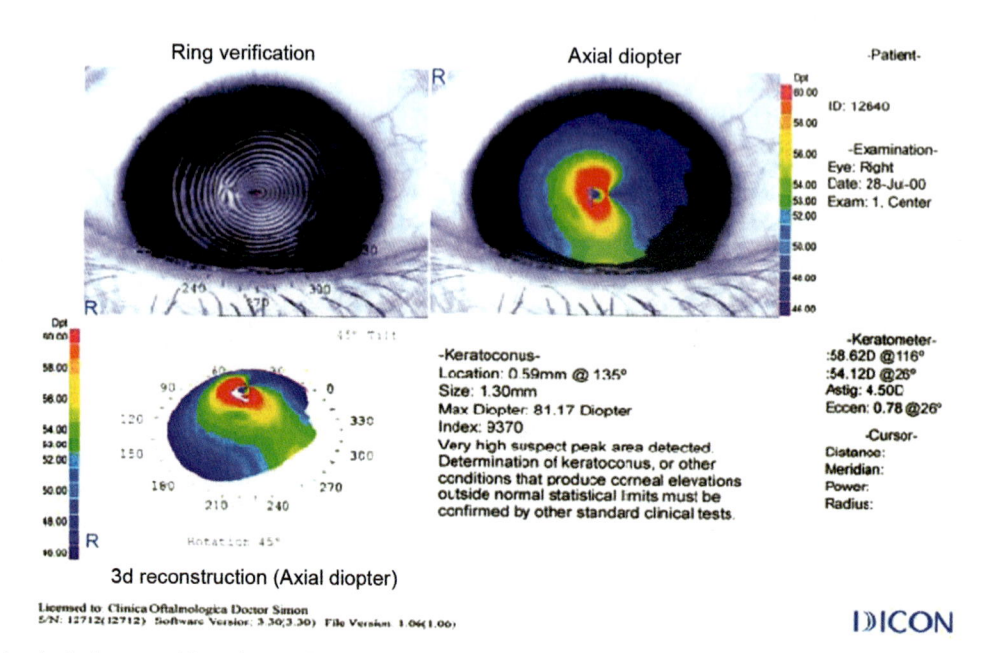

Figure 2.5 A quadruple display map of the right eye of a 55-year-old man suffering from progressive bilateral corneal central ectasia. Notice the distortion of the mires in the ring verification map (up and left), the enormous "red" central and paracentral elevation in the axial diopter map (up and right). Statistical information is displayed following the peak detection, identifying the location, size, maximum power, peak index and probability statement (very high suspect peak area detected). One such high index (index = 9370) always means that we face a keratoconus or another kind of corneal ectasia. The ectasia was clearly visible at the slit-lamp

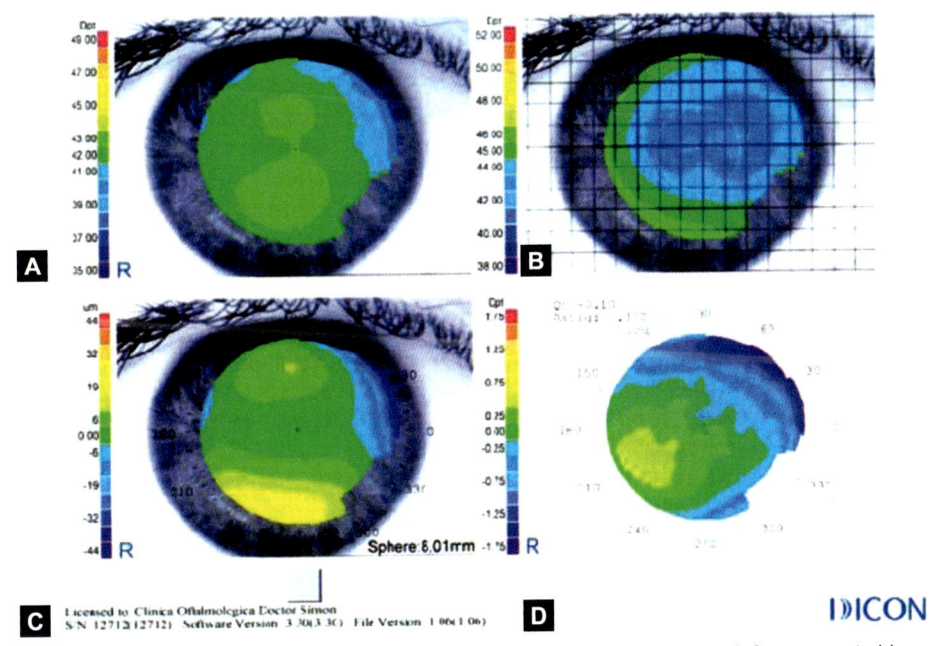

Figures 2.6A to D The "Single Analysis" menu option of the Dicon® CT-200™ displays a single exam with four customisable map views (A) axial diopter, (B) refractive diopter (shown with a square grid overlay), (C) spherical height and (D) irregularity (shown without the eye overlay). The irregularity map (D) reports an index (Q = –0.10) that measures eccentricity (a measure of asphericity) and the amount of astigmatism that has been subtracted from the original ideal spherical corneal data (in this case, 1.12 D)

DICON® CT-200™ Technical Specifications

Videokeratoscope

Tested area	
Keratoscope cone	Big cone, 16 bright Placido rings and 16 dark rings
Measured points	11,500
Corneal coverage	Total, by means of different fixation targets with standard software (optional Multiview™ software provides total corneal coverage)
Range of dioptric powers	
Resolution	
Focusing	Autofocus, autoalignment for X, Y and Z
Camera	High-resolution videosystem
Voltage	110 or 230 V, 50/60 Hz

Computer — Included with the system (may vary), separate

Processor	Intel® PENTIUM™
Main memory	32 Mb RAM (minimum)
Hard disk	4.3 Gb (minimum)
Floppy disk drive	3½"-1.44 Mb
Monitor	Color 14" Super VGA
Video mode	Up to 1024 × 768 and 256 colors
Mouse	included, 100% Microsoft compatible
Printer	Any color printer running under Windows
Modem	Internal (in some countries)
Software	32-bit programs (Eye 3.40 and Backup software on CD), running under Windows™ 95

Contd...

Contd...

Color maps

Color scales	Absolute, normalized, adjustable, mm or D
Keratometric data	Simulated K-reading, mm or D
Pupil	Edge mapping, diameter and offset
Available maps	Axial, Spherical height, Tangential, Refractive, Numerical display, Meridional, 3-D reconstruction map, Elliptical elevation
Printouts	Full color, customisable reports
Special functions	Profile, Map difference, Map comparison, PRK-LASIK simulation
	Simultaneous screen displays for rapid analysis and ease of use
	Keratoconus detection
	Irregularity index to measure corneal distortion which affects quality of vision
	Delta map to determine changes between exams
Surgical modules	Advanced surgical module for healing trend analysis with difference maps (optional)
	VISX® STAR S2™ Ablation Planner
On-line help	Available
Contact lens fitting	Fluorescein simulation of any RGP CL geometry or major CL producers (customisable lens design)
	Mandell contact lens module "Easy-Fit™" (standard)
	Mandell contact lens module "Advanced-Fit™" (optional)
Internet connection	Possible
Direct faxing	Possible as standard for contact lens ordering or sending reports, through operating system
LAN operations	Possible, through operating system

EYESYS® 2000

Topographers from Premier Laser Systems, EyeSys Corneal Analysis System 2000 and EyeSys Vista Hand-held corneal topographer, have been the leading topographers in the USA for years but might have been discontinued at the moment you may read this chapter due to Premier Laser Systems' bankruptcy. We have included them to honor the topographers we learned with, as most topographic texts still refer to them. We hope that new partners in early future or potential buyers help to guarantee the survival of EyeSys topographers in this hard market place.

KERATRON™ CORNEAL TOPOGRAPHER (OPTIKON 2000® SPA, ITALY-EUROPE)

The Keratron™ topographer **(Figure 2.7)** is one of our preferred systems: It is a must, if you are in refractive surgery. The Keratron topographers offer automatic image capture. A patented corneal vertex detector system is housed inside a slight protrusion on either side of the cone. If you position the Keratron™ too close or too far, image capture just will not happen. Only when the system detects the vertex in the exact right position, image is automatically captured, thus obtaining more reproducible maps.

Introduced in 1994, the Keratron™ was the first hardware platform designed to get the most of an arc-step surface reconstruction, achieving accuracy and sensitivity, without smoothing of data or extrapolating to fill in topographic shadows. The Keratron's own method of arc-step mapping accurately maps aspheric surfaces. It uses a small Placido cone of rings.

Its patented infrared vertex detector sensor determines the exact position of the corneal vertex and begins constructing a web of "Arcs" between the intersections of 26 rings and 256 meridians, from the vertex to the periphery. Defining corneal vertex position and starting measurements from it provide this topographer with high accuracy. Curvature and height are simultaneously derived from the length and shape of each arc. Mapping beginning at the corneal vertex, this instrument easily detects central islands or minor defects. Each data point of the "web" is related to another one, thus eliminating inaccuracies of traditional Placido "concentric rings method" which take measurement of each point independently from one another, resulting in possible errors.

While most topographers first create an axial map and then convert the axial data into different maps, every Keratron's map is calculated separately without conversions, thus decreasing probability of errors. Since, the Keratron does not convert data, map error is minimal in all maps.

True corneal elevation (height) in microns as well as the traditional curvature maps are created. This system enables to map the image of a patient with bad fixation-through mathematics reconstruction. The system is fast and easy to use, working under MS Windows™ environment. The powerful software is the gem of the system novice will find some difficulty but once you master it you will not want to get rid of this topographer.

You can design unique lenses for each cornea (personalized designs) and send the data directly to the manufacturer (via modem). A recently developed software by Jim Edwards, OD (*patents pending*) called wave uses a unique but logical approach to contact lens design by effectively creating a mirror image of the peripheral cornea in the lens design process. Contact lenses designed with Wave drape the cornea in a manner similar to a soft lens. As the lens periphery matches the peripheral cornea, lens centration should be unsurpassed, even with reverse geometry lenses.

Optikon 2000® has made a small portable topographer called Scout Portable Topographer with the same features as

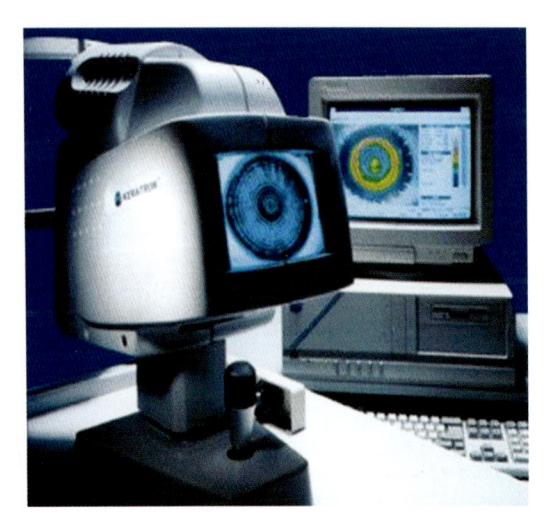

Figure 2.7 Keratron™ corneal topographer (Optikon 2000® SpA, Italy-Europe)

KERATRON™ Corneal Topographer Technical Specifications

Videokeratoscope

Tested area	10 × 14 mm (visible on the monitor)
Keratoscope cone	28 equally spaced borders of black and bright Placido rings
Tested points	More than 80,000
Measured points	7,168
Corneal coverage	From 0.33 mm (first ring) to about 90% of a normal cornea
Range of dioptric powers	From I to 127 D
Resolution	+/−0.01D; 1 micron
Focusing	Infrared automatic, Eye Position Control System (patented)
Camera	High-resolution (CCIR system)
Monitor	6" black and white

Contd...

Contd...

Computer (Minimal Requirements)	
Processor	Intel™ PENTIUM®
Main memory	32 Mb RAM (minimum)
Hard disk	2 Gb (minimum)
Floppy disk drive	3½"-1.44 Mb
Monitor	Color 14" Super VGA
Video Mode	Up to 1280 × 1024 and up to 16 million colors
Mouse	Any 100% Microsoft compatible
Printer	Any color printer running under Windows™
Software	Microsoft® Windows™ 3.11, '95 or '98
Color Maps	
Color scales	Absolute, normalized, adjustable, spherical offset, mm or D
Keratometry	K-reading, Meridians, Emi-meridians, Maloney indices
Pupil	Edge mapping, Diameter and offset
Zones	3, 5 and 7 mm
Maps representations	Local True Curvature, Axial and Refractive powers. (All with arc-step algorithm)
Eye/map orientation	Video-keratoscope axis, or moved to the entrance pupil or to any chosen axis
Printouts	Large and small size with the patient's form, list of the filed examinations
Special functions	Profile, Map difference, Map comparison, PRK simulation
On-line help	Available from any screen
Contact lens fitting	Simulation of any RGP CL geometry or major CL producers
	Tilting and displacement of the lens
	Eccentricity and apical radius measurements at 6/8 mm of the main axes, or locally on any axis
	Autofit programs (Curvature Classical and Height fitting) with personalized protocols
	Adjustable clearance scale
	Optional Wave Contact Lens Design software (available in the USA)
Internet connection	Possible with personalized template letter
LAN operations	Possible
Image capture	Possible from an external slit-lamp TV camera, with KeraCap software (included) and a generic frame capture board

the full size device: At the moment as these lines are written it suffers from some youth design defects that will be soon addressed by Opticon 2000®. It is available as slit-lamp model, hand-held model, table top model or surgical microscope model.

ET-800 CORNEAL TOPOGRAPHY SYSTEM

Euclid Systems Corporation® ET-800 CTS is another interesting product in this round-up, since it uses a completely different method of topography called **Fourier profilometry**.

The technique uses the projection of 2 identical sine wave patterns onto the surface of the eye. The projection is done using filtered blue light that induces fluorescence of a liquid (fluorescein) that has been applied to the tear film before the examination. The resulting image is captured by a CCD camera. Two dimensional Fourier transform mathematics are used to calculate the phase shift of the projected wave pattern. The phase shift is directly related to the height information. This method analyzes over 300,000 data points to achieve true elevation coordinates, with each point accurate to approximately the thickness of the tear film (about one micron). The problem is that thickness of the tear film varies with daytime, and is not the same for each patient.

The system uses no rings or Placido's disk. It is quite fast (processing time: 4 seconds). The focusing mechanism is a live TV camera. It provides full scleral and corneal coverage up to 22 – 17 mm (useful to assess pterygium evolution). It is sold as the "only" topographer to measure true corneal elevation. Let's observe again that most topographers measure corneal elevation by extrapolating from corneal reflex (thus, interfered by tear film layer quality). It might well be the most precise method, each of the 300,000 data points being accurate to about 1 micron, but unfortunately it is not widespread enough to become a reference system. It still needs clinical validation.

This projection technique visualizes the surface directly while a reflection technique amplifies the corneal topographic distortions. It measures with low light level, offering full K analysis, "e" value analysis, cross sections, ellipsoidal difference map, full patient and radiological histories, and a easy to use four click exam wizard.

EYE MAP EH-290 ALCON® CORNEAL TOPOGRAPHY SYSTEM

Alcon® EH-290 Eye Map corneal Topography System is a large 23 narrow modified Placido's disk system. The modified patented Placido cone design is supposed to be very accurate

Alcon® EH-290 Eye Map Corneal Topography System Technical Specifications

Measuring System:
- Aspheric measuring system
- Placido's disk images
- Over 8,000+ data reference points
- 23 non-linear rings
- Fully Automated (centring/focusing/image capture), with 20 step image focusing process
- Microsoft™ Windows™ operating system -produces a graph in less than 30 seconds
- Linear analysis verification graph
- True Tangential Measuring algorithms
- 3D data calculations
- Large image view

System Hardware:

Separate optical head and computer system (computer system may vary in different countries). Storage capacity of over 31,000 + patient files (w/o images).

Contd...

Contd...

Eye Map EH-290 Specifications

- Power requirements: 110/120 volts AC, 60 HZ, 220/250 volts AC, 50 HZ
- Processing time: 7 seconds
- Fixation point distance: Optical infinity/on axis
- Area of coverage: < 4.6 mm diameter to 10 > mm diameter depending on the surface curvature
- Photokeratoscope: patented Visioptic design (US Patent No. 4,978,213)
- Optical Head: 23 non-linear spaced rings
- Positioning system: EyeMap EH-290 software driven autoposition system
- Camera: High resolution CCD Video Camera
- Monitor: Color monitor
- Keyboard: 101 Key Enhanced Keyboard
- Hard disk: 540 Megabytes
- Removable hard disk: 1.5 Gigabytes
- Floppy disk: 1,44 Megabytes

and sensitive. Easy and intuitive to use (software runs under Windows™), it offers advanced contact lens software, keratoconus detection, corneal statistics information and advanced communication software.

TOMEY® AUTOTOPOGRAPHER

Tomey® autotopographer is a cheap, small and portable fully automatic self-topographer that requires no operator alignment. The patient places his or her face on an ergonomically designed face rest and the automated topographer is activated by proximity sensors, automatically taking the measurements. The software, that can be installed in a preowned PC, runs under Windows™ operating system. The software is very complete and comprehensive, and includes a contact lens wizard with interactive fluorescein displays. Optional software packages include: Height and Height Change Maps, Klyce Corneal Statistics, Keratoconus Screening and the Contact Lens Wizard. The low level lights is intended to produce minimal glare and disturbance for the patient.

TOMEY™ AUTOTOPOGRAPHER
Technical Specifications

Area measured	: 0.19 to 11.5 mm
Dioptric range	: 9 to 101.5 Diopters
Number of rings	: 31, low level light
Evaluated points	: 7.936
Dimensions	: 384 (height) × 230 (width) × 358 (depth) mm
Power	100/120/220/240 VAC, 50/60 Hz
Weight	: 5.5 kg/12 lbs
PC minimum requirements	: Intel® Pentium™ 133 Microsoft® Windows™ 95 or better, 32 MB RAM, 100 MB hard disk drive free space 800 × 640 SVGA color monitor bidirectional parallel port 3.5" floppy disk drive

OCULUS® KERATOGRAPH™ AND HAAG-STREIT® KERATOGRAPH CTK 922

Oculus® Keratograph **(Figure 2.8)** and Haag-Streit® Keratograph CTK 922 **(Figure 2.9)** are very similar instruments sold under different brand names and different packaging. They are compact systems that can fit any refractive unit and include built-in keratometer in connection with the topography system. The software runs under Windows™ operating system and is easy to use, with automatic measurement. The Oculus® can be an integrated computerized system (Keratograph C, in the Figure) or an independent system linked to a preowned computer. A noncontact measurement large Placido system with 22 rings in a hemisphere and 22,000 measuring points try to guarantee a high resolution.

The working distance of 80 mm is enough to make the patient feel comfortable. The light system (warm colored) is intended to produce minimal glare and disturbance for the patient.

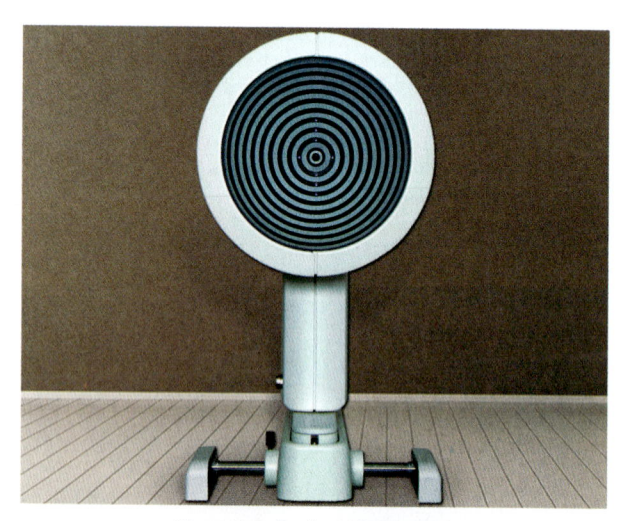

Figure 2.8 Oculus® Keratograph

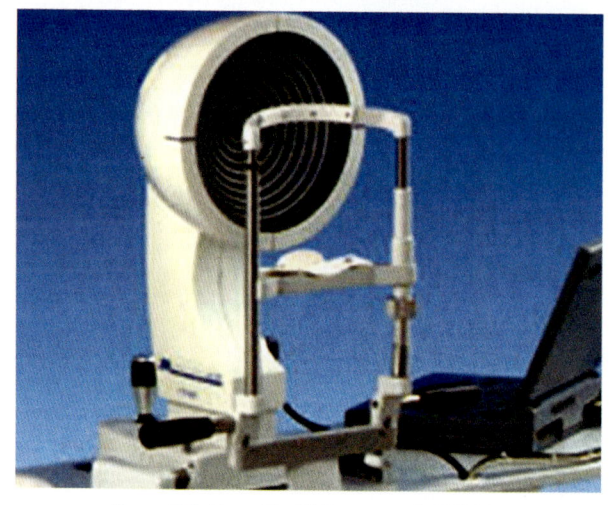

Figure 2.9 Haag-Streit® Keratograph CTK 922

Chapter 2: Topographic Machines 29

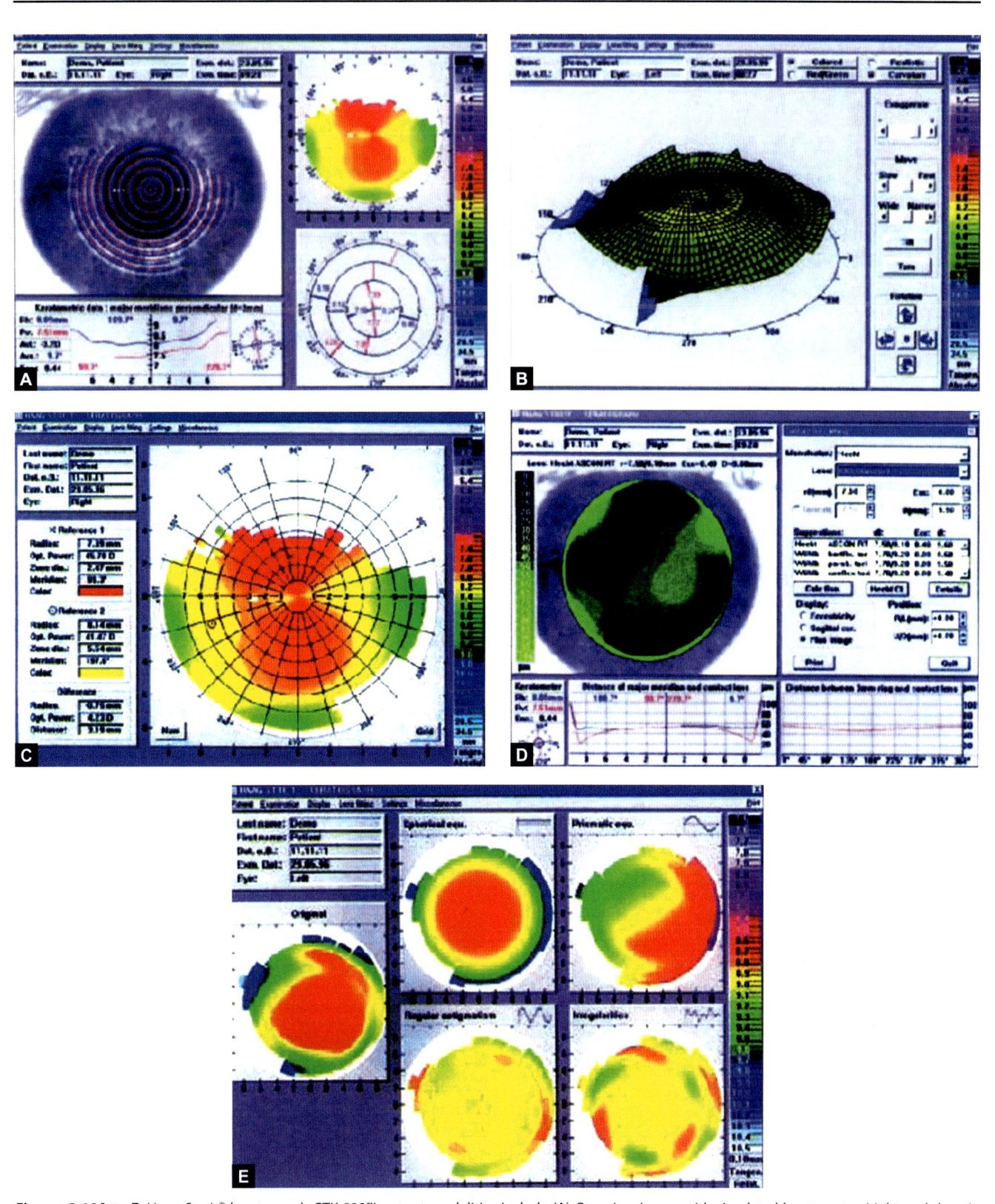

Figures 2.10A to E Haag-Streit® keratograph CTK 922™ output modalities include (A) Overview image with simulated keratometer (right and down), (B) Comprehensive kinetic three-dimensional (3-D) analysis of corneal topography for simple explanation to the patient, (C) Zoom-up image of a map, (D) Fluorescein image simulation for contact lens fitting, and (E) Fourier expressive analysis (Published with permission from Haag Streit® AG International)

Section I: Introduction to Corneal Topography and Orbscan

They have an interesting software that allows contact lens-fitting in three simple steps: Automated contact lens recommendation with a database that includes 20,000 lens geometries from all major contact lens manufacturers, and can be easily enlarged, and realistic fluo-image simulation of contact lens adaptation **(Figures 2.10A to E)**. There is a possibility of measuring the back surface of rigid gas permeable contact lens through optional Lens Check software.

There is also an optional statistics software package called Datagraph, intended for refractive surgeons.

This systems allows wonderful comprehensive kinetic three-dimensional analysis of corneal topography for simple explanation to the patient **(Figure 2.11A)**. Fourier surface analysis **(Figure 2.11B)** is available and new software is under development for refractive surgery and contact lens fitters.

Also optional is the Topolink software, that integrates the corneal topography data and some but not all excimer laser software.

OCULUS® KERATOGRAPH™ and HAAG-STREIT® KERATOGRAPH™ CTK 922 *Technical specifications*	
Measuring	: 3 to 38 mm / 9 to 99 Diopters
Accuracy	: ± 0,1 D
Reproducibility	: ± 0,1 D
Number of rings	: 22
Evaluated points	: 22.000
Dimensions	: 510 (height) × 300 (width) × 280 (depth) mm 2,3 kg
Weight	: Intel® Pentium™ 100
PC requirements	: Windows 3.1 or higher / 16 MB of RAM memory / 1 MB graphics VGA card with at least 256 colors

ORBSCAN IIZ™ -BAUSCH AND LOMB® SURGICAL, INC. (USA)

This is a truly revolutionary instrument for the study of the cornea **(Figure 2.12)**. It combines a slit scanning system and a Placido's disk (with 40 rings) to measure the anterior elevation and curvature of the cornea and the posterior elevation and curvature of the cornea. It offers a full corneal pachymetry map with white to white measurements **(Table 2.1)**.

Orbscan IIz™ takes a series of slit-beam images of two scanning slit-lamps beams projected at 45 degrees, to the right or left of the instrument axis. During the exam, the patient fixates on a blinking red light coaxial with the imaging system. Forty images are taken by the system, 20 with slit beams projected from the right and 20 from the left. The 20 images are acquired in 0.7 seconds each. Simultaneously, a tracking system measures the nonvoluntary movements of the eye during the exam.

Orbscan IIz™ is able to measure anterior chamber depth, angle kappa, pupil diameter, simulated keratometry readings (3 and 5 central mm of the cornea), and the thinnest corneal pachymetry reading **(Figures 2.13 and 2.14)**. It offers every traditional map apart form those of posterior corneal surface. Elevation topography of the anterior cornea enables clinicians to more accurately visualize the shape of abnormal corneas, which should lead to more accurate diagnoses and better surgical results. It has proven to be an extraordinary tool for research and for the refractive surgeon.

The system is able to acquire over 9000 data points in 1.5 seconds, which is fast, but not enough for the patient to feel comfortable. Not every patient can avoid blinking, and in some cases measurements have to be repeated. A faster processing speed would be desirable, although we feel very comfortable with the system.

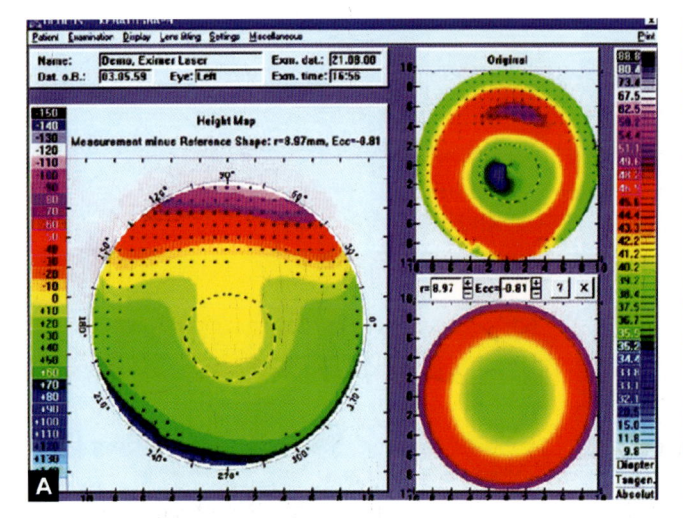

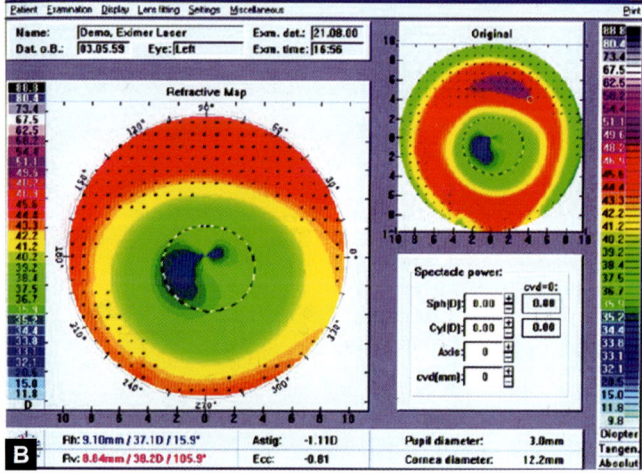

Figures 2.11A and B Oculus® Keratograph™ screen shots with elevation (height) map and refractive map that will be included in 2001 software version (latest review). A new algorithm method for increased precision (Published with permission from Oculus Optikgeraete GmbH)

Chapter 2: Topographic Machines 31

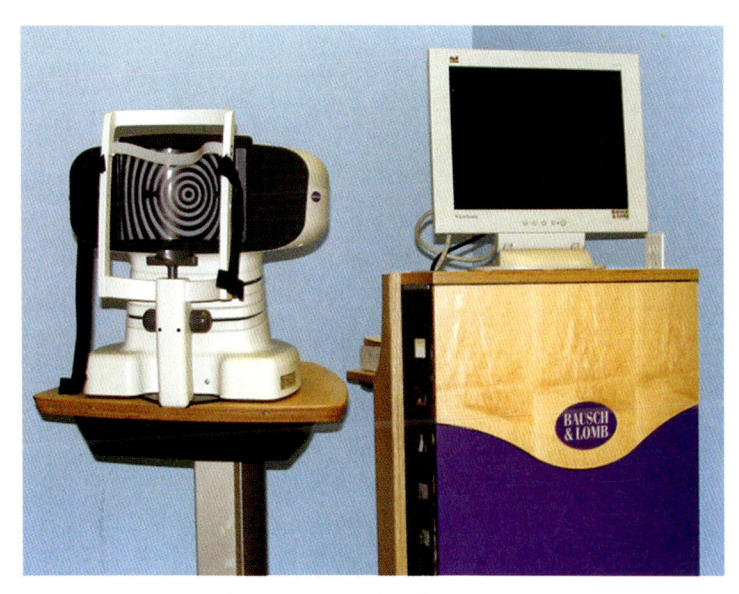

Figure 2.12 Orbscan IIz™ -Bausch and Lomb® Surgical, Inc. (USA)

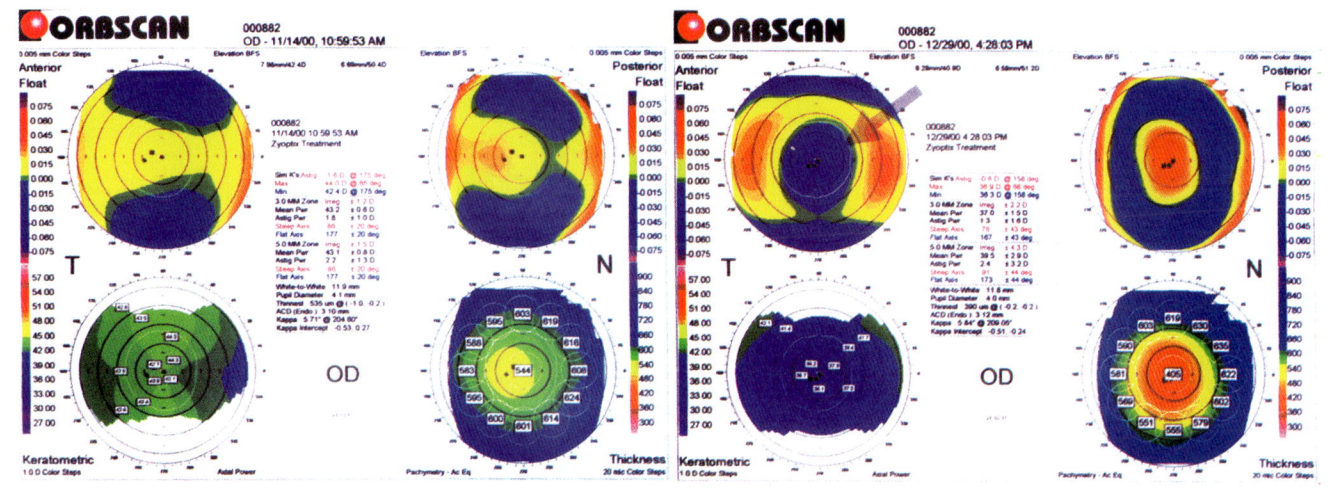

Figure 2.13 Displays different preoperative and postoperative maps of the right eye of a patient who underwent a refractive myopic Zyoptics™ LASIK procedure. Images were taken with Orbscan IIz™ - Bausch and Lomb® Surgical, Inc. (USA) topographer. The Anterior Best Fit Sphere (BFS) is calculated to best match the anterior corneal surface. The elevation BFS map subtracts the calculated best fit sphere size against the eye surface in millimeters (mm). The difference between the sphere and the eye surface is expressed in distance, in a radial way, from the center of the sphere as shown in the figure (map anterior float BFS). The shape of a sphere being easily imagined by the explorer, deviation from that spherical surface in a special case helps to appreciate the true shape of the eye and its deviation from symmetry (asymmetry). The map has 35 default color steps, the size of each step being measured at the bottom of each color. (Five microns is the default for the BFS map). The best fit between eye surface and sphere is represented in green. Areas under this spherical ideal surface are represented in blue, while warmer colors (orange-red) identify areas above this ideal sphere. The box in the middle of the displays shows patient information of interest like patient's name, examination date, diameter (mm) and power (D) of the ideal sphere, diagnosis, simulated keratometry readings, white to white distance, pupil diameter, thinnest measurement for that cornea, anterior chamber depth (either from epithelium or endothelium), angle Kappa, and Kappa intercept. The Posterior Best Fit Sphere (BFS) is calculated to best match the posterior corneal surface. The Keratometric simulates keratometric values at special areas. The Thickness Map (Pachymetry map) shows the differences in elevation between the anterior and posterior surfaces of the cornea. By moving the mouse over the map, explorer can obtain measurements of the thickness at each point. This map can be overlaid by the average measurements that would be taken with a traditional ultrasound pachymeter (encircled values). This map is invaluable for preoperative assessment of the refractive patient, and to determine the true ablated tissue depth in the postoperative period of PRK and refractive patients. Thickness maps clearly demonstrate that ablation zone (arrow) has decreased in thickness form 544 to 405 microns. Notice that corneal thickness increases as we get closer to the limbus. (*Courtesy*: Dr Andreu Coret, Institut Oftalmològic de Barcelona, Barcelona - Spain)

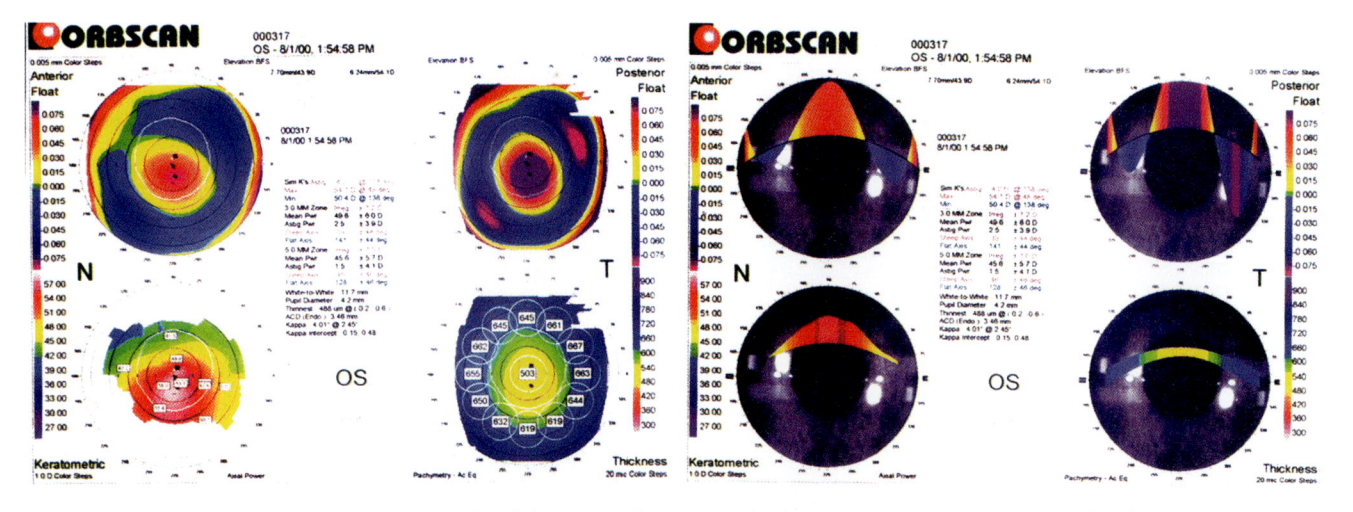

32   Section I: Introduction to Corneal Topography and Orbscan

Figure 2.14 Keratoconus: Displays different maps of the left (OS) eye of a patient with a keratoconus. Images were taken with Orbscan IIz™ - Bausch and Lomb® Surgical, Inc. (USA) topographer. Notice the central elevation in both anterior and posterior surfaces of the cornea, with reduced corneal thickness (comparing to a normal eye) and high astigmatism. The four inferior maps display different cross-section along the 0°-180° meridian that demonstrate how the cornea is higher than the best fit sphere centrally (reddish central mountain overlaid on the corneal display) and lower in the mid-periphery (bluish depression at both sides of the mountain). (*Courtesy*: Dr Andreu Coret, Institut Oftalmològic de Barcelona, Barcelona-Spain)

Table 2.1 Measurable parameters with Bausch and Lomb surgical® ORBSCAN IIz™

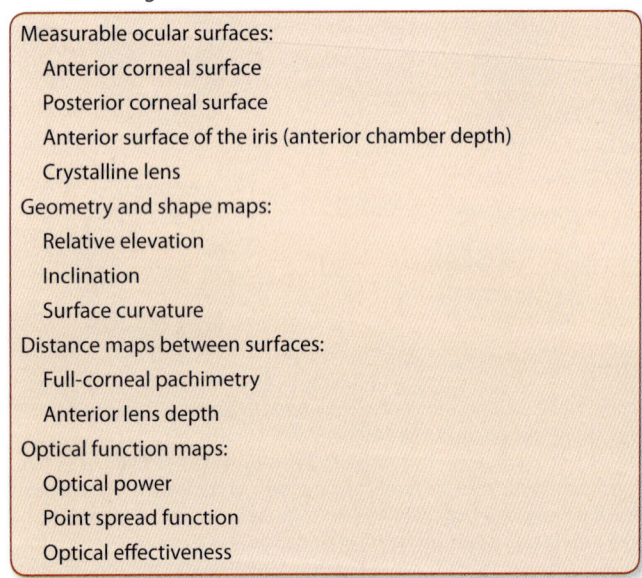

Measurable ocular surfaces:
Anterior corneal surface
Posterior corneal surface
Anterior surface of the iris (anterior chamber depth)
Crystalline lens
Geometry and shape maps:
Relative elevation
Inclination
Surface curvature
Distance maps between surfaces:
Full-corneal pachimetry
Anterior lens depth
Optical function maps:
Optical power
Point spread function
Optical effectiveness

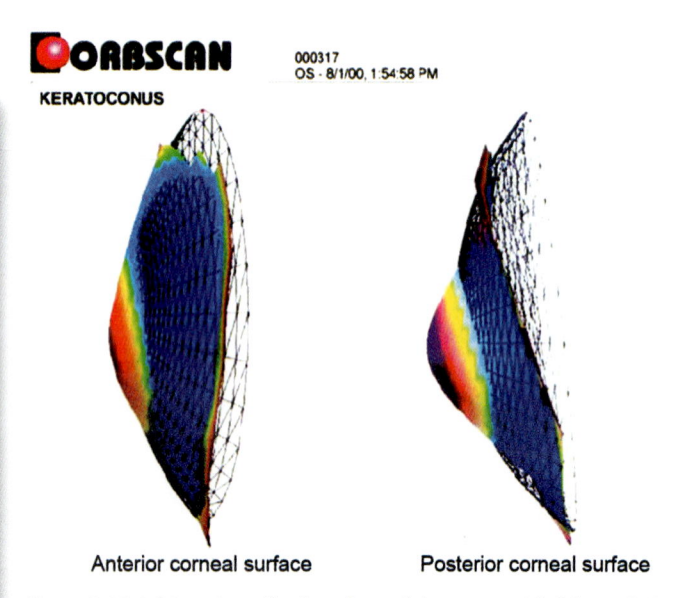

Figure 2.15 3-D imaging of both surfaces of the cornea with Orbscan IIz™ software is really meaningful for the patient. Notice that central protrusion is higher in posterior than in anterior surface of the cornea: in between, corneal thickness is reduced. (*Courtesy*: Dr Andreu Coret, Institut Oftalmològic de Barcelona, Barcelona-Spain)

Easy to use and running under Microsoft® Windows™ NT 4.0 operating system, the major disadvantage is the high price, that makes it not affordable for most ophthalmologists. Any color printer running under NT 4.0 can be used. Three dimensional views of the different maps are available **(Figure 2.15)**.

Chapter 3

Corneal Topography and the Orbscan

Amar Agarwal (India), Athiya Agarwal (India)

INTRODUCTION

Keratometry and corneal topography with Placido's disk systems were originally invented to measure anterior corneal curvature.[1-3] Computer analysis of the more complete data acquired by the latter in recent years has been increasingly more valuable in the practice of refractive surgery. The problem in the Placido's disk systems is that one cannot perform a slit scan topography of the cornea. This has been solved by an instrument called the Orbscan that combines both slit scan and Placido images to give a very good composite picture for topographic analysis. Bausch and Lomb manufacture this.

PARAXIAL OPTICS

Spectacle correction of sight is designed only to eliminate defocus errors and astigmatism. These are the only optical aberrations that can be handled by the simplest theory of imaging, known as paraxial optics, which excludes all light rays finitely distant from a central ray or power axis. Ignoring the majority of rays entering the pupil, paraxial optics examines only a narrow thread-like region surrounding the power axis. The shape of any smoothly rounded surface within this narrow region is always circular in cross-section. Thus from the paraxial viewpoint, surface shape is toric at most. Only its radius may vary with meridional angle. As a toric optical surface has sufficient flexibility to null defocus and astigmatism, only paraxial optics is needed to specify corrective lenses for normal eyes. Paraxial optics is used in keratometers and two-dimensional topographic machines.

RAYTRACE OR GEOMETRIC OPTICS

The initial objective of refractive surgery was to build the necessary paraxial correction into the cornea. When outcomes are less than perfect, it is not just because defocus correction is inadequate. Typically, other aberrations (astigmatism, spherical aberration, coma, etc.) are introduced by the surgery. These may be caused by decentered ablation, asymmetric healing, biomechanical response, poor surgical planning, and inadequate or misinformation. To assess the aberrations in the retinal image all the light rays entering the pupil must properly be taken in account using raytrace (or geometric) optics. Paraxial optics and its hypothetical toric surfaces must be abandoned as inadequate, which eliminates the need to measure surface curvature. Raytrace optics does not require surface curvature, but depends on elevation and especially surface slope. The Orbscan uses raytrace or geometric optics.

ELEVATION

Orbscan measure elevation, which is not possible in other topographic machines. Elevation is especially important because it is the only complete scalar measure of surface shape. Both slope and curvature can be mathematically derived from a single elevation map, but the converse is not necessarily true. As both slope and curvature have different values in different directions, neither can be completely represented by a single map of the surface. Thus, when characterizing the surface of non-spherical test objects used to verify instrument accuracy, elevation is always the gold standard.

Curvature maps in corneal topography (usually misnamed as power or dioptric maps) only display curvature measured in radial directions from the map center. Such a presentation is not shift-invariant, which means its values and topography change as the center of the map is shifted. In contrast, elevation is shift-invariant. An object shifted with respect to the map center is just shifted in its elevation map. In a meridional curvature view it is also described. This makes elevation maps more intuitively understood, making diagnosis easier.

To Summarize

1. Curvature is not relevant in raytrace optics.
2. Elevation is complete and can be used to derive surface curvature and slope.
3. Elevation is the standard measure of surface shape.
4. Elevation is easy to understand.

The problem we face is that there is a cost in converting elevation to curvature (or slope) and visa versa. To go from elevation to curvature requires mathematical differentiation, which accentuates the high spatial frequency components of the elevation function. As a result, random measurement error or noise in an elevation measurement is significantly multiplied

34 Section I: Introduction to Corneal Topography and Orbscan

in the curvature result. The inverse operation, mathematical integration used to convert curvature to elevation, accentuates low-frequency error. The Orbscan helps in good mathematical integration. This makes it easy for the ophthalmologist to understand as the machine does all the conversion.

ORBSCAN I AND II

Previously, Orbscan I was used. This had only slit scan topographic system. Then the Placido's disk was added in Orbscan I. Hence, Orbscan II came into the picture.

SPECULAR VS BACK-SCATTERED REFLECTION

The keratometer eliminates the anterior curvature of the pre-corneal tear film. It is an estimate because the keratometer only acquires data within a narrow 3 mm diameter annulus. It measures the anterior tear-film because it is based on specular reflection (**Figure 3.1**), which occurs primarily at the air-tear interface. As the keratometer has very limited data coverage, abnormal corneas can produce misleading or incorrect results.

Orbscan can calculate a variety of different surface curvatures, and on a typical eye, these are all different. Only on a properly aligned and perfectly spherical surface are the various curvatures equal. The tabulated SimK values (magnitudes and associated meridians) are the only ones designed to give keratometer-like measurements. Therefore, it only makes sense to compare keratometry reading with SimK values.

Orbscan uses slit-beams and back-scattered light (**Figure 3.2**) to triangulate surface shape. The derived mathematical surface is then raytraced using a basic keratometer model to produce simulated keratometer (SimK) values. So it is the difficulty of calculating curvature from triangulated data, the repeatability of Orbscan I SimK values is usually not as good as a clinical keratometer. But when several readings of the same eye are averaged, no diskernable systematic error is found.

So if one reading is taken and a comparison is made, the difference may be significant enough to make you believe the instrument is not working properly. So when the Placido illuminator was added to Orbscan II to increase its anterior curvature accuracy, it also provided reflected data similar to that obtained with a keratometer. This reflective data is now used in SimK analyses, resulting in repeatabilities similar to keratometers and other Placido based corneal topography instruments.

Keratometry measures the tear-film, while slit-scan triangulation (**Figure 3.3**) as embodied in Orbscan sees through the tear-film and measures the corneal surface directly. Thus, an abnormal tear film can produce significant differences in keratometry but not in Orbscan II.

Curvature measures the geometric bending of a surface, and its natural unit is reciprocal length, like inverse millimeters (1/mm). When keratometry was invented this unfamiliar unit was replaced by a dioptric interpretation, making keratometry

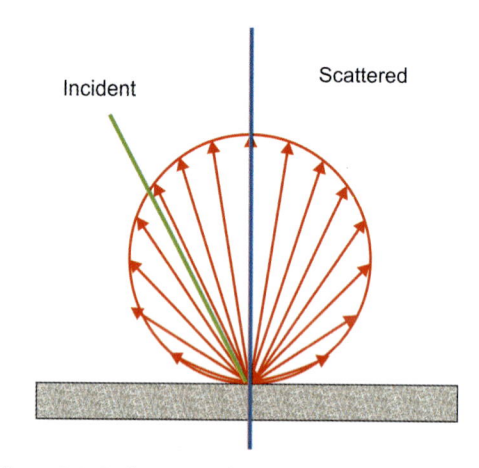

Figure 3.2 Back-scatter reflection. This is used in Orbscan. This is omni-directional

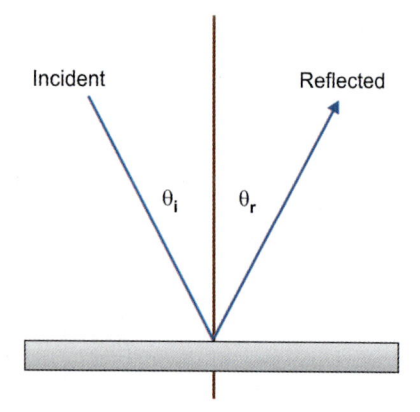

Figure 3.1 Specular reflection. This is used in keratometers. This is angle dependent

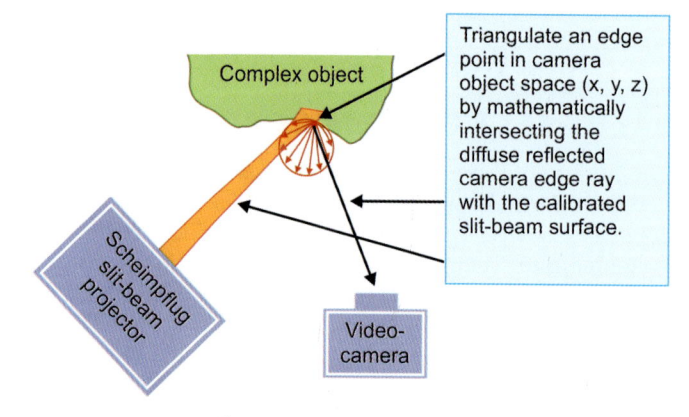

Figure 3.3 Direct triangulation

values equivalent on average (i.e. over the original population) to the paraxial back-vertex power of the cornea. As it has become increasingly more important to distinguish optical from geometric properties, it is now more proper to evaluate keratometry in "keratometric diopters". The keratometric diopter is strictly defined as a geometric unit of curvature with no optical significance. One inverse millimeter equals to 337.5 keratometric diopters.

IMAGING IN THE ORBSCAN

In the Orbscan, the calibrated slit, which falls on the cornea, gives a topographical information, which is captured and analyzed by the video camera **(Figure 3.4)**. Both slit-beam surfaces are determined in camera object space. Object space luminance is determined for each pixel value and framegrabber setting. Forty slit images are acquired in two 0.7-second periods. During acquisition, involuntary saccades typically move the eye by 50 microns. Eye movement is measured from anterior reflections of stationary slit-beam and other light sources. Eye tracking data permits saccadic movements

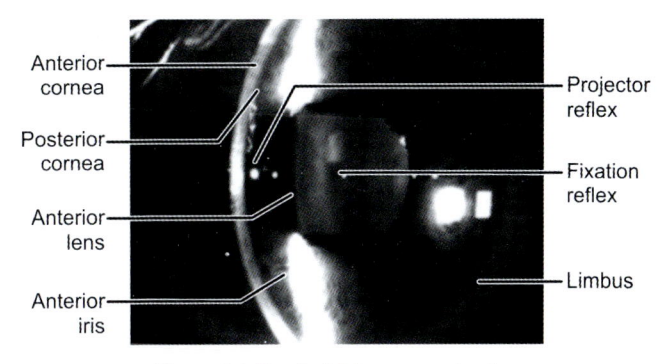

Figure 3.6 Detailed Orbscan examination

to be subtracted from the final topographic surface. Each of the 40 slit images triangulates one slice of ocular surface **(Figure 3.5)**. Before an interpolating surface is constructed, each slice is registered in accordance with measured eye movement. Distance between data slices averages 250 microns in the coarse scan mode (40 slits limbus to limbus). So, Orbscan exam consists of a set of mathematical topographic surfaces (x, y), for the anterior and posterior cornea, anterior iris and lens and backscattering coefficient of layers between the topographic surfaces (and over the pupil) **(Figure 3.6)**.

MAP COLORS CONVENTIONS

Color contour maps have become a standard method for displaying 2-D data in corneal and anterior segment topography. Although there are no universally standardized colors, the spectral direction (from blue to red) is always organized in definite and intuitive way.

Blue = Low, level, flat, deep, thick, or aberrated.
Red = High, steep, sharp, shallow, thin, or focused.

ANALYSIS OF THE NORMAL EYE BY THE ORBSCAN MAP

The general quad map in the Orbscan of a normal eye **(Figure 3.7)** shows 4 pictures. The upper left is the anterior float, which is the topography of the anterior surface of the cornea. The upper right shows the posterior float, which is the topography of the posterior surface of the cornea. The lower left map shows the keratometric pattern and the lower right map shows the pachymetry (thickness of the cornea). The Orbscan is a three-dimensional slit scan topographic machine. If we were doing topography with a machine, which does not have slit scan imaging facility, we would not be able to see the topography of the posterior surface of the cornea. Now, if the patient had an abnormality in the posterior surface of the cornea, for example as in primary posterior corneal elevation

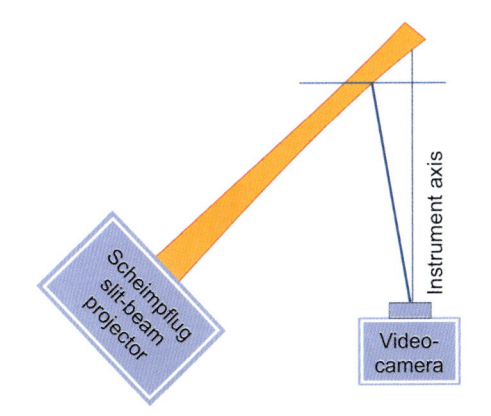

Figure 3.4 Beam and camera calibration in the Orbscan

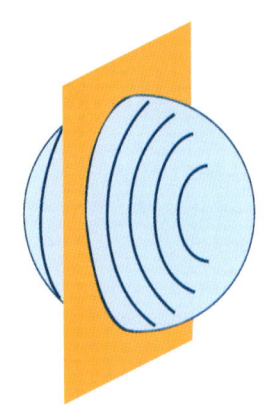

Figure 3.5 Ocular surface slicing by the Orbscan slit

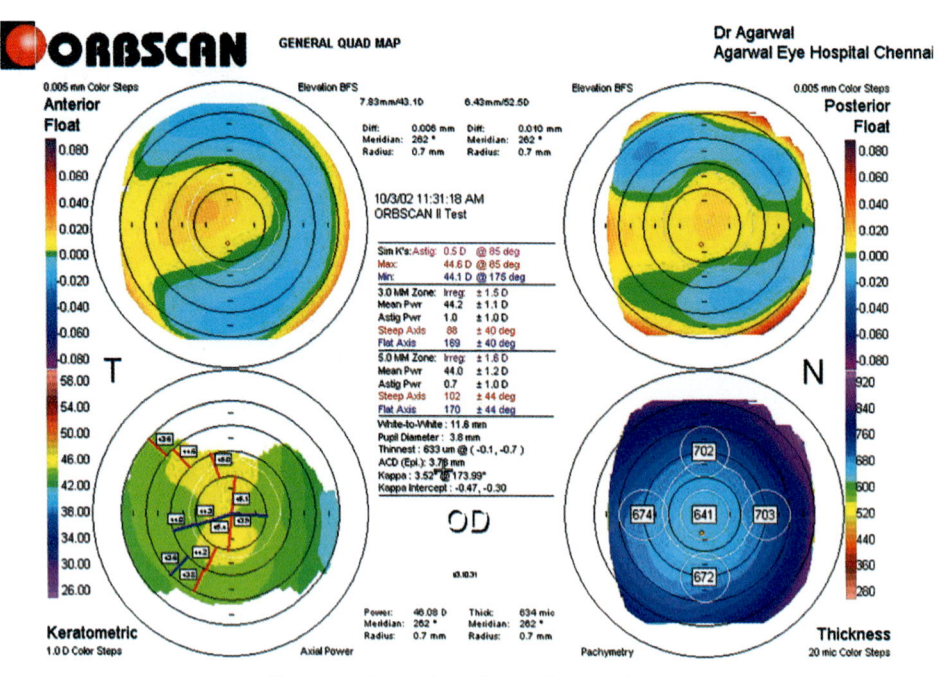

36   Section I: Introduction to Corneal Topography and Orbscan

Figure 3.7 General quad map of a normal eye

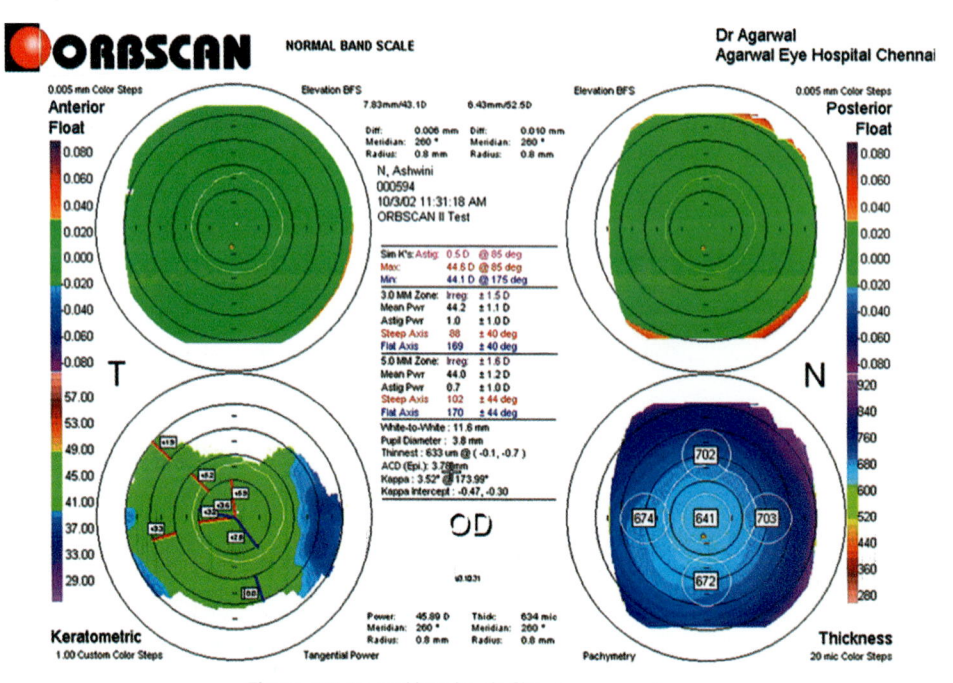

Figure 3.8 Normal band scale filter on a normal eye

this would not be diagnosed. Then, if we perform Lasik on such a patient we would create an iatrogenic keratectasia. The Orbscan helps us to detect the abnormalities on the posterior surface of the cornea.

Another facility, which we can move onto once we have the general quad map, is to put on the normal band scale filter **(Figure 3.8)**. If we are in suspicion of any abnormality in the general quad map then we put on the normal band scale filter. This highlights the abnormal areas in the cornea in orange to red colors. The normal areas are all shown in green. This is very helpful in generalized screening in preoperative examination of a LASIK patient.

Chapter 3: Corneal Topography and the Orbscan 37

CLINICAL APPLICATIONS

Let us now understand this better in a case of a primary posterior corneal elevation. If we see the general quad map of a primary posterior corneal elevation (**Figure 3.9**) we will see the upper left map is normal. The upper right map shows abnormality highlighted in red. This indicates the abnormality in the posterior surface of the cornea. The lower

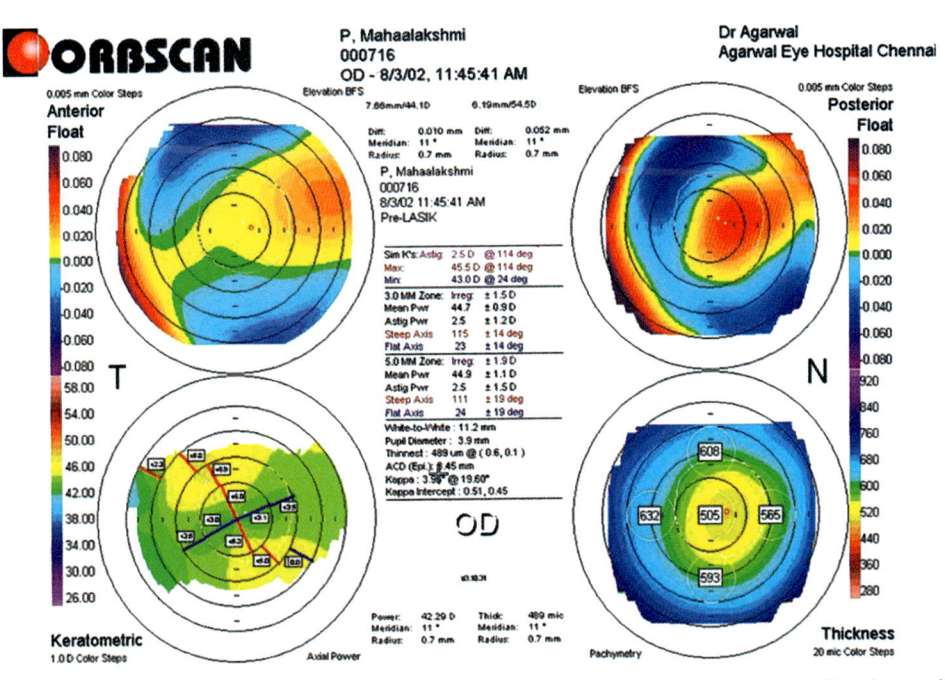

Figure 3.9 General quad map of a primary posterior corneal elevation. Notice the upper right map has an abnormality whereas the upper left map is normal. This shows the anterior surface of the cornea is normal and the problem is in the posterior surface of the cornea

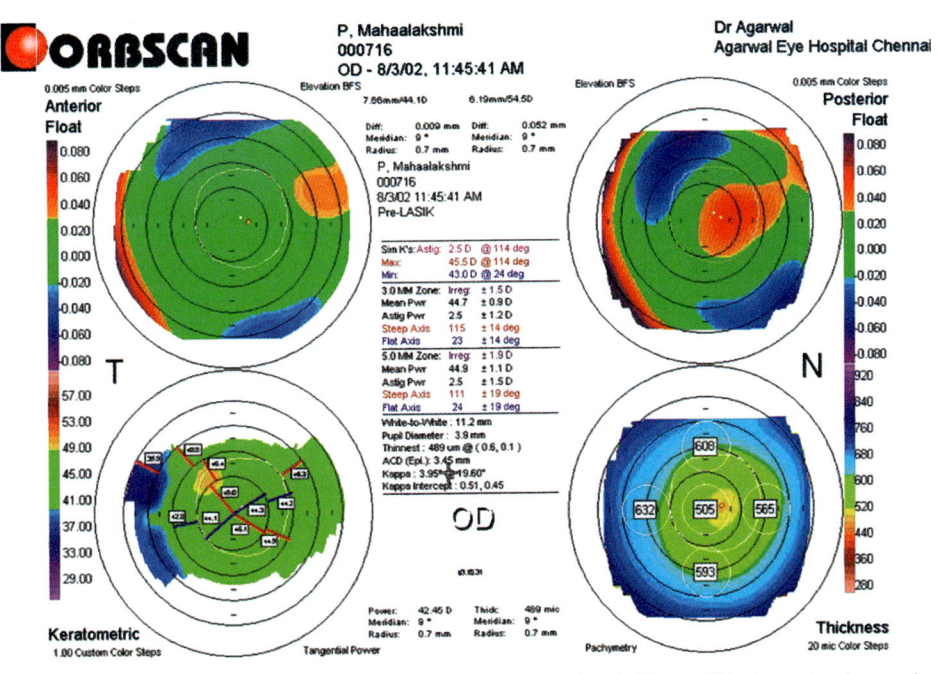

Figure 3.10 Quad map of a primary posterior corneal elevation with the normal band scale filter on. This shows the abnormal areas in red and the normal areas are all green. Notice the abnormality in the upper right map

left keratometric map is normal and if we see the lower right map, which is the pachymetry map one will see slightly, thin cornea of 505 microns but still one cannot diagnose the primary posterior corneal elevation only from this reading. Thus, we can understand that if not for the upper right map, which denotes the posterior surface of the cornea, one would miss this condition. The Orbscan can only diagnose this.

Now, we can put on the normal band scale filter on **(Figure 3.10)** and this will highlight the abnormal areas in red. Notice in **(Figure 3.10)** the upper right map shows a lot of abnormality denoting the primary posterior corneal elevation. One can also take the three-dimensional map of the posterior surface of the cornea **(Figure 3.11)** and notice the amount of elevation in respect to the normal reference sphere shown as a black grid. In a case of a keratoconus **(Figure 3.12)** all four maps show an abnormality, which confirms the diagnosis.

If we take a LASIK patients topography we can compare the pre- and the post-LASIK **(Figure 3.13)**. This helps to understand the pattern and amount of ablation done on the cornea. The picture on the upper right is the preoperative topographic picture and the one on the lower right is the post-LASIK picture. The main picture on the left shows the difference between the pre- and post-LASIK topographic patterns. One can detect from this any decentered ablations or any other complication of LASIK surgery.

Corneal topography is extremely important in cataract surgery. *The smaller the size of the incision lesser the astigmatism and earlier stability of the astigmatism will occur.* One can reduce the astigmatism or increase the astigmatism of a patient after cataract surgery. The simple rule to follow is that-*wherever you make an incision that area will flatten and wherever you apply sutures that area will steepen.* One can use the Orbscan to analyze the topography before and after cataract surgery.

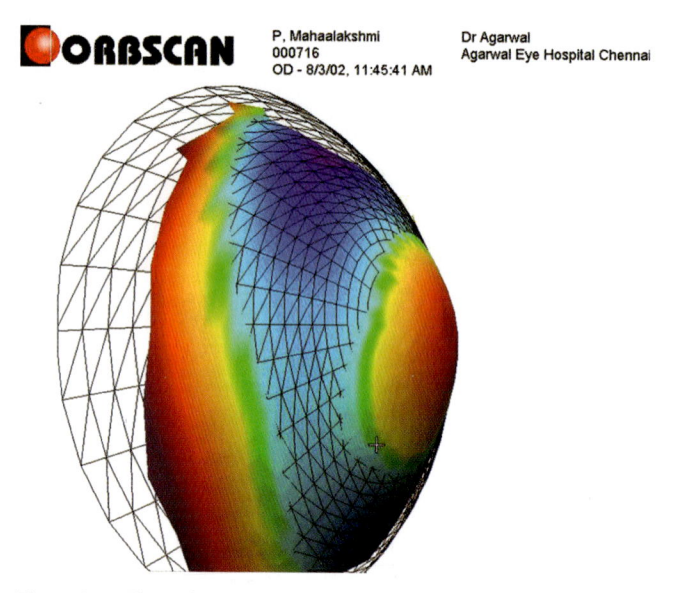

Figure 3.11 Three-dimensional map of primary posterior corneal elevation. This shows a marked elevation in respect to a normal reference sphere highlighted as a black grid. Notice the red color protrusion on the black grid This picture is of the posterior surface of the cornea

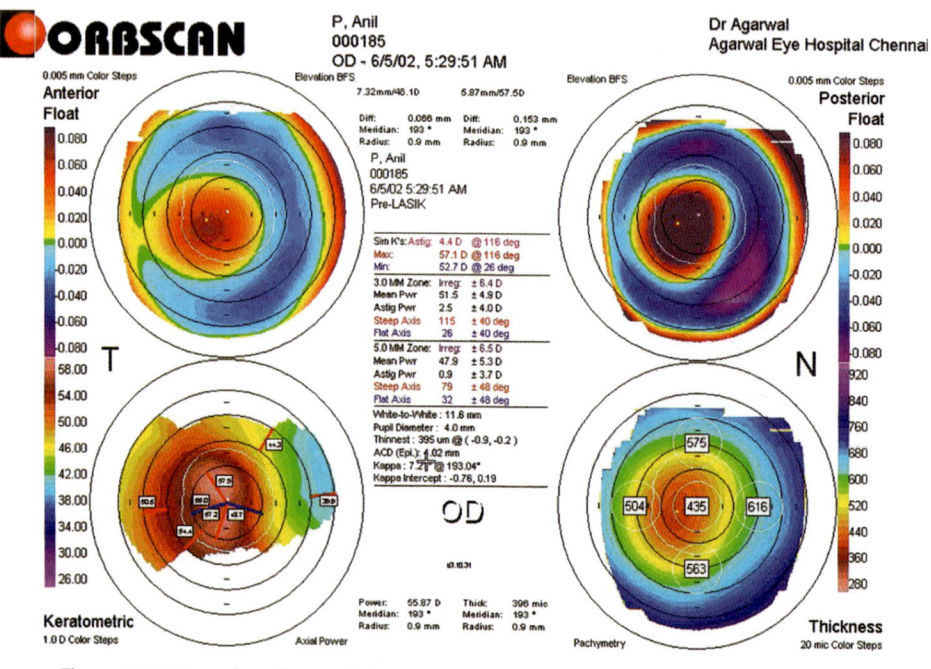

Figure 3.12 General quad map of a keratoconus patient showing abnormality in all four maps

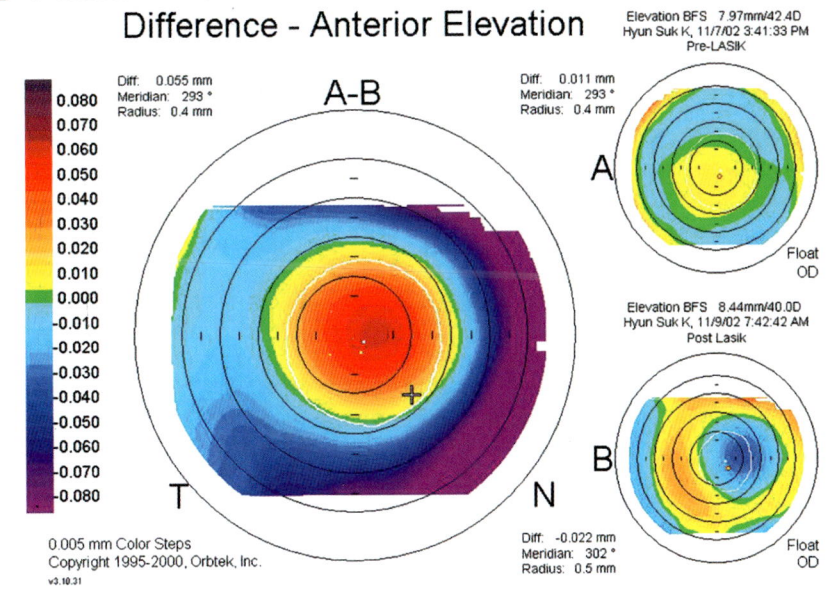

Figure 3.13 Difference of pre- and post-LASIK

For instance in an extracapsular cataract extraction one can check to see where the astigmatism is most and remove those sutures. In a phaco the astigmatism will be less and in Phakonit where the incision is sub 1.5 mm the astigmatism will be the least.

We can use the Orbscan to determine the anterior chamber depth and also analyze where one should place the incision when one is performing astigmatic keratotomy. The Orbscan can also help in a good fit of the contact lens with a fluorescein pattern.

SUMMARY

The Orbscan has changed the world of topography as it gives us an understanding of a slit scan three-dimensional picture. One can use this in understanding various conditions.

REFERENCES

1. Agarwal S, Agarwal A, Agarwal A. Four volume textbook of ophthalmology; Jaypee Brothers Medical Publishers 2000; India.
2. Agarwal A. Handbook of ophthalmology; Slack Inc, 2005, USA.
3. Agarwal A. Refractive surgery nightmares: Conquering refractive surgery catastrophes; Slack Inc, 2007, USA.

Chapter 4

The Orbscan IIz Diagnostic System and Zywave Wavefront Analysis

*Gregg Feinerman (USA), N Timothy Peters (USA), Hoo Yeun Kim (USA),
Marcus Solorzano (USA), Shiela Scott (USA)*

INTRODUCTION

The combination of topographic and wavefront data is the foundation for customized ablation. The Zyoptix™ Diagnostic Workstation seamlessly integrates wavefront and topographical data for customized treatments **(Figure 4.1)**. It is ergonomic and easy to use, and provides surgeons with a platform for comprehensive diagnosis and treatment. The ORBSCAN® IIz uses slit scanning technology to measure corneal curvature. It also provides true three-dimensional elevation based on triangulation and curvature of both anterior and posterior surfaces of the cornea. The ZYWAVE™ II ABERROMETER provides wavefront measurements based on Hartmann-Shack technology. It measures higher order aberrations (HOAs) up to the 5th order.

ORBSCAN

Corneal topography has evolved overtime from a manual keratometer to simple Placido's disk topographers, to the Orbscan. The Orbscan uses a combination of Placido's disk images with 20 slit scans to the left and 20 slits scan to the right. This allows for forty overlapping scans in the central 5 mm zone that then allows for the four basic measurements listed below. The Orbscan measures four essential elements:
1. Corneal power
2. Corneal thickness
3. Anterior corneal elevation
4. Posterior corneal elevation.

QUAD MAP

The quad map is the most common and useful way to get an overall view of the cornea. It combines anterior elevation, posterior elevation, corneal power and pachymetry into one view **(Figures 4.2 and 4.3)**.

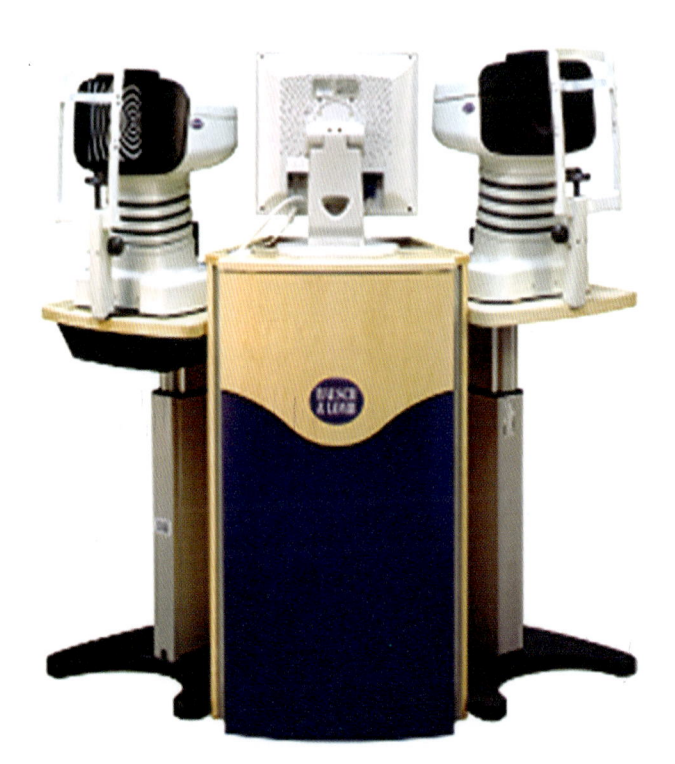

Figure 4.1 The Zyoptix™ diagnostic workstation

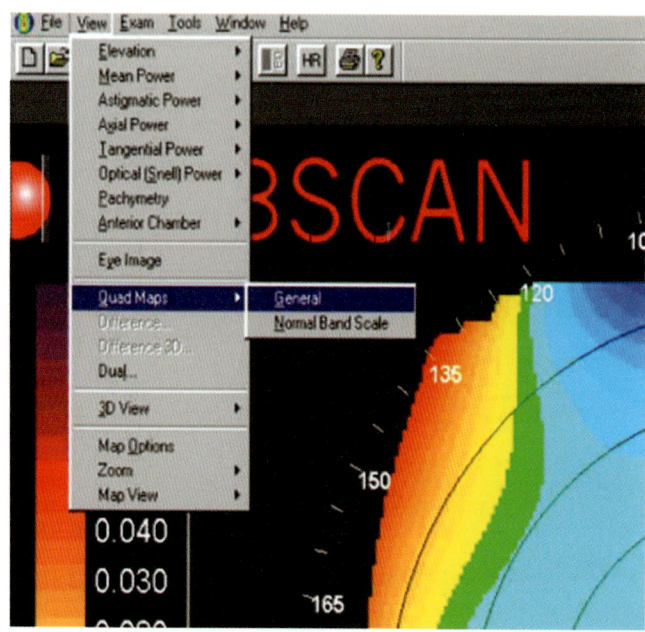

Figure 4.2 Selecting the quad map

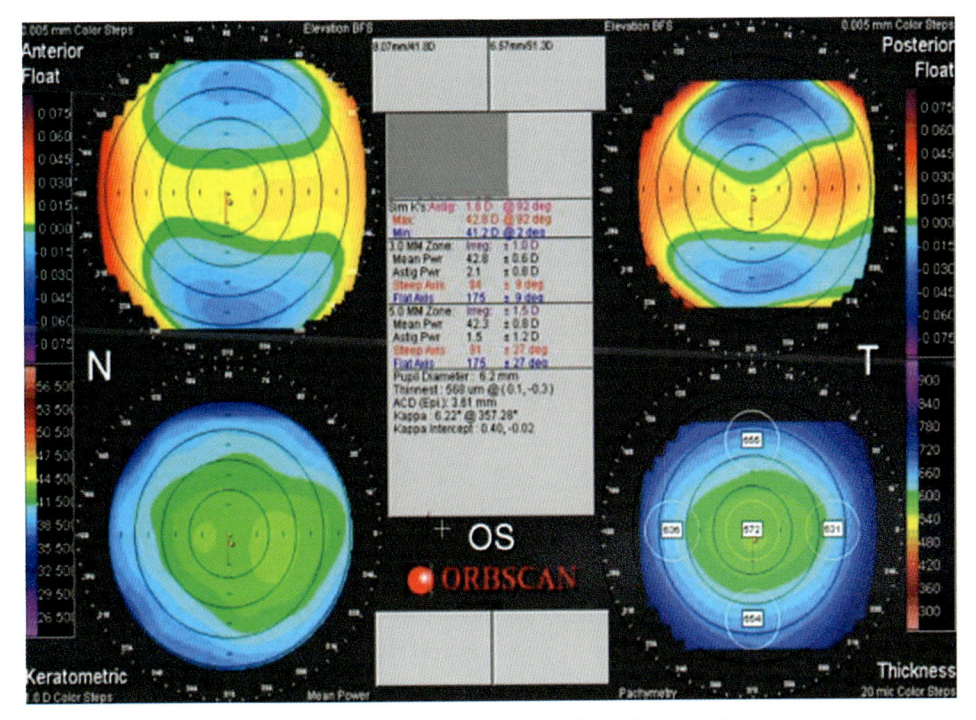

Chapter 4: The Orbscan IIz Diagnostic System and Zywave Wavefront Analysis

Figure 4.3 Normal quad map showing typical with the rule astigmatism

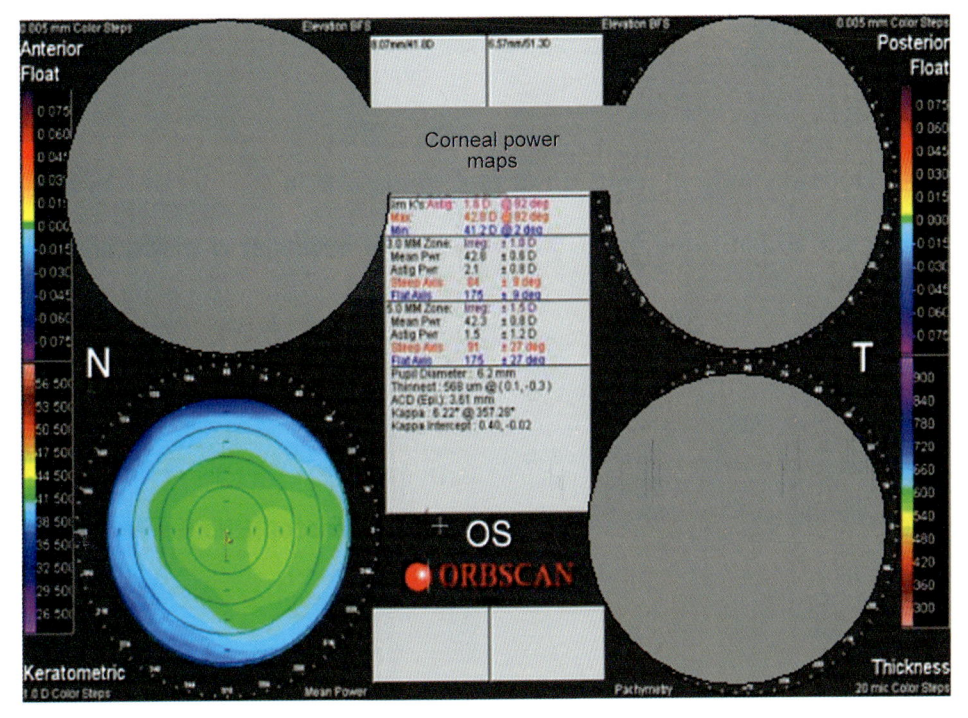

Figure 4.4 Mean power map

POWER MAPS

One of the most confusing tasks in refractive diagnostic testing is deciding which corneal power maps to interpret. The Orbscan offers multiple ways to measure corneal power. The type of corneal power map to choose depends on what you are trying to interpret. The default setting is the mean power map **(Figures 4.4 to 4.6)**. It is most useful for eyes with extreme abnormalities. The mean power map determines the location of a surface abnormality. The axial power map is a familiar sagittal map from Placido systems **(Figures 4.7 and 4.8)**. It provides a comfortable transition for new Orbscan users; but only uses Placido rings. Normal astigmatism appears in a classic bow-tie pattern.

PACHYMETRY MAP

The pachymetry map **(Figures 4.9 to 4.11)** unquestionably makes the Orbscan diagnostic system unique. The Orbscan measures thickness from the tear film layer to Descemet's membrane, thus its pachymetry readings are thicker than those obtained with ultrasound pachymetry. However, the Orbscan has an adjustment factor called the acoustic factor, which can be set to replicate ultrasound pachymetry. The default setting is 92%, but each user may adjust this percentage to mimic what their own ultrasound reading show. The Orbscan not only provides a central pachymetry reading, but it also provides a superior, inferior, nasal, and temporal reading at the 6 mm zone. It also provides a reading showing the thinnest part of the cornea that may not necessarily be the central reading. The extra reading allows for the subtle interpretation of variable corneal thickness in conjunction with other topographic abnormalities, to aid in the detection of forme-fruste keratoconus as well as other corneal disease processes.

READING CORNEAL ELEVATION MAPS

Global Perspective

The map in the upper left of the quad maps **(Figure 4.12)** is the anterior elevation map. Understanding the usefulness of the map requires some background perspective. Think first from a global perspective. If we view the surface of the earth from a great distance it losses all of its relevant features and appears totally smooth, but if we change the scale then we can perceive significant height discrepancies. The cornea is the same way. When looking at a proper scale we can see height differences. To understand these differences we have to compare the height of the actual cornea to the heights of a best-fit sphere.

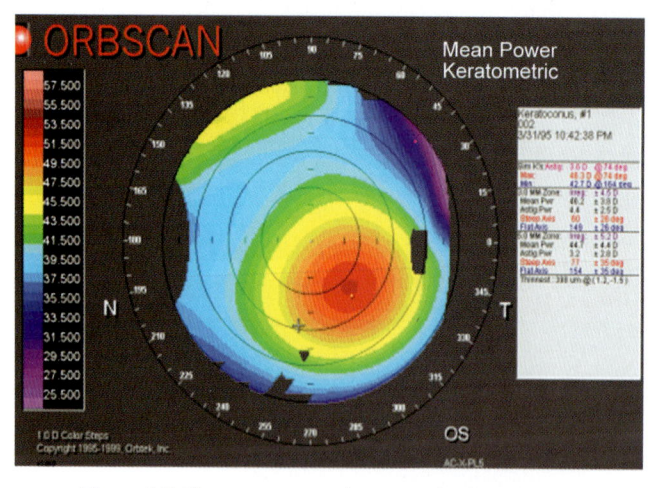

Figure 4.5 Mean power map demonstrating keratoconus

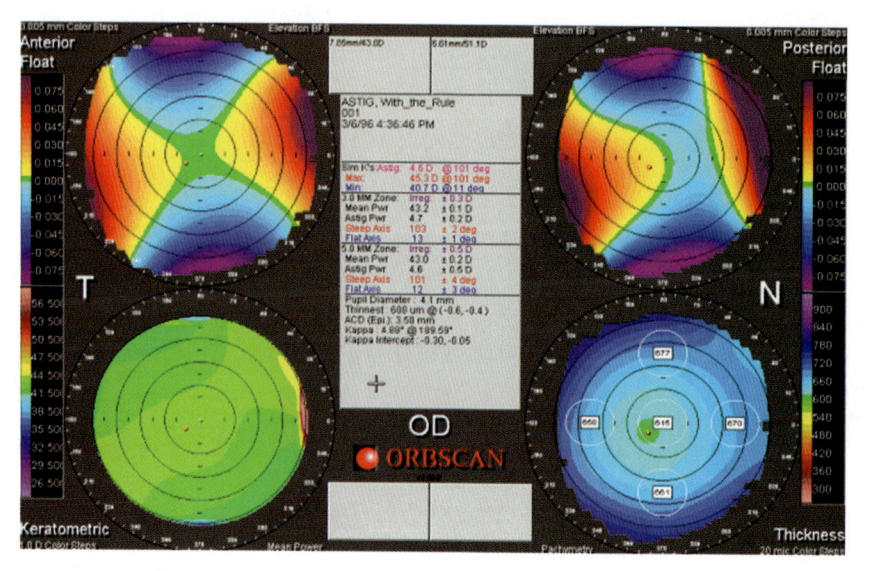

Figure 4.6 Mean power map demonstrating regular astigmatism

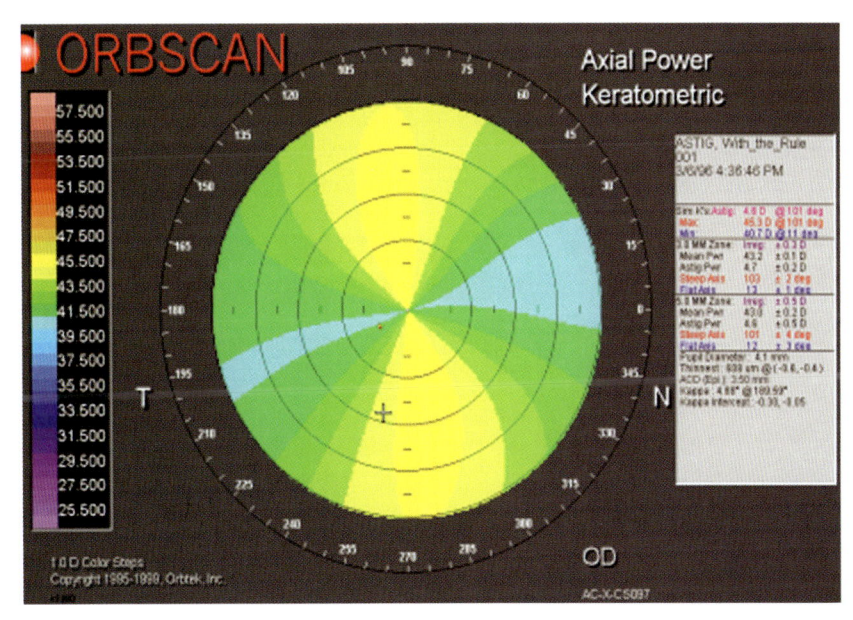

Chapter 4: The Orbscan IIz Diagnostic System and Zywave Wavefront Analysis 43

Figure 4.7 Axial power map

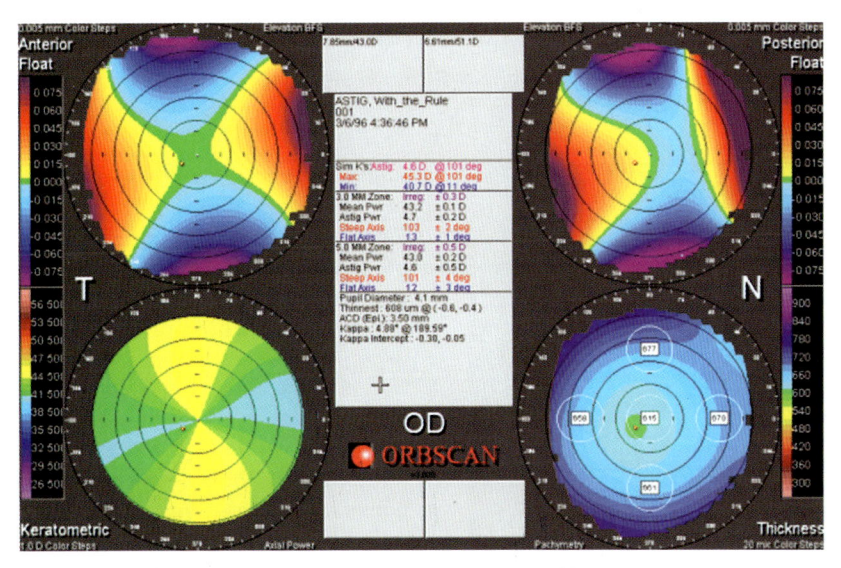

Figure 4.8 Axial power map demonstrating regular astigmatism

A normal prolate cornea is steep in the center, and flat in the periphery **(Figures 4.13 and 4.14)**. When this is overlayed with a best-fit sphere the center of the normal cornea is steeper than the best-fit sphere. Steep colors are red ones, and thus the central cornea is red on a normal elevation map. The mid-periphery of a normal cornea is flatter than our reference best-fit sphere and thus appears blue on an elevation map. Now consider a post-LASIK elevation profile on a previously myopic patient **(Figure 4.15)**. The reference sphere is best fit to the postablation shape, but the post-LASIK cornea is now oblate with a flatter center. This will appear as a blue central zone. The mid-periphery is now steeper than the reference sphere and appears as a red ring. The untouched peripheral cornea again then becomes flatter than the reference sphere and appears blue on our scale in a normal postmyopic LASIK elevation map. The anterior corneal elevation take home message is that:

- Elevation is measured relative to a "Best-fit Sphere"
- The elevation "is what it is" but may appear different depending how we look at it in relation to the best-fit sphere.

POSTERIOR CORNEAL ELEVATION MAPS

The posterior corneal elevation is another unique and defining feature of the Orbscan. As we recall from basic science, the

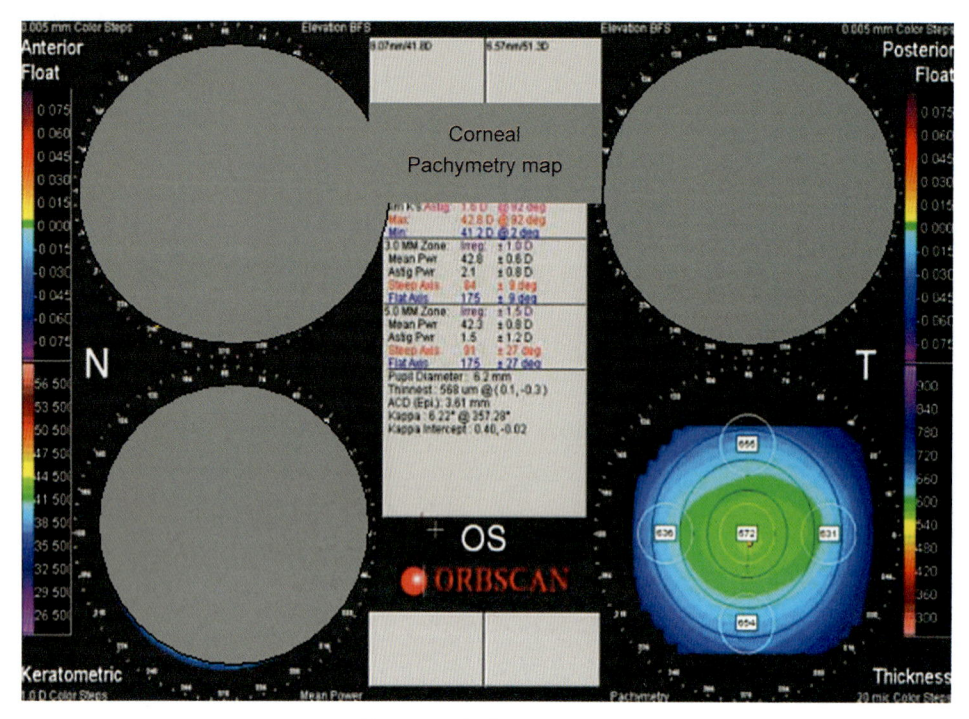

Figure 4.9 Pachymetry map

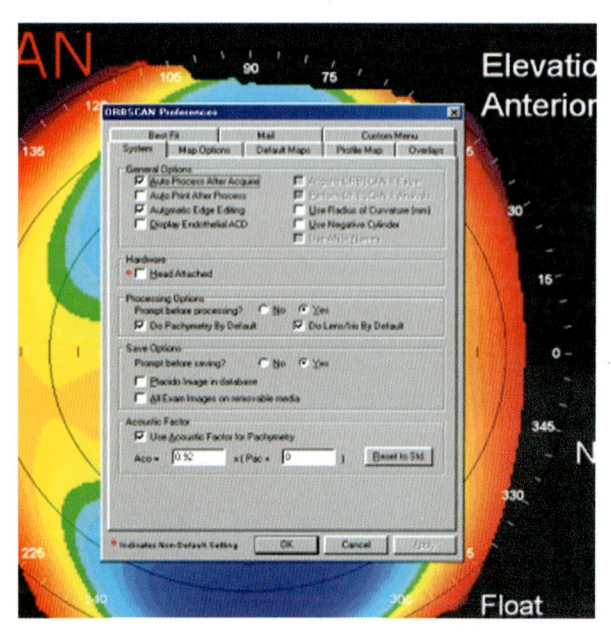

Figure 4.10 Adjusting the acoustic factor for pachymetry

posterior corneal power is negative and much smaller than anterior corneal power **(Figure 4.16)**. Thus, the posterior surface reduces corneal power.

There has been no prior experience with this information, and this surface is simply assumed to be normal by all other topographic systems. When interpreting the posterior float we need to put the posterior cornea in context. It is important to look for pattern recognition, and to look for related changes on other maps. Similar to the anterior elevation map, the posterior elevation map is related to a best-fit sphere. When reading this map two features are of greatest importance. One is the location of the steepest part of the posterior float. This should be relatively central, but is a more concern should it be located away from the center and in an area of corneal thinning. The second is the posterior float difference. This number is given in microns and is the difference between the steepest and flattest part of the posterior elevation. Much debate has centered over the magnitude that constitutes an abnormal reading, but 45 to 50 microns seems to be the maximum difference that is widely accepted. It is also important to keep in mind that while the posterior float difference appears to be clinically relevant, that isolated findings have limited value.

THREE STEP RULE

Dr Karpecki and Moyes have developed what they refer to as the three step rule when interpreting the posterior elevation. If there is one abnormal map **(Figure 4.17)** then it is okay to perform LASIK with caution. If there are two abnormal maps **(Figure 4.18)**, then it is still okay to proceed, but with concern, and if there are three abnormal maps **(Figure 4.19)** the LASIK is contraindicated. Below are some quad maps demonstrating the different levels of concern.

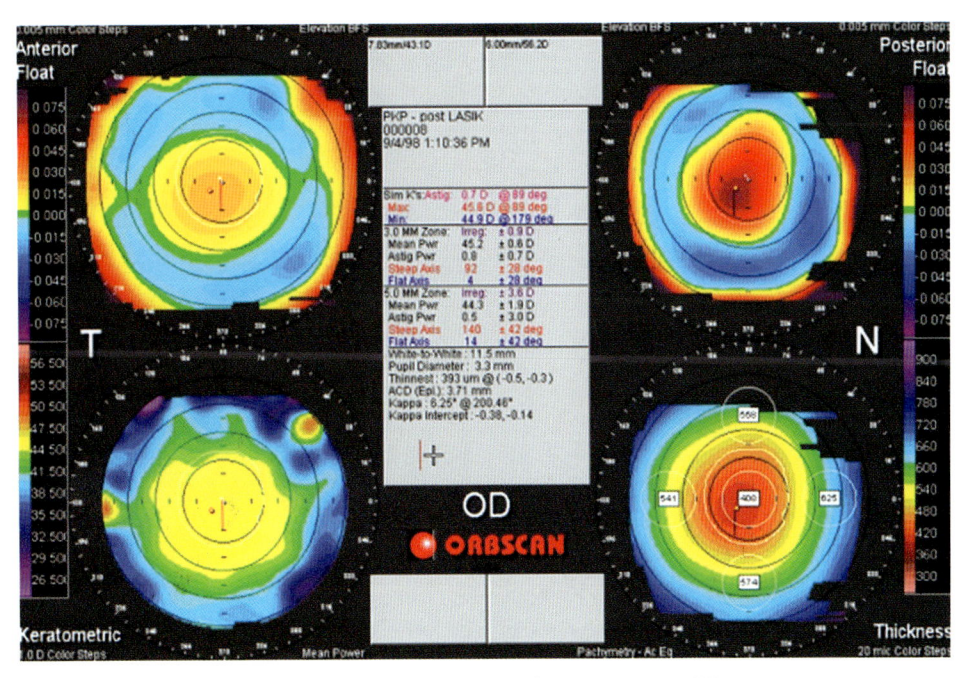

Chapter 4: The Orbscan IIz Diagnostic System and Zywave Wavefront Analysis 45

Figure 4.11 Pachymetry map of postoperative LASIK

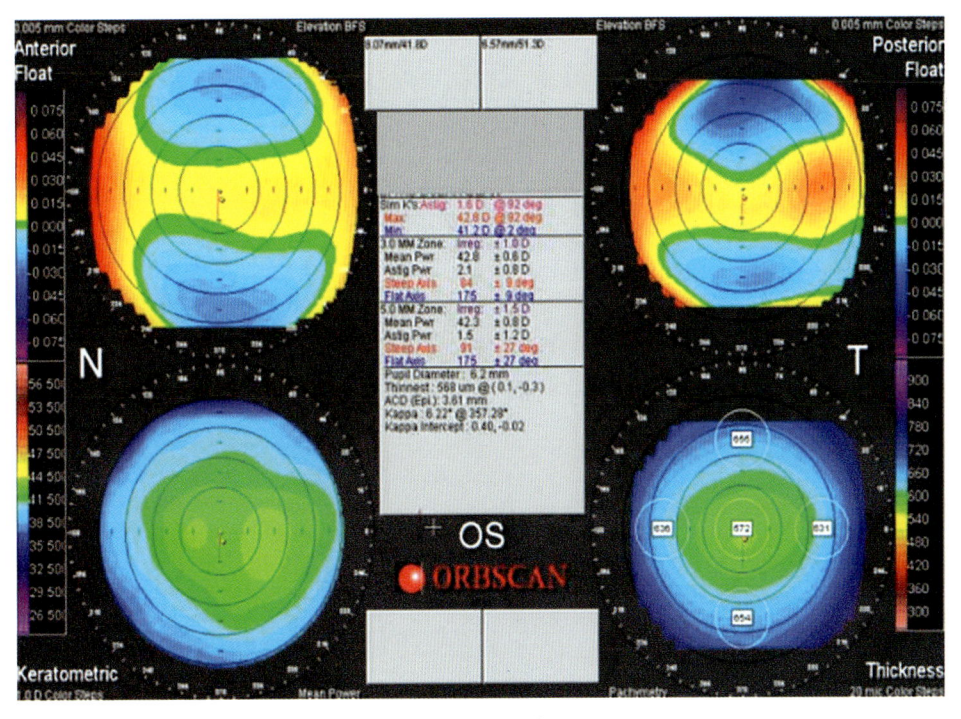

Figure 4.12 Quad map

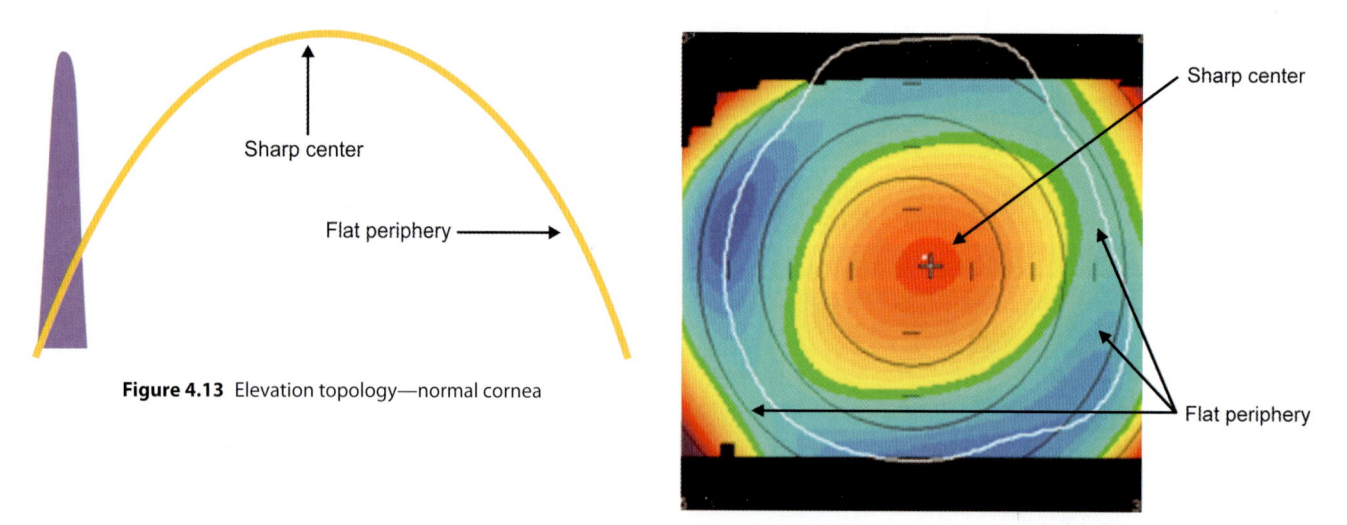

Section I: Introduction to Corneal Topography and Orbscan

Figure 4.13 Elevation topology—normal cornea

Figure 4.14 Anterior corneal elevation map

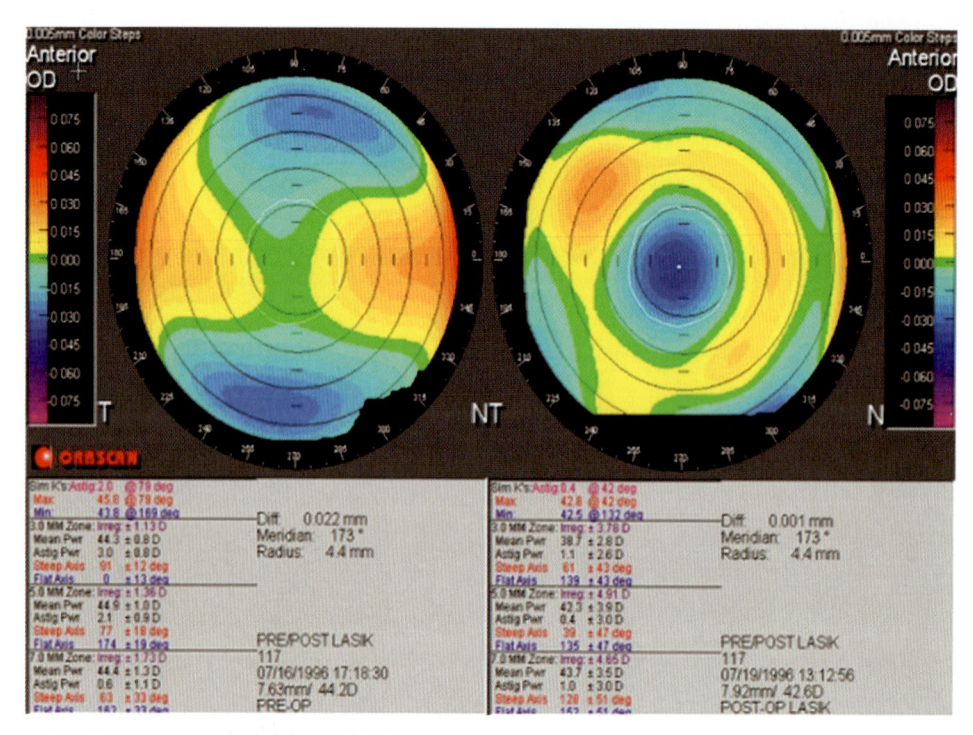

Figure 4.15 Elevation map pre- and postoperative LASIK

PREOPERATIVE LASIK SCREENING

Three Step Rule

- One abnormal map: Caution
- Two abnormal maps: Concern
- Three abnormal maps: Contraindication.

This quad map shows three normal maps, but the posterior float is abnormal because the difference reading is greater than 50 microns.

This quad map shows two normal maps, but the posterior difference is again over 50 microns. This quad map, however, also shows an abnormally thin central pachymetry. This thinning has good correlation with the steepest location of the posterior elevation map.

This quad map has three abnormal maps. The posterior difference is greater then 50 microns, there is a well-correlated steep area on the anterior elevation map, and a well-correlated area of high power on the mean power map. This is an absolute contraindication for LASIK.

MIDDLE BOX

When reading the quad maps try not to forget the information in the middle box **(Figure 4.20)**. This box provides standard keratometric readings, white-to-white distance in millimeters, angle kappa readings, and more. The thinnest area of the cornea is displayed here as well as the amount of corneal irregularity within the central 3 and 5 mm zones. These irregularity indices are considered abnormal if they exceed 1.5 and 2 diopters respectively. This extra information combined with the quad maps provides the most complete screening tool available to detect preoperative corneal abnormalities to reduce the risk of iatrogenic induced keratoectasia. Dr(s) Karpecki and Moyes have compiled a list of Orbscan risk factors for keratoectasia based on extensive retrospective case reviews. This is a guideline that other users may want to consider when screening LASIK candidates.

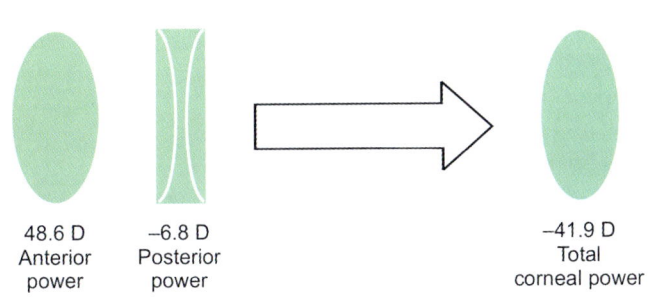

Figure 4.16 The posterior corneal surface reduces corneal power

48.6 D Anterior power — −6.8 D Posterior power → −41.9 D Total corneal power

ORBSCAN RISK OF ECTASIA INDICES

- Number of abnormal maps
- Posterior surface float (difference) >0.050 D
- 3 and 5 mm irregularity
- Peripheral thickness changes
- Astigmatism variance between eyes
- Steep K's—mean power map.

The first item is the number of abnormal maps. As stated earlier in the three-step rule, one abnormal map is a caution sign, two is of concern, and three is an absolute contraindication. The second item is the posterior float difference **(Figure 4.21)**. A difference of greater than 50 is generally accepted as abnormal, but other physicians have suggested that 50 is the limit in normal corneas, but in corneas that are thinner than normal to start with a difference over 40 should be considered abnormal.[1] The third item is the amount of irregularity in the central 3 and 5 mm zones **(Figures 4.22A and B)**. Greater than 1.5 and 2.0 diopters respectively is considered abnormal and cause for concern. The fourth item is how the central pachymetry reading compares to the peripheral 6 mm reading and to the thinnest reading **(Figure 4.23)**. These numbers are considered abnormal if the peripheral 6 mm readings are not at least 20 microns thicker than the central reading, especially if they are correlated with abnormalities on other quad maps. The thinnest reading is also considered abnormal if it is less than 30 microns thinner than the central reading, again if it is also correlated with an abnormality on another quad map. The fifth item is a difference of greater than

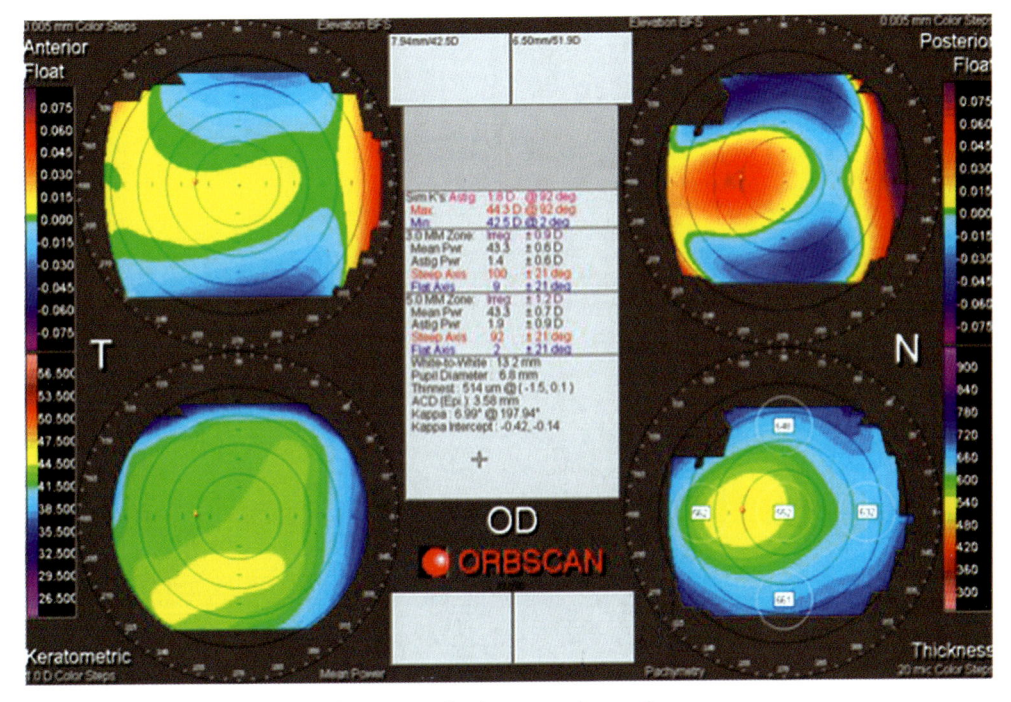

Figure 4.17 Caution—one abnormal map

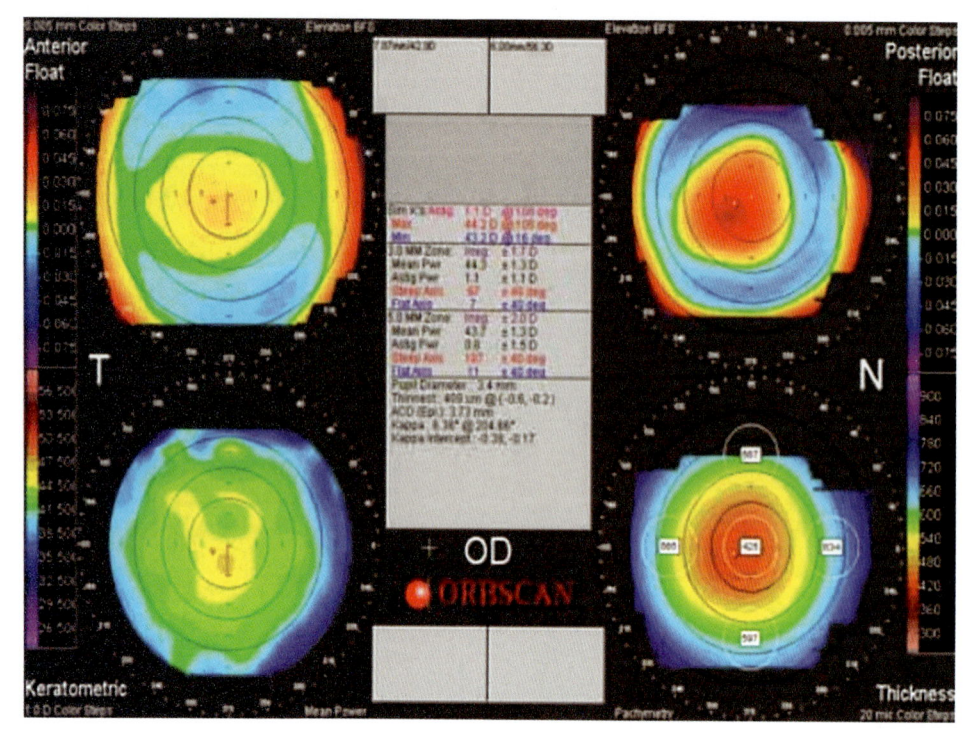

48 Section I: Introduction to Corneal Topography and Orbscan

Figure 4.18 Concern—two abnormal maps

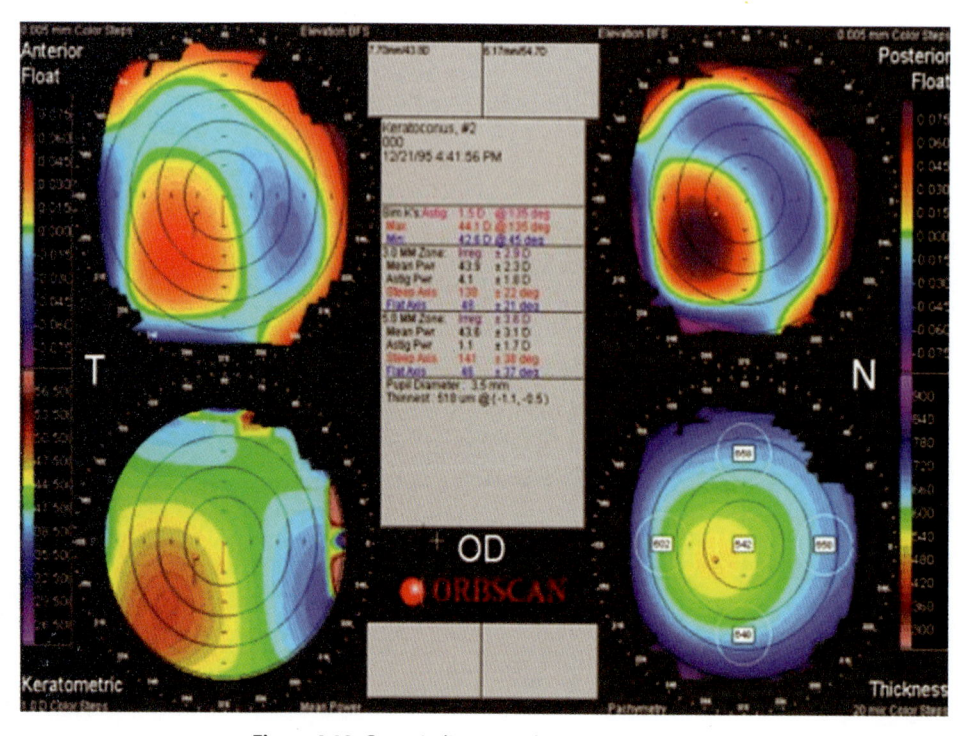

Figure 4.19 Contraindication—three abnormal maps

Chapter 4: The Orbscan IIz Diagnostic System and Zywave Wavefront Analysis

1.00 diopter in the amount of corneal astigmatism between eyes (**Figures 4.24 and 4.25**). The last item is a localized steep area on the mean power map, especially if correlated with other abnormalities (**Figure 4.26**).

These guidelines are meant to help alert the clinician to a poor candidate. The example below is an actual patient who preoperatively had a steep posterior difference, a thinnest spot of the cornea greater than 30 microns thinner than the central reading, and a higher amount of irregularity in the central 3 and 5 mm zones (**Figure 4.27**). As you follow this patient's course postoperatively you can see progressive steepening and topographic irregular astigmatism at the 4 and 17 month visits indicating keratoectasia (**Figures 4.28 and 4.29**).

CLINICAL EXAMPLES

As with all topographies, an abnormal tear film layer can significantly distort the readings. Below is an example of normal topography on a patient, and then a repeat topography taken after 3 minutes of drying (**Figures 4.30 and 4.31**). Note the significant change is surface quality and validity of the dry eye reading. The next example is that of a keratoconus patient (**Figure 4.32**). Note the larger posterior float difference, the well-correlated steep anterior float, the well-correlated steep power reading on the mean power map, the thinnest spot of the cornea not being central and being greater than 30 microns thinner than the central reading, and the large amounts of irregularity in the central 3 and 5 mm zones. The final example is of pellucid marginal degeneration (**Figure 4.33**). Note the classic large amount of against the rule astigmatism, the large posterior float difference,

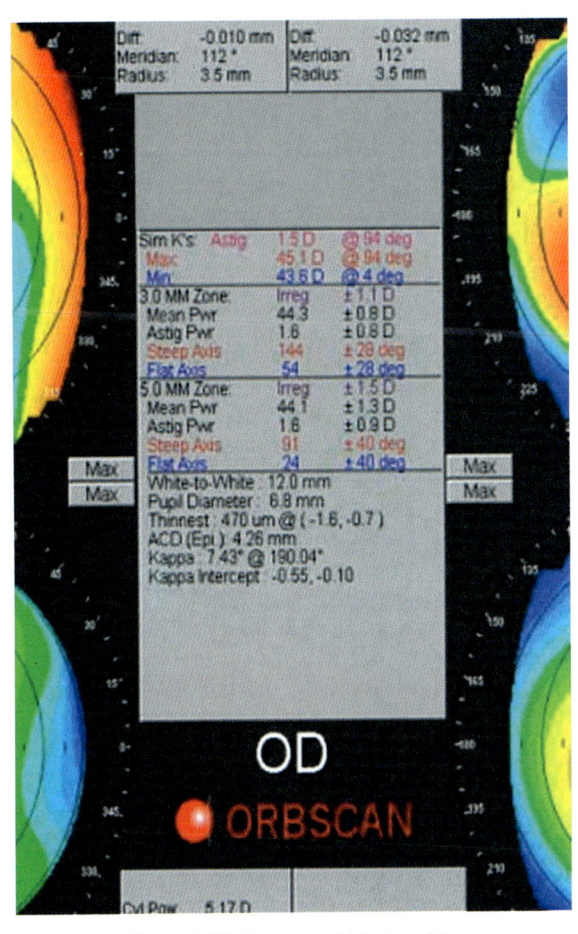

Figure 4.20 Orbscan middle box data

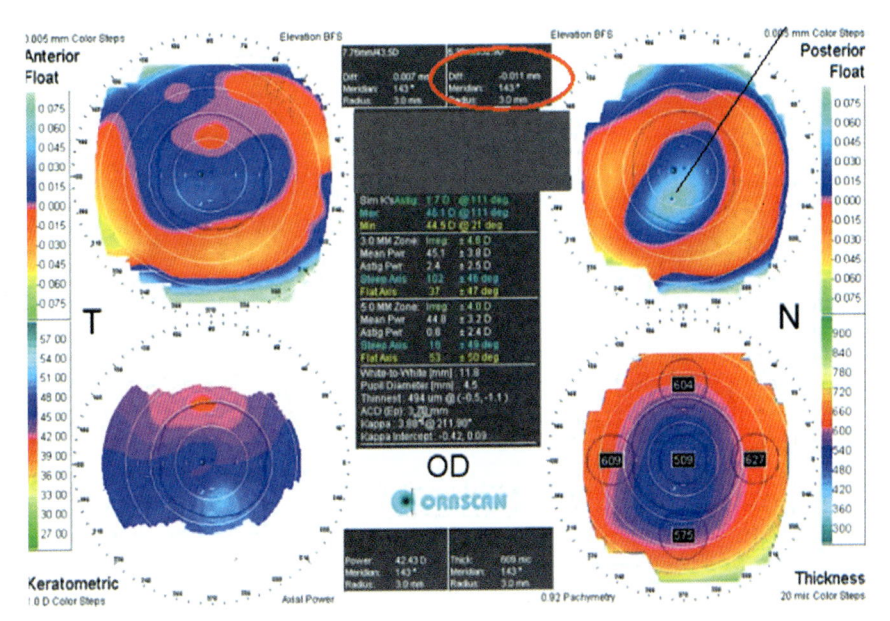

Figure 4.21 Posterior float difference

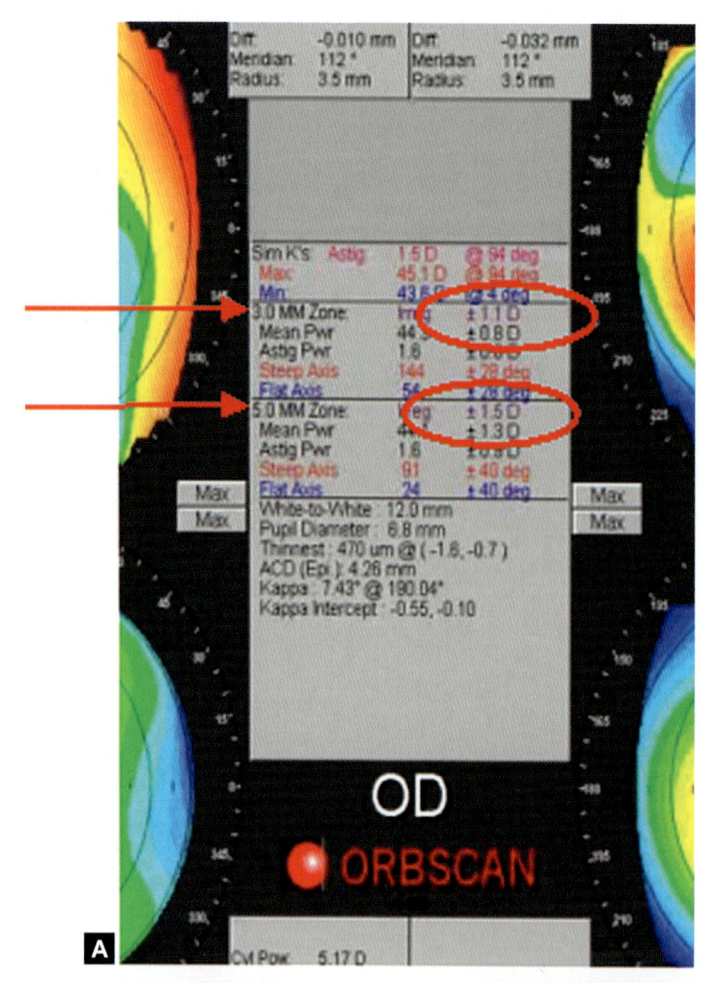

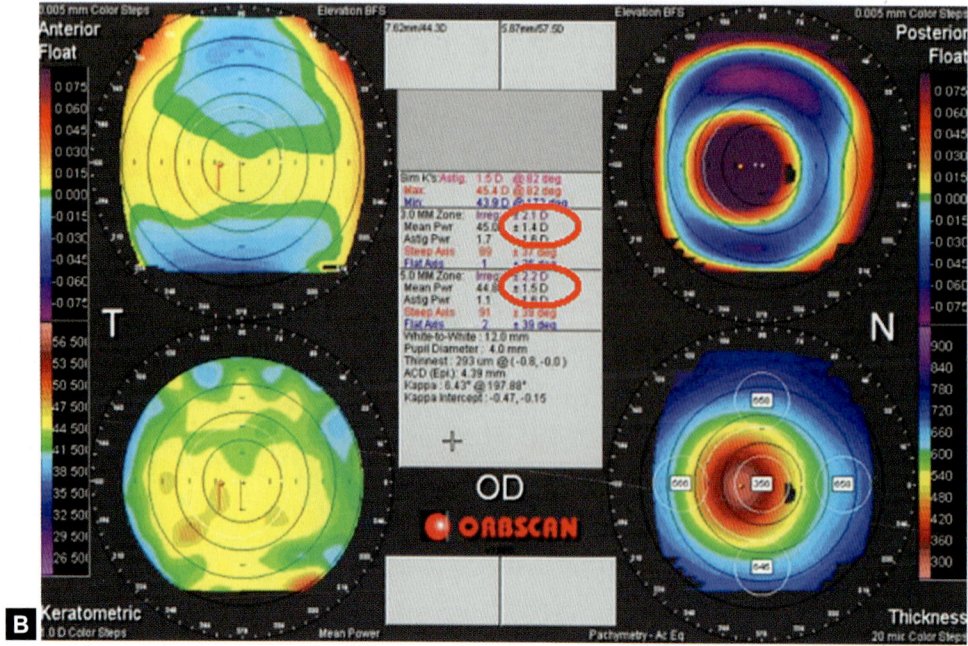

50 Section I: Introduction to Corneal Topography and Orbscan

Figures 4.22A and B 3 and 5 mm irregularity

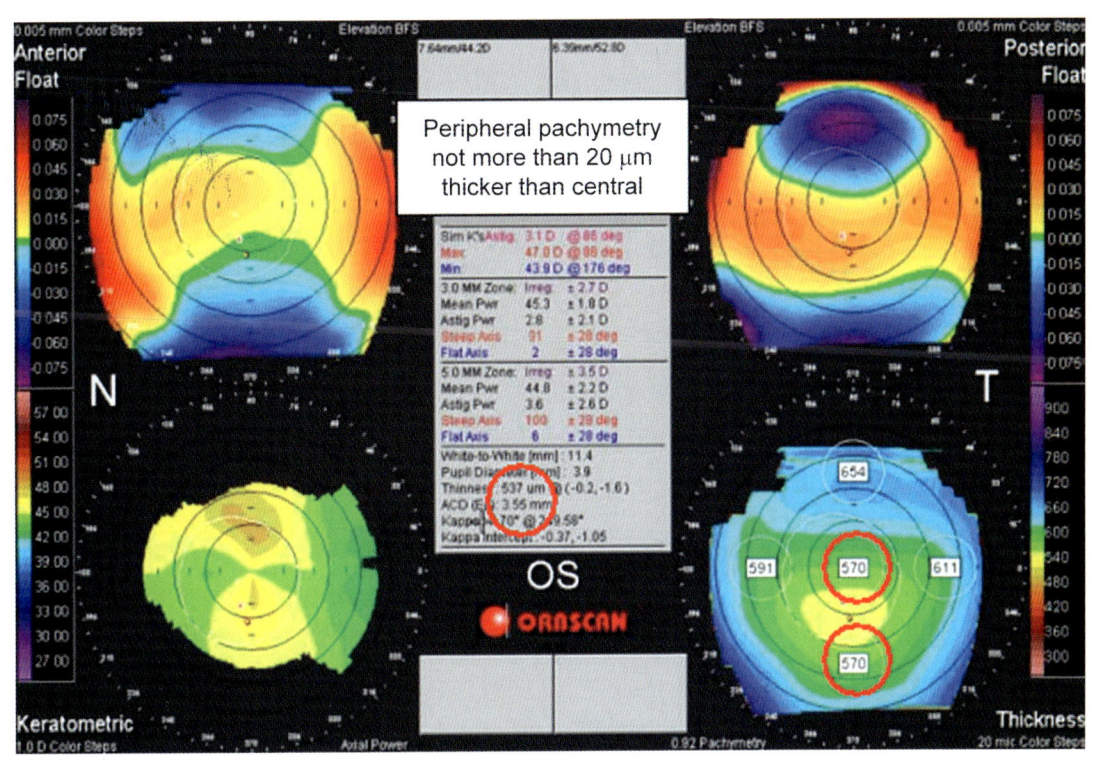

Chapter 4: The Orbscan IIz Diagnostic System and Zywave Wavefront Analysis 51

Figure 4.23 Peripheral thickness comparison

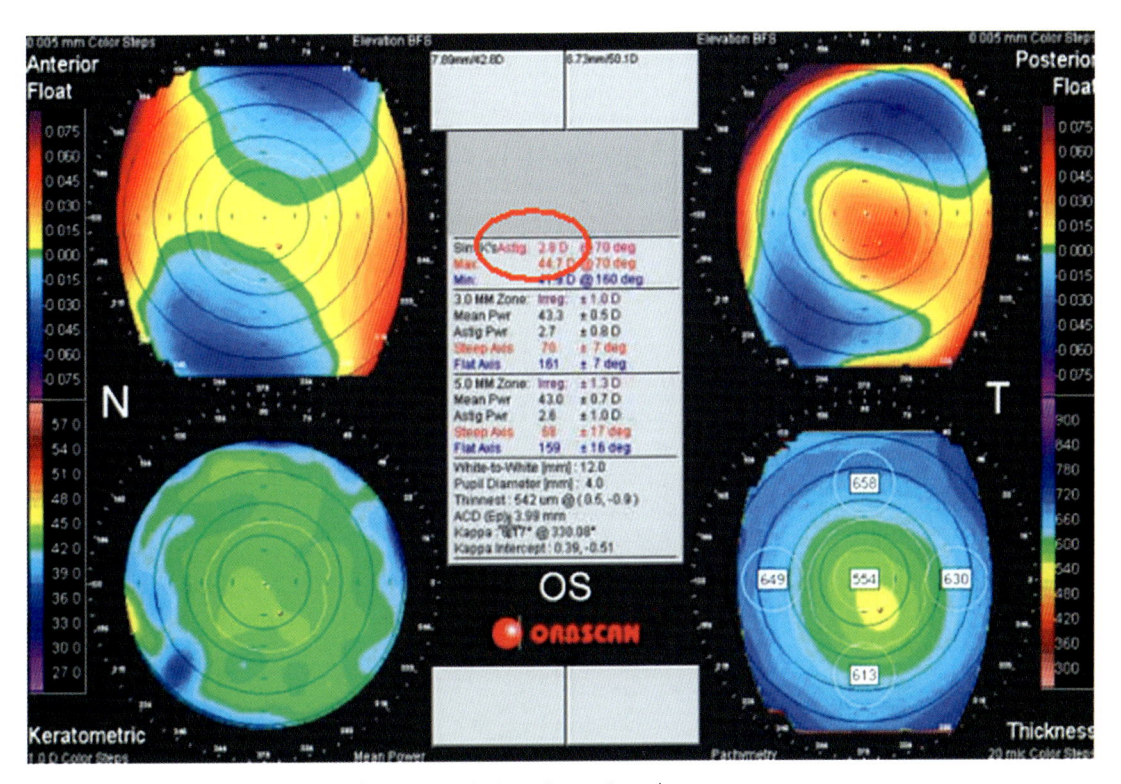

Figure 4.24 Astigmatism variance between eyes

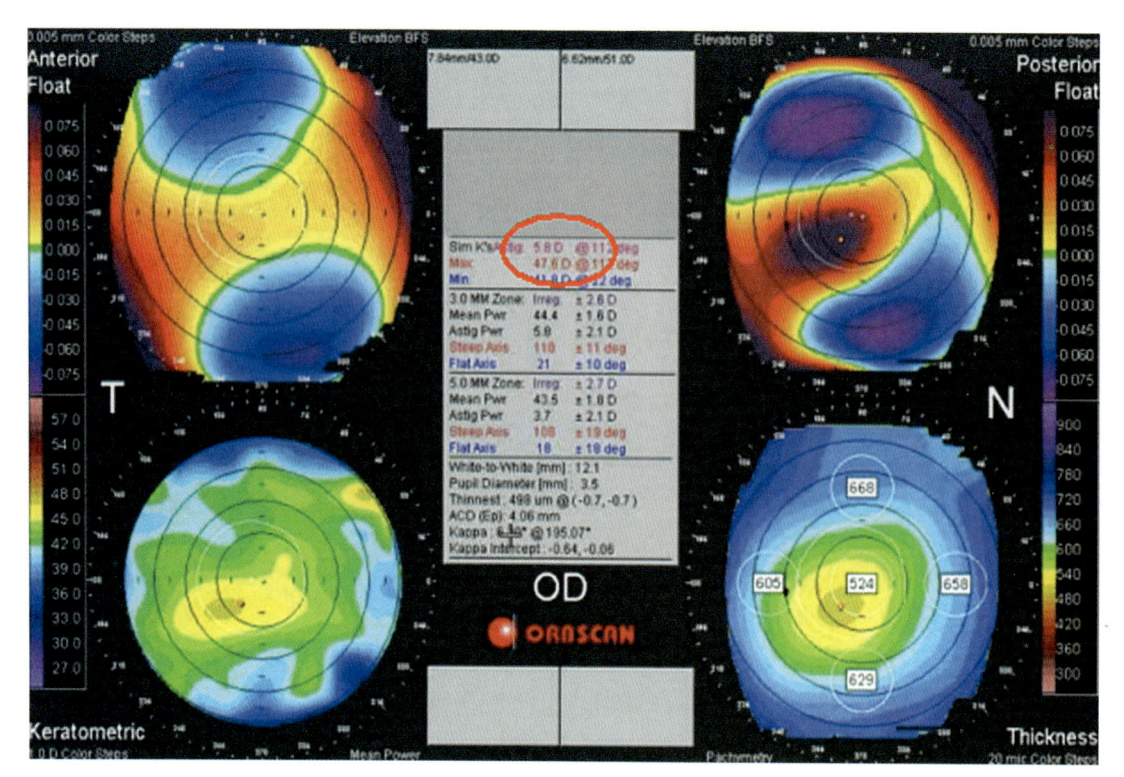

52   Section I: Introduction to Corneal Topography and Orbscan

Figure 4.25 Astigmatism variance between eyes

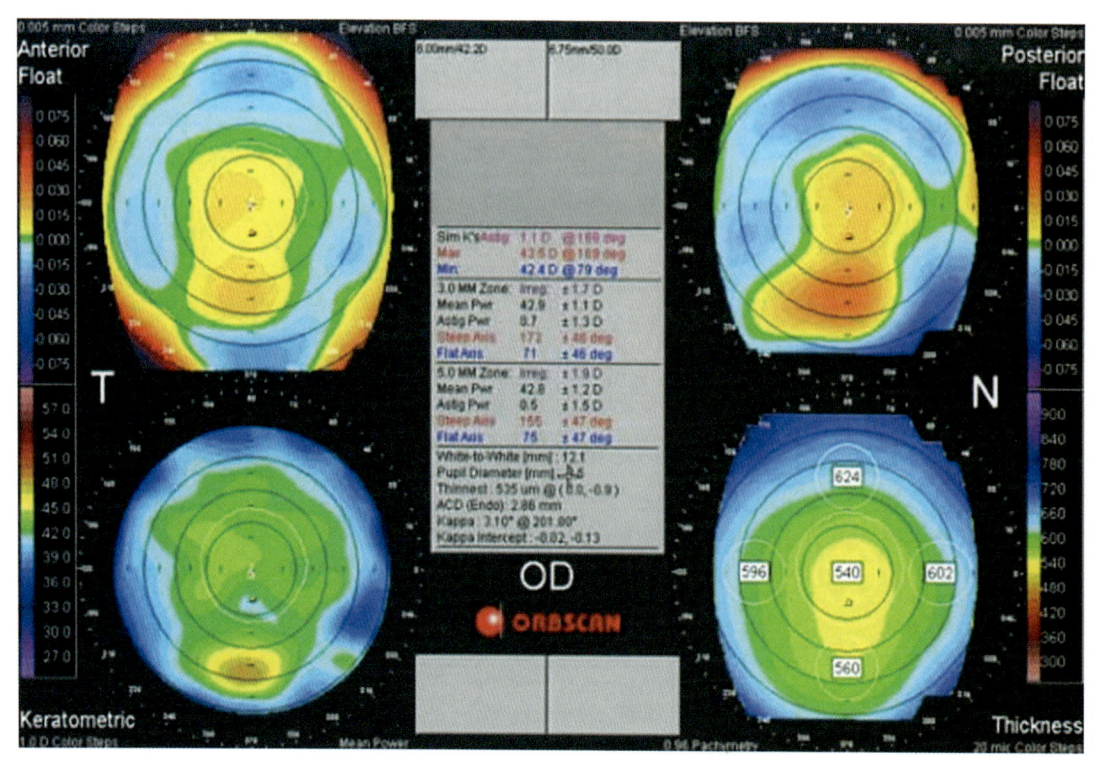

Figure 4.26 Steep keratometry on mean power map

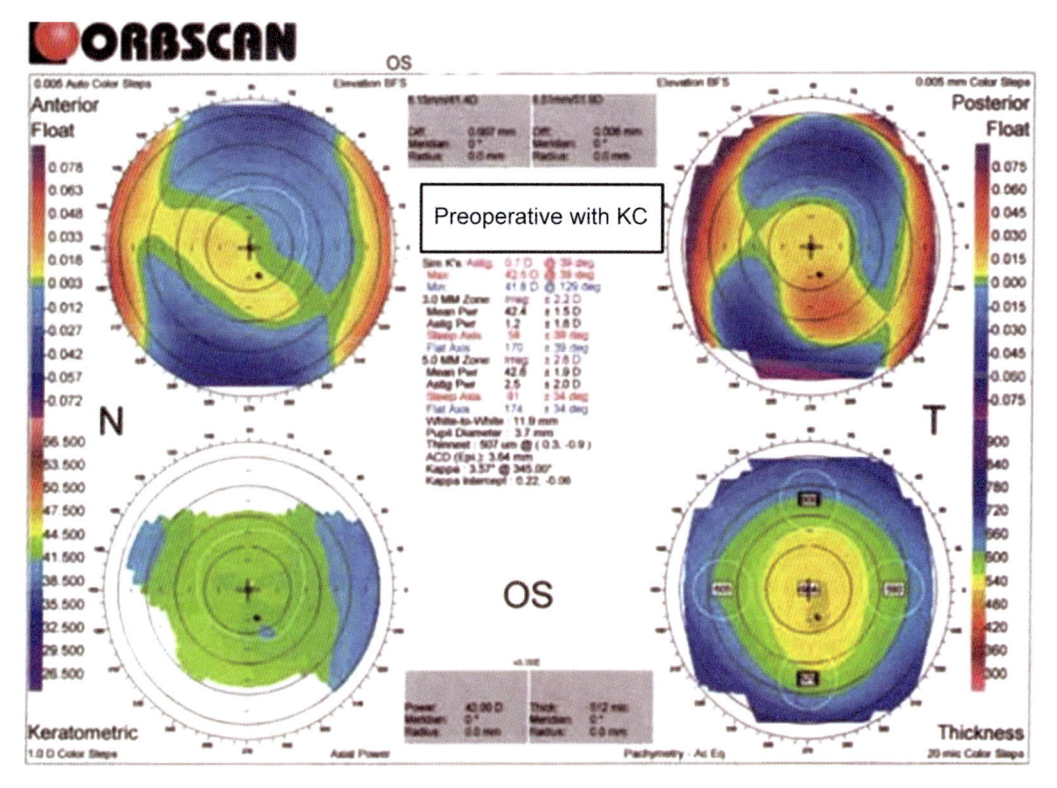

Chapter 4: The Orbscan IIz Diagnostic System and Zywave Wavefront Analysis 53

Figure 4.27 Preoperative patient with keratoconus

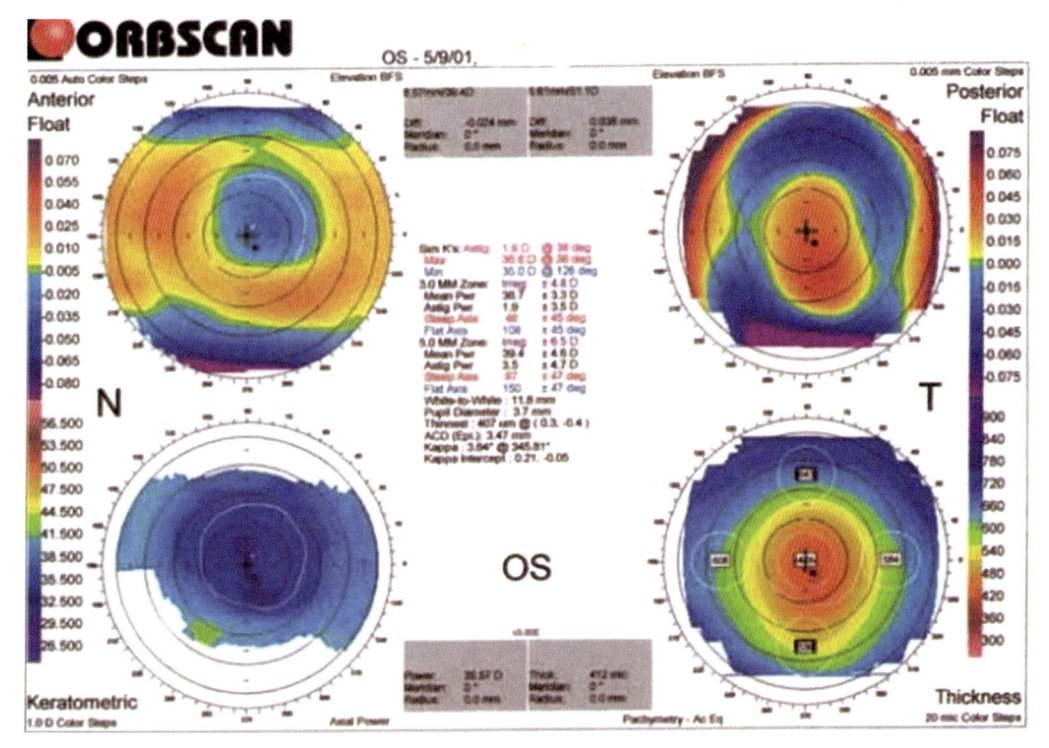

Figure 4.28 Four months postoperative LASIK with keratoconus

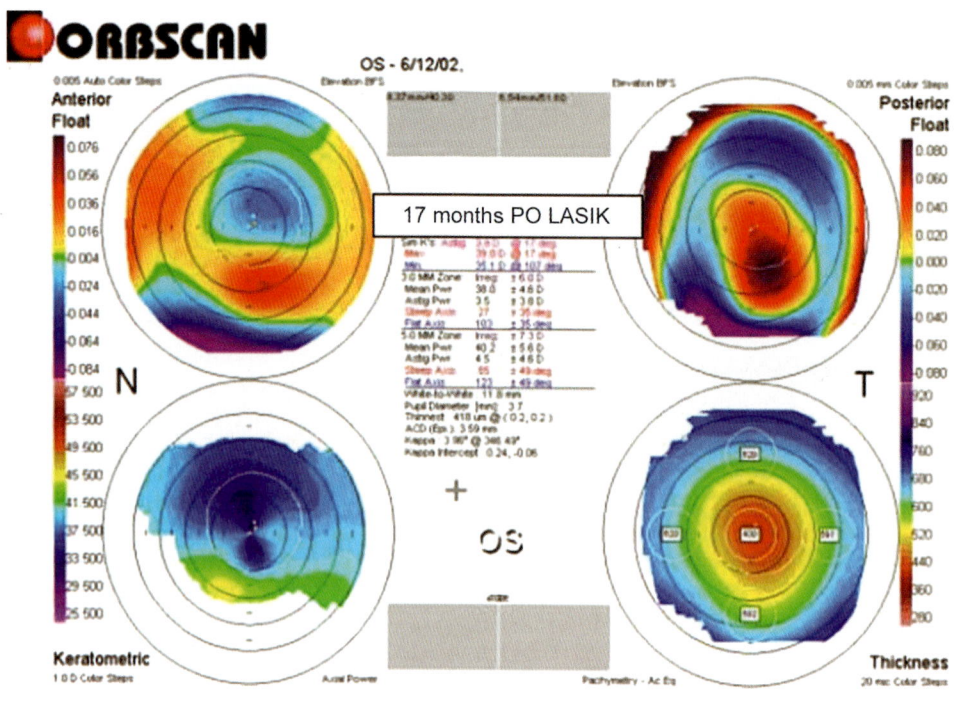

54 Section I: Introduction to Corneal Topography and Orbscan

Figure 4.29 Seventeen months postoperative LASIK

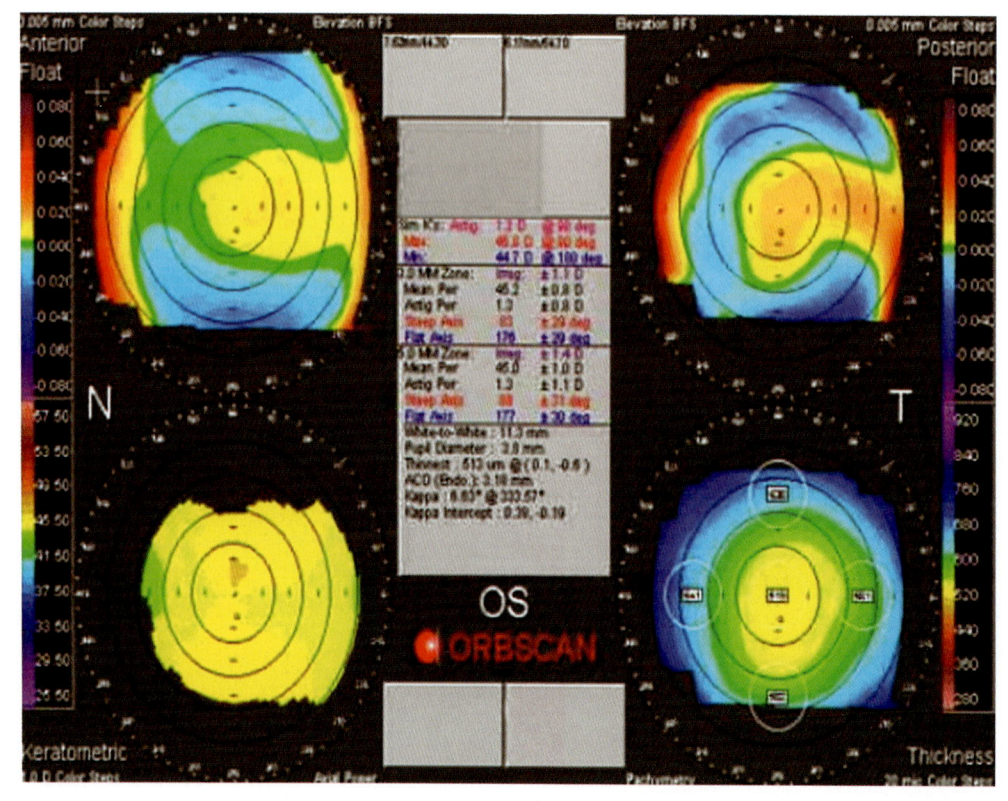

Figure 4.30 Normal Orbscan

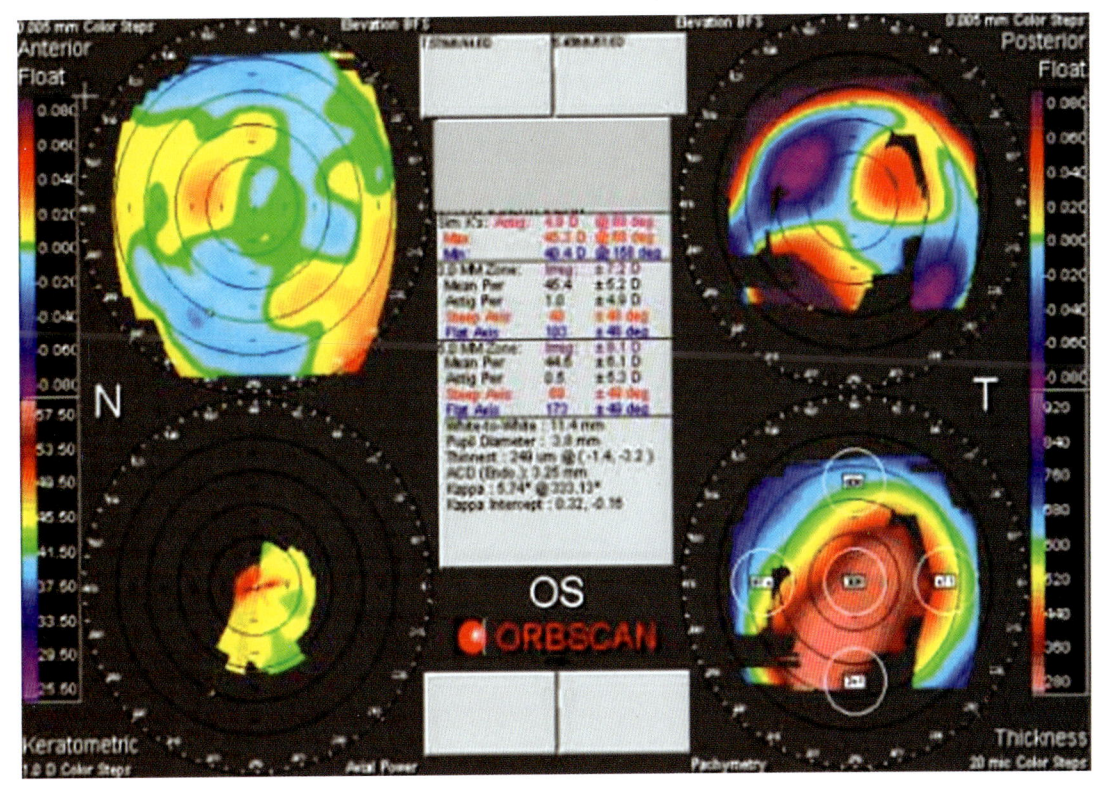

Chapter 4: The Orbscan IIz Diagnostic System and Zywave Wavefront Analysis

Figure 4.31 Orbscan after 3 minutes of desiccation

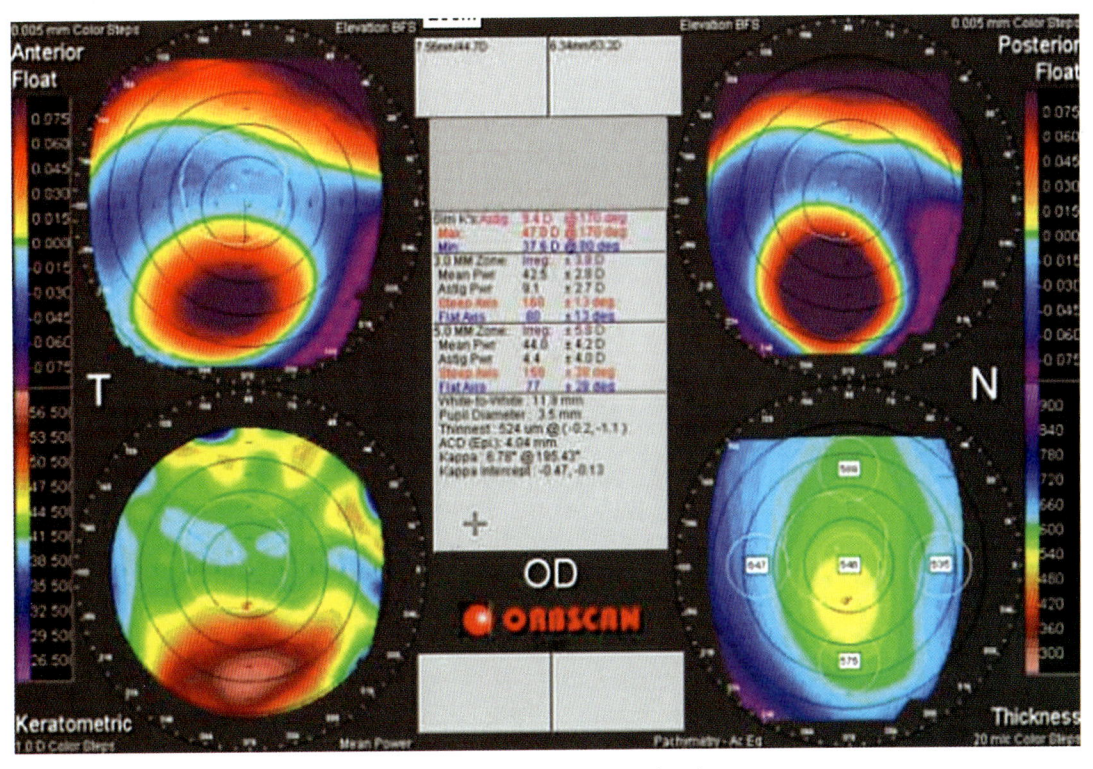

Figure 4.32 Keratoconus with normal pachymetry

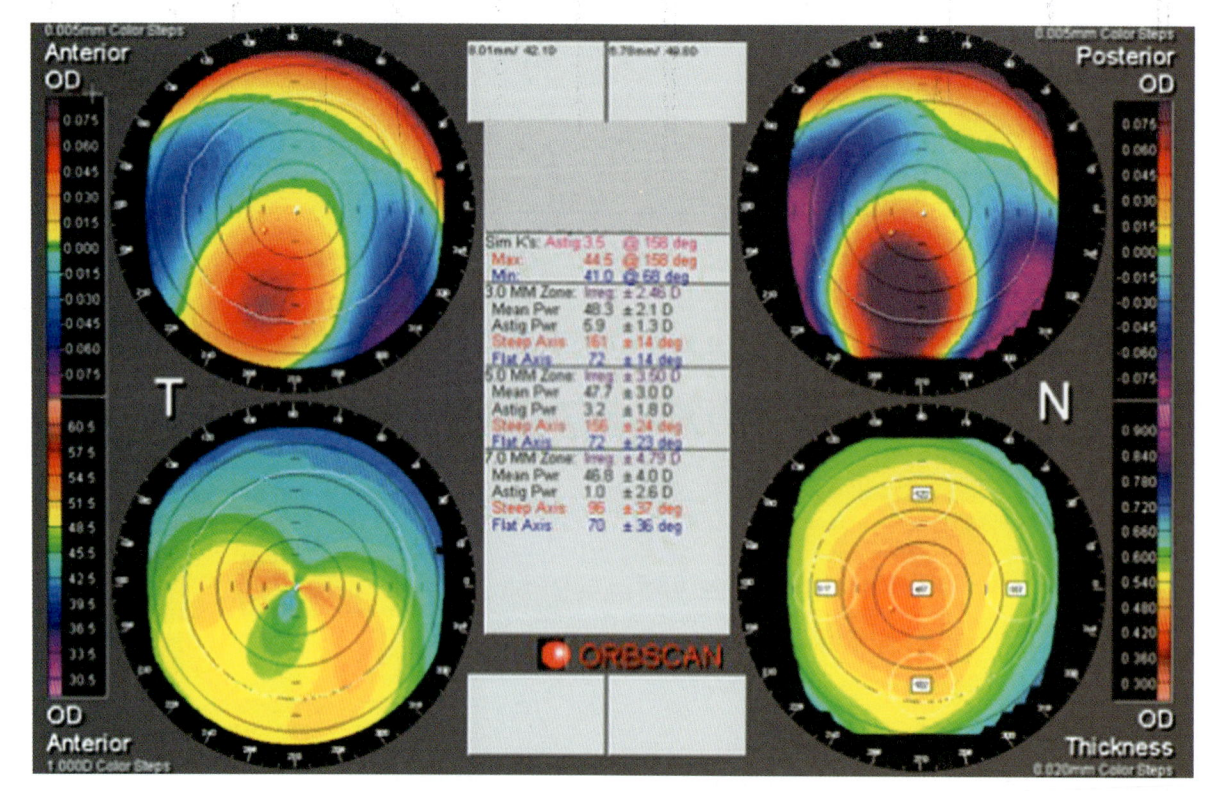

56 Section I: Introduction to Corneal Topography and Orbscan

Figure 4.33 Pellucid marginal degeneration

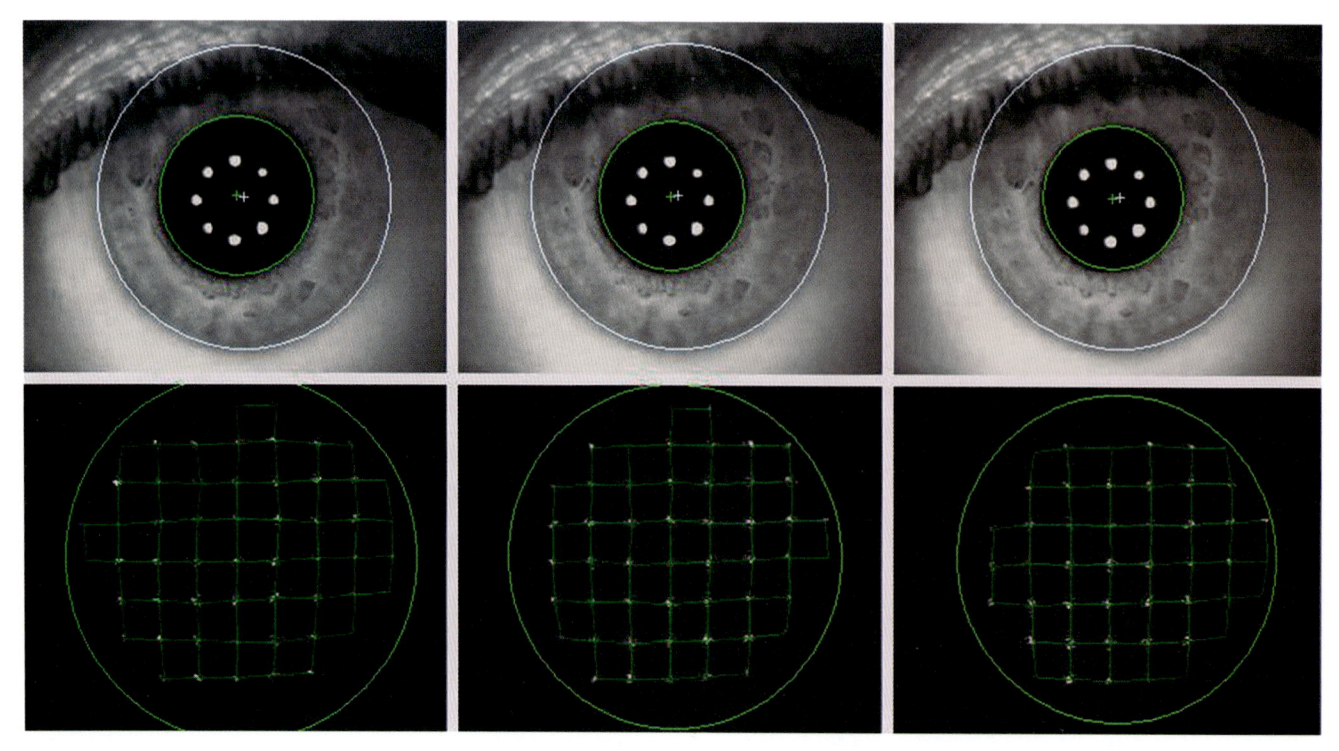

Figure 4.34 Zywave raw data *(Courtesy: Dr Agarwal's Eye Hospital)*

the well-correlated anterior elevation abnormality, and the large amounts of irregularity in the central 3 and 5 mm zones.

ZYOPTIX

The Zyoptix wavefront diagnostic system version 2.38 is a Hartmann-Schack wavefront aberrometer developed by Bausch and Lomb. This system is combined with the information obtained from the Orbscan to form the basis for wavefront-guided ablations through the Zylink platform and Technolas 21Z excimer laser.

The first step in any aberrometer is data acquisition. In the dual workstation system patient demographics are entered into the Orbscan, including manifest refraction, and this information is simply exported into the Zywave database. The current FDA indications are myopia less than 7.00 diopters and astigmatism less than 3.00 diopters. This information can be entered in plus or minus format and there is a quick conversion button on the Zywave screen. The patient status (i.e. preoperative dilated or undilated, postoperative, etc.) is entered and then testing can begin.

It is recommended that an undilated Zywave be taken and then an anterior segment exam is performed. The Zywave will use Hartmann-Schack technology and its lenslet array to capture up to 9000 data points. These are then analyzed using Zernike polynomials and the data is displayed up to 5th order Zernike terms. It is crucial that the raw data received at this stage be verified for good quality before proceeding. The Zywave will obtain five scans and the best three sets of raw data will be automatically selected for analysis. The examiner needs to verify proper centration of the scans, good quality of the scans, and good accuracy of the scans before proceeding **(Figure 4.34)**. Centration of the Zywave scans is verified be looking at the three sets of raw data to see that the central "x" is near pupil center, and that the outer ring around the raw data is green. If it is not centered the outer ring will be yellow and the Zywave needs to be repeated **(Figure 4.35)**. The Zywave system comes with an alignment aid, which greatly improves the ease of acquisition and verification of centration. This aid has color bars and rings that change in size and color until optimally centered and crisp, and then the scan can be taken. The next item is to verify that the raw data is of good quality. The examiner must look at the three sets of raw data and see that all the centroids are sharp, and that the lines from other centroids connect them all. If the lines are broken around the extreme edges it is still okay, but any break in the central areas denotes poor quality and needs to be repeated.

Lastly, the Zywave will display all five sets of predicted phoropter refractions (PPRs). Three will be highlighted and checked as the best three chosen by the computer for analysis **(Figure 4.36)**. It is our practice to not only verify the tight deviations among the chosen three, but to verify that all five PPRs correlate tightly with each other and with the subjective refraction. A range greater than 0.75 diopters on sphere, 0.50 diopters on cylinder and 0.15 degree on axis is considered unacceptable. An examination summary screen will display the subjective refraction, the PPR at the 3.5 mm zone, and the differences between them. It will highlight in red any deviation larger than the amounts mentioned.

If the undilated pupil size is large enough to allow for the desired optical zone for the individual patient, then no further testing is required. If, however, the pupil size is not large enough, then dilation should be performed with 2.5% phenylephrine and 0.5% mydriacyl. A full 20 minutes should be allowed for dilation to ensure that there is no asymmetrical shift to the pupil during mid dilation that might then alter the centration of the captured Zywave over the actual physiologic pupil center during treatment.

After successful data capture the surgeon has the ability to review the wavefront data at three different pupil sizes **(Figure 4.37)**. The data can be viewed at a 5 mm zone, a more standard 6 mm zone, or at the size of the captured pupil.

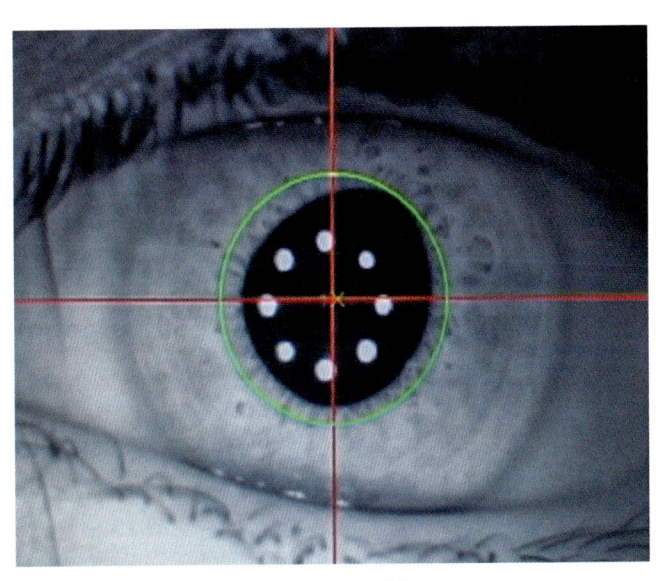

Figure 4.35 Well-centered Zywave scan
(Courtesy: Dr Agarwal's Eye Hospital)

No.	Exam Dia. (mm)	PPR	OK
1.	4.62	-0.41 / -0.35 / 22°	✓
2.	4.56	-0.56 / -0.15 / 174°	✓
3.	4.31	-0.63 / -0.20 / 164°	✓
4.	4.47	-0.57 / -0.50 / 33°	✗
5.	4.55	-0.58 / -0.33 / 131°	✗

Figure 4.36 Predicted phoropter refractions (PPRs)
(Courtesy: Dr Agarwal's Eye Hospital)

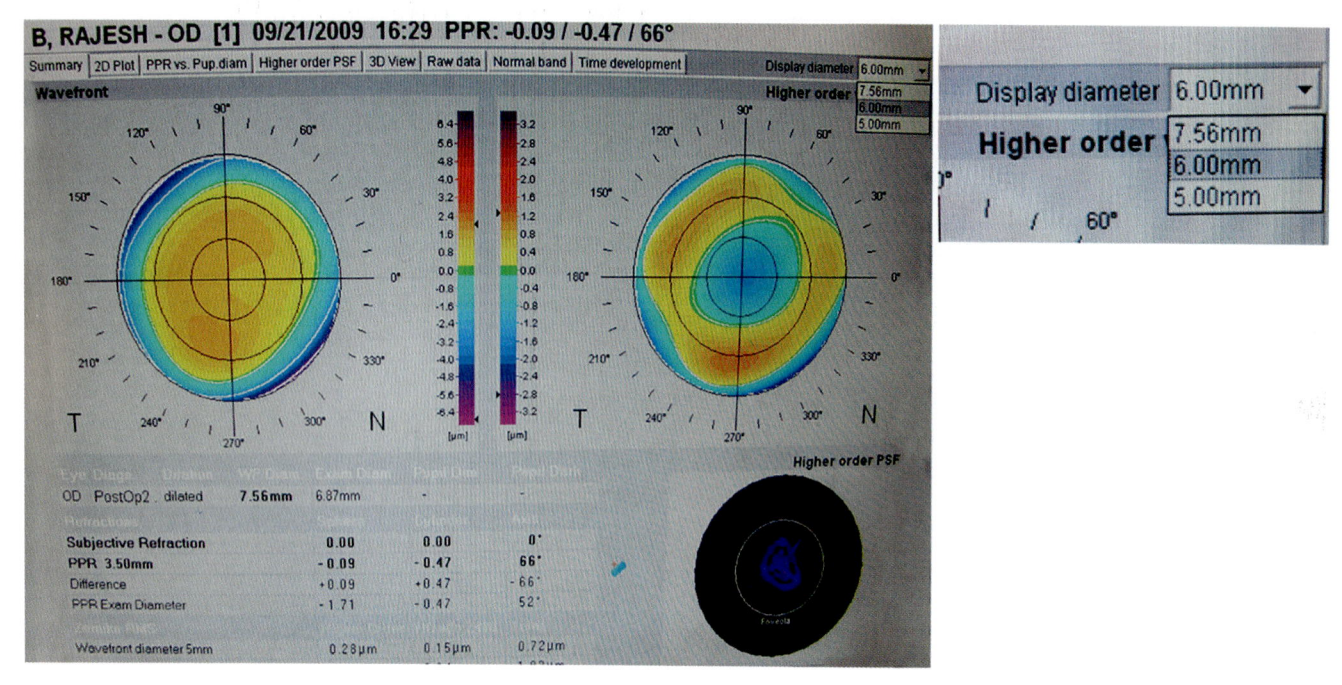

Figure 4.37 Examination summary (*Courtesy: Dr Agarwal's Eye Hospital*)

This can be viewed in a higher-order point spread function showing a graphic splay of how light is scattered based on HOAs only. It can be viewed graphically broken down by each individual type of HOA at the 5 or 6 mm zones and have the graphs displayed over a normal amount of each of these aberrations for the given zone size. Or it can be displayed as a color map of the HOA's similar to the color topographic maps we are accustom to viewing. One of the most useful features of these displays is the ability to choose a standard viewing zone (not related to treatment zone) for examining the three mentioned displays of HOAs. This allows the surgeon, overtime, to be able to use pattern recognition for different types and amount of HOAs similar to how pattern recognition is used in topographic maps today. It would be impossible to do this if all HOA maps were displayed at different zone sizes as opposed to displaying them all at the same zone size. Again as a reminder the 6 mm zone chosen to display the HOA data does not then mandate that the treatment be at a 6 mm zone. The surgeon may still choose any zone desired for treatment from 5.5 to 7.0 mm.

After capturing and reviewing the Zywave data the surgeon may then comfortably discuss the benefits of wavefront treatment with each patient. Individual markers for custom treatment vary from surgeon-to-surgeon, but generally patients with larger pupil sizes, higher prescriptions, residual bed issues, higher amounts of HOAs to begin with, and higher quality of vision expectations are good candidates for wavefront treatments.

ACKNOWLEDGMENT

Orbscan Figures, *Courtesy* Andrew L Moyes, MD and Paul M Karpecki, OD.

REFERENCE

1. Rao SN, Raviv T, Majumdar PA, Epstein RJ. Role of Orbscan II in screening keratoconus suspects before refractive corneal surgery. Ophthalmology. 2002;109(9):1642-6.

Section II

Orbscan and Refractive Surgery

CHAPTERS

5. Orbscan Corneal Mapping in Refractive Surgery
6. Anterior Keratoconus
7. Posterior Corneal Changes in Refractive Surgery
8. Corneal Ectasia Post-LASIK: The Orbscan Advantages

Chapter 5

Orbscan Corneal Mapping in Refractive Surgery

Francisco Sánchez León (Mexico)

INTRODUCTION

Today corneal topography plays several critical roles in different refractive surgery decisions. Conventional axial and tangential topography maps are not enough to demonstrate a healthy cornea and sometimes it is decided whether LASIK surgery, surface ablation refractive procedure, Phakic IOLs or intracorneal rings is suitable for any case based only on surface topographic evaluation.

Inability to analyze the posterior float or corneal thinning preoperatively may lead to corneal post-LASIK ectasia even in cases of mild to moderate myopia.[1]

Bausch and Lomb's Orbscan® IIz is a fully integrated multidimensional diagnostic system that elevates diagnostics beyond mere topography. Unlike current topography systems which scan the surface of the eye at standard points, the Orbscan II acquires over 9000 data points in 1.5 seconds to meticulously map the entire corneal surface (11 mm), and analyze elevation and curvature measurements on both the anterior and posterior surfaces of the cornea.

The Orbscan® system (Bausch & Lomb, Rochester, NY) uses the principle of projection. Forty scanning slit beams (20 from the left and 20 from the right with up to 240 data points per slit) are used to scan the cornea from limbus to limbus and to measure independently the X, Y, and Z locations of several thousand points on each surface. The images captured are then used to construct the anterior corneal surface, posterior corneal surface, and anterior iris and anterior lens surfaces. Data regarding the corneal pachymetry and anterior chamber depth are also displayed. In the newer version of the Orbscan® system, a Placido disc has been mounted to this device in order to improve the accuracy of the curvature measurements.

An advantage of this device is that it measures all surfaces of the anterior segment. Scanning time (1.2–1.5 seconds) is required, this device use a tracking system to track the eye movements in order to minimize the influence of involuntary eye movement.

By providing more comprehensive preoperative diagnostics and planning, exclusionary criteria such as keratoconus, prekeratoconus, and corneal thinning can be identified to optimize outcomes in both primary treatments and enhancements. The Orbscan II may help explain decreased visual acuity postoperative, and is designed to allow the surgeon to more accurately prescribe retreatments, if necessary. This technology is capable of detecting and analyzing posterior corneal abnormalities where corneal anomalies first appear.

ORBSCAN CORNEAL MAPPING FOR REFRACTIVE SURGERY DIAGNOSTICS

The Orbscan II **(Figure 5.1)**, together with other diagnostic tools such as aberrometry, pupillometry and pachymetry, provides us with an unprecedented opportunity to select patients for an appropriate technique (LASIK, LASEK, PRK, Phakik IOL, Intracorneal Rings), minimizing complications such as long-term corneal posterior ectasia.

Posterior ectasia has been identified after refractive surgery techniques such as LASIK, where insufficient corneal tissue has been left behind postoperatively.[2] It has manifested itself as a forward 'bulging' of corneal tissue **(Figure 5.2)**, developing from the posterior corneal surface. Research indicates that up to 90% of keratoconus developing in the untreated eye appear first from the posterior surface. This is thought to be related to leaving the cornea with too little tissue postoperatively; and indeed although this is established, there are other indicators which could also put a patient at risk. The Orbscan II provide us additional information to predict these risk.

It has become a universally accepted standard to leave at least 250 microns residual stromal bed as a safety measure in LASIK, and the Orbscan II has played its part to make this happen. However, the true validity of this limit is in some doubt.[4] The average cornea can range in thickness from 490–600 microns, so it is not logical to leave a standard 250 micron in all cases.

A number of surgeons support the view that a percentage thickness of the cornea should remain instead, and/or that a minimum of at least 260 to 280 micron is a more realistic standard. To facilitate this, intraoperative pachymetry (corneal thickness measurement) can be performed to provide a more accurate idea of how much tissue will remain after a procedure.[5] This in itself has limitations, but gives an additional safety criterion, rather than merely relying on manufacturers' estimations of flap thickness.

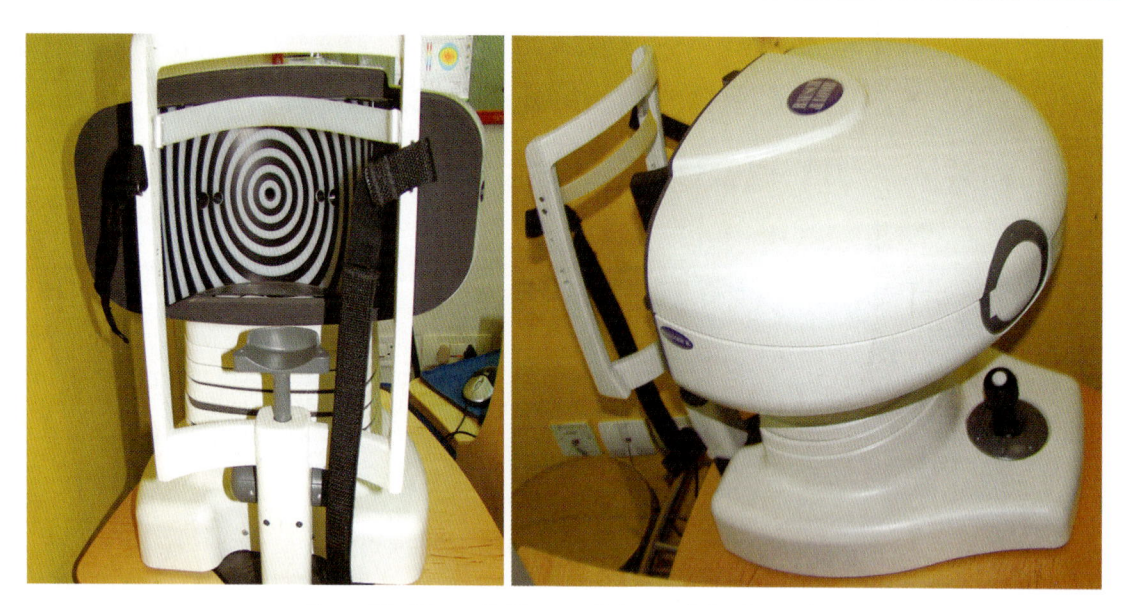

Figure 5.1 Orbscan IIz (*Courtesy:* Dr Agarwal's Eye Hospital)

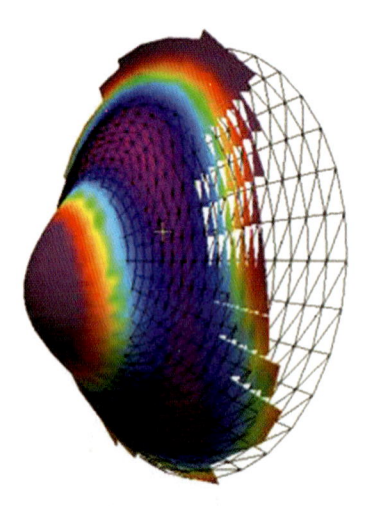

Figure 5.2 Ectasia

In summary, the residual stromal bed is by far from our clinical perspective the only indicator for safe preoperative screening. So, how does the Orbscan II influence decisions on whether or not to treat? It is important to understand that selection criteria for refractive surgery never stands alone, and it is the clinician's responsibility to bring together all the information gathered in the screening process, before deciding whether it is safe to proceed. The Orbscan influences this decision in a number of ways.

Unlike other modern topography systems, the Orbscan is based on slit scanning technology in addition to traditional Placido-based techniques **(Figure 5.3)**.

The Placido image gives us information on axial keratometric readings, by converting distortion of the rings into topographical data. A series of illuminated annular rings are projected onto the cornea. Using the corneal tear film as a mirror, the reflected image of the rings is captured by a digital video camera. The captured image is then subjected to an algorithm to detect and identify the position of the rings in relation to the video keratographic axis. Once these borders are detected, the digital image is 'reconstructed' to show anterior corneal curvature.

Orbscan goes much further than this; slit-beam scanners and triangulation are used to derive the actual spatial location of thousands of points on the surface. Each beam sweep across the cornea gives information on corneal elevation, or height, from the anterior corneal surface, posterior surface and iris. To represent the corneal surface data in a way that is easily understood, the computer calculates a hypothetical sphere that matches as close as possible to the actual corneal shape being measured. This is called the best-fit sphere (BFS). It then compares the real surface to the hypothetical sphere, showing areas 'above' the surface of the sphere in warm colors, and areas 'below' the surface in cool colors.

This has many uses, but for the purposes of refractive surgery selection, 'bulges' in both the posterior and anterior surface can indicate patients who may be at risk of ectasia development. This enables the surgeon to screen them out early in the selection process.

A "quad map" can be produced, which gives four different maps each portraying different information about the cornea **(Figure 5.4)**. The bottom left hand map is the axial keratometry map, based on Placido technology. This is similar to maps produced from the majority of commercially available

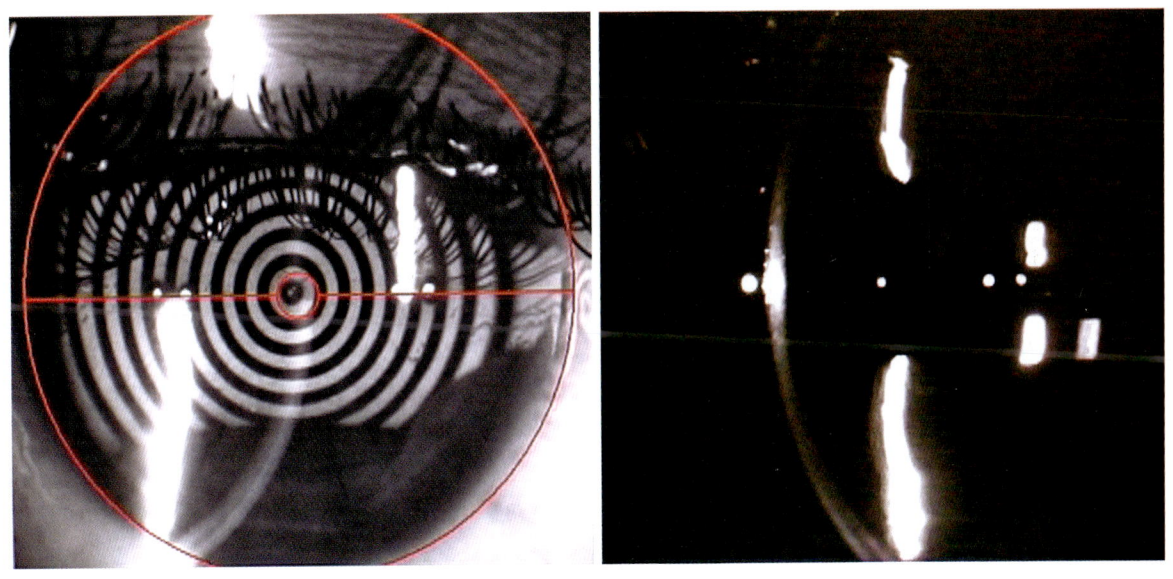

Chapter 5: Orbscan Corneal Mapping in Refractive Surgery 63

Figure 5.3 Slit scanning technology in the Orbscan (*Courtesy:* Dr Agarwal's Eye Hospital)

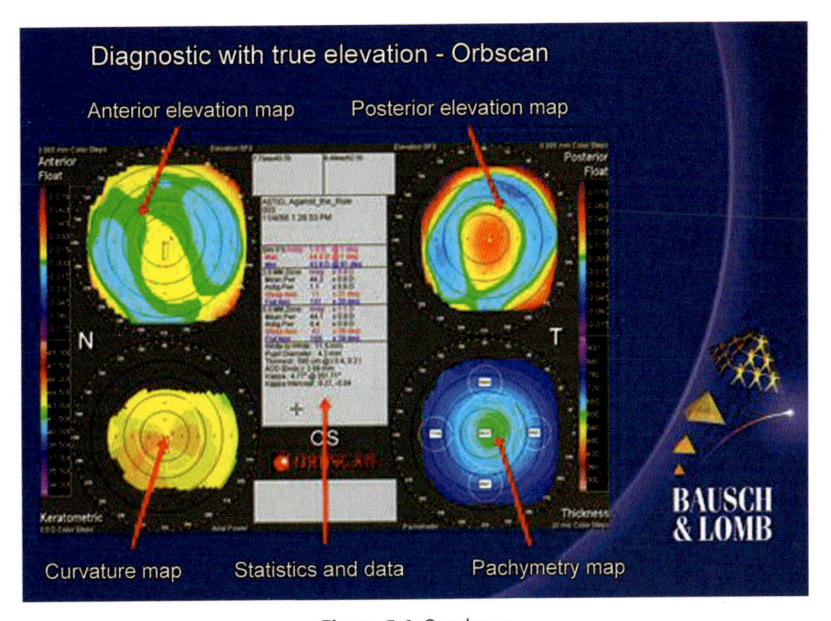

Figure 5.4 Quad map

topography systems, and provides detailed keratometric information across the diameter of the cornea.

For LASIK selection, this information is important for a number of reasons. The 'K' readings are important, because normal limits of K readings are between certain values; the cornea must be neither too steep nor too flat. It is difficult for the microkeratome (blade designed for flap cutting), to create a good quality corneal flap in LASIK if either of these extremes is the case, as this can lead to surgical flap complications.

In addition, K readings of more than 48 D are an indication of potential keratoconus, particularly where this is decenterd inferonasally. Details of the K readings can be found in the stats and data information in the center of the quad map.

The top left hand map of **Figure 5.4** is the anterior elevation map, and as with the top right hand posterior elevation map, slit scanning provides the means of creating the information. As mentioned before, slit scanning provides elevation data, and this also can create a 3 D interpretation of the cornea. Looking at both elevation maps, if it is imagined that the green tissue is at sea level, then the warmer colors are above sea level, or towards the viewer, and the cooler colors are below, or further away from the viewer.

64 Section II: Orbscan and Refractive Surgery

A 3 D interpretation of both elevation maps can be seen in **Figure 5.5**. The meshwork affect indicates how the cornea would appear if it were entirely spherical and is referred to as the reference sphere.

This elevation data can be interpreted usefully in a number of ways. First the difference between the highest and lowest points is a potential kerataconus indicator, if over 100 microns; Rousch criteria[6] **(Figure 5.6)**.

In addition, on the posterior map, the highest elevation value can again be interpreted as a keratoconus indicator, or at least as a screen for those patients who may be at risk of developing kerectasia postoperatively. This provides safety criteria to avoid treating patients at risk. From the work of Vukich[7] and Potgeiter,[8] 55D elevation has been recommended as an absolute cut-off. As can be seen from **Figures 5.5 and 5.6**, the elevation on the right hand side (posterior elevation) is more advanced than that on the left (anterior elevation), indicating that 'bulges' develop from the posterior surface of the cornea in the first instance.

From studying the relationship between the two elevation maps, further information can be gleaned. A ratio can be calculated between the posterior and anterior surfaces, which

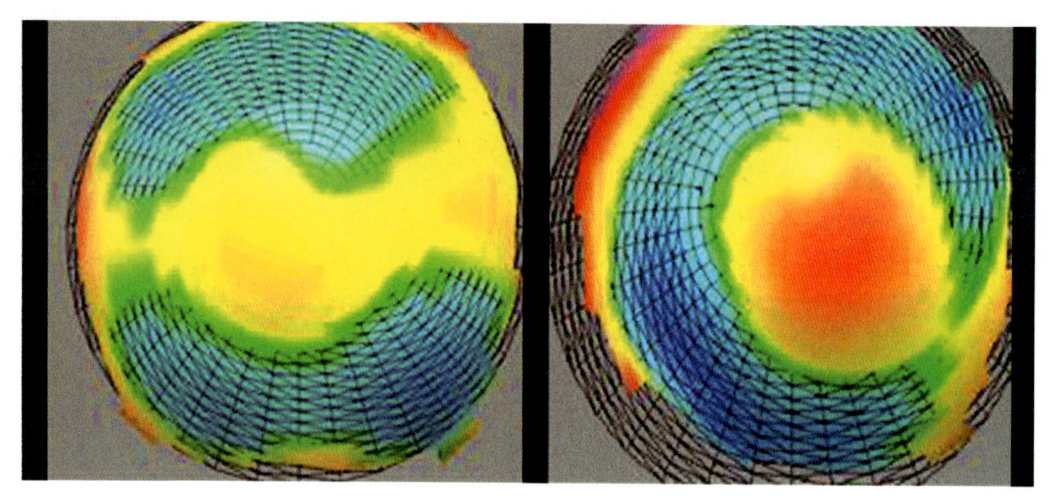

Figure 5.5 Elevation map

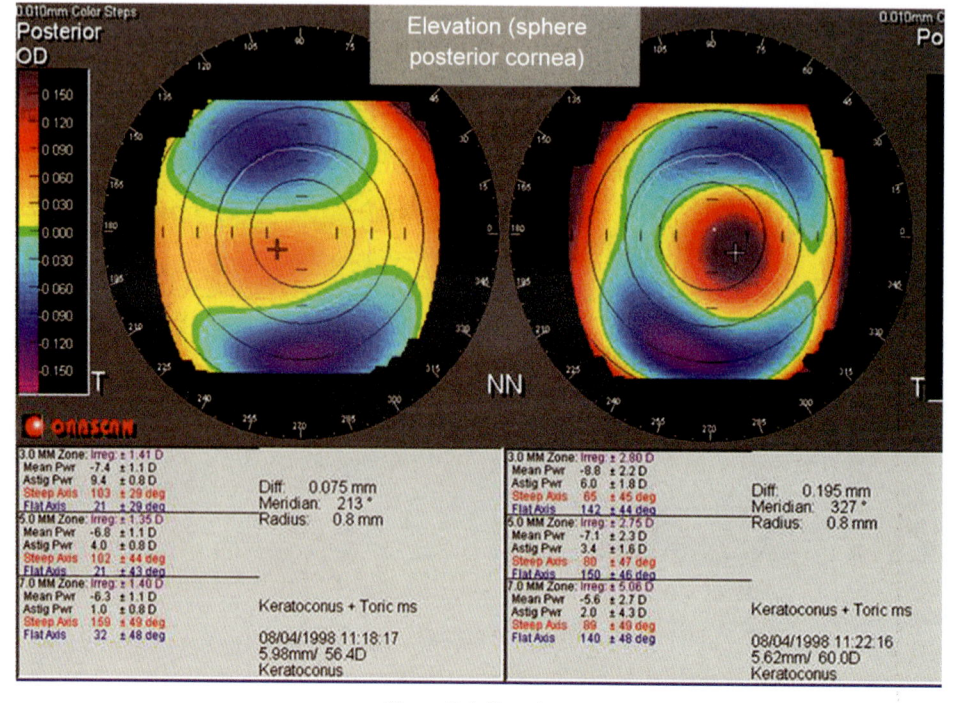

Figure 5.6 Elevation

Chapter 5: Orbscan Corneal Mapping in Refractive Surgery 65

gives an indication of the relative difference in curvature between the two maps.[9] **Figures 5.7A and B** shows two corneal cross-sections.

This very simplistic diagram **(Figures 5.7A and B)** shows us that the same elevation data for the posterior surface can have a different impact on the stability of the cornea. In diagram B where the ratio is high at 1.27, it can be seen that a weak area (indicated by the arrow) develops which is not apparent in A, even though posterior elevation data is the same for both. This information on elevation and ratio would rarely be used as exclusion criteria alone, but by considering these together, more conclusive information can be obtained. For example, a high ratio of say 1.26 would be far more concerning if the posterior elevation was high at 55 D, the cornea was of borderline thickness, and the preoperative prescription high.

The final map to study is the pachymetry map. This is map four of our quad map in **Figure 5.4**. Traditionally, pachymetry has been measured using ultrasound, which provides a reading of corneal thickness from Bowman's membrane to Descemet's membrane. Through slit scanning technology, Orbscan provides us with a pachymetry reading from the precorneal tear film to the endothelium, therefore slightly thicker readings can be expected.[10] The Orbscan can, however, be calibrated to take this into consideration when comparing readings. The true advantage of the pachymetry map is that it provides us with thickness information across the cornea from limbus to limbus, not just in single points as with ultrasound. This once again gives the opportunity to detect areas of weakness, thinning or scarring. Auffarth et al[11] state that the relationship between the highest point on anterior and posterior elevation maps, and the thinnest point (shown by a yellow dot) is an indicator of kerataconus.

The relationship between pachymetry readings can be looked at, and it has been suggested that 100 microns should be a cut-off criteria between thickness regions on the map. **Figure 5.8** shows the relationship between the central reading in the white circle, and the four peripheral readings, indicated by the arrows. Once again these criteria would be used alongside other information, but alone would not exclude a patient. The readings within the circles are averages of measurements within the area, but the Orbscan also flags the thinnest point, indicated by a yellow dot.

In conclusion, it can be seen that much information can be obtained from analysis of Orbscan maps, and this information does not have the scope to cover it all. The most important

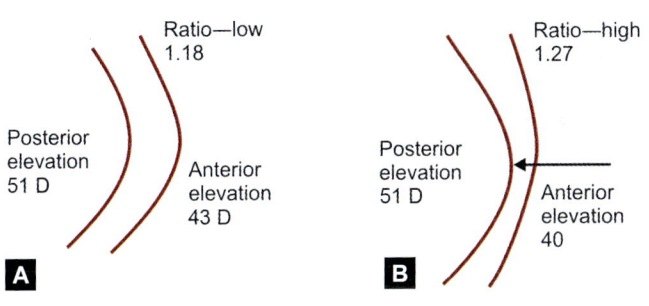

Figures 5.7A and B Corneal cross-sections

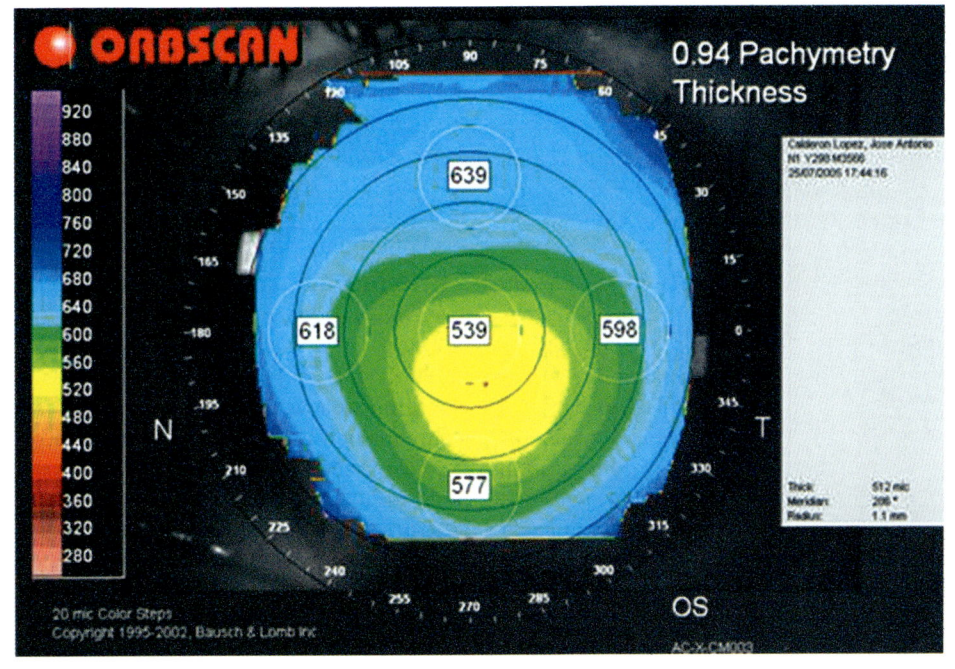

Figure 5.8 Pachymetry

message is that the criteria does not stand alone, and by looking at all the maps together along with other information, an informed decision can be made as to whether it is safe to proceed to surgery.

SELECTION CRITERIA

The diagnosis of keratoconus proper, seldom proves to be problematic, and represents the undisputed black end of the spectrum, as would be the case for the patient with simple with the rule astigmatism who would be on the white end of the spectrum. However, in between a large grey area exists, consisting of against-the-rule astigmatism, asymmetric astigmatism, nonorthogonal astigmatism, irregular astigmatism and forme fruste keratoconus.

Over the past number of years since true elevation corneal topography became available, a set of criteria (**Tables 5.1 and 5.2**)[6,8,9] were developed to distinguish to among these entities. Although corneal topography provides us with the most clues for the diagnosis of early keratoconus, other clinical criteria also need to be considered.

These would include the patient's age, a family history of keratoconus, history of systemic or local pathology, associated with keratoconus, refractive stability, as well as whether a good and crisp endpoint could be achieved on refractive testing of the subject.

Table 5.1 Rousch's Orbscan criteria for subclinical keratoconus detection

1. Elevation difference superior of 100 microns at the central optical zone of 7 mm
2. Clinical difference superior of 100 microns at the central optical zone of 7 mm
3. Anterior elevation superior of 40 microns at the central optical zone of 7 mm from BFS
4. Posterior elevation superior of 50 microns at the central optical zone of 7 mm from BFS

Table 5.2 Efkarpides's Orbscan criteria for subclinical keratoconus detection

1. Anterior/Posterior BFS of reference difference in μm superior to 1.25 to 1.27
2. Morphological difference between anterior and posterior face (warpage)
3. Remarkable convergence of points (highest point on anterior elevation, highest point on posterior elevation, thinnest point in pachymetry, steepest curvature on the power map)
4. Inferotemporal displacement of these remarkable points
5. Color code statistical analysis (Normal band scale). Elevation values, curvature, pachymetry of more than 2 standard deviations from controls.

No single cornea topographic sign is on its own right diagnostic of forme fruste keratoconus, but rather a combination of a set of criteria. One might look at each of these criteria as an "alarm sign" noted, with the probability for early keratoconus proportionate to the number of alarms present.

These criteria can be divide into the following categories:
a. Power map changes
b. Posterior elevation maps
c. Pachymetry
d. Composite/integrated topography information.

Power Maps

A. Mean corneal curvature >45 diopters. Mean corneal curvature measuring in excess of 45 diopters is a wells-established feature of keratoconus.
B. Bow-tie/broken-tie pattern. In addition to steep corneal curvatures, the bow-tie or broken bow-tie appearance of astigmatic pattern might be indicative of early keratoconus, and also a well-known criteria.
C. Central corneal asymetry. A change within the central 3 mm optical zone of the cornea of more than 3 diopters from superior or inferior can be correlated with the presence of vertical coma. However, this may be merely a sign of asymetrical astigmatism, and is not necessarily an indicator of pathology.

Posterior Elevation

The elevation map displays corneal height or elevation relative to a reference plane, which may be a spherical or aspherical surface depending on the topographer. It is important to note that the elevation display depends on reference surface size, shape, alignment, and fitting zone. This map shows the three-dimensional shape of the cornea and is useful in measuring the amount of tissue removed by a procedure, assessing postoperative visual problems, or planning/monitoring surgical procedures.

Many surgeons think the first sign of keratectasia appears on the posterior surface of the cornea, not on the anterior topography map. Considering this, the importance of recognizing a change in the posterior surface deserves special emphasis.[1-3] While one would not perform corneal laser surgery on eyes with keratoconus, keratoconus suspects or posterior ectasia defined by technologies with the capability of posterior corneal float analysis, it might prove useful to look at the criteria for early form of keratoconus in order to define those cases, and distinguish them from eyes that would be suited to laser refractive surgery.

Laser clinics had shown that 5 to 8% of patients screened for refractive procedure are not good candidates because of keratoconus detection by simple axial topography, however, a Mexican study demostrated that 3.13% of population screened for Laser eye surgery had posterior ectasia criteria by

Orbscan, despite having axial topography classified as normal (unpublished data).[3]

We have found four different posterior float patterns in patients screened for Laser eye surgery: Complete positive band 71.87%, incomplete positive band 18.75%, butterfly wings common in patients with high astigmatism 6.25%, and central island 3.13% **(Figure 5.9)**. In other words, if we do not know posterior float features from every case, we have at least 3% risk of unstable LASIK result or iatrogenic ectasia in the worst case.[3]

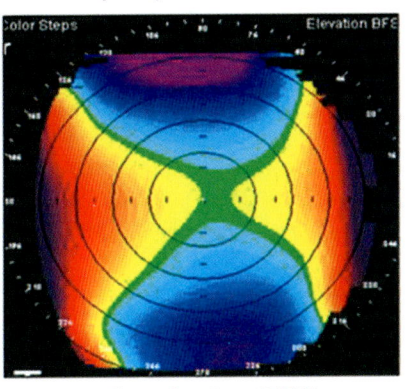

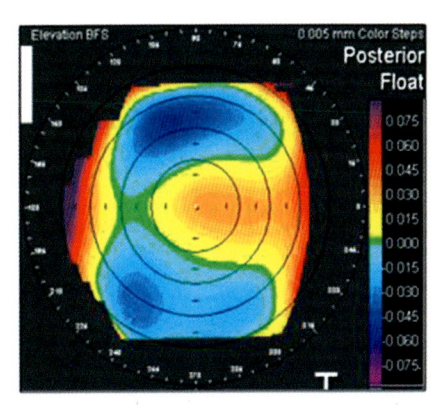

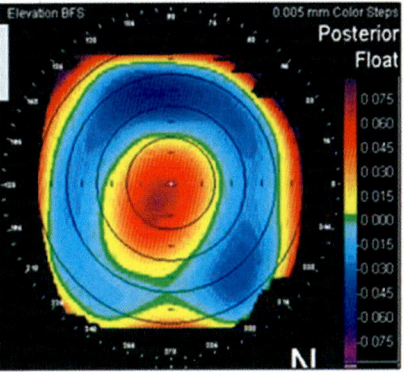

Best fit sphere > 55 diopters. The most common reference surface for viewing elevation maps is the "best fit sphere". This geometric surface is constructed by fitting a spherical plane with the least square of difference values though the three dimensional elevation data from the cornea, whether it be the anterior or posterior profile. The sphere can thus be employed to judge the average profile of the surface in question. A best fit sphere (BFS) with the power of 55 diopters or more on the posterior profile, could be indicative of posterior ectasia. This criterion is not diagnostic as a sign of early keratoconus per se, as this sign may also be seen in small diameter corneas.

Posterior high point >50 micron above BFS. Early keratoconus is often seen first on the posterior corneal profile. Whenever a localized elevation above BFS on the posterior surface measures more than 50 micron in elevation, this might be indicative of an early posterior ectasia.

Many authors have reviewed the posterior surface's response to LASIK, and Orbscan is a unique technology to evaluate this changes.[11-15] Increased forward shift of the posterior corneal surface is common after myopic LASIK and correlates with the residual corneal thickness and ablation percentage per total corneal thickness.[12]

An excessively thin residual cornea bed or a large ablation percentage may increase the risk of iatrogenic complications, such as ectasia. Others have considered that even if a residual corneal bed of 300 microns or thicker is preserved, anterior bulging of the cornea after LASIK can occur. Eye with thin corneas and high myopia requiring greater laser ablation are more predisposed to an anterior shift of the posterior central cornea.[13,14]

Roberts[15] with the help of Orbscan proposes a new theory to explain the increased posterior elevation post-LASIK, she suggests that the mild ectasia appearance may be due to a

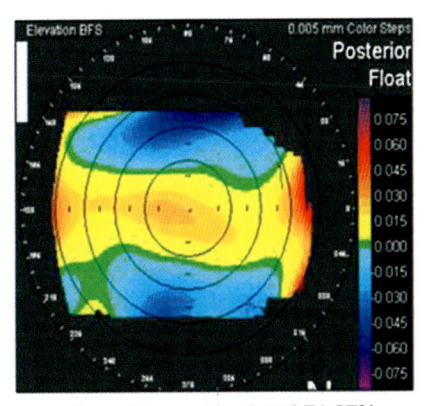

Figure 5.9 Posterior float patterns

68 Section II: Orbscan and Refractive Surgery

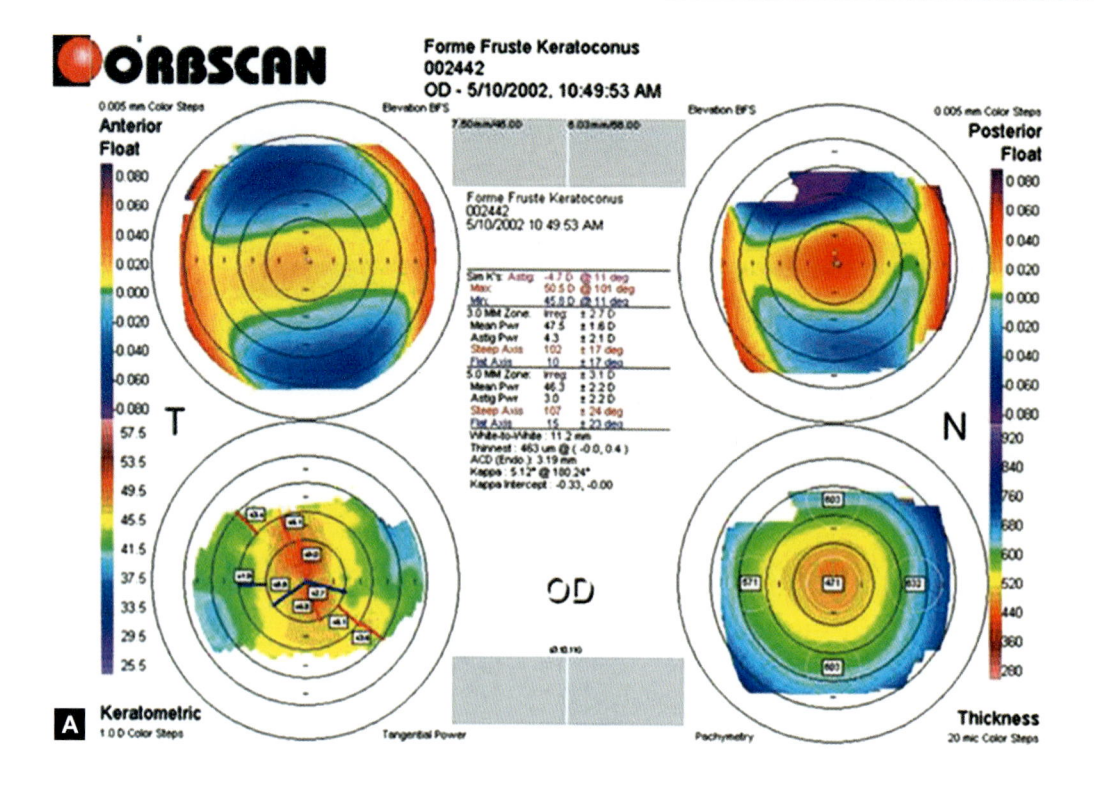

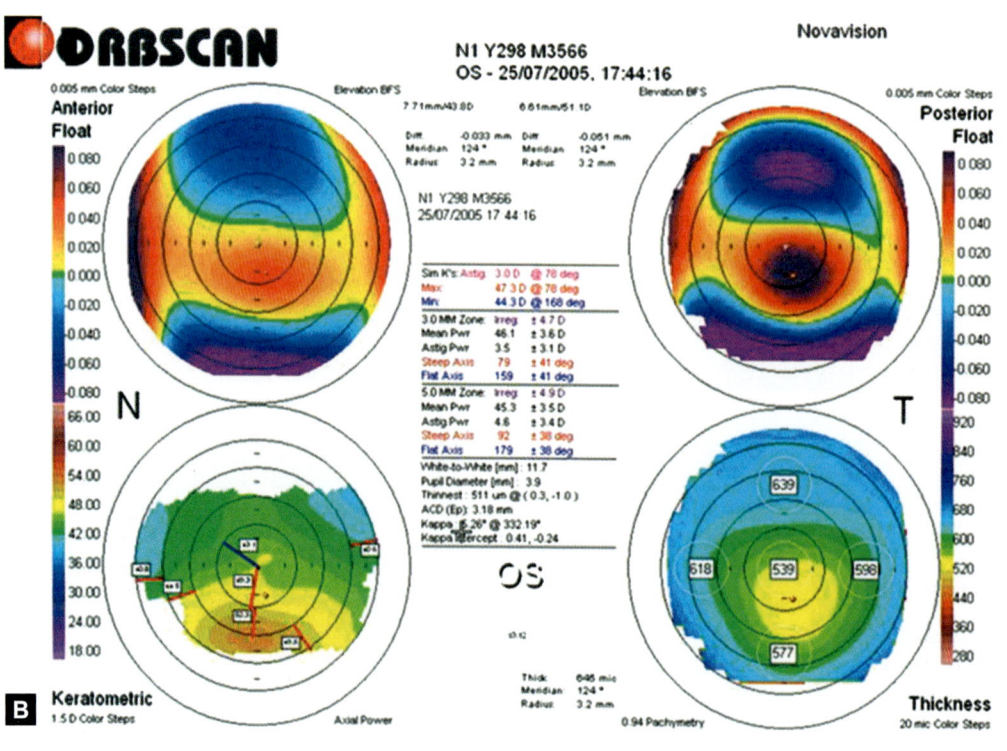

Figures 5.10A and B Keratoconus

backward swelling of the peripheral redistributed cornea rather than a pathological forward bulging of the central cornea.

Pachymetry

Thinnest point < 470 micron. This constitutes an absolute contraindication to corneal refractive surgery. In pathological corneas, this thinnest point is often displaced inferotemporal.

Difference of > 100 microns at 7 mm optical zone. A difference of more than 100 microns from the thinnest point to the values at the 7 mm optical zone implies a steep gradient of thinning from the midperiphery towards the thinnest point. These, in conjunction with other signs, can be indicative of early pathology.[9]

Composite/Integrated Information

As a default, four corneal maps are routinely presented by the Orbscan II (Bausch & Lomb, Orbtek, Salt Lake City, Utha). Elevation topography system.[16] These include the anterior elevation profile, posterior elevation profile, power map, and a total pachymetry map. Through integration of the information provided on these maps, one is able to detect subtle, but powerful signs not present on any individual map. These signs include the following:

Bent/Warped Cornea

Similarity between anterior and posterior profiles implies a forward bending of those areas shown above the BFS. If this bending is in association with the thinnest point on the cornea, it could be related to structural weakness in the cornea, irrespective of whether the thinnest point still shows an adequate pachymetry. This sign has to be evaluated within the context of other signs above.

Inferotemporal displacement of the highest point on the anterior as well as the posterior elevation profile can be indicative of early keratoconus, but must also be seen in context **(Figure 5.10A)**.

Correlation of Signs of the Highest Point on the Posterior Elevation

This is probably the strongest topographic sign indicative of early keratoconus. If the highest point on the posterior elevation coincides with the highest point of anterior elevation, the thinnest point on pachymetry, and the point of steepest curvature on the power map, one has to very careful regarding one's decision to operate. This signs implies that the thinnest point represents an structural weakness, which cause a forward bending of the cornea (as is noted on the posterior and anterior

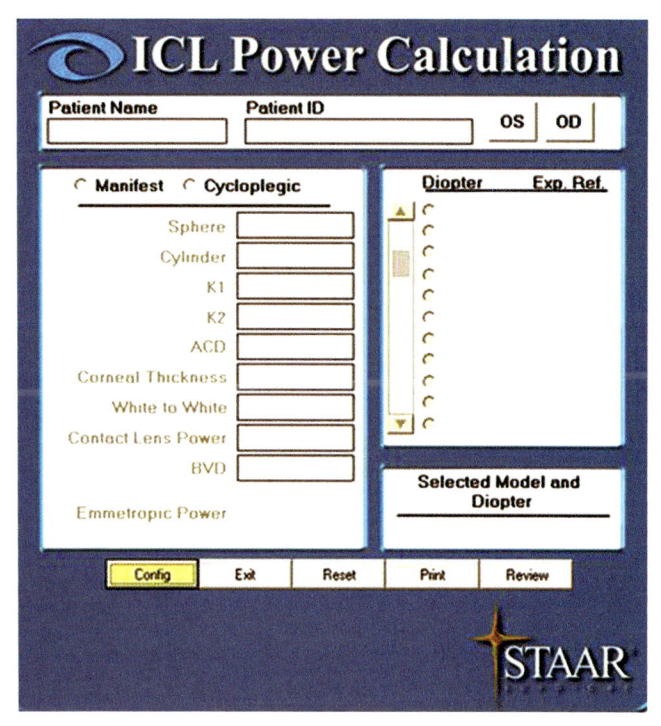

Figure 5.11 ICL power calculation for phakic IOL (STAAR)

elevation maps), further supported by the curvature change on the power map **(Figure 5.10B)**.

Recognizing keratoconus and the other forms of corneal pathology like pellucid marginal degeneration that contraindicate corneal laser refractive surgery is central to safe clinical practice.

Finally, if some criteria of unhealthy cornea or posterior ectasia have been found, other refractive surgical techniques can be attempted such as phakic IOL in the case of forme fruste keratoconus or thin cornea for a high myopia patient **(Figure 5.11)**; or in the scenario of a keratoconus, intracorneal rings can be attempted, Orbscan helps to make this decision and helps in following up.

REFERENCES

1. Maw R. Avoiding Postoperative LASIK Ectasia. Cataract and Refractive Surgery Today. Nov-Dec 2003.
2. Seiler T, Koufala K, Richter G. Iatrogenic keratectasia after laser in situ keratomileusis. J Cataract Refrac Surg. 1998;14: 312-7.
3. Vaca, Oscar. Posterior Float Features in Population Screened for Laser Eye Surgery. Mexican Cornea and Refractive Surgery Society 1999.
4. Ambrosio R, Klyce SD, Wilson SE. Corneal topographic and pachymetric screening of keratorefractive patients. J Refractive Surg. 2003;19:24-9.
5. Ou RJ, Shaw EL, Glasgow BJ. Keratectasia after laser in situ keratomileusis (LASIK): Evaluation of the calculated residual stromal bed thickness. Am J Ophthalmol. 2002;134 (5):771-3.

6. Roush C. Orbscan II Manual (Salt Lake City, Utha. Orbtek)
7. Vukich J, et al. Early spatial changes in the posterior corneal surface after laser in situ keratomileusis. J Cataract Refract Surg 2003;29:778-84.
8. Potgeiter F. Custome LASIK Surgical Techniques and Complications. Buranto L, Brint S Slack; 2004. pp. 435-37.
9. Assouline M. Chirugie Ceil-Le Kératocone. De nouveaux critéres de detection de kératocone infraclinique. www.inclo.com/le-keratocone.php
10. Fakhry M, Artola A, Belda J, et al. Comparison of corneal pachymetry using ultrasound and Orbscan II . J Cataract Refract Surg. 2002; 28:248-52.
11. Auffarth GU, Tetz MR, Biazid Y, et al. Keratoconus evaluation using the Orbscan Topography System. J Cataract Refract Surg. 2002;26:222-8.
12. Lee DH, Seo S, Jeong KW, et al. Early spatial changes in the posterior corneal surface after laser in situ keratomileusis. J Cataracy Refract Surg. 2003;29;778-84.
13. Twa MD, Roberts C, Mahmound AM, et al. Response of the posterior corneal surface to laser in situ Keratomileusis for myopia. J Cataract Refract Surg. 2003;31:61-71.
14. Miyata K, Tokunaga T, Nakahara M, et al. Residual bed thickness and corneal forward shift after laser in situ Keratomileusis. J Cataract Refract Surg. 2004;30:1067-72.
15. Grzybowski DM, Roberts CJ, Mahmound AM, et al. Model for nonectatic in posterior corneal elevation after ablative procedures. J Cataract Refract Surg. 2005;31:72-81.
16. Cairns G, McGhee NJ, Collins MJ, et al. Accuracy of Orbscan II slit scanning elevation topography. J Cataract Refract Surg. 2002;28:2181-7.

Chapter 6

Anterior Keratoconus

Amar Agarwal (India), Athiya Agarwal (India)

INTRODUCTION

Keratoconus is characterized by noninflammatory stromal thinning and anterior protrusion of the cornea. Keratoconus is a slowly progressive condition often presenting in the teen or early twenties with decreased vision or visual distortion. Family history of keratoconus is seen occasionally. Patients with this disorder are poor candidates for refractive surgery because of the possibility of exacerbating keratectasia.[1] The development of corneal ectasia is a well recognized complication of LASIK and attributed to unrecognized preoperative forme fruste Keratoconus.

ORBSCAN

The Orbscan (Bausch and Lomb) corneal topography system uses a scanning optical slit scan that is fundamentally different from the corneal topography that analyzes the reflected images from the anterior corneal surface. The high-resolution video camera captures 40 light slits at 45 degrees angle projected through the cornea similarly as seen during slit lamp examination. It has an acquisition time of 4 seconds.[2] The diagnosis of keratoconus is a clinical one and early diagnosis can be difficult on clinical examination alone. Orbscan has become a useful tool for evaluating the disease, and with the advent of its use, morphology and any subtle changes in the topography can be detected in early keratoconus. We always use the Orbscan system to evaluate our potential LASIK candidates preoperatively to rule out anterior keratoconus.

TECHNIQUE

All eyes to undergo LASIK are examined by Orbscan. Eyes are screened using quad maps with the normal band (NB) filter turned on. Four maps included:
a. *Anterior corneal elevation:* NB = ± 25 μ of best-fit sphere.
b. *Posterior corneal elevation:* NB = ± 25 μ of best-fit sphere.
c. *Keratometric mean curvature:* NB = 40 to 48 D, K.
d. *Corneal thickness (pachymetry):* NB = 500 to 600 μ.

Map features within normal band are colored green. This effectively filters out variation falling within normal band. When abnormalities are seen on the normal band quad map screening, a standard scale quad map is examined. For those cases with anterior keratoconus, we also generate three-dimensional views of anterior and posterior corneal elevation. The following parameters are considered to detect anterior keratoconus (a) Radii of anterior and posterior curvature of the cornea, (b) posterior best-fit sphere, (c) difference between the thickest corneal pachymetry value in 7 mm zone and thinnest pachymetry value of the cornea, (d) normal band (NB) scale map, (e) elevation on the anterior float of the cornea, (f) elevation on the posterior float of the cornea, (g) location of the cone on the cornea.

ANTERIOR KERATOCONUS

On Orbscan analysis in patients with anterior keratoconus the average ratio of radius of the anterior curvature to the posterior curvature of cornea is 1.25 (range 1.21 to 1.38), average posterior best-fit sphere is –56.98 Dsph (range –52.1 Dsph to –64.5), average difference in pachymetry value between thinnest point on the cornea and thickest point in 7 mm zone on the cornea is 172.7 μm (range 117 μm to 282 μm), average elevation of anterior corneal float is 55.25 μm (range 25 μm to 103 μm), average elevation of posterior corneal float is 113.6 μm (range 41 μm to 167 μm). **Figures 6.1 to 6.6** show the various topographic features of an eye with anterior keratoconus. In **Figure 6.1** (general quad map) upper left corner map is the anterior float, upper right corner map is posterior float, lower left corner is keratometric map while the lower right is the pachymetry map showing a difference of 282 μm between the thickest pachymetry value in 7 mm zone of cornea (597 μm) and thinnest pachymetry value (315 μm). In **Figure 6.2**, normal band scale map of anterior surface shows significant elevation on the anterior and posterior float with abnormal keratometric and pachymetry maps. **Figure 6.3** is three-dimensional representation of the anterior float with reference sphere 64 μm. **Figure 6.4** shows three-dimensional representation of posterior float with reference sphere. **Figure 6.5** shows amount of elevation (color coded) of the anterior corneal surface in microns (64 μm). **Figure 6.6** shows amount of elevation (color coded) of the posterior corneal surface in microns (167 μm).

DISCUSSION

Topography is valuable for preoperative ophthalmic examination of LASIK candidates. Three-dimensional imaging

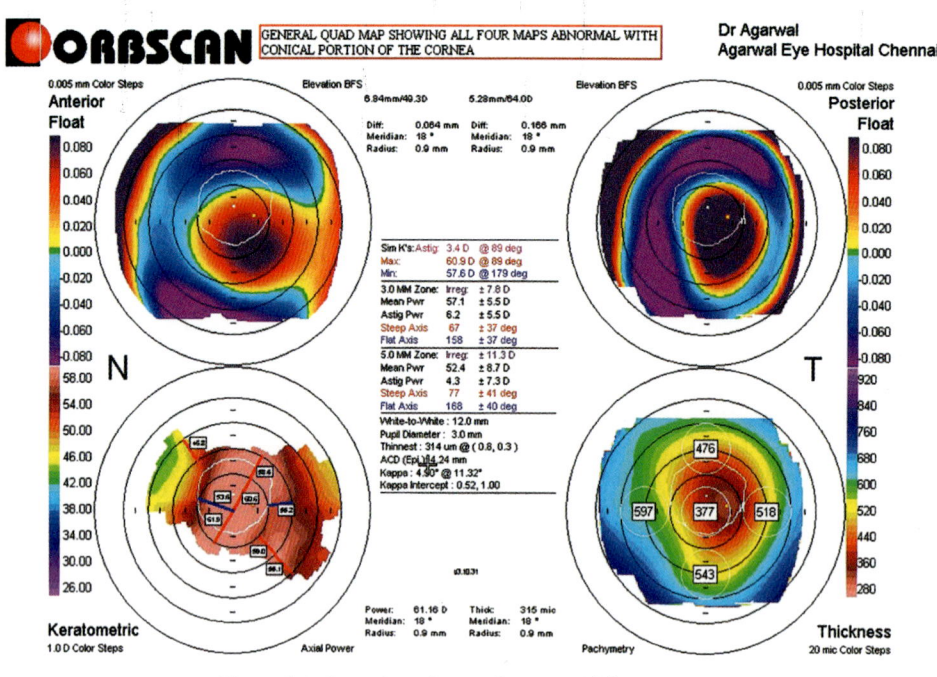

Figure 6.1 General quad map of an eye with keratoconus

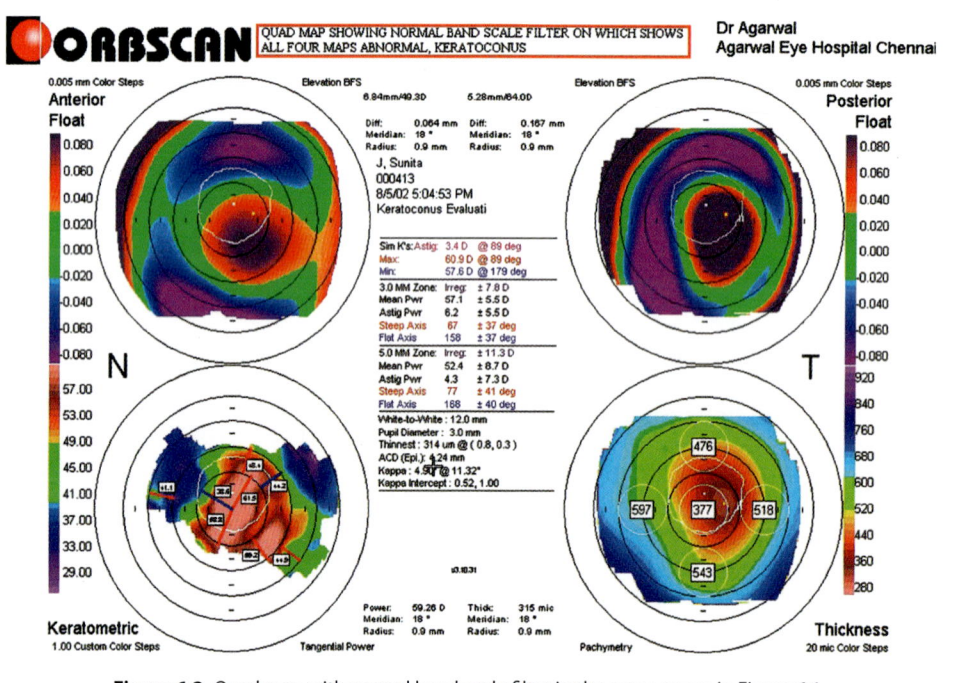

Figure 6.2 Quad map with normal band scale filter in the same eye as in Figure 6.1

allows surgeons to look at corneal thickness, as well as the corneal anterior and posterior surface and can predict the shape of cornea after LASIK surgery. Topographic analysis using three dimensional slit scan system allows us to predict which candidates would do well with LASIK and also confers the ability to screen for subtle configurations which may be contraindication to LASIK.[3] It is known that corneal ectasias and keratoconus have posterior corneal elevation as the earliest manifestation. In addition Wang et al have shown that the posterior corneal elevation increases after LASIK, and the

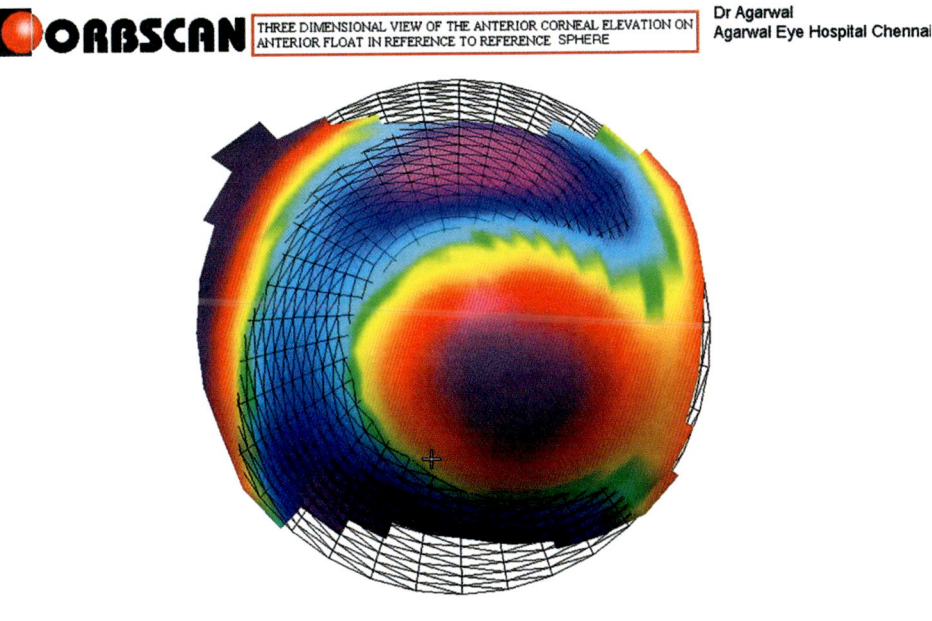

Figure 6.3 Three-dimensional anterior float

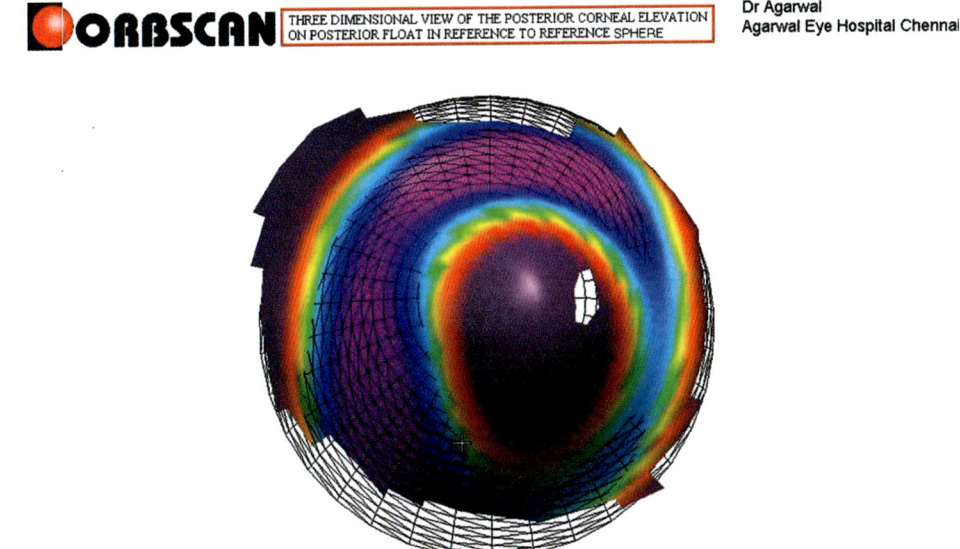

Figure 6.4 Three-dimensional posterior float

increase is correlated with residual corneal bed thickness.[4] We found that patients with positive keratoconus have higher posterior and anterior elevation on Orbscan II topography.

Elevation is not measured directly by Placido based topographers, but certain assumptions allow the construction of elevation maps. Elevation of a point on the corneal surface displays the height of the point on the corneal surface relative to a spherical reference surface. Reference surface is chosen to be a sphere. Best mathematical approximation of the actual corneal surface called best-fit sphere is calculated. Posterior corneal surface topographic changes after LASIK are known. Increased negative keratometric diopters and oblate asphericity of the PCC are common after LASIK leading to mild keratectasia.[5,6] Lamellar refractive surgery reduces the biomechanical strength of cornea that may lead to mechanical instability and keratectasia. Iatrogenic keratectasia represents

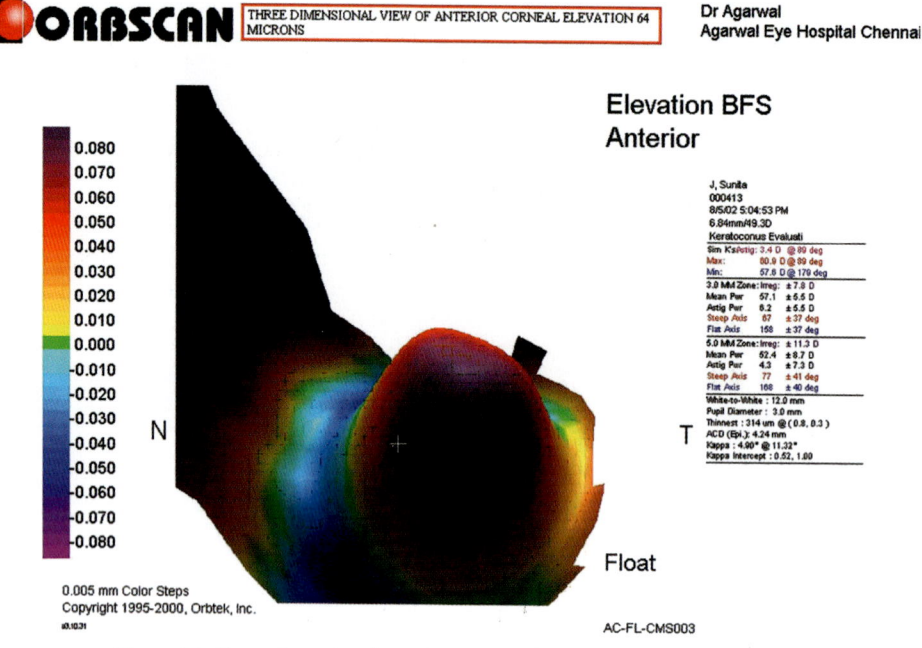

Figure 6.5 Three-dimensional anterior corneal elevation measured in microns

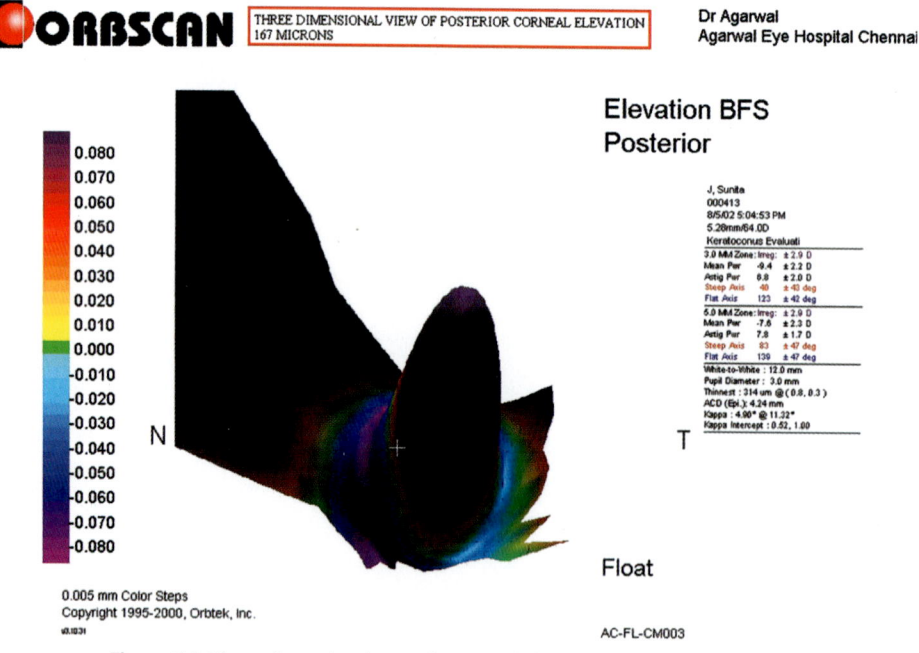

Figure 6.6 Three-dimensional posterior corneal elevation measured in microns

a complication after LASIK that may limit the range of myopic correction.[7] Corneal ectasia has also been reported after LASIK in cases of forme fruste keratoconus.[8] Posterior corneal bulge may be correlated with residual corneal bed thickness. The risk of keratectasia may be increased if the residual corneal bed is thinner than 250 μm.[9] Age, attempted correction and the optical zone diameter are other parameters that have to be considered to avoid post-LASIK ectasia.[10,11]

CONCLUSION

The Orbscan provides reliable, reproducible data of the anterior corneal surface; posterior corneal surface, keratometry, and pachymetry values with three-dimensional presentations and all LASIK candidates must be evaluated by this method preoperatively to detect an "early keratoconus". We suggest that Orbscan II is an important preoperative investigative tool to decide the suitable candidate for LASIK and thus avoiding any complication of LASIK surgery and helping the patient out by contact lens or keratoplasty. The following parameters must be analyzed in all LASIK candidates to rule out keratoconus (a) ratio of radii of anterior to posterior curvature of cornea: > 1.21 and < 1.27 (b) posterior best fit sphere: > –52.0 Dsph (c) difference between thickest corneal pachymetry value at 7 mm zone and thinnest pachymetry value: > 100 μm (d) posterior corneal elevation > 50 μm.

REFERENCES

1. Seiler T, Quurke AW. Iatrogenic keratectasia after LASIK in a case of forme fruste keratoconus. J Cataract Refract Surg. 1998;24:1007-9.
2. Fedor P, Kaufman S. Corneal topography and imaging. eMedicine Journal. 2001;2(6).
3. McDermott G K Topography's benefits for LASIK. Review of Ophthalmology. Editorial, vol no: 9:03 issue.
4. Wang Z, Chen J, Yang B. Posterior corneal surface topographic changes after laser in situ keratomileusis are related to residual corneal bed thickness. Ophthalmology. 1999;106:406-9; discussion 409-10.
5. Seitz B, Torres F, Langenbucher A, et al. Posterior corneal curvature changes after myopic laser in situ keratomileusis. Ophthalmology. 2001;108 (4):666-72.
6. Geggel HS, Talley AR. Delayed onset keratectasia following laser in situ keratomileusis. J Cataract Refract Surg. 1999;25(4):582-6.
7. Seiler T, Koufala K, Richter G. Iatrogenic keratectasia after laser in situ keratomileusis. J Refract Surg. 1998;14(3):312-7.
8. Seiler T, Quurke AW. Iatrogenic keratectasia after laser in situ keratomileusis in a case of Forme Fruste keratoconus. J Refract Surg. 1998;24(7):1007-9.
9. Wang Z, Chen J, Yang B. Posterior corneal surface topographic changes after laser in situ keratomileusis are related to residual corneal bed thickness. Ophthalmology. 1999;106(2):406-9.
10. Pallikaris IG, Kymionis GD, Astyrakakis NI. Corneal ectasia induced by laser in situ keratomileusis. J Cataract Refract Surg. 2001;27(11):1796-802.
11. Argento C, Cosentino MJ, Tytium A, et al. Corneal ectasia after laser in situ keratomileusis. J Cataract Refract Surg. 2001;27(9):1440-810.

Chapter 7

Posterior Corneal Changes in Refractive Surgery

Amar Agarwal (India), Soosan Jacob (India), Athiya Agarwal (India)

INTRODUCTION

The development of corneal ectasia is a well-recognized complication of LASIK and amongst other contributory factors, unrecognized preoperative forme fruste keratoconus is also an important one. Patients with this disorder are poor candidates for refractive surgery because of the possibility of exacerbating keratectasia. It is known that posterior corneal elevation is an early presenting sign in keratoconus, and hence, it is imperative to evaluate posterior corneal curvature (PCC) in every LASIK candidate.

TOPOGRAPHY

Topography is valuable for preoperative ophthalmic examination of LASIK candidates. Three-dimensional imaging allows surgeons to look at corneal thickness, as well as the corneal anterior and posterior surface and it can also predict the shape of the cornea after LASIK surgery. Topographic analysis using three dimensional slit scan system allows us to predict which candidates would do well with LASIK and also confers the ability to screen for subtle configurations which may be a contraindication to LASIK.

ORBSCAN

The orbscan slits are projected onto the anterior segment of the eye: the anterior cornea, the posterior cornea, the anterior iris and anterior lens. The data collected from these four surfaces are used to create a topographic map. Each surface point from the diffusely reflected slit beams that overlap in the central 5 mm zone is independently triangulated to x, y, and z coordinates, providing three-dimensional data.

This technique provides more information about the anterior segment of the eye, such as anterior and posterior corneal curvature, elevation maps of the anterior and posterior corneal surface and corneal thickness. It has an acquisition time of 4 seconds.[1] This improves the diagnostic accuracy. It also has passive eye-tracker from frame-to-frame and 43 frames are taken to ensure accuracy. It is easy to interpret and has good repeatability.

PRIMARY POSTERIOR CORNEAL ELEVATION

The diagnosis of frank keratoconus is a clinical one. Early diagnosis of forme fruste can be difficult on clinical examination alone. ORBSCAN has become a useful tool for evaluating the disease, and with its advent, abnormalities in posterior corneal surface topography have been identified in keratoconus. Posterior corneal surface data is problematic because it is not a direct measure and there is little published information on normal values for each age group. In the patient with increased posterior corneal elevation in the absence of other changes, it is unknown whether this finding represents a manifestation of early keratoconus. The decision to proceed with refractive surgery is therefore more difficult.

Posterior Corneal Topography

One should always use the ORBSCAN system to evaluate potential LASIK candidates preoperatively to rule out primary posterior corneal elevations. Eyes are screened using quad maps with the normal band (NB) filter turned on. Four maps include (a) anterior corneal elevation: NB = ± 25 μ of best-fit sphere; (b) posterior corneal elevation: NB = ± 25 μ of best fit sphere; (c) Keratometric mean curvature: NB = 40 to 48 D; (d) Corneal thickness (pachymetry): NB = 500 to 600 μ. Map features within normal band are colored green. This effectively filters out variations falling within the normal band. When abnormalities are seen on normal band quad map screening, a standard scale quad map should be examined. For those cases with posterior corneal elevation, three-dimensional views of posterior corneal elevation can also be generated. In all eyes with posterior corneal elevation, the following parameters are generated (a) radii of anterior and posterior curvature of the cornea, (b) posterior best fit sphere, (c) difference between the corneal pachymetry value in 7 mm zone and thinnest pachymetry value of the cornea.

Pre-existing Posterior Corneal Abnormalities

Figures 7.1 to 7.6 show the various topographic features of an eye with primary posterior corneal elevation detected

Chapter 7: Posterior Corneal Changes in Refractive Surgery

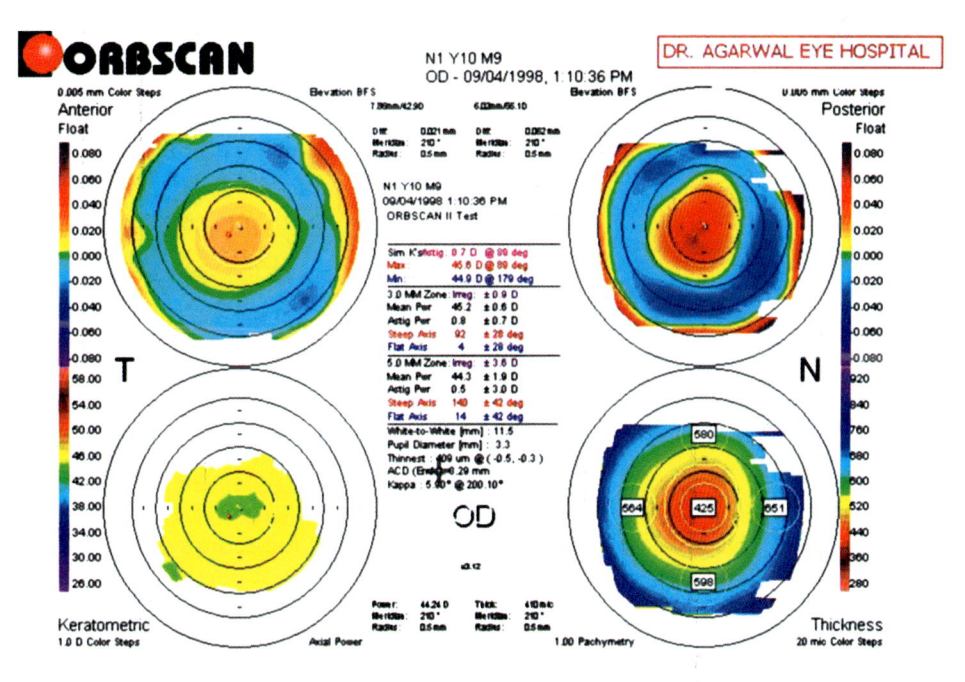

Figure 7.1 General quad map of an eye with primary posterior corneal elevation. Notice the red areas seen in the top right picture showing the primary posterior corneal elevation

during pre-LASIK assessment. In **Figure 7.1** (general quad map) upper left corner map is the anterior float, upper right corner map is posterior float, lower left corner is keratometric map while the lower right is the pachymetry map showing a difference of 100 μm between the thickest pachymetry value in 7 mm zone of cornea and thinnest pachymetry value. In **Figure 7.2**, normal band scale map of anterior surface shows "with the rule astigmatism" in an otherwise normal anterior surface (shown in green), the posterior float shows significant elevation inferotemporally. In **Figure 7.2** only the abnormal areas are shown in red for ease in detection. **Figure 7.3** is three-dimensional representation of the maps in **Figure 7.2**. **Figure 7.4** shows three-dimensional representation of anterior corneal surface with reference sphere. **Figure 7.5** shows three-dimensional representation of posterior corneal surface showing a significant posterior corneal elevation. **Figure 7.6** shows amount of elevation (color coded) of the posterior corneal surface in microns (50 μm).

In the light of the fact that keratoconus may have posterior corneal elevation as the earliest manifestation, preoperative analysis of posterior corneal curvature to detect a posterior corneal bulge is important to avoid post LASIK keratectasia. The rate of progression of posterior corneal elevation to Frank keratoconus is unknown. It is also difficult to specify that exact amount of posterior corneal elevation beyond which it may be unsafe to carry out LASIK. Atypical elevation in the posterior corneal map more than 45 μm should alert us against a post LASIK surprise. Orbscan provides reliable, reproducible data of the posterior corneal surface and all LASIK candidates must be evaluated by this method preoperatively to detect an "early keratoconus".

Elevation is not measured directly by Placido based topographers, but certain assumptions allow the construction of elevation maps. Elevation of a point on the corneal surface displays the height of the point on the corneal surface relative to a spherical reference surface. Reference surface is chosen to be a sphere. Best mathematical approximation of the actual corneal surface called best-fit sphere is calculated. One of the criteria for defining forme fruste keratoconus is a posterior best fit sphere of > 55.0 D.

Ratio of radii of anterior to posterior curvature of cornea ≥ 1.21 and ≤ 1.27 has been considered as a keratoconus suspect. Average pachymetry difference between thickest and the thinnest point on the cornea in the 7 mm zone should normally be less than 100 μm.

Agarwal Criteria to Diagnose Primary Posterior Corneal Elevation

1. Ratio of the radii of anterior and posterior curvature of the cornea should be more than 1.2. In **Figure 7.2** note the radii of the anterior curvature is 7.86 mm and the radii of the posterior curvature is 6.02 mm. The ratio is 1:3.
2. Posterior best fit sphere should be more than 52 D. In **Figure 7.2** note the posterior best fit sphere is 56.1 D.
3. Difference between the thickest and thinnest corneal pachymetry value in the 7 mm zone should be more than 100 microns. The thickest pachymetry value as seen

78 Section II: Orbscan and Refractive Surgery

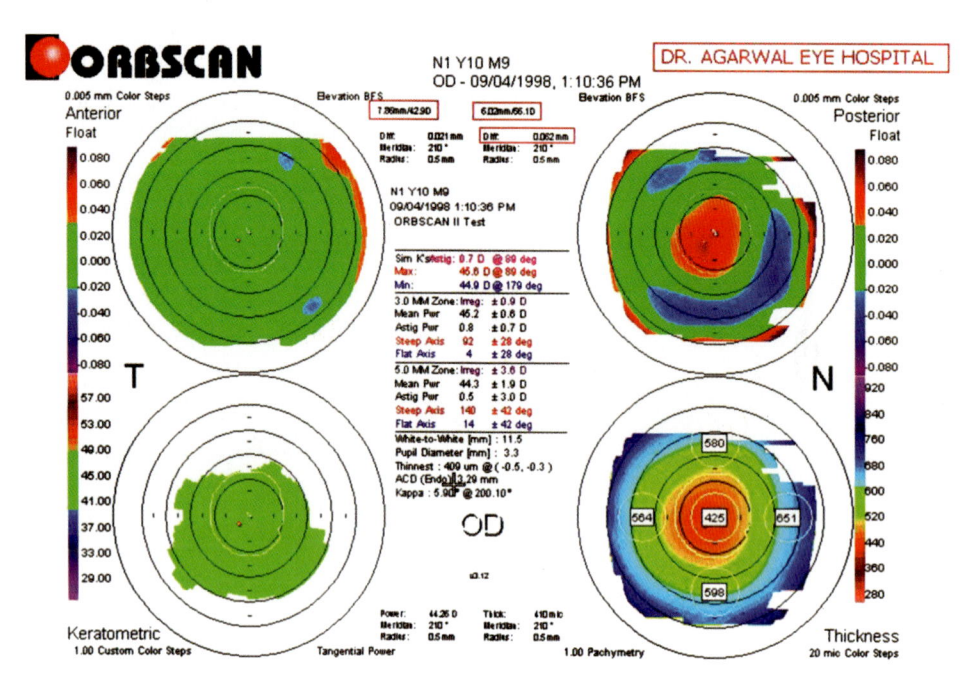

Figure 7.2 Quad map with normal band scale filter on in the same eye as in **Figure 7.1**

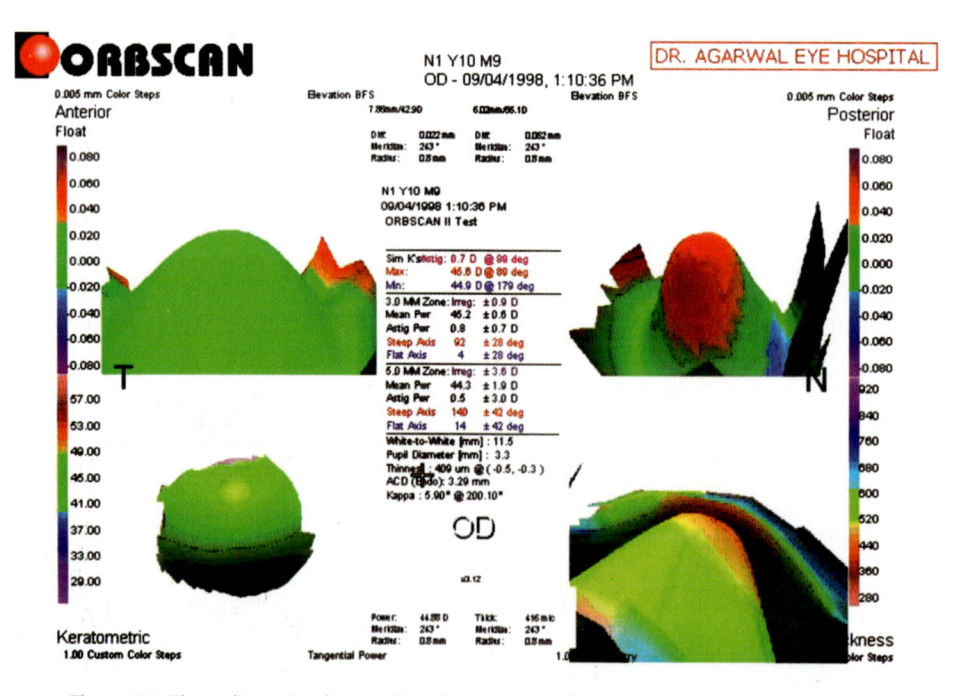

Figure 7.3 Three-dimensional normal band scale map. In the top right note the red areas which shows the elevation on the posterior cornea. The anterior cornea is normal

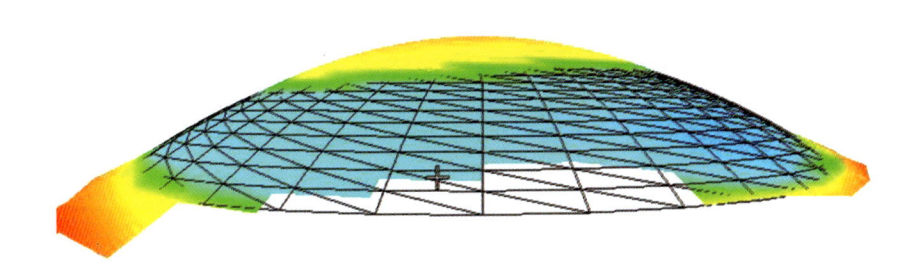

Figure 7.4 Three-dimensional anterior float. Notice it is normal

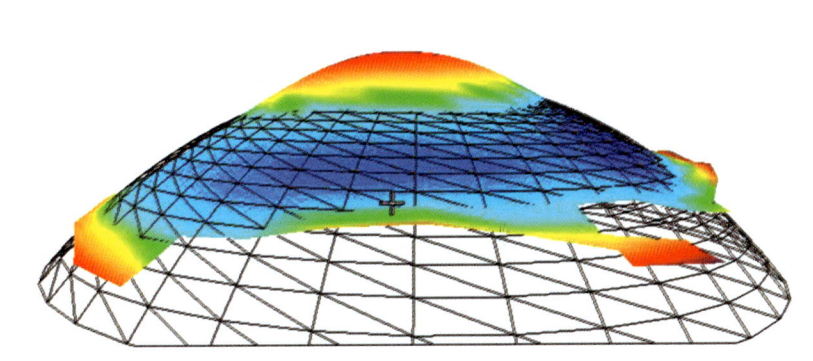

Figure 7.5 Three-dimensional posterior float. Notice in this there is marked elevation as seen in the red areas

in **Figure 7.2** is 651 microns and the thinnest value is 409 microns. The difference is 242 microns.

4. The thinnest point on the cornea should correspond with the highest point of elevation of the posterior corneal surface. The thinnest point as seen in **Figure 7.2** bottom right picture is seen as a cross. This point or cursor corresponds to the same cross or cursor in **Figure 7.2** top right picture which indicates the highest point of elevation on the posterior cornea.

5. Elevation of the posterior corneal surface should be more than 45 microns above the posterior best fit sphere. In **Figure 7.2** you will notice it is 0.062 mm or 62 microns.

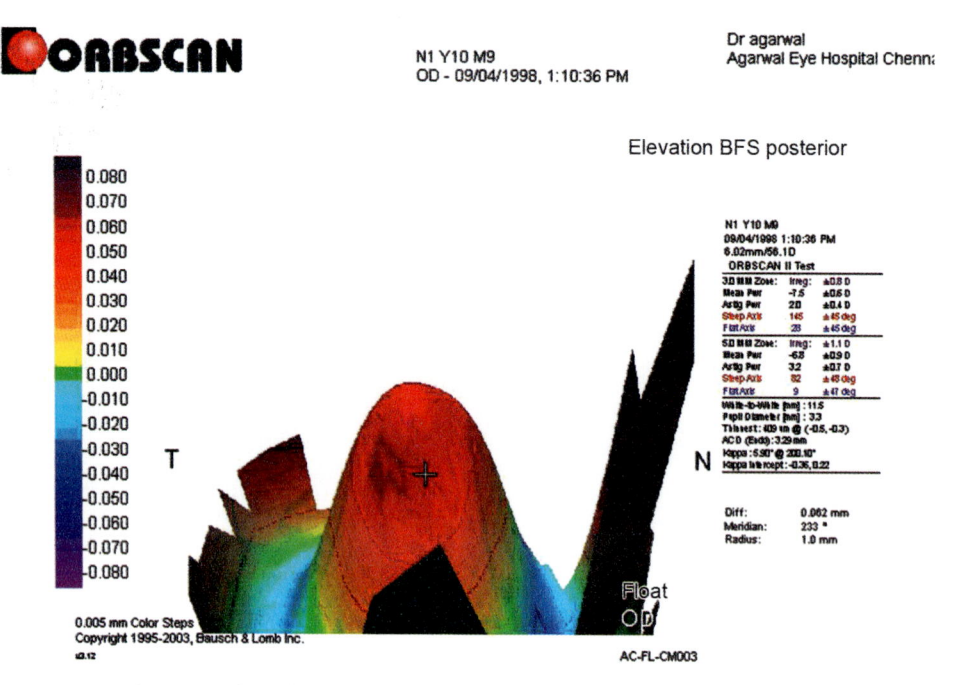

Figure 7.6 Three-dimensional posterior corneal elevation measured in microns

IATROGENIC KERATECTASIA

Iatrogenic keratectasia may be seen in some patients following ablative refractive surgery **(Figures 7.7 and 7.8)**. The anterior cornea is composed of alternating collagen fibrils and has a more complicated interwoven structure than the deeper stroma and it acts as the major stress-bearing layer. The flap used for LASIK is made in this layer and thus results in a weakening of that strongest layer of the cornea which contributes maximum to the biomechanical stability of the cornea.

The residual bed thickness (RBT) of the cornea is the crucial factor contributing to the biomechanical stability of the cornea after LASIK. The flap as such does not contribute much after its repositioning to the stromal bed. This is easily seen by the fact that the flap can be easily lifted up even up to 1 year after treatment. The decreased RBT as well as the lamellar cut in the cornea both contribute to the decreased biomechanical stability of the cornea. A reduction in the RBT results in a long-term increase in the surface parallel stress on the cornea. The intraocular pressure (IOP) can cause further forward bowing and thinning of a structurally compromised cornea. Inadvertent excessive eye rubbing, prone position sleeping, and the normal wear and tear of the cornea may also play a role. The RBT should not be less than 250 μm to avoid subsequent iatrogenic keratectasias.[2-4] Reoperations should be undertaken very carefully in corneae with RBT less than 300 μm. Increasing myopia after every operation is known as "dandelion keratectasia".

The ablation diameter also plays a very important role in LASIK. Postoperative optical distortions are more common with diameters less than 5.5 mm. Use of larger ablation diameters implies a lesser RBT postoperatively. Considering the formula: Ablation depth $[\mu m] = 1/3 \cdot (\text{diameter } [mm])^2 \times (\text{intended correction diopters } [D])$,[4,5] it becomes clear that to preserve a sufficient bed thickness, the range of myopic correction is limited and the upper limit of possible myopic correction may be around 12 D.[6]

Detection of a mild keratectasia requires knowledge about the posterior curvature of the cornea. Posterior corneal surface topographic changes after LASIK are known. Increased negative keratometric diopters and oblate asphericity of the PCC, which correlate significantly with the intended correction are common after LASIK leading to mild keratectasia.[6,7] This change in posterior power and the risk of keratectasia was more significant with a RBT of 250 μm or less.[8] The difference in the refractive indices results in a 0.2 D difference at the back surface of the cornea becoming equivalent to a 2.0 D change in the front surface of the cornea.[6] Increase in posterior power and asphericity also correlates with the difference between the intended and achieved correction 3 months after LASIK. This is because factors like drying of the stromal bed may result in an ablation depth more than that intended.[6] Reinstein et al predict that the standard deviation of uncertainty in predicting the RBT preoperatively is around 30 μm. [Invest Ophthalmol Vis Sci 40 (Suppl): S403, 1999]. Age, attempted correction, the optical zone diameter and the flap thickness are other parameters that have to be considered to avoid post-LASIK ectasia.[9,10]

The flap thickness may not be uniform throughout its length. In studies by Seitz et al, it has been shown that the Moris Model One microkeratome and the Supratome cut deeper

Chapter 7: Posterior Corneal Changes in Refractive Surgery 81

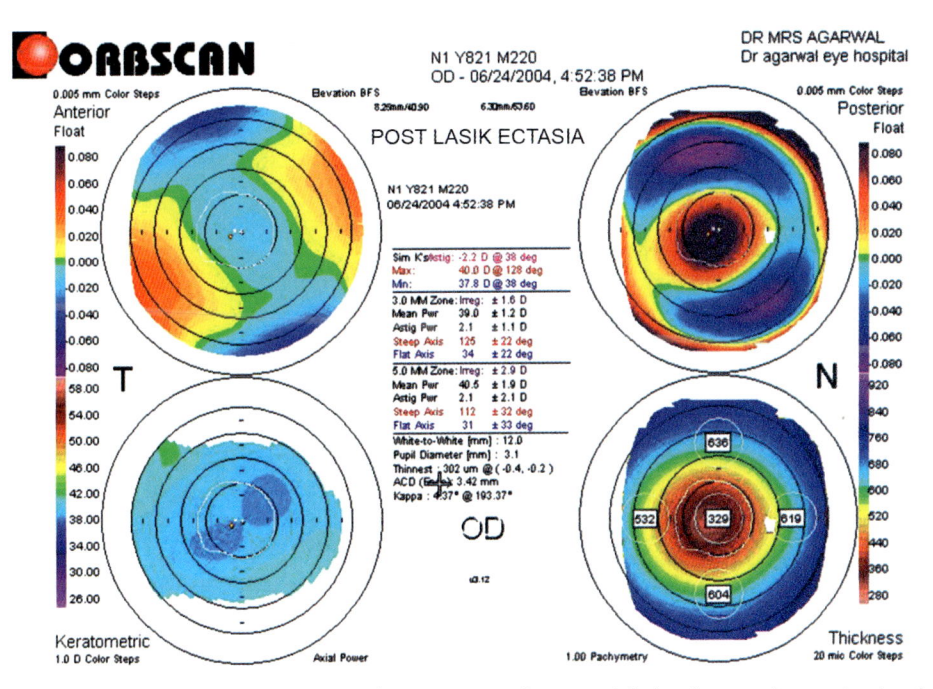

Figure 7.7 A patient with iatrogenic keratectasia after LASIK. Note the upper right hand corner pictures showing the posterior float has thinning and this is also seen in the bottom right picture in which pachymetry reading is 329

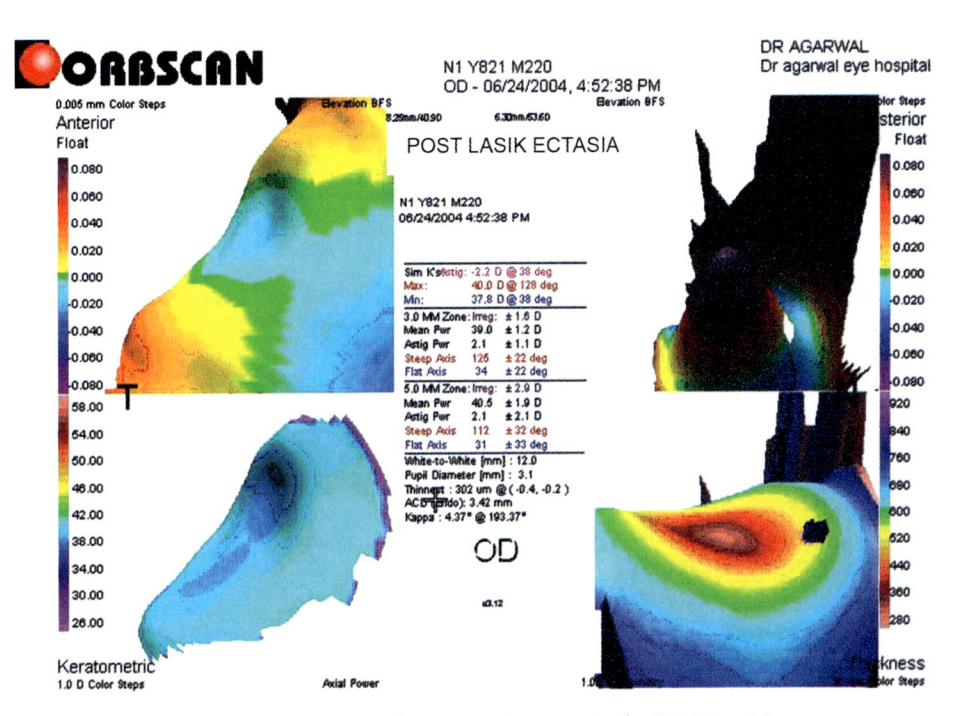

Figure 7.8 The same patient with iatrogenic keratectasia after LASIK in a 3 D pattern. Notice the ectasia seen clearly in the bottom right picture

towards the hinge, whereas the Automated Corneal Shaper and the Hansatome create flaps that are thinner towards the hinge. Thus, accordingly, the area of corneal ectasia may not be in the center but paracentral, especially if it is also associated with decentered ablation. Flap thickness has also been found to vary considerably, even upto 40 μm, under similar conditions and this may also result in a lesser RBT than intended.[11-17]

It is known that corneal ectasias and keratoconus have posterior corneal elevation as the earliest manifestation.[18] The precise course of progression of posterior corneal elevation to frank keratoconus is not known. Hence it is necessary to study the posterior corneal surface preoperatively in all LASIK candidates.

EFFECT OF POSTERIOR CORNEAL CHANGE ON INTRAOCULAR LENS CALCULATION

Intraocular lens power calculation in post-LASIK eyes is different because of the inaccuracy of keratometry, change in anterior and posterior corneal curvatures, altered relation between the two and change in the standardized index of refraction of the cornea. Irregular astigmatism induced by the procedure, decentered ablations and central islands also add to the problem.

Routine keratometry is not accurate in these patients. Corneal refractive surgery changes the asphericity of the cornea and also produces a wide range of powers in the central 5 mm zone of the cornea. LASIK makes the cornea of a myope more oblate so that keratometry values may be taken from the more peripheral steeper area of the cornea, which results in calculation of a lower than required IOL power resulting in a hyperopic "surprise". Hyperopic LASIK makes the cornea more prolate, thus resulting in a myopic "surprise" post cataract surgery.

Post-PRK or LASIK, the relation between the anterior and posterior corneal surface changes. The relative thickness of the various corneal layers, each having a different refractive index also changes and there is a change in the curvature of the posterior corneal surface. All these result in the standardized refractive index of 1.3375 no longer being accurate in these eyes.

At present there is no keratometry, which can accurately measure the anterior and posterior curvatures of the cornea. The Orbscan also makes mathematical assumptions of the posterior surface rather than direct measurements. This is important in the LASIK patient because the procedure alters the relation between the anterior and posterior surfaces of the cornea as well as changes the curvature of the posterior cornea.

Thus, direct measurements such as manual and automated keratometry and topography are inherently inaccurate in these patients. The corneal power is therefore calculated by the calculation method, the contact lens overrefraction method and by the CVK method. The flattest K reading obtained by any method is taken for IOL power calculation (the steepest K is taken for hyperopes who had undergone LASIK). One can still aim for 1.00 D of myopia rather than emmetropia to allow for any error, which is almost always in the hyperopic direction in case of pre LASIK myopes. Also, a third or fourth generation IOL calculating formula should be used for such patients.

REFERENCES

1. Fedor P, Kaufman S. Corneal topography and imaging. eMedicine Journal, 2001;vol 2, no 6.
2. Seiler T, Koufala K, Richter G. Iatrogenic keratectasia after laser in situ keratomileusis. J Refract Surg. 1998;14(3):312-7.
3. Seiler T, Quurke AW. Iatrogenic keratectasia after laser in situ keratomileusis in a case of Forme Fruste keratoconus. J Refract Surg. 1998;24(7):1007-9.
4. Probost LE, Machat JJ. Mathematics of laser in situ keratomileusis for high myopia. J Cataract Refract Surg. 1998;24:5.
5. Mc Donnell PJ. Excimer laser corneal surgery: new strategies and old enemies {review}. Invest Ophthalmol Vis Sci. 1995;36; 4-8.
6. Seitz B, Torres F, Langenbucher A, et al. Posterior corneal curvature changes after myopic laser in situ keratomileusis. Ophthalmology. 2001;108(4):666-72.
7. Geggel HS, Talley AR. Delayed onset keratectasia following laser in situ keratomileusis. J Cataract Refract Surg. 1999;25(4):582-6.
8. Wang Z, Chen J, Yang B. Posterior corneal surface topographic changes after laser in situ keratomileusis are related to residual corneal bed thickness. Ophthalmology. 1999;106(2):406-9.
9. Pallikaris IG, Kymionis GD. Astyrakakis NI. Corneal ectasia induced by laser in situ keratomileusis. J Cataract Refract Surg. 2001;27(11):1796-802.
10. Argento C, Cosentino MJ, Tytium A, et al. Corneal ectasia after laser in situ keratomileusis. J Cataract Refract Surg. 2001;27(9): 1440-8.
11. Binder PS, Moore M, Lambert RW, et al. Comparison of two microkeratome systems. J Refract Surg. 1997;13:142-53.
12. Hofmann RF, Bechara SJ. An independent evaluation of second generation suction microkeratomes. Refract Corneal Surg. 1992;8:348-54.
13. Schuler A, Jessen K, Hoffmann F. Accuracy of the microkeratome keratectomies in pig eyes. Invest Ophthalmol Vis Sci . 1990;31: 2022-30.
14. Behrens A, Seitz B, Langenbucher A, et al. Evaluation of corneal flap dimensions and cut quality using a manually guided microkeratome [published erratum appears in J Refract Surg. 1999;15:400]. J Refract Surg. 1999;15:118-23.
15. Behrens A, Seitz B, Langenbucher A, et al. Evaluation of corneal flap dimensions and cut quality using the Automated Corneal Shaper microkeratome. J Refract Surg. 2000;16:83-9.
16. Behrens A, Langenbucher A, Kus MM, et al. Experimental evaluation of two current generation automated microkeratomes: The Hansatome® and the Supratome®. Am J Ophthalmol. 2000;129:59-67.
17. Jacobs BJ, Deutsch TA, Rubenstein JB. Reproducibility of corneal flap thickness in LASIK. Ophthalmic Surg Lasers. 1999;30:350-3.
18. McDermott GK. Topography's benefits for LASIK. Review of Ophthalmology. Editorial, vol no:9:03 issue.

Chapter 8

Corneal Ectasia Post-LASIK: The Orbscan Advantages

Erik L Mertens (Belgium), Arun C Gulani (USA), Paul Karpecki (USA)

INTRODUCTION

With the advent of corneal topography and its increasing application in practice, our knowledge about the shape of the cornea has rapidly accumulated.[1] Determination of the ability of the cornea to undergo laser refractive surgery is of the utmost importance. The purpose is to avoid corneal ectasia and visual impairment in otherwise healthy eyes. First reported by Prof Theo Seiler[2] this condition is characterized by progressive protuberance and steepening, increasing myopia and or astigmatism with distorted and decreased best corrected vision in the involved eye. Some of the reported cases can be traced back to the preoperative evaluations and lack of recognition for risk factors (Gulani AC: Corneal Topography and Wavefront Instructional Course, ASCRS San Diego, May 2004).

CORNEAL ECTASIA

Postrefractive surgical ectasia was a planned event in automated lamellar keratomileusis for hyperopia where the corneal flap was created at 70% depth to allow for a controlled steepening. This phenomenon has been seen not only with LASIK surgery where the creation of the corneal flap is an additional contributing factor but also with surface photorefractive keratectomy wherein the depth of ablation and repetitive or multiple ablative patterns add to the risk. The most important diagnosis in this direction is that of forme fruste keratoconus.

Over several years data collected in retrospective analysis of post-LASIK ectasias underscores the importance of this diagnosis. These thoughts have been repeatedly addressed but not solved (Gulani AC and Nordan LT–Personal Correspondence). We shall need to strive to introduce newer and effective measurement criterias and combination technologies to further assist us in this field of Obscure clinical findings but drastic postoperative outcomes. Through the years the Orbscan II and Orbscan IIz (Bausch & Lomb Orbtek, Salt Lake City, Utah) became more and more the standard for preoperative screening amongst refractive surgeons. It is an important diagnostic tool to help separate cases of corneal ectatic disorders like keratoconus and pellucid marginal degeneration as well as identify preclinical cases of corneal instability and forme fruste keratoconus (Gulani AC: Advanced Diagnostics Course: B & L—AAO, Washington DC, April 2005).

SELECTION CRITERIA

A lot of these criteria are published throughout the years. Most of the parameters were empirically established by studying the unexpected postoperative ectasia patients. Some surgeons were able to find correlations with preoperative corneal maps and could even quantify abnormal preoperative corneal map findings.[3] This chapter will give you an overview of the most useful and important of these parameters.

Besides the topographical parameters never forget to look at the clinical signs (fluctuation of subjective refraction, younger patients, history of keratoconus, steep/distorted keratometry readings,...) and analyze the Orbscan maps on the Orbscan IIz system, *not on the Orbscan printout!!!*

The decision to continue with refractive laser surgery is not based on a single clue, but rather on a combination of a set of criteria. When looking at the Orbscan's Quad Map you can find so called 'red flags' or 'yellow flags'. A 'red flag' definitively means a no-go situation and a 'yellow flag' is suspicious and will drive our attention to look very closely into the other corneal maps. On a typical Quad Map four corneal maps are routinely presented by the Orbscan II (Bausch and Lomb Orbtek, Salt Lake City, Utah). You will find the anterior elevation map in the upper left quadrant and the posterior elevation map in the upper right quadrant. The keratometric curvature map (power map) is located in the lower left quadrant and the pachymetry[4] map in the lower right quadrant **(Figure 8.1)**. In the center of these four maps a lot of statistics and useful data are displayed.

Pachymetry[5]

An absolute contraindication for lamellar corneal laser surgery is a thinnest point of < 470 microns. When pathological, this point is often displaced inferotemporal **(Figure 8.2)**. A difference of < 30 microns (yellow flag) or < 20 microns (red flag) between the central pachymetry and the peripheral thickness indicators can be seen in abnormal corneas **(Figure 8.3)**. A difference of > 100 microns from the thinnest point to the values at the 7 mm optical zone implies a steep

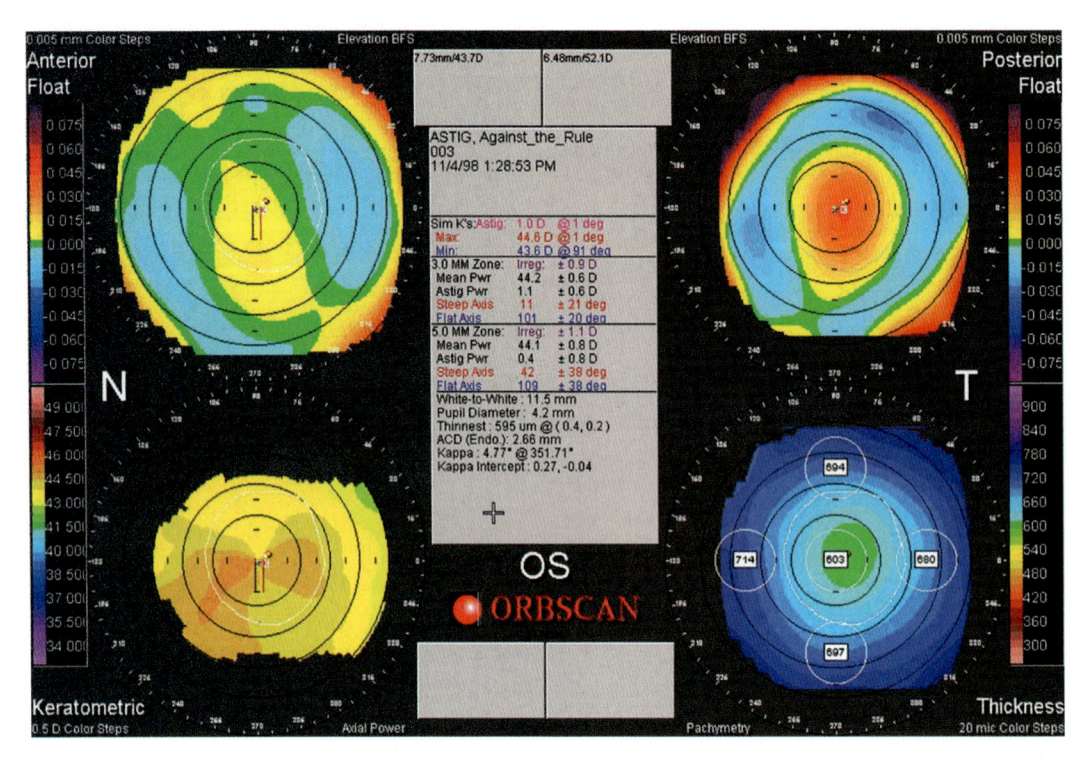

Figure 8.1 Typical quad map (Orbscan II)

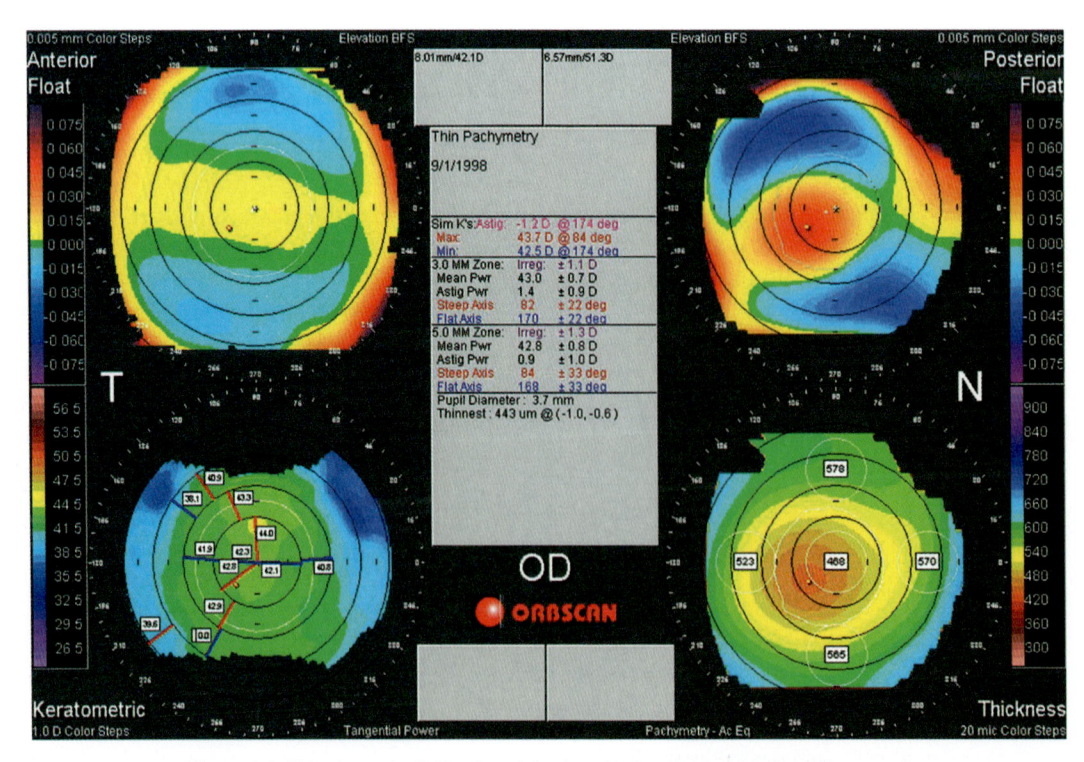

Figure 8.2 Thinnest point (443 micron) displaced inferotemporal and a difference of >100 microns from the thinnest point to the values at the 7 mm zone

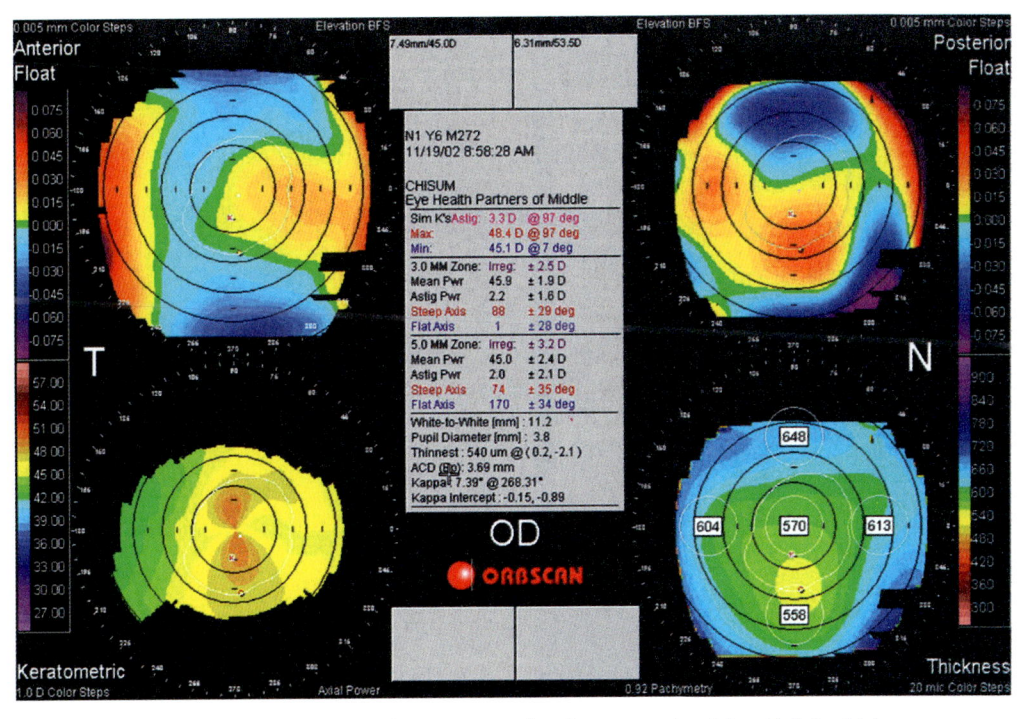

Figure 8.3 Less than 20 microns between central pachymetry and peripheral inferior thickness

gradient of thinning from the midperiphery towards the thinnest point (yellow flag) **(Figure 8.3)**.

Posterior Elevation Map (Figure 8.4)

1. The most common reference surface for viewing elevation maps is the "best fit sphere" (BFS). A posterior high point > 50 microns above BFS might be indicative of an early posterior ectasia. However, in cylindrical corneas with an astigmatism > 2.5 D, this elevation can be induced by the astigmatism and needs to be checked with the other corneal maps **(Figure 8.5)**.

   A posterior high point > 35 microns above BFS with corresponding thinning on the pachymetry map is a red flag for LASIK, but not for PRK, LASEK or epiLASIK.

2. The power of the posterior best-fit sphere (BFS) is in normal corneas around 51 D. A BFS with a power of more than 55 diopters **(Figure 8.4)** on the posterior profile, could be indicative of early keratoconus. This criterion is not diagnostic as a sign of early ectasia[6] per se, as this may also be seen in small corneas (WTW < 11 mm), very steep corneas or in Asian eyes.

   A power between 53 and 54 diopters can be suspicious, and needs to be correlated with other signs and/or symptoms.

3. *Roush criterion:* Indicative of early keratoconus is a relative difference > 100 microns between the highest and lowest point on the posterior elevation map **(Figure 8.4)**. A relative difference > 70 microns is a yellow flag, except when the cornea is very symmetrical and when it is caused by a regular astigmatism.

Power Map

1. Steep corneal curvatures are always suspicious. Keratometric mean power map > 46 diopters or total mean power map > 45 diopters are definitely red flags **(Figure 8.6)**.
2. Bow-tie/broken bow-tie pattern. The so-called "lazy-C" on the axial power map is very suspicious when the astigmatism shifts > 20° from a straight line **(Figure 8.7)**.
3. Central corneal asymmetry. A change within the central 3 mm optical zone of the cornea of more than 3 diopters from superior to inferior (yellow flag) can be correlated with the presence of vertical coma **(Figure 8.7)**. However, this may be merely a sign of asymmetric astigmatism, and is not necessarily indicative of pathology.

COMPOSITE/INTEGRATED INFORMATION

1. Correlation of signs with the highest point on the posterior elevation. This is probably the *strongest topographic sign* indicative of early keratoconus.[7] If the highest point on the posterior elevation coincides with the highest point on the anterior elevation, the thinnest point on pachymetry,

86   Section II: Orbscan and Refractive Surgery

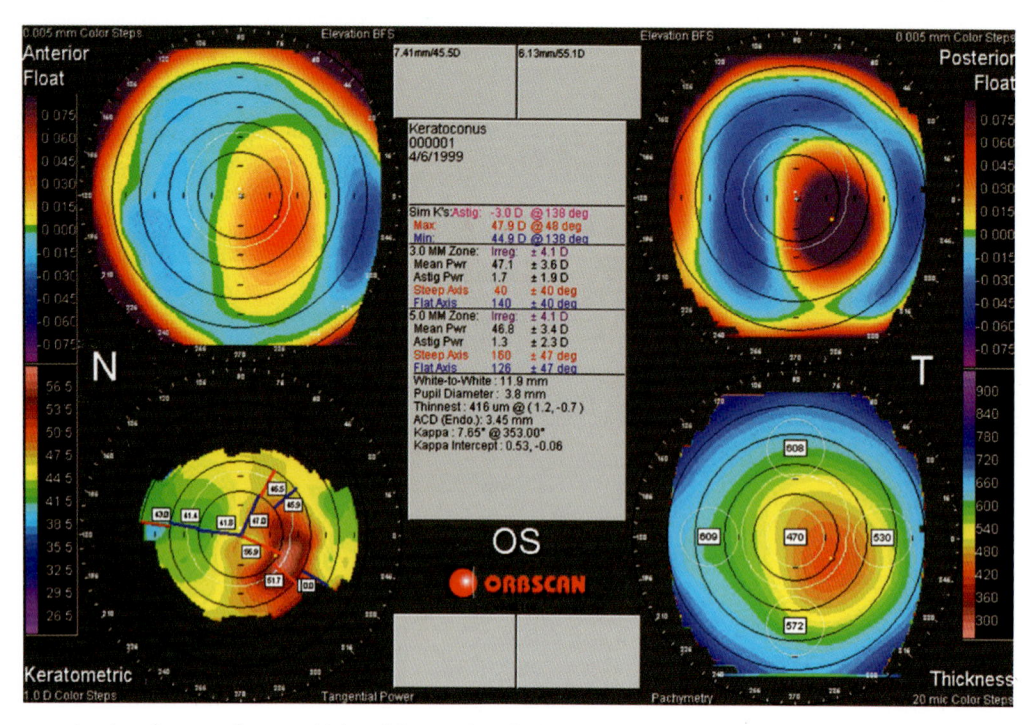

Figure 8.4 The posterior elevation map shows multiple red flags as described in the text. The highest point on the posterior elevation coincides with the highest point on the anterior elevation, the thinnest point on pachymetry, and the point of steepest curvature on the power map

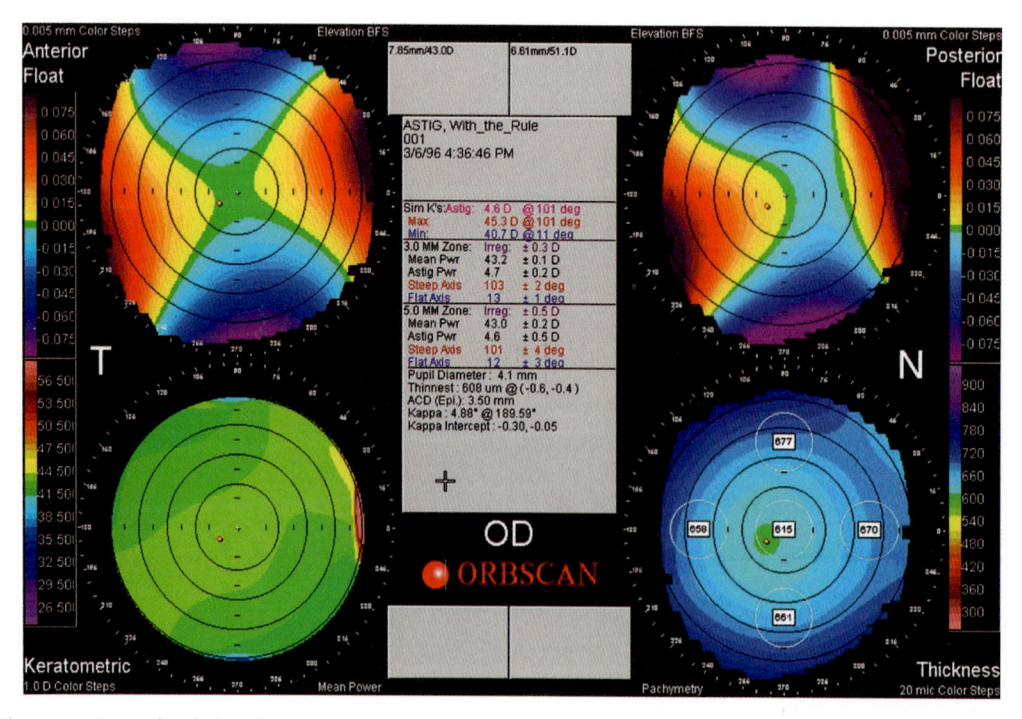

Figure 8.5 Normal with the rule astigmatism. However, the highest point on the posterior elevation map is > 50 microns

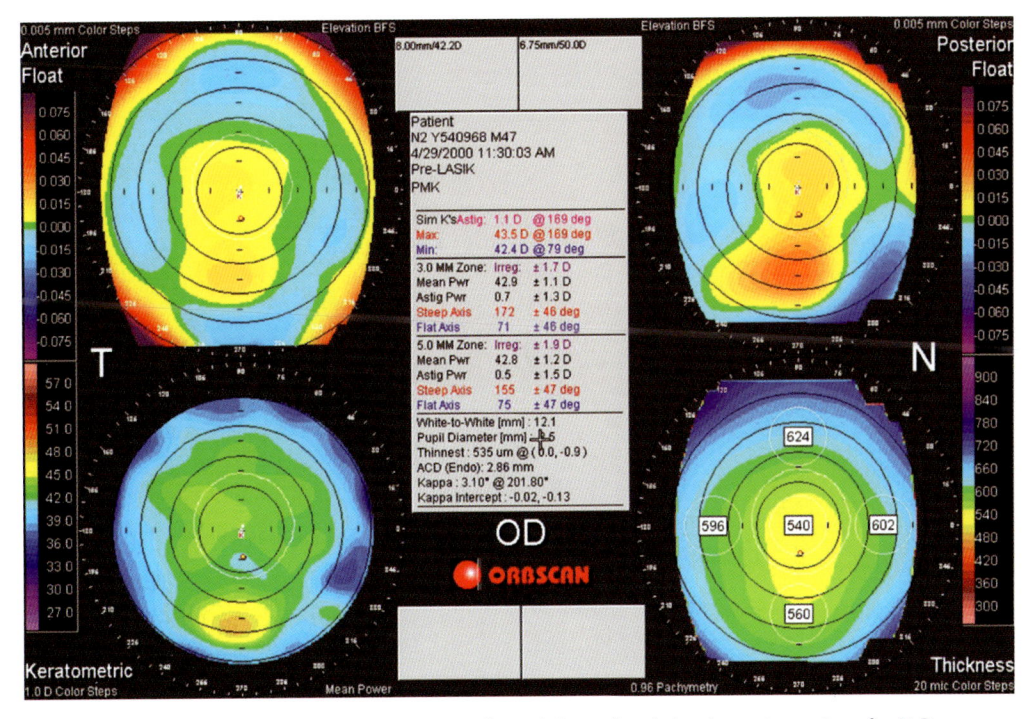

Chapter 8: Corneal Ectasia Post-LASIK: The Orbscan Advantages

Figure 8.6 Keratometric mean power map (lower left quadrant) showing a steepening of > 46 D

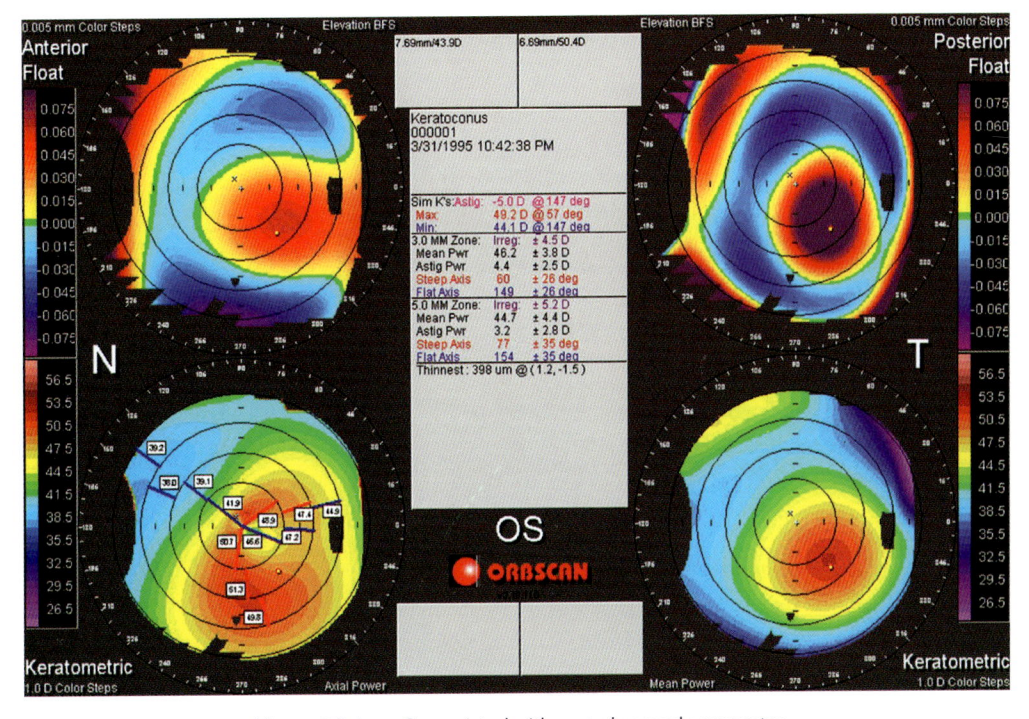

Figure 8.7 Lazy-C associated with central corneal asymmetry

Section II: Orbscan and Refractive Surgery

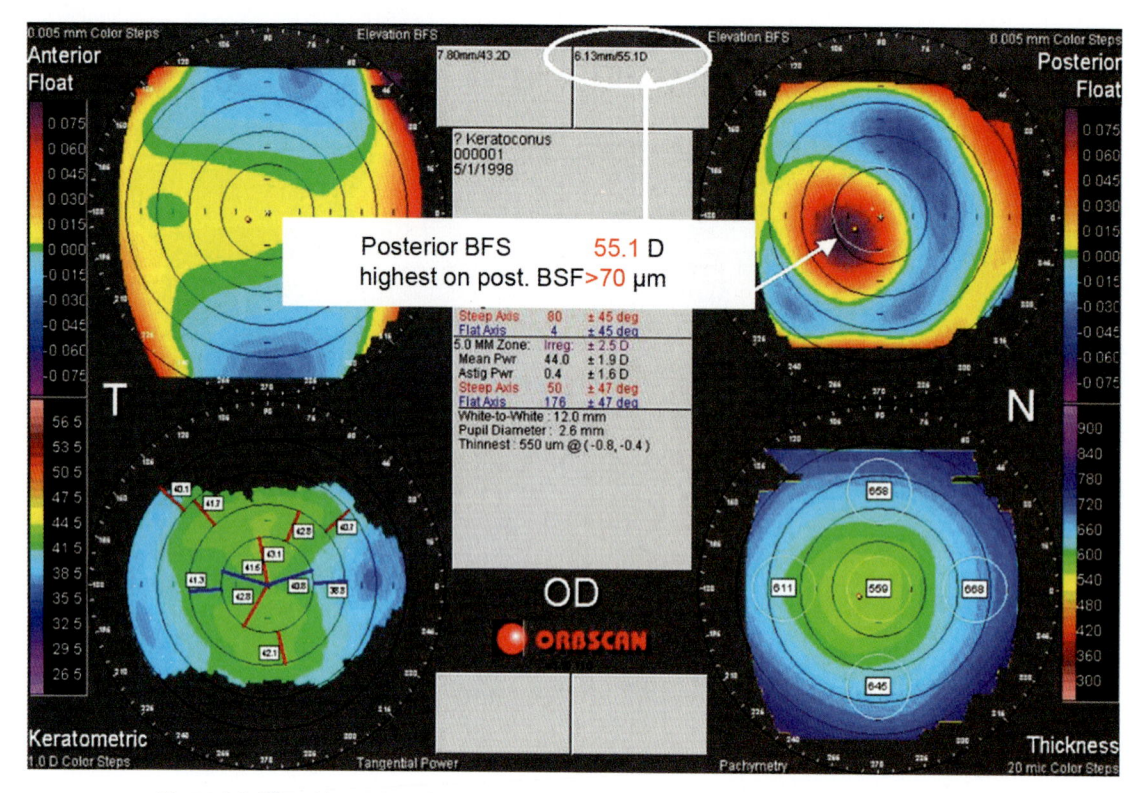

Figure 8.8 Efkarpides : 7.8 mm/6.13 mm = 1.273. In this obvious case also other red flags appear

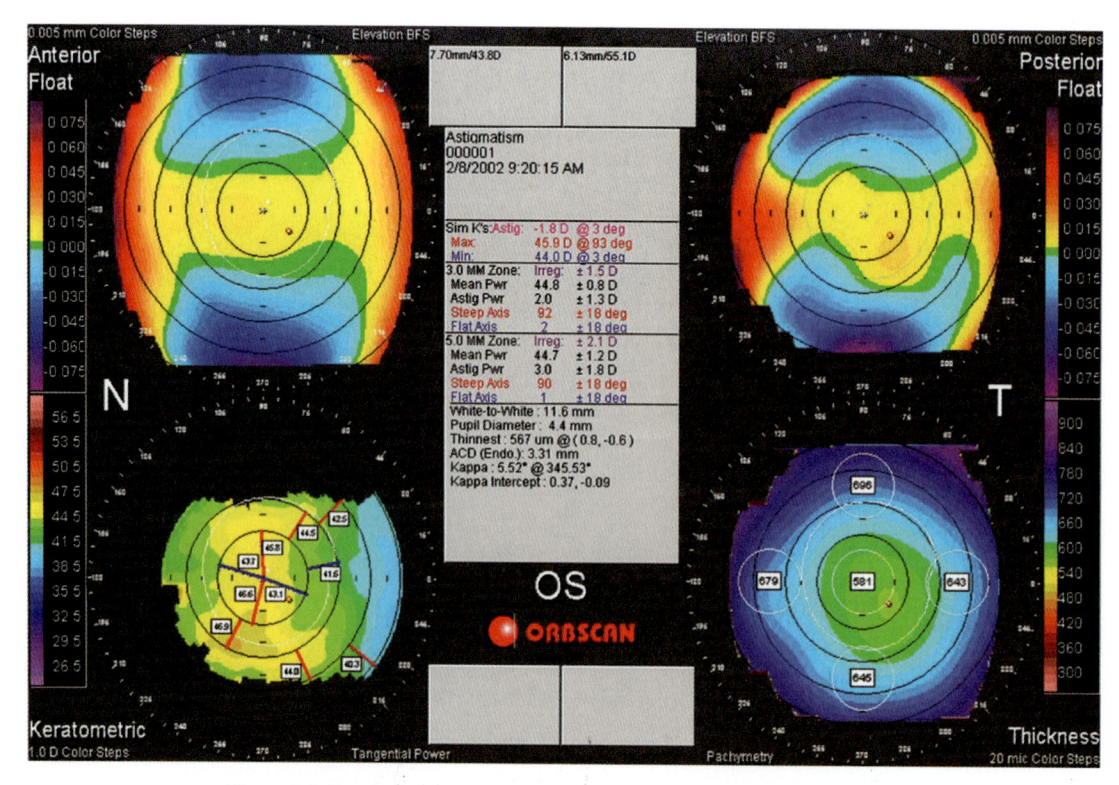

Figure 8.9 Bent/warped cornea: Symmetry of anterior and posterior elevation

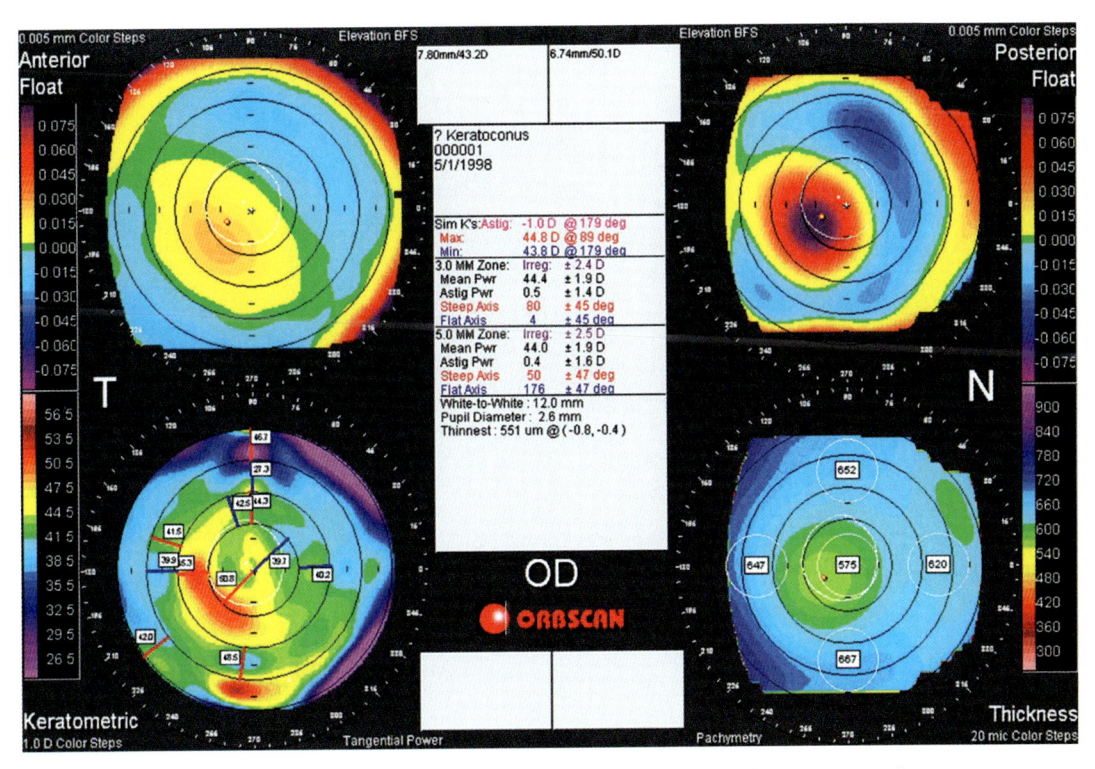

Chapter 8: Corneal Ectasia Post-LASIK: The Orbscan Advantages

Figure 8.10 Inferotemporal displacement of the highest point on the anterior as well as the posterior elevation profile can be indicative of early keratoconus

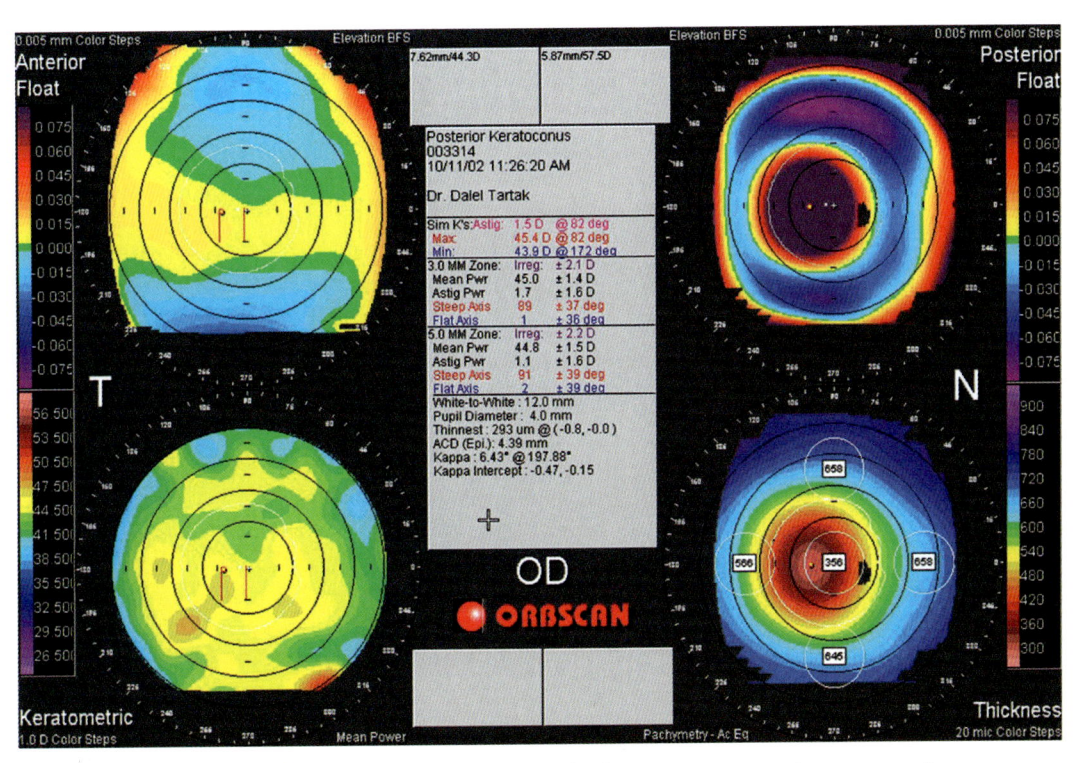

Figure 8.11 An irregularity of >1.5 D in the 3 mm central zone and of > 2.0 D in the 5 mm central zone should alert us. This sign is probably the weakest of all, but should not be ignored

90 Section II: Orbscan and Refractive Surgery

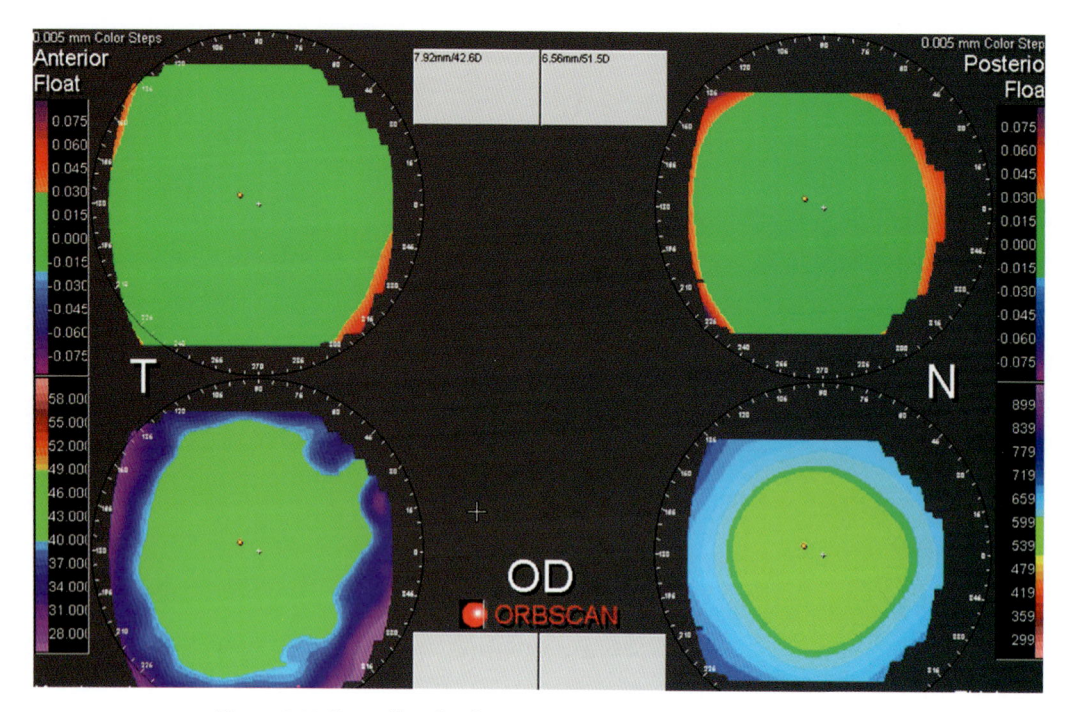

Figure 8.12 Normal band scale: No pop-ups—cornea within normal band

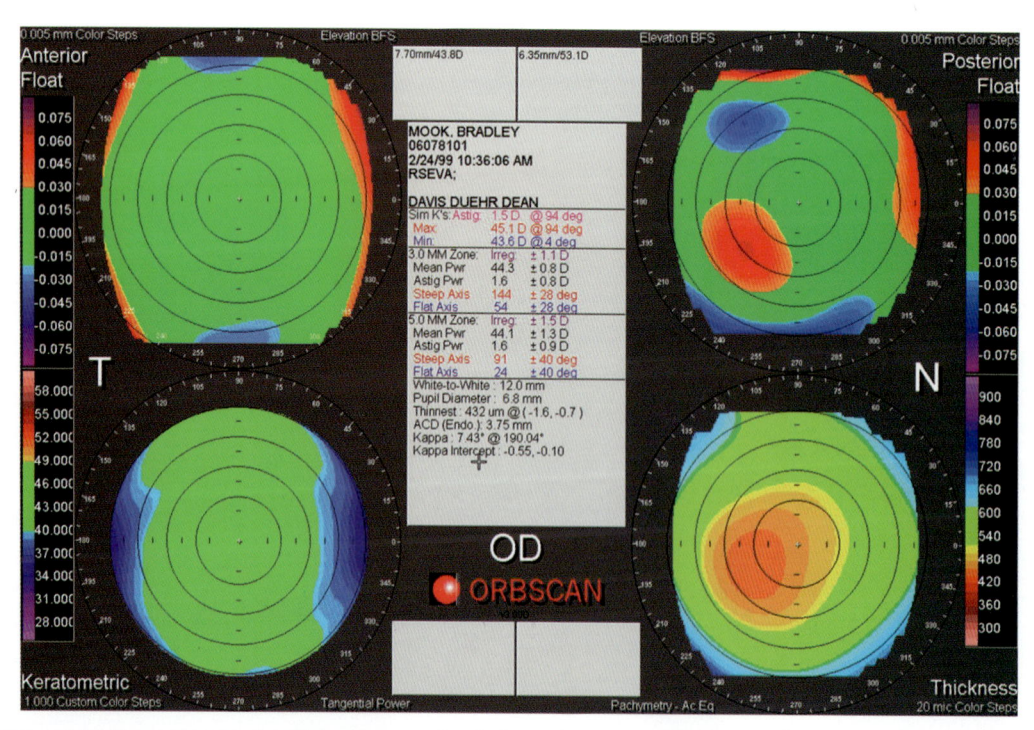

Figure 8.13 Normal band scale with two pop-ups: One in the pachymetry map and one in the posterior elevation map—there is great concern about this corneas ability to undergo lamellar refractive surgery

and the point of steepest curvature on the power map, never perform laser refractive surgery. This implies that the thinnest point represents a structural weakness, which causes a forward bending on the cornea **(Figure 8.4)**.

2. Efkarpides criteria. The ratio of the radius in mm of the anterior BFS divided by the radius in mm of the posterior BFS. Surprisingly in normal corneas this ratio will be around 1.21. Between 1.23 and 1.27 we should be suspicious and look for other abnormalities. But when this ratio is 1.27 or higher this cornea should never be treated with laser **(Figure 8.8)**.
3. Bent/warped cornea. Similarity between the anterior and posterior profiles implies a forward bending of those areas shown above BFS. If this bending is in association with the thinnest point on the cornea, it could relate to a structural weakness in the cornea. This sign needs to be evaluated within the context of the other parameters[8] **(Figure 8.9)**.
4. Inferotemporal displacement of the highest point on the anterior as well as the posterior elevation profile can be indicative of early keratoconus **(Figure 8.10)**.
5. Nature is surprisingly often very symmetrical, also our corneas. When a difference of more than 1 D of astigmatism between two eyes is detected, there exists a higher risk of ectasia postoperatively.
6. Never forget to look at the information in the center of the quad maps. An irregularity of >1.5 D in the 3 mm central zone and of > 2.0 D in the 5 mm central zone should alert us (R Lindstrom, MD). This sign is probably the weakest of all, but should not be ignored **(Figure 8.11)**.
7. Normal band scale. For the anterior and posterior elevation maps a normal band means an elevation within +/- 0.25 microns of the best-fit sphere (BFS). The normal band for the total corneal power map is 40–48 diopters and for corneal thickness is between 500 and 600 microns. One pop-up means caution, two means concern and three pop-ups means a no-go situation **(Figures 8.12 to 8.14)**.
8. *If one eye fails on the indices but the other eye does not: Never Treat Either Eye*

The above mentioned indices can become useful in the armamentarium of preoperative evaluations for potential LASIK candidates towards safe and effective outcomes.

With newer technology integration using wavefront guidance (Zywave- B and L) we can detect higher order aberrations in the form of Coma and increased RMS values (Gulani AC. Wavefront principles: Simplified and Applied. Instructional course, ESCRS, Paris, Sept 2004) aiding earlier detection of keratoconus and other potential ectatic corneal conditions. Pellucid marginal degeneration is mostly the cause of corneal topographic changes when correlated with higher levels of trefoil. Keratoconus will induce most likely higher levels of coma.

FUTURE THOUGHTS

I (Gulani AC, MD) would suggest moving in a direction that will incorporate a dynamic corneal imaging system (Dynamic corneal imaging: Prof Gunther Grabner et al: University Eye Clinic, Paracelsus Private Medical University, Salzburg,

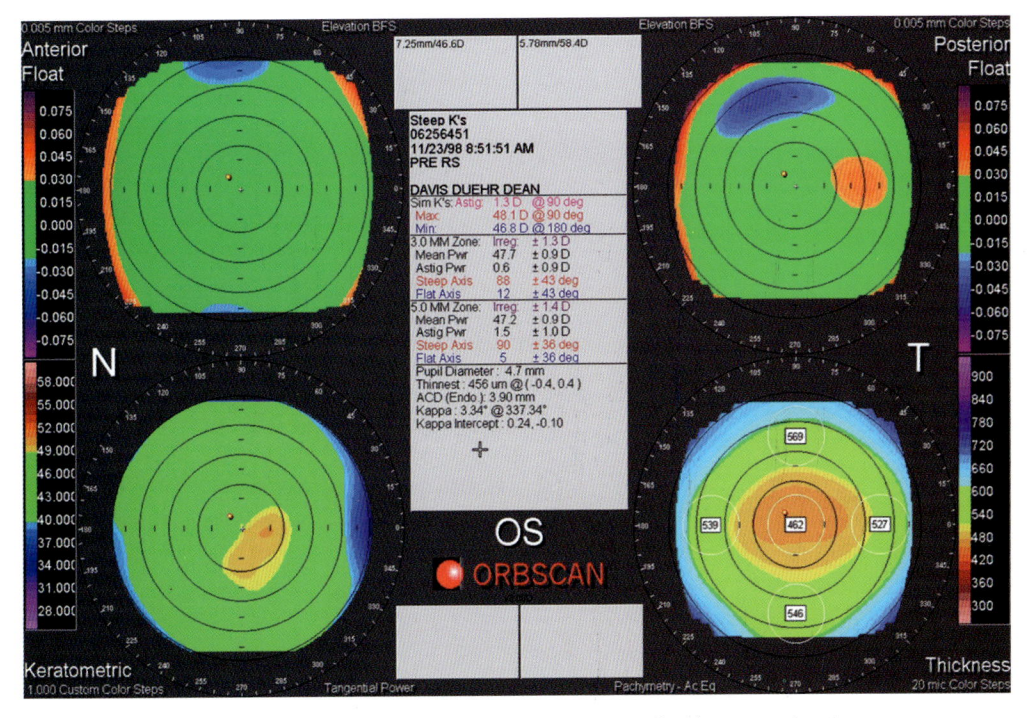

Figure 8.14 Normal band scale with three pop-ups: Definitely a no-go situation

Austria), video-topography for measurement of the tear film and its contour (Janos Nemeth, et al. from the First Department of Ophthalmology, Semmelweis University, Budapest, Hungary; the Computer and Automation Research Institute, Hungarian Academy of Sciences, Budapest, Hungary; and the Department of Statistics, National Health Insurance Fund Administration, Budapest, Hungary). Wavefront incorporation[9] to rule out other internal optical elements keeping corneal measurement precise and noncontaminated. We could even consider confocal visualization along with posterior corneal analysis to give clinical relevance to our findings besides artifactual assumptions.

Thus, a technology that would combine, biomechanical forces, elasticity modules, wavefront analysis, confocal imaging, high-speed videography and dynamic testing even during the refractive surgery in real time would be my Gold Standard in corneal refractive surgery. I am privileged to be involved presently in this direction and shall look forward to sharing my insights in the next generation of this textbook.

ACKNOWLEDGMENTS

The work presented above was not the achievement of any single individual, but is the result of support and encouragement by many colleagues and friends. Those who played an important role, include Dr Frederik Potgieter, Dr John Vukich, and our good friend, Philippe Dumarey from Bausch and Lomb, Belgium. Without their input and support, this work would not be possible.

REFERENCES

1. Charles N, Charles M, Croxatto JO, Charles DE, Wertheimer D. Surface and Orbscan II slit-scanning elevation topography in circumscribed posterior keratoconus. J Cataract Refract Surg. 2005;31(3):636-9.
2. Seiler T, Quurke AW. Iatrogenic keratectasia after LASIK in a case of forme fruste keratoconus. J Cataract Refract Surg. 1998; 24(7):1007-9.
3. Rao SN, Raviv T, Majmudar PA, Epstein RJ. Role of Orbscan II in screening keratoconus suspects before refractive corneal surgery. Ophthalmology. 2002;109(9):1642-6.
4. Pflugfelder SC, Liu Z, Feuer W, Verm A. Corneal thickness indices discriminate between keratoconus and contact lens-induced corneal thinning, Ophthalmology. 2002;109(12):2336-41.
5. Ghergel D, Hosking SL, Mantry S, Banerjee S, Naroo SA, Sha S. Corneal pachymetry in normal and keratoconic eyes: Orbscan II versus ultrasound. J Cataract Refract Surg. 2004;30(6):1272-7.
6. Arntz A, Duran JA, Pijoan JI. Subclinical keratoconus diagnosis by elevation topography: Arch Soc Esp Oftalmol. 2003;78(12):659-64.
7. Auffarth GU, Wang L, Volcker HE. Keratoconus evaluation using the Orbscan Topography System. J Cataract Refract Surg. 2000;26(2):222-8.
8. Cairns G, McGhee CN. Orbscan computerized topography: Attributes, applications and limitations. J Cataract Refract Surg. 2005;31(1):205-20.
9. Gulani AC, Probst L, Cox I, Veith R. Wavefront in LASIK: The Zyoptix. Platform. Ophthalmol Clin N Am. 2004;17:173-81.

Section III

Pentacam and Anterior Segment Optical Coherence Tomography

CHAPTERS

9. Pentacam
10. Evaluation of Patients for Refractive Surgery with Visante Anterior Segment OCT and the Combined Data Link with ATLAS Corneal Topographer
11. Corneal Inflammation and Optical Coherence Tomography
12. Optical Coherence Tomography in Corneal Ectasia
13. Spectral-domain Anterior Segment Optical Coherence Tomography in Refractive Surgery

Chapter 9

Pentacam

Tracy Schroeder Swartz (USA)

INTRODUCTION

The Pentacam ocular scanner is a specialized camera which utilizes Scheimpflug imaging to accomplish a variety of ophthalmic applications. Scheimpflug imaging was patented by Theodor Scheimpflug in 1904 after he discovered that when the planes within a camera intersect rather than be placed in parallel, the depth of focus extended.

In a typical camera, three imaginary surfaces exist: The film plane, lens plane and sharp image plane. These are parallel to each other such that the image of the object placed in the plane of sharp focus will pass through the lens plane perpendicular to the lens axis, and fall on to the film plane. The depth of focus is limited in such a camera.

In a Scheimpflug camera, the three planes are not parallel but intersect in a line, called the '*Scheimpflug line*'. When the lens is tilted such that it intersects the film plane, the plane of sharp focus also passes through the Scheimpflug line, extending the depth of focus. Note that this results in mild image distortion, which is then corrected by the Pentacam system.[1]

A two-dimensional cross-sectional image results, as shown in **Figure 9.1**. When performing a scan, two cameras are used to capture the image. One centrally located camera detects pupil size and orientation, and controls fixation. The second rotates 180 degrees to capture 25 or 50 images of the anterior segment up to the level of the iris, and through the pupil to evaluate the lens. Five hundred true elevation data points are generated

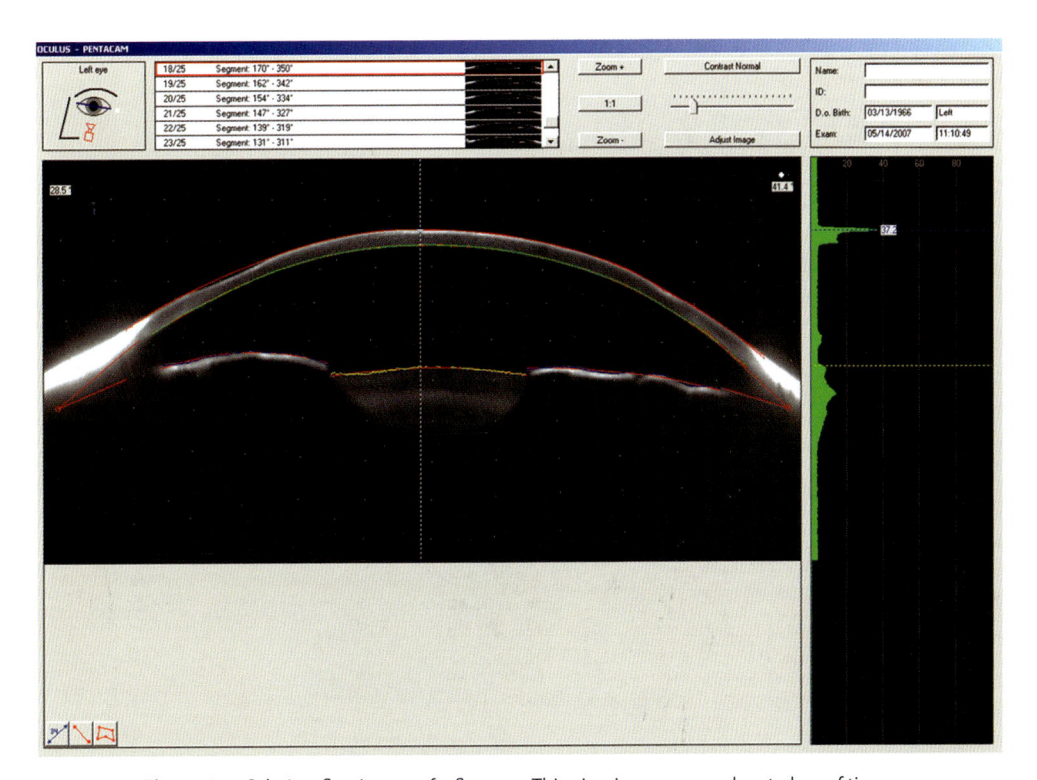

Figure 9.1 Scheimpflug image of a flap tear. Thinning is seen secondary to loss of tissue where the flap was rotated away from the bed

per image to yield up to 25,000 points for each surface. Data points are captured for the center of the cornea, an area that placido disc topographers and slit-scanning devices are unable to evaluate.

Elevation data measured using this technique has several advantages. Because it is independent of axis, orientation and position, it yields a more accurate representation of true corneal shape. Thus, the Pentacam's curvature map, because it is not sensitive to position, is theoretically more accurate. The elevation maps are created using one of three reference bodies: A best-fit sphere, an ellipse of revolution, and toric. The best-fit sphere calculation approximates the sphere as accurately as possible to the true nature of the cornea. This facilitates comparison between other topographers but is not the best-fit for the aspheric cornea.

The ellipsoid of revolution is calculated from the keratometry eccentricity and the mean central radius. This reference shape correlates well with the true shape of the normal cornea.

The toric is based on the central radii and keratometry eccentricity as well. The flat and steep radii are automatically used. The toric is a good estimation for astigmatic corneas. The toric ellipsoid float display best facilitates pattern recognition of abnormalities on the front and back surfaces, such as found in keratoconus.[2] **Figures 9.2 to 9.4** show the same astigmatic eye mapped using the three different reference bodies. The cone is easily detected using the toric ellipse reference body.

Displays

The default view presented following data capture is the "Overview display", which includes the Scheimpflug image, three-dimensional model, an additional map, keratometry, pupil, anterior chamber measurements, and pachymetry. An example of an overview display in a patient with a history of conductive keratoplasty is shown in **Figure 9.5**. From here, other displays are typically chosen relative to the reason for scanning: surgical vision correction, keratoconus evaluation, cataract or anterior chamber evaluation, etc.

Topography and Keratometry

The refractive and topographic displays for the patient in **Figure 9.5** are shown in **Figures 9.6 and 9.7**. Single maps can also be viewed by selecting the preferred single display. Several indices, listed in **Table 9.1**, are presented to aid in clinical diagnosis, and system set-up guidelines to facilitate pattern recognition of pathology are listed in **Table 9.2. Table 9.3** lists the examination quality measures used to determine, if the map is of sufficient quality or needs to be repeated. The "Quality Score", listed as QS on the printout, will be highlighted in yellow for caution and red when the map should be repeated. Note that even with the talented operators, highly irregular corneas may show QS values. Clicking on this value opens the Examination Quality Specification screen which details errors.

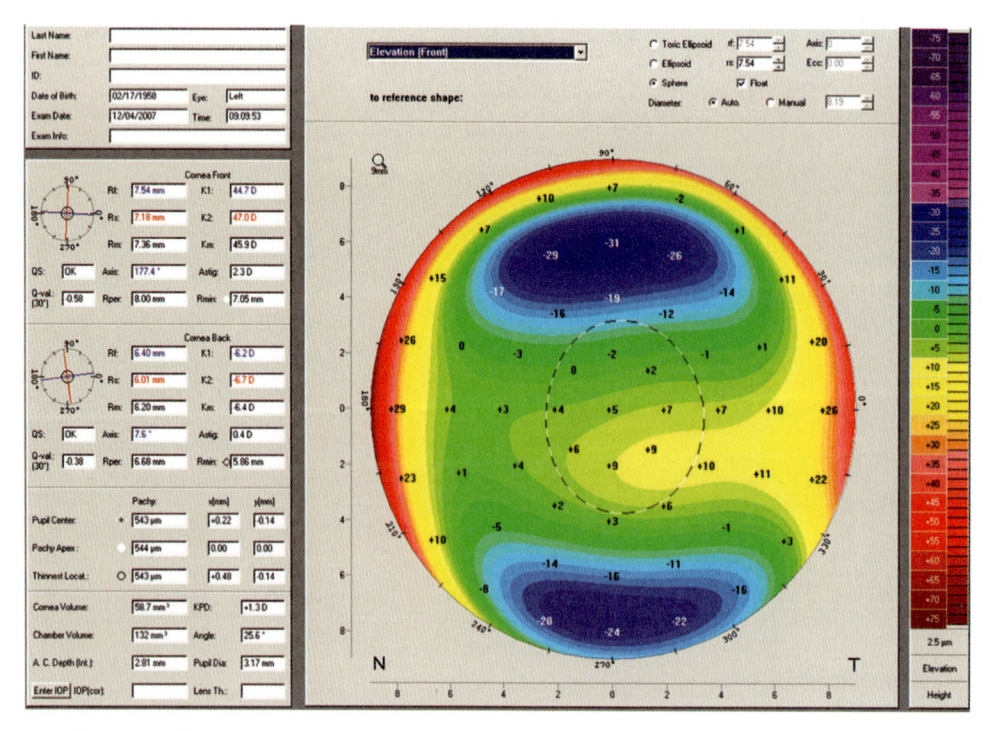

Figure 9.2 Elevation map using the best-fit sphere reference body. The astigmatism appears to be a "saddle" without a significant cone

Chapter 9: Pentacam 97

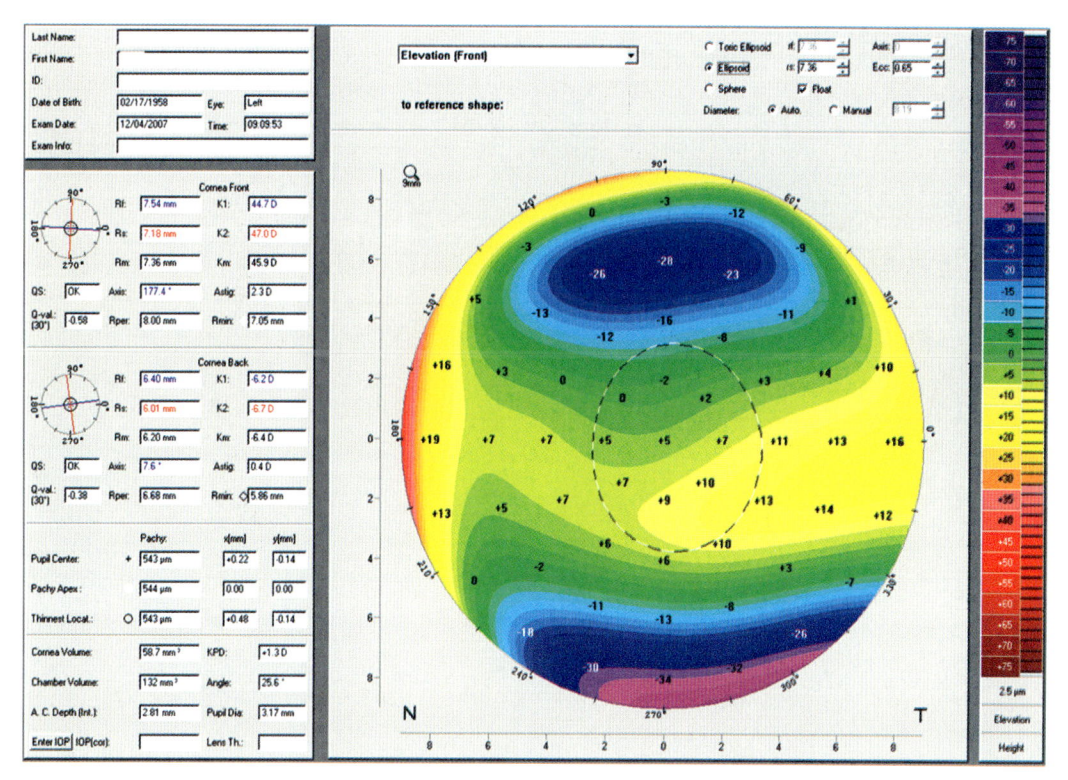

Figure 9.3 Elevation map using the ellipse reference body

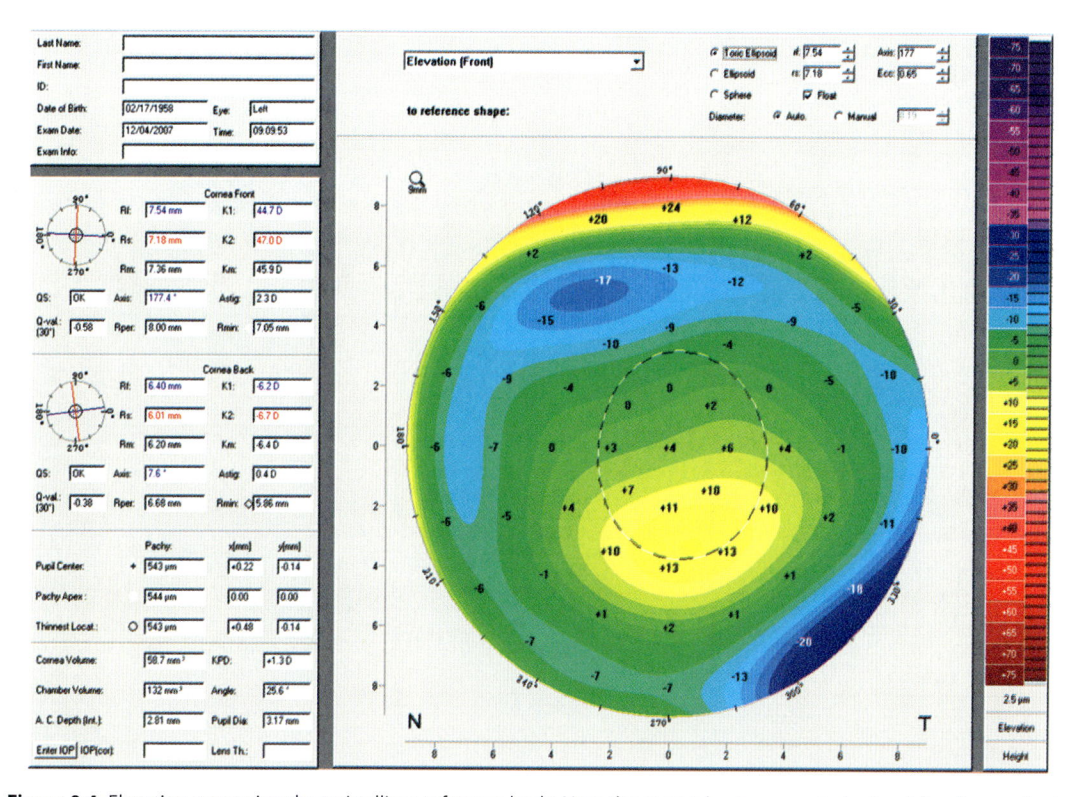

Figure 9.4 Elevation map using the toric ellipse reference body. Note the cone is best represented using this reference body

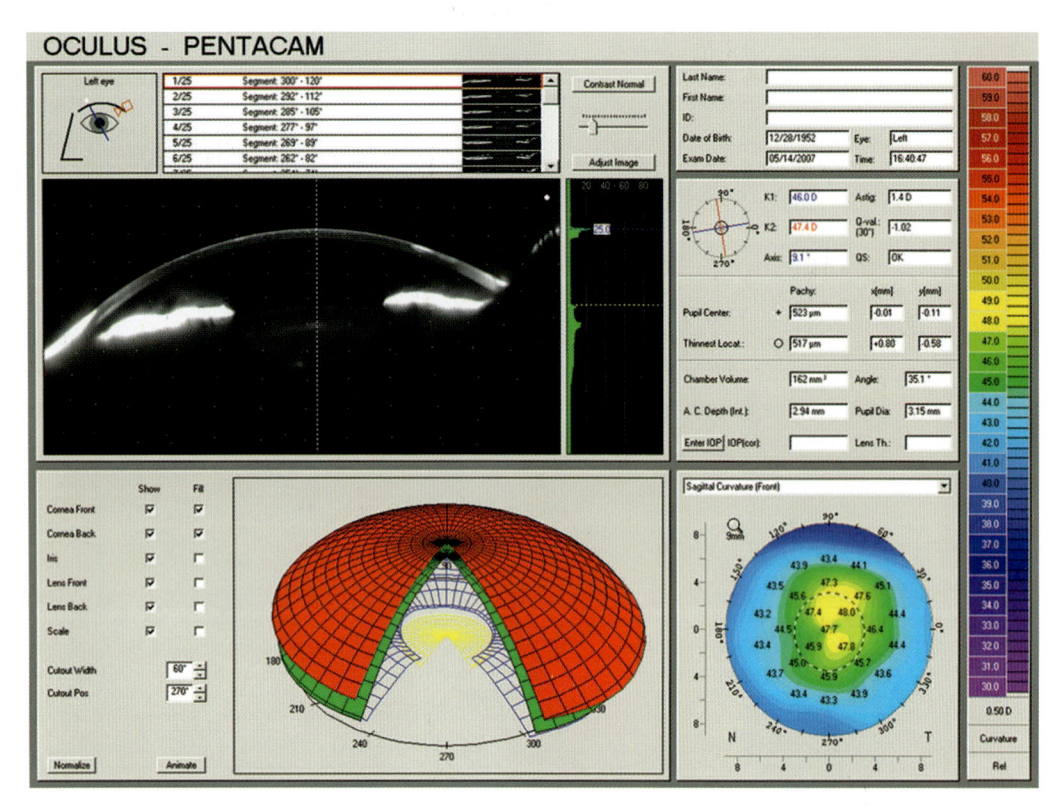

98 Section III: Pentacam and Anterior Segment Optical Coherence Tomography

Figure 9.5 Overview display from a patient with a history of conductive keratoplasty and cataract

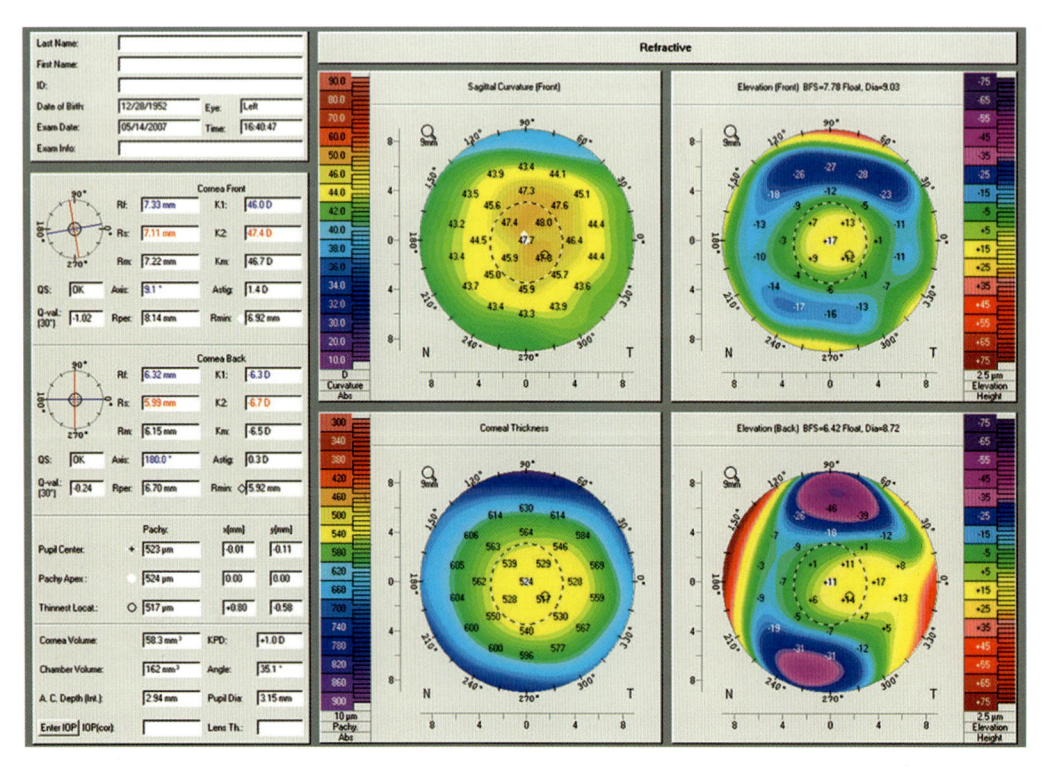

Figure 9.6 Refractive display for the patient in Figure 9.5. It is commonly used when evaluating patients for elective vision correction

Chapter 9: Pentacam

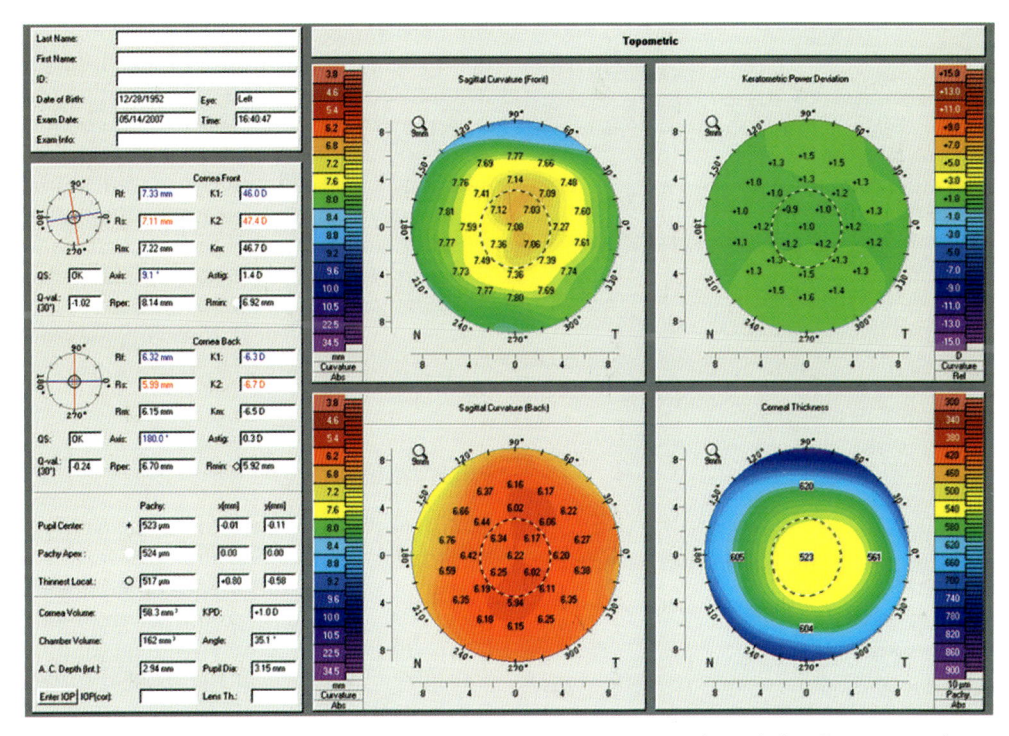

Figure 9.7 Topographic display for the patient in Figure 9.5. It is most commonly used when fitting contact lenses

Table 9.1 Topographic indices

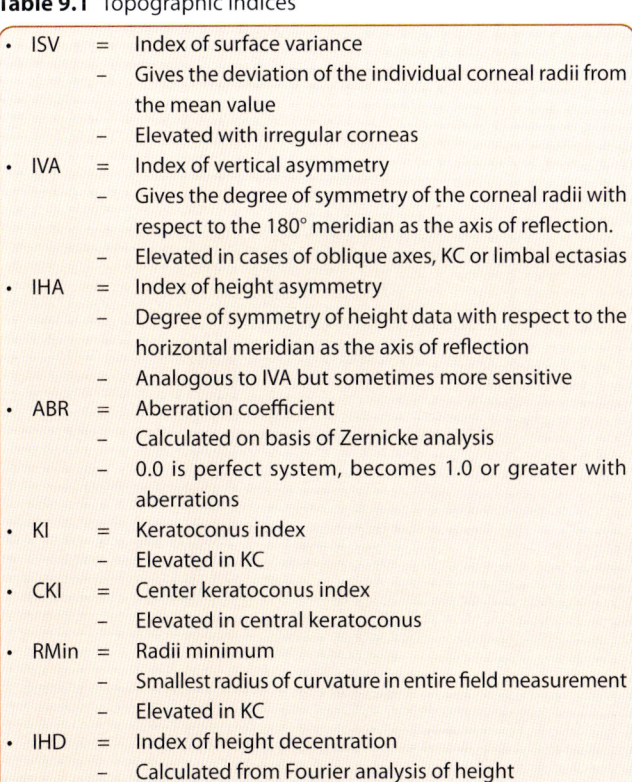

- ISV = Index of surface variance
  - Gives the deviation of the individual corneal radii from the mean value
  - Elevated with irregular corneas
- IVA = Index of vertical asymmetry
  - Gives the degree of symmetry of the corneal radii with respect to the 180° meridian as the axis of reflection.
  - Elevated in cases of oblique axes, KC or limbal ectasias
- IHA = Index of height asymmetry
  - Degree of symmetry of height data with respect to the horizontal meridian as the axis of reflection
  - Analogous to IVA but sometimes more sensitive
- ABR = Aberration coefficient
  - Calculated on basis of Zernicke analysis
  - 0.0 is perfect system, becomes 1.0 or greater with aberrations
- KI = Keratoconus index
  - Elevated in KC
- CKI = Center keratoconus index
  - Elevated in central keratoconus
- RMin = Radii minimum
  - Smallest radius of curvature in entire field measurement
  - Elevated in KC
- IHD = Index of height decentration
  - Calculated from Fourier analysis of height
  - Gives degree of vertical decentration
  - Steeper in KC

Table 9.2 Guidelines for system set-up to aid in pattern recognition

- *Scans*: 25
- *Elevation map*: Sphere fitted in float, automatic diameter
- *Keratometer*: Rstp/Rflat, diameter automatic
- *Corneal form factor asphericity Q*:
  - Q < 0, indicates an untreated case
  - Q > 1, indicates a treated cornea (LASIK, PRK, RK)
- *Color scale*:
  - Pachymetry step width normal: 10 μm
  - Topography step width normal: 1 D
  - Elevation step with minimum 2.5 μm
- *4 maps refractive*: Similar to Orbscan Quad map layout

The two major meridians, determined using the 3 mm ring are at 90 degrees from each other, are listed as K_1 (flat) and K_2 (steep), with corresponding radii R_1 and R_2. The mean radius and mean keratometry are the arithmetic average of the corresponding measures. "Astig" describes the central corneal astigmatism. The mean radii of the 7 and 9 mm rings are described as the "Rper".

The Q-value describes the corneal shape factor, or the eccentricity of the cornea. A value of –0.26 is ideal. Highly prolate corneas with significantly higher negative values may suggest keratoconus or hyperopic treatment. Positive values suggest oblate corneas, such as those with a history of myopic treatment.

The presentation of the now widely accepted "Quad map" includes the sagittal curvature, anterior and posterior elevation,

Section III: Pentacam and Anterior Segment Optical Coherence Tomography

Table 9.3 Examination quality measures

- Yellowed comments in the *quality score* (QS) box alert the technician to retake the examination due to suspect quality. This may read "Fix!" (Fixation) or "Model!" (severely irregular shape) to indicate the nature of the problem.
- *Analyzed area* decreases, if the eye is not opened widely, and the map should be corrected by instructing patient to open the eye widely. This must be higher than 60% for the anterior surface, and 50% for the posterior.
- *Valid data* considers lighting conditions. It should be 95% for the anterior surface and 90% for the posterior.
- *Lost segments* represents loss of image and subsequently, data. If the number of Scheimpflug images lost due to blinking exceeds three, the image needs to be repeated.
- If the number of continuous segments exceeds two, the scan must be repeated.
- Model evaluation considers the deviation between the corneal height data points and the smooth calculation of the 3 D model. The difference must be lower than 10 for the anterior surface and 14 for the posterior surface.
- Alignment (XY) describes the horizontal (X) and vertical (Y) alignment, and must be less than 1000.
- Alignment (Z) describes the distance between the patient's eye and the Pentacam, and must be less than 1000.
- *Eye movement* indicates the stability of the eye during acquisition. High values indicate excessive movement, and value should be less than 150.

and pachymetry maps. When examining the Pentacam quad map to determine candidacy for elective vision correction, the relationship between the maps must be assessed. Since the posterior surface is the first to manifest ectatic changes, inspect this map first. Elevated areas noted on the posterior surface map may correspond to a displaced "thinnest area" on the pachymetry map, elevated area on the anterior elevation map, and irregular astigmatism on the curvature map. Examples are shown in **Figures 9.8 to 9.10**. Astigmatism often manifests as a "saddle" on the posterior surface as seen in **Figure 9.11** and may not be pathological. Checking the elevation map using the toric ellipse is an excellent method to ruling out ectasia in these eyes.

Pachymetry

Optical pachymetry is calculated from direct measurement of the anterior and posterior surface elevations. While ultrasound remains the standard for pachymetry measurement, optical pachymetry has been reported to be reproducible and reliable in the literature. [3,4] One advantage of optical pachymetry is display of values over the corneal surface **(Figure 9.12)**. It is important to inspect the pachymetry values relative to those around it as well as the thinnest value. One study found Pentacam provided measurements that were slightly but systematically lower than the measurements provided by

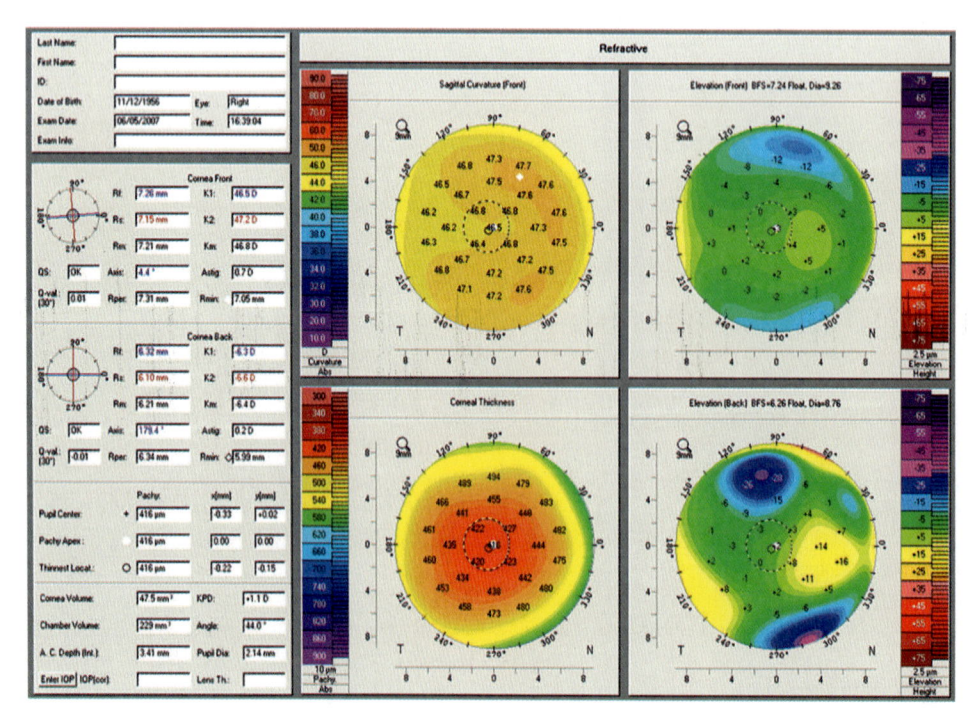

Figure 9.8 When considering a patient for refractive surgical correction, look at the relationship between the four maps on the refractive display. This illustrates a suspicious "two point touch" where the posterior elevation corresponds to a mild anterior elevation. This patient had low pachymetry, but the pachymetry map was otherwise normal, symmetrical around the center

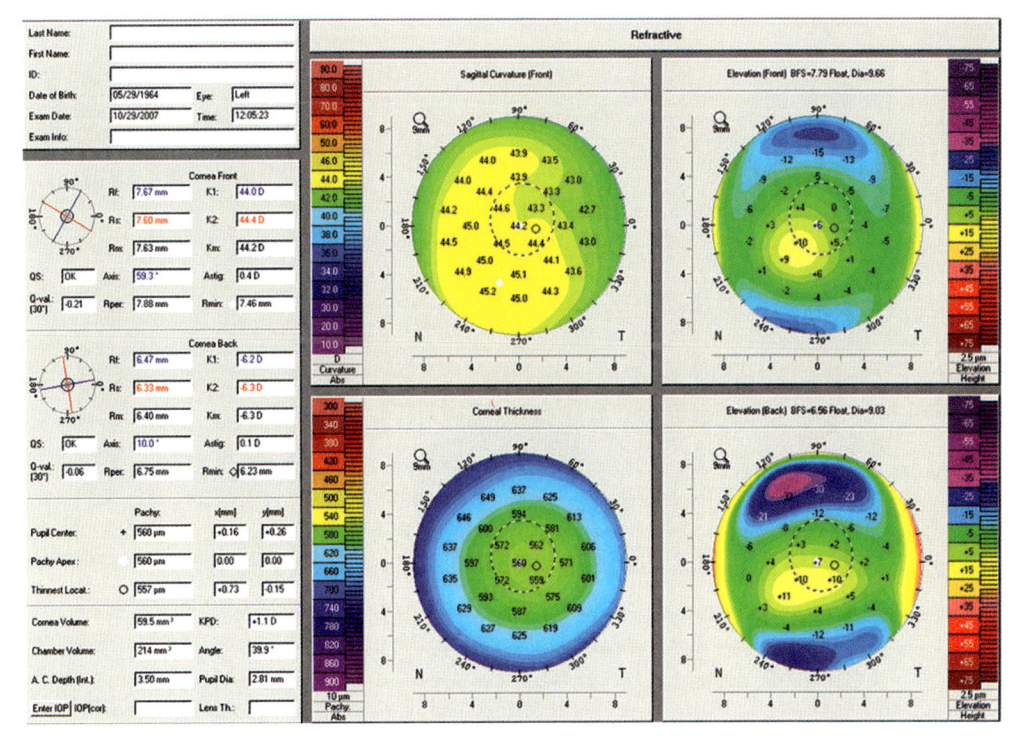

Figure 9.9 This is an example of a "three point touch" where the elevation on the posterior and anterior surface corresponds to a steep area on the curvature map

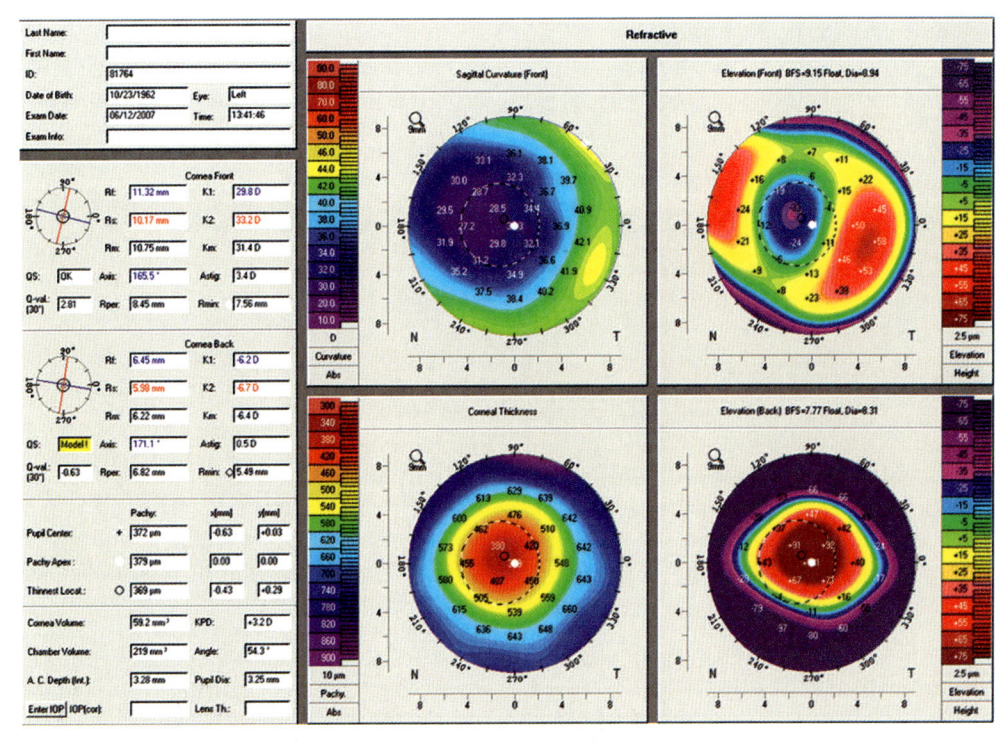

Figure 9.10 This is an example of a classic ectasia following excimer ablation for high myopia, where all four maps show characteristic signs of ectasia

Figure 9.11 Astigmatism manifests as a "saddle" pattern on the posterior surface

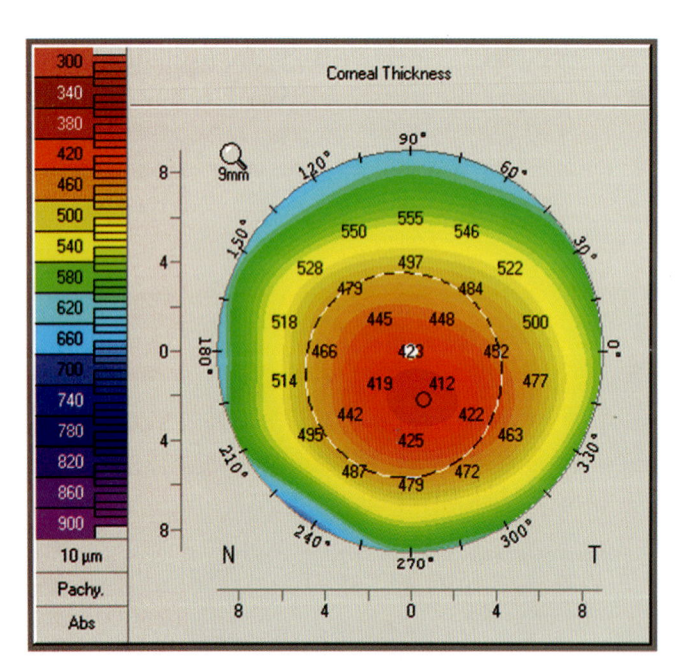

Figure 9.12 A pachymetry map of a patient with keratoconus. Note the displacement of the thinnest point, and the overall reduction of corneal thickness

Pachymetry after PRK has been shown to be problematic for slit-scanning devices.[11,12] Corneal thickness was measured using Pentacam, Orbscan II, and ultrasonic pachymetry in unoperated eyes, and in those after myopic PRK. Authors reported following myopic PRK, the Pentacam measurement were comparable to ultrasonic pachymetry, while Orbscan measurements were thinner.[13] Pachymetry after LASIK has been shown to be variable as well.[14,15] Several studies have been published, with reports of good repeatability in pachymetry measurements[16,17] and strong correlation[18] such that authors suggested Pentacam pachymetry may be substituted for ultrasound in the post-LASIK patient.[19]

Posterior Surface

As a tomographer, the Pentacam measures the posterior surface directly, as shown in **Figure 9.13A**. Calculations are based on the Gull-Strand eye model. Values are negative, due to the negative refractive index of the cornea and aqueous humor. **Table 9.4** lists the values suggested for clinical ectasia.

Literature reports suggest good repeatability for the posterior Best-fit sphere (BSF),[20,21] with significant differences when compared to Orbscan **(Figure 9.13B)**. Hashemi et al studied LASIK patients using the Orbscan and Pentacam pre- and postoperatively. They reported that, the Orbscan II yielded larger posterior elevation values before and after surgery, and significant postoperative changes in posterior corneal elevation and posterior maximum elevation compared to the Pentacam.[22]

Ciolino found no statistically significant difference in posterior corneal displacement between LASIK and PRK

ultrasonic pachymetry in normal corneas[5], and another found measurements obtained with the Orbscan II (CF) are thinner than those obtained with the Pentacam in normal eyes.[6] Most essentially reported significant agreement with one another, but these methods may not be simply interchangeable.[7-10]

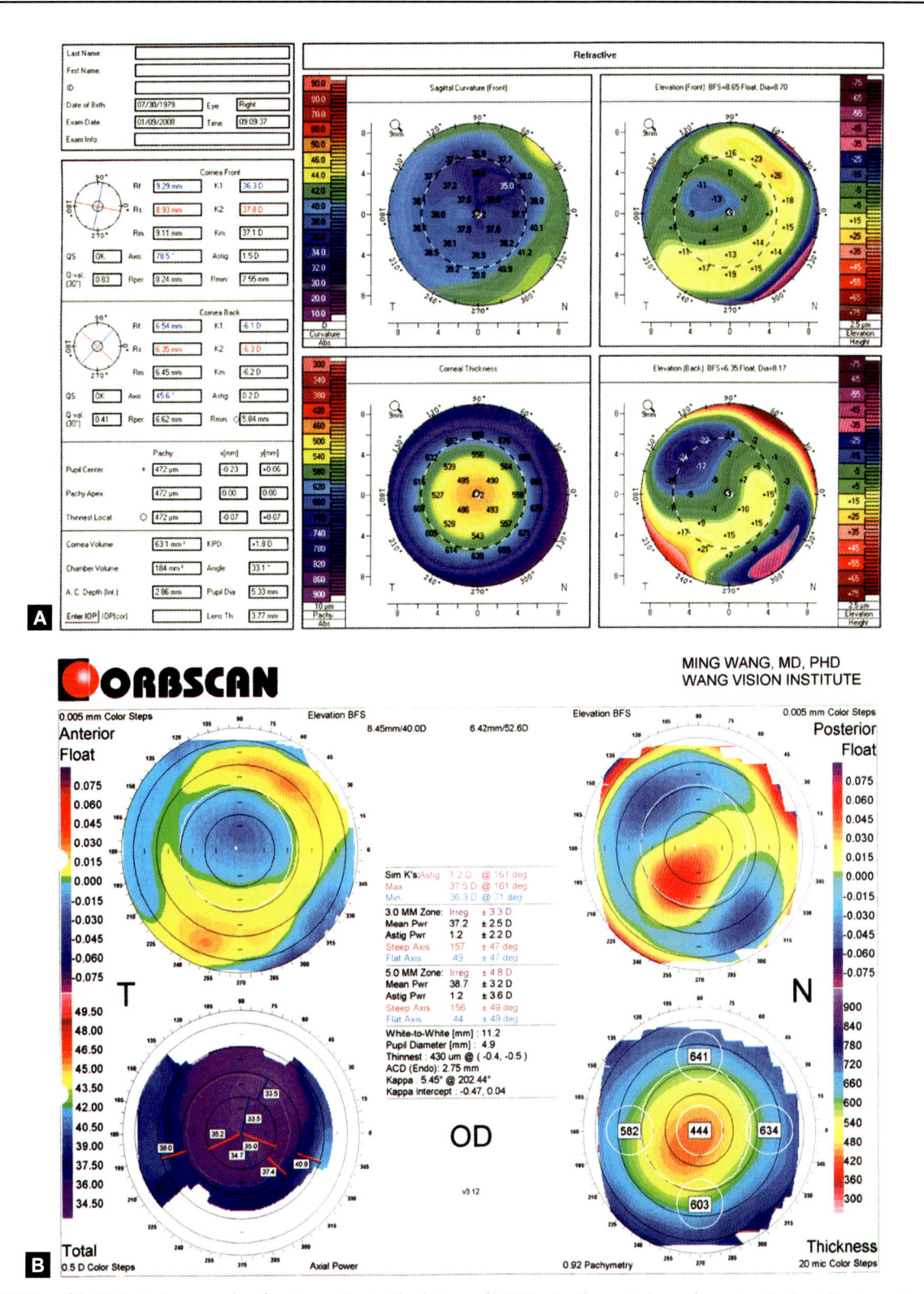

Figures 9.13A and B (A) Posterior corneal surface in a patient with a history of LASIK using the posterior surface using the best-fit sphere. No significant ectasia was noted on the Pentacam, and pachymetry was similar to ultrasound value (480 microns); (B) Orbscan quad map of the eye shown in Figure 9.13A. Note the difference in the appearance of the posterior float map, which indicates ectasia. The pachymetry was 444 microns, significantly different from 472 of Pentacam and ultrasound (480 microns)

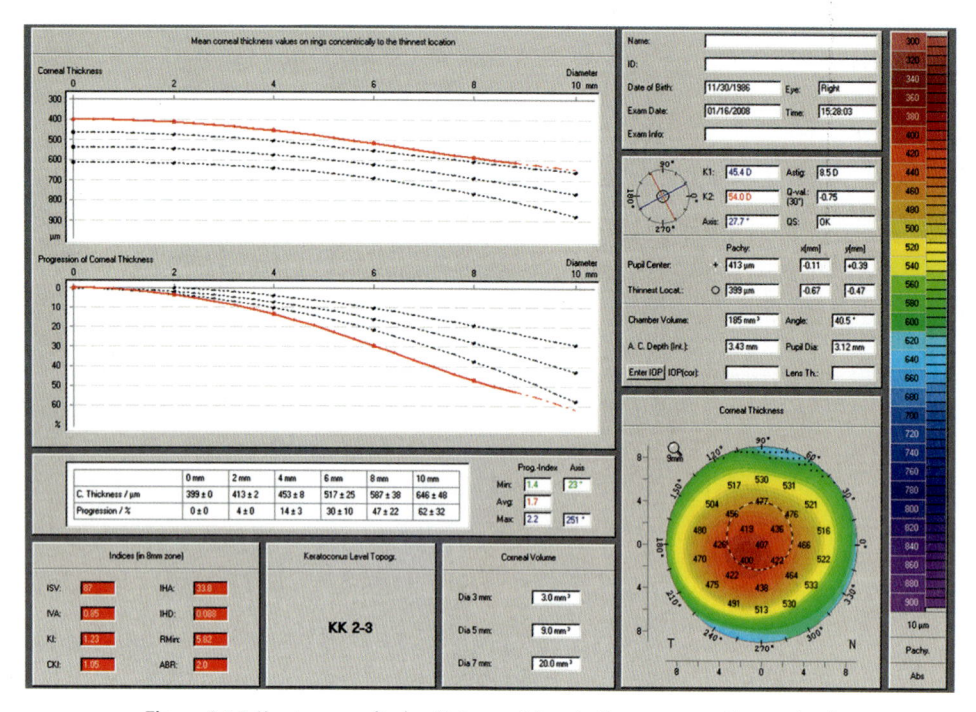

Figure 9.14 Keratoconus display. Note suspicious indices appear yellow and red

patients as measured by the Pentacam and suggested ectasia may not routinely occur after LASIK.[23] Quisling et al found the Pentacam and Orbscan IIz measure similar thinnest points but differ in posterior elevations above the best-fit sphere, despite similar radii of curvature. They were not able to determine, if the Pentacam underestimated posterior vault, or if Orbscan overestimates the height.[24]

Keratoconus Screening

The *keratoconus screening display* incorporates the keratometry, pachymetry, anterior chamber information, corneal volume, and thickness assessment relative to the thinnest point. "Rings" with diameters of 1, 2, 3, 4, and 5 mm around the thinnest point are created, and mean corneal thickness and corneal thickness progression are illustrated in graphical displays, as shown in **Figure 9.14**. Various indices, described in **Table 9.4** are used to determine the level of KC risk, and suspect values appear in red, as shown in **Figure 9.15**. Note these indices are calculated using *only* the anterior surface. Numerical values describing normal, suspect and pathological values for these indices are listed in **Table 9.5**. The KC index describes the risk of keratoconus using a 4 stage classification based on those of Amsler and Muckenhirm. Selecting "keratoconus level topography" opens the table which describes classical signs of keratoconus used by the KC index. Clinical assessment must be incorporated as these should not be used for diagnosis alone.

Parameters listed on the KC display are based on studies indicating differences exist among those with KC and healthy corneas. Emre et al found that with progression of disease, total corneal thickness and anterior chamber depth were statistically different and there were statistically significant differences in anterior chamber angle and corneal volume measurements between the mild keratoconus and severe keratoconus groups.[25]

Table 9.4 KC screening guidelines for anterior and posterior elevation

	Normal	Suspect	Pathological
Anterior	Less than 12 μm	12 to 15 μm	Greater than 15 μm
Posterior	Less than 17 μm	17 to 20 μm	Greater than 20 μm

Figure 9.15 Various indices, described in Table 9.5, are used to determine the level of KC risk, and suspect values appear in red

Ambrosio et al studied mild-to-moderate keratoconic eyes compared with normal eyes using the Pentacam. Corneal-thickness spatial profile, corneal-volume distribution, percentage increase in thickness, and percentage increase in volume were different between keratoconic corneas and normal corneas.[26]

Cataract Evaluation

Evaluation of cataracts can be objectively performed using Densometry, shown in **Figure 9.16**. The tomography display

Table 9.5 KC index levels

Index	Abnormal (Yellow)	Pathological (Red)
Index of surface variance (ISV)	≥ 37	≥ 41
Index of vertical asymmetry (IVA)	≥ 0.28	≥ 0.32
Keratoconus index (KI)	>1.07	>1.07
Center keratoconus index (CKI)	≥ 1.03	≥ 1.03
Radii Minimum (R_{min})	< 6.71	< 6.71
Index of height asymmetry (IHA)	≥ 19	≥ 21
Index of height decentration (IHD)	≥ 0.014	≥ 0.016
Aberration coefficient (ABR)	≥ 1	≥ 1

(Figure 9.17) can also be used to educate patients on the level of cataract development, and is tremendously valuable for patients presenting for elective vision correction with mild cataracts. Pentacam imaging has been reported to be helpful in the evaluation of penetrating eye injury and intralenticular foreign body,[27] as well as diagnosis and management of CBDS, posterior capsular haze,[28] and subclinical manifestations of electric cataract injuries.[29] Note that when the goal of the examination is densitometry, the 'enhanced dynamic examination scanning mode should be selected. This lengthens the exposure time per Scheimpflug image during the scan. Progress may be monitored when the same number of images during the scans is selected upon the patient's subsequent visits.

IOL Calculation

The Holladay Report **(Figure 9.18)** was developed to assist surgeons in calculation of IOL power in patient with a history of refractive surgery. Changes in the central topography may produce "refractive surprise", an unwanted result in this age of high patient expectation. Typical keratometry fails to estimate the true corneal power in patients with surgically altered topography. Errors result because keratometers assume the ratio of power between the anterior and posterior cornea is 82%, as in a virgin eye. They calculate corneal power using an

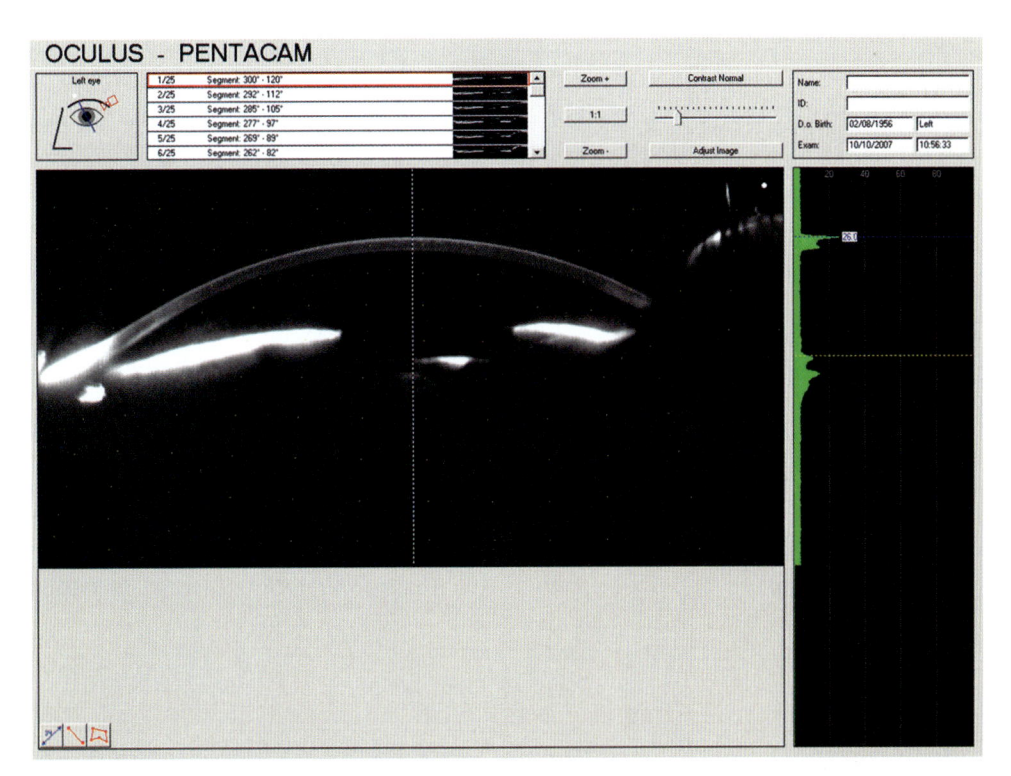

Figure 9.16 Densitometry in a patient with an ASC. The spike in the level of opacification corresponds directly to the placement of the cursor, and allows the clinician numerical assessment of the lens to track progression of cataracts

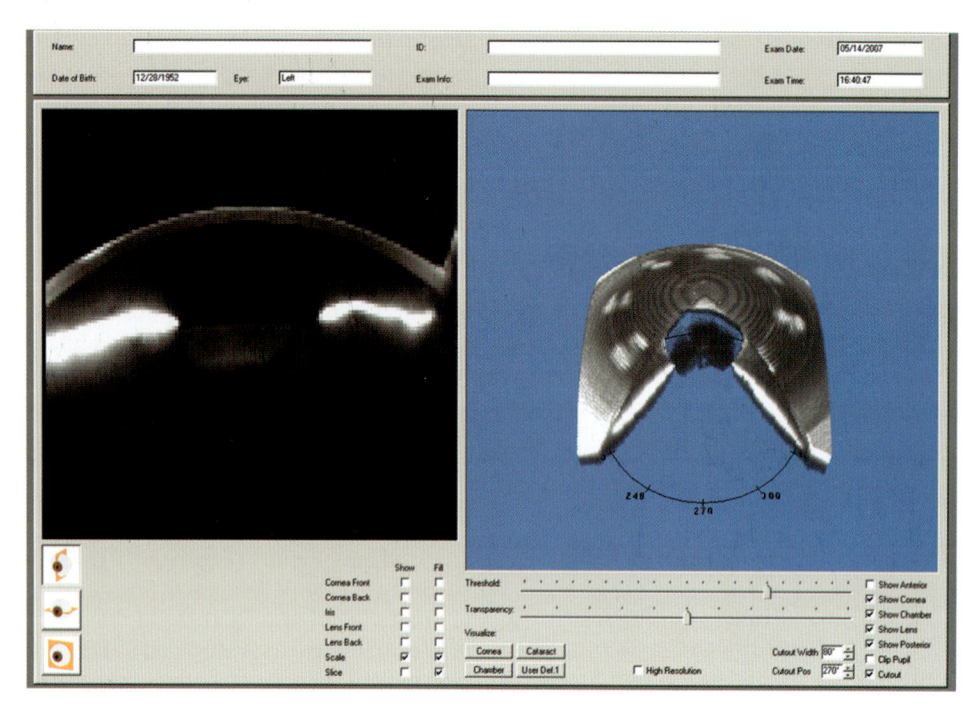

Figure 9.17 The tomography display can also be used to educate patients on the level of cataract development, and is especially valuable for patients presenting for enhancement following keratorefractive correction with mild cataracts. This patient had a history of conductive keratoplasty and presented with complaints of decreased reading vision. Cataract surgery was recommended rather than additional refractive surgery

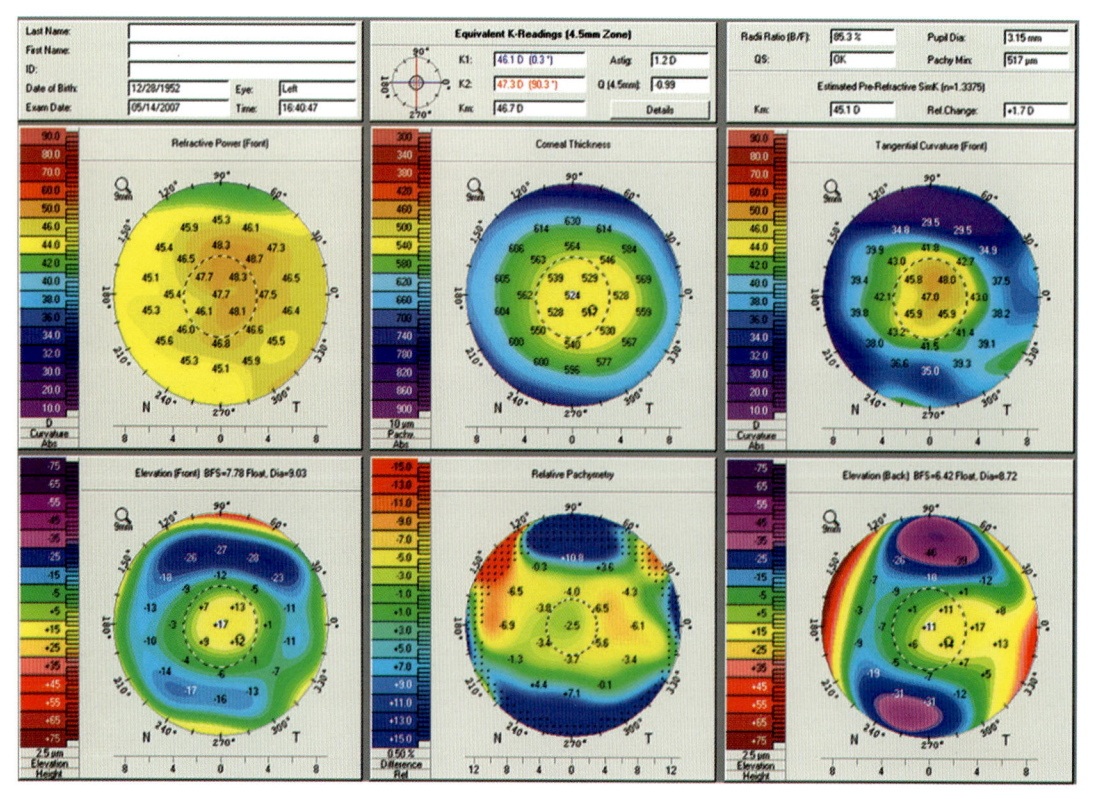

Figure 9.18 The Holladay report is useful when calculating intraocular lens power in patients with a history of refractive surgery

index of 1.3375. Because excimer treatment alters this ratio, the calculation is inaccurate, and the lens implant power fails to properly correct the refractive error. The Pentacam calculates the front and back surface power, and produces the "equivalent K readings" or EKRs. The EKRs are used with IOL calculation formulas to obtain correct IOL powers for patients with surgically altered corneas.

The calculation of EKRs is related to the pupil center rather than the corneal apex as in keratometry, and utilizes the refractive power map rather than the curvature map. The calculation is based on the ratio of the anterior and posterior surface radii within the 4.5 mm zone, shown to be the most pertinent for patients with a history of excimer treatment.

The detailed report **(Figure 9.19)** shows the EKRs for manually selected zone measurements, and may be of value when other zones may be better options, such as in patients with a history of radial keratotomy (RK), trauma, or severe irregular astigmatism.

Anterior Chamber Evaluation

The Pentacam presents data regarding anterior chamber depth and volume, as well as assessment of the chamber angle. The anterior chamber display is shown in **Figures 9.20A and B**.

The chamber volume is calculated directly, while the distance between the cornea's posterior surface and the iris are integrated in a 12 mm diameter around the corneal apex. The angle should not be evaluated while the pupil is dilated, and may be used to evaluate patients for glaucoma risk due to narrow angles. Anterior chamber information can also be used when evaluating patients for phakic lens implants.

Nemeth et al compared the ultrasound and Pentacam Anterior Chamber Depth (ACD) measurements in phakic and pseudophakic eyes. They reported similar ACD measurements with the Pentacam and ultrasound in phakic eyes, with significantly lower measurements using the Pentacam in pseudophakes, however.[30] Elbaz et al compared ACD measurements taken from Pentacam, ultrasound A-scan and IOLMaster (Carl Zeiss Meditach, Jena, Germany). Measurements of ACD by the Pentacam differed significantly from those of ultrasound and IOLMaster. Authors concluded measurements of ACD and corneal curvature using these machines may not be interchangeable.[31] In contrast, when comparing Pentacam and Orbscan ACD measurements. Lackner et al studied the differences of ACD values as well as inter- and intraobserver variability measured with Orbscan and Pentacam were such that the two modalities can be regarded as interchangeable.[32] Angle anatomy relative to

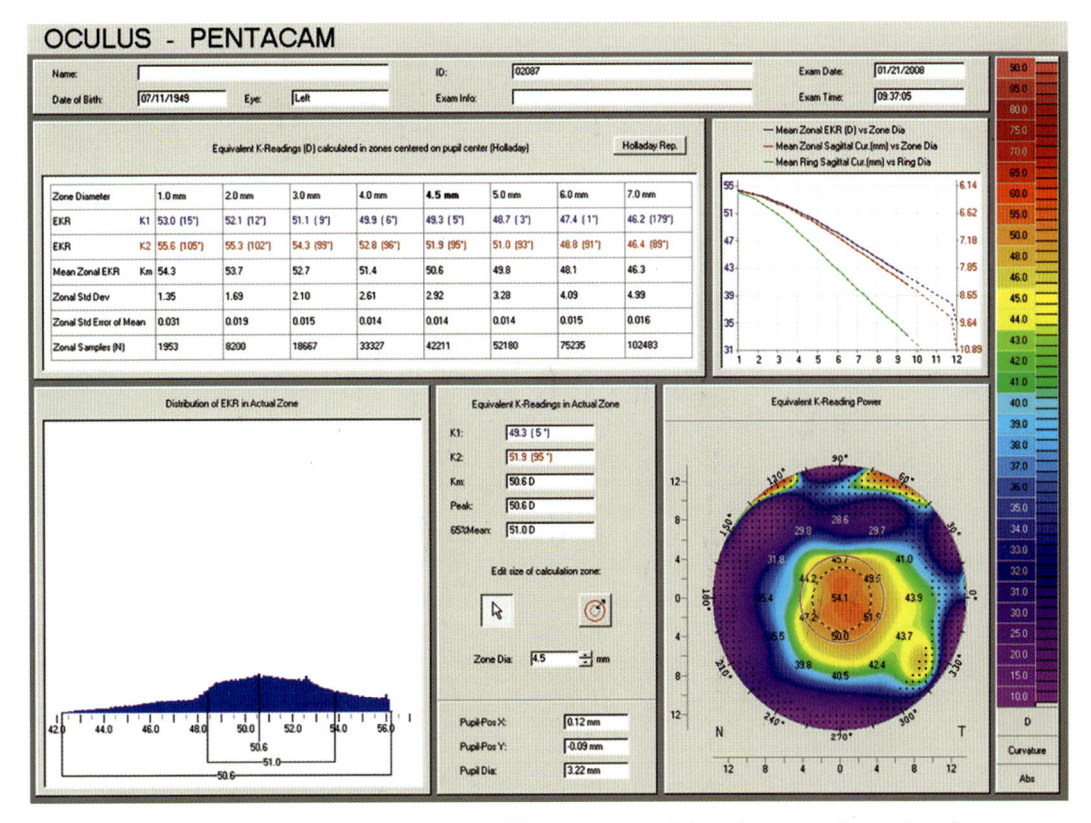

Figure 9.19 Various optical zones may be needed for cases of severely irregular astigmatism, such as shown in the EKR Detail Report in a patient with a history of repeated LASIK surgeries and central corneal scarring

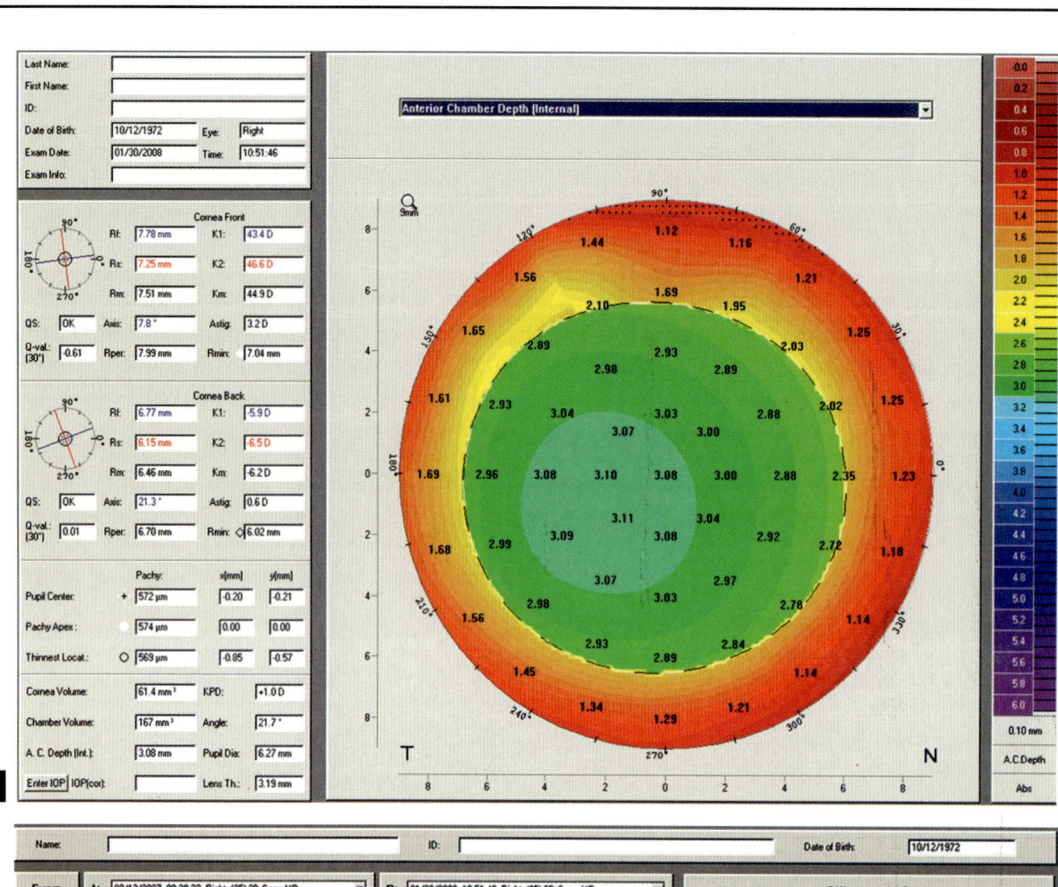

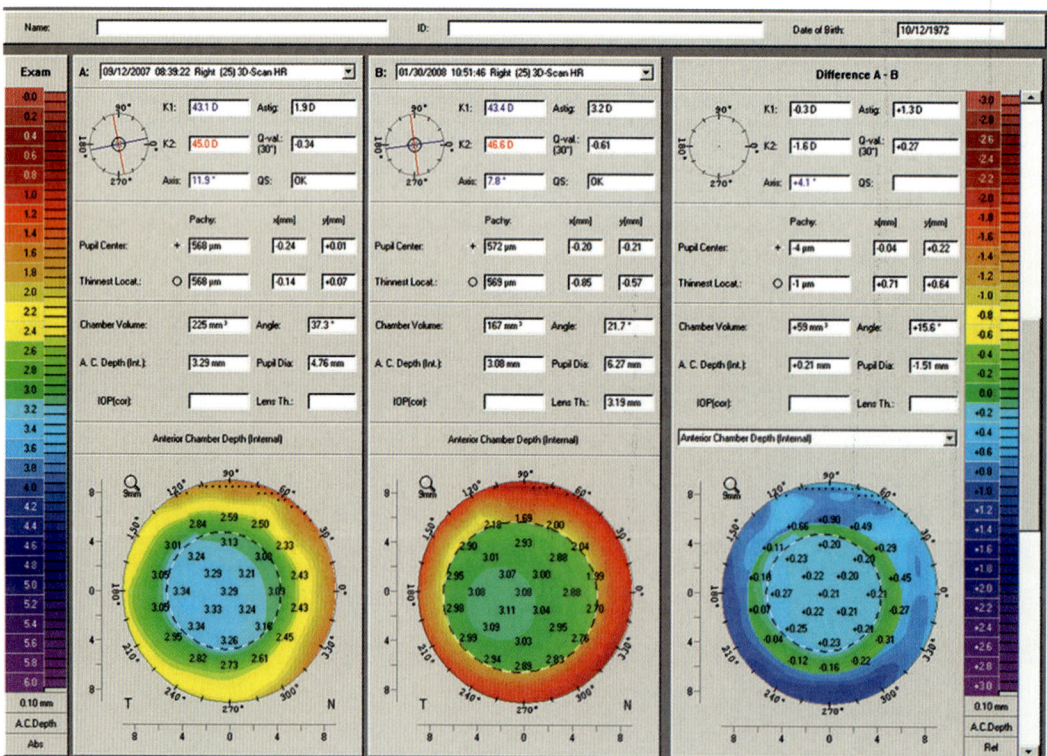

108 Section III: Pentacam and Anterior Segment Optical Coherence Tomography

Figures 9.20A and B (A) Anterior chamber display in a patient evaluated for increased IOP after Visian lens (Staar, Irvine, CA) implantation; (B) A difference map showing the AC information preoperatively, and after a Visian lens implantation. The plateau iris and physical bowing of the iris cause a mid-dilated pupil block, and increased pressure. The Scheimpflug image demonstrated the architecture of the iris was the cause of the pupil block. Note the decrease in the chamber angle

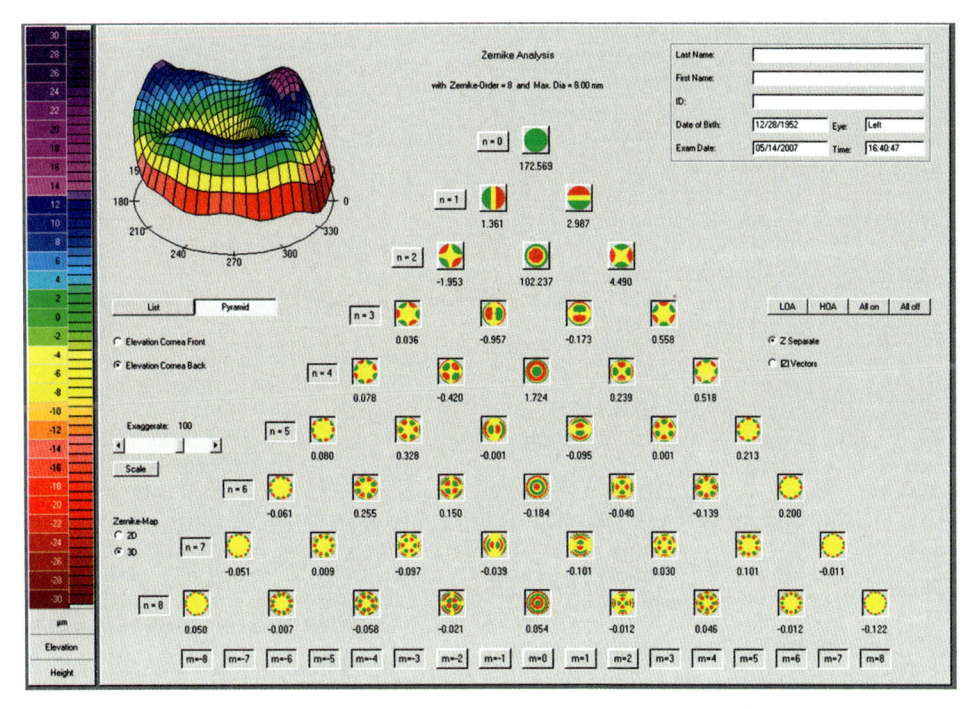

Figure 9.21 Corneal wavefront maps for the patient in Figure 9.5 with a history of CK

angle-closure glaucoma may be assessed using the Pentacam as well. Rabsiber et al found the good reliability with anterior chamber assessment, and suggested the Pentacam may be used to classify the potential risk for angle-closure glaucoma.[33]

Corneal Wavefront Evaluation

Pentacam describes the wavefront errors based on height data for the anterior and posterior surface. Note this is different from a wavefront aberrometer, which measures the whole eye wavefront error. Zernicke analysis is performed without a reference body, but rather compared to normative data (from healthy eyes). Abnormal values are highlighted for ease of detection. An example is shown in **Figure 9.21**. The Zernicke coefficients are used to calculate the aberration coefficient. A value of 0 denotes no aberration. Values greater than 1.0 may be visually significant.

Anterior Chamber Phakic Lens Simulation

The software simulation was created to assist surgeons with implantation of phakic lenses into the anterior chamber. Posterior chamber lenses cannot be imaged, as the Pentacam is not able to image structures behind the iris. Lens type and power can be chosen from the database, and software calculates the refractive lens power based on the manifest refraction entered by the clinician. Distances between the phakic lens, crystalline lens, and endothelium are displayed, and aging simulations are also available. The software assumes the crystalline lens grows at a rate of 18 microns per year, which overtime would cause the iris to move toward the cornea with age, crowding the anterior chamber and putting the endothelium at risk.

CONCLUSION

The Pentacam serves many purposes for the refractive surgeon: Elevation topography, cataract and anterior chamber evaluation, high resolution corneal imaging, corneal wavefront, pachymetry, and tomography. Applications include clinical diagnosis of ectasia, cataracts, glaucoma risk, etiology of reduced best corrected vision, and keratoconus, as well as aids for patient education. Its versatility makes it beneficial for the corneal and refractive surgeon.

REFERENCES

1. Maus M, Krober S, Swartz T, Belin M, Michaelson M, Sutphin J, Wang M. Pentacam. Wang M (Ed): Corneal Topography in the Wavefront Era, Slack, Inc; Thorofare, NJ 2006.
2. Holladay J. Tomography and Tomography Course Handout, AAO November 5, 2007. New Orleans, LA. http://www.docholladay.com/handouts/Topography%20&%20Tomography%20Course%20Handout%20Color%20Nov07.pdf accessed 2008.
3. Lackner B, Schmidinger G, Pieh S, Funovics MA, Skorpik C. Repeatability and reproducibility of central corneal thickness measurement with Pentacam, Orbscan, and ultrasound. Optom Vis Sci. 2005;82(10):892-9.

4. Barkana Y, Gerber Y, Elbaz U, Schwartz S, Ken-Dror G, Avni I, Zadok D. Central corneal thickness measurement with the Pentacam Scheimpflug system, optical low-coherence reflectometry pachymeter, and ultrasound pachymetry. J Cataract Refract Surg. 2005;31(9):1729-35.
5. O'Donnell C, Maldonado-Codina C. Agreement and repeatability of central thickness measurement in normal corneas using ultrasound pachymetry and the oculus Pentacam. Cornea. 2005;24(8):920-4.
6. Rosa N, Lanza M, Borrelli M, Polito B, Filosa ML, De Bernardo M. Comparison of central corneal thickness measured with Orbscan and Pentacam. J Refract Surg. 2007;23(9):895-9.
7. Amano S, Honda N, Amano Y, Yamagami S, Miyai T, Samejima T, Ogata M, Miyata K. Comparison of central corneal thickness measurements by rotating Scheimpflug camera, ultrasonic pachymetry, and scanning-slit corneal topography. Ophthalmology. 2006;113(6):937-41.
8. Fujioka M, Nakamura M, Tatsumi Y, Kusuhara A, Maeda H, Negi A. Comparison of Pentacam Scheimpflug camera with ultrasound pachymetry and noncontact specular microscopy in measuring central corneal thickness. Curr Eye Res. 2007;32(2):89-94.
9. Barkana Y, Gerber Y, Elbaz U, Schwartz S, Ken-Dror G, Avni I, Zadok D. Central corneal thickness measurement with the Pentacam Scheimpflug system, optical low-coherence reflectometry pachymeter, and ultrasound pachymetry. J Cataract Refract Surg. 2005;31(9):1729-35.
10. Al-Mezaine HS, Al-amro SA, Kangave D, Sadaawy A, Wehaib TA, Al-Obeidan S. Comparison between central corneal thickness measurements by Oculus Pentacam and ultrasonic pachymetry. Int ophthalmol. 2007;26. DOI10.1007/s 10792-007-9143-9.
11. Mohamed A Fakhry, Alberto Artola, José I Belda, Ma José Ayala, Jorge L Alio. Comparison of corneal pachymetry using ultrasound and Orbscan II. J Cataract Refract Surg. 2002;28:248-52.
12. Francesco Boscia, Maria Gabriella La Tegola, Giovanni Alessio, Carlo Sborgia. Accuracy of Orbscan optical pachymetry in corneas with haze. J Cataract Refract Surg. 2002;28:253-8.
13. Kim SW, Byun YJ, Kim EK, Kim TI. Central corneal thickness measurements in unoperated eyes and eyes after PRK for myopia using Pentacam Orbscan II, and ultrasonic pachymetry. J Refract Surg. 2007;23(9):888-94.
14. Chakrabarti HS, Craig JP, Brahma A, et al. Comparison of corneal thickness measurements using ultrasound and Orbscan slit-scanning topography in normal and post-LASIK eyes. J Cat Refract Surg. 2001:27;1823-8.
15. Iskander NG, Anderson Penno E, Peters NT, et al. Accuracy of Orbscan pachymetry measurements and DHG ultrasound pachymetry in primary laser *in situ* keratomileusis and LASIK enhancement procedures. J Cat Refract Surg. 2001;27;681-5.
16. Jain R, Dilraj G, Grewal SP. Repeatability of corneal parameters with Pentacam after laser *in situ* keratomileusis. Indian J Ophthalmol. 2007;55(5):341-7.
17. Hashemi H, Mehravaran S. Central corneal thickness measurement with Pentacam, Orbscan II, and ultrasound devices before and after laser refractive surgery for myopia. J Cataract Refract Surg. 2007;33(10):1701-7.
18. Ho T, Cheng AC, Rao SK, Lau S, Leung CK, Lam DS. Central corneal thickness measurements using Orbscan II, Visante, ultrasound, and Pentacam pachymetry after laser *in situ* keratomileusis for myopia. J Cataract Refract Surg. 2007;33(7):1177-82.
19. Ciolino JB, Khachikian SS, Belin MW. Comparison of corneal thickness measurements by ultrasound and Scheimpflug photography in eyes that have undergone laser *in situ* keratomileusis. Am J Ophthalmol. 2008;145(1):75-80.
20. Chen D, Lam AK. Intrasession and intersession repeatability of the Pentacam system on posterior corneal assessment in the normal human eye. J Cataract Refract Surg. 2007;33(3):448-54.
21. Jain R, Dilraj G, Grewal SP. Repeatability of corneal parameters with Pentacam after laser *in situ* keratomileusis. Indian J Ophthalmol. 2007;55(5):341-7.
22. Hashemi H, Mehravaran S. Corneal changes after laser refractive surgery for myopia: Comparison of Orbscan II and Pentacam findings. J Cataract Refract Surg. 2007;33(5):841-7.
23. Ciolino JB, Belin MW. Changes in the posterior cornea after laser *in situ* keratomileusis and photorefractive keratectomy. J Cataract Refract Surg. 2006;32(9):1426-31.
24. Quisling S, Sjoberg S, Zimmerman B, Goins K, Sutphin J. Comparison of Pentacam and Orbscan IIz on posterior curvature topography measurements in keratoconus eyes. Ophthalmology 2006;113(9):1629-32.
25. Emre S, Doganay S, Yologlu S. Evaluation of anterior segment parameters in keratoconic eyes measured with the Pentacam system. J Cataract Refract Surg. 2007;33(10):1708-12.
26. Ambrósio R Jr, Alonso RS, Luz A, Coca Velarde LG. Corneal-thickness spatial profile and corneal-volume distribution: Tomographic indices to detect keratoconus. J Cataract Refract Surg. 2006;32(11):1851-9.
27. Grewal SP, Jain R, Gupta R, Grewal D. Role of Scheimpflug imaging in traumatic intralenticular foreign body. Am J Ophthalmol. 2006;142(4):675-6.
28. Jain R, Grewal D, Gupta R, Grewal SP. Scheimpflug imaging in late capsular bag distention syndrome after phacoemulsification. Am J Ophthalmol. 2006;142(6):1083-5.
29. Grewal DS, Jain R, Brar GS, Grewal SP. Unilateral electric cataract: Scheimpflug imaging and review of the literature. J Cataract Refract Surg. 2007;33(6):1116-9.
30. Nemeth G, Vajas A, Kolozsvari B, Berta A, Modis L Jr. Anterior chamber depth measurements in phakic and pseudophakic eyes: Pentacam versus ultrasound device. J Cataract Refract Surg. 2006;32(8):1331-5.
31. Elbaz U, Barkana Y, Gerber Y, Avni I, Zadok D. Comparison of different techniques of anterior chamber depth and keratometric measurements. Am J Ophthalmol. 2007;143(1):48-53. Epub 2006 Sep 29.
32. Lackner B, Schmidinger G, Skorpik C. Validity and repeatability of anterior chamber depth measurements with Pentacam and Orbscan. Optom Vis Sci. 2005;82(9):858-61.
33. Rabsilber TM, Khoramnia R, Auffarth GU. Anterior chamber measurements using Pentacam rotating Scheimpflug camera. J. Cataract Refract Surg. 2006;32(3):456-9.

Chapter 10

Evaluation of Patients for Refractive Surgery with Visante Anterior Segment OCT and the Combined Data Link with ATLAS Corneal Topographer

Amin Ashrafzadeh (USA), Roger F Steinert (USA)

Optical coherence tomography (OCT) is a technique that uses light to create a two dimensional cross-section image of the eye. This technique allows for imaging of either the anterior segment or the posterior segment of the eye. Decision-making for refractive surgery is aided by evaluations in either the preoperative or postoperative stages.[1-4] The main focus of this chapter is to discuss the Visante Anterior Segment OCT, its properties, capabilities and functions in evaluation of patients being considered for excimer laser treatment and phakic intraocular lens implantation. Although one of the most common refractive surgery procedures is cataract extraction, that topic is outside the scope of this chapter.

The newest software version 3.0 of the Visante has created a datalink with the ATLAS Corneal Topographer. The capacity to combine the anterior surface data from the ATLAS with the pachymetric mapping of the Visante creates the capacity to calculate the posterior surface data. This posterior surface data plays an increasingly important role in consideration of excimer laser refractive surgery.

VISANTE ANTERIOR SEGMENT OPTICAL COHERENCE TOMOGRAPHY

Optical coherence tomography (OCT) is a noncontact, real-time technique that uses low energy infrared laser to image structures. The more commonly used retinal OCT uses 820 nm light which allows for excellent tissue penetration to the level of the retina. The Visante Anterior Segment OCT (Carl Zeiss Meditec, Dublin, California, USA) utilizes 1310 nm light which has greater absorption resulting in limited penetration. This allows for increased intensity of the light as decreased amounts reach the retina. As such, in the Visante, the light is 20 times more intense, giving a much greater signal to noise ratio. This increased intensity allows for increasing the speed in imaging by twenty times, yet retaining similar signal to noise ratio levels as the retinal OCT, but with resultant decreased motion artifact. Additionally, the 1310 nm light has reduced scattering and therefore better penetration through opaque tissue such as an opaque cornea and sclera. This results in better evaluation of the anterior segment and visualization of the angle and to a lesser degree, the ciliary body.

There are two modes to the Visante OCT: Standard resolution imaging and high resolution imaging. Standard resolution imaging provides a broader view of the anterior segment with a 16 mm width and 6 mm depth image. This provides a full overview of the anterior segment including cornea, anterior chamber, iris and both angles. The high resolution imaging mode (High Res Mode) provides a more detailed image with dimensions of 10 mm width with 3 mm depth. The High Res Mode is more appropriate for imaging of the cornea and any segment in need of detailed evaluation.

In the standard resolution mode the Visante performs 256 scans assessing the 16 by 6 mm area in 0.125 seconds. In the High Res Mode, the Visante performs 512 scans to assess the 10 by 3 mm area in 0.250 seconds. The resolution of the Visante images is limited by the spacing between the scans performed. The resolution of the Visante reaches 18 microns axially and 60 microns transversally.

In addition to a single scan, the operator has the option of selecting automatic dual or quad scans. The dual scan mode performs two scans—one at a selected orientation between 20° and 200° and the second scan between 160° and 340°. The quad scan mode performs four scans between the 0° and 180°, 45° and 225°, 90° and 270° and 135° and 315° axes. All scans in all modes can be rotated manually to any of the 180 axis lines at the discretion of the operator performing the imaging.

The Pachymetric Corneal Mapping (Pachy Map) module in the standard software performs 8 modified high resolution scans of the cornea in preset radial axis lines starting at 0° axis and rising at 22.5° intervals. The High Res Mode allows for the Pachy Map to be performed in 0.5 seconds with little artifactual distortions. The Pachy Map produces a 10 by 10 mm pachymetric map of the cornea, revealing the corneal thickness in all locations. The preset grid separates the cornea into the central 0 to 2 mm area along with eight radial regions at 2 to 5 mm, 5 to 7 mm, and 7 to 10 mm concentric to the central region. All areas produce 3 numbers, the thinnest area, noted as the top number, the average, noted as the middle number, and the thickest area, noted as the bottom number. The Global Pachy Map in the Visante 2.0 software performs 16 modified high resolution scans of the cornea in 1.0 second. The preset radial axis lines start at the 0° and rise at 11.25°

intervals. The Global Pachy Map is able to provide twice as many data points and therefore a more detailed evaluation. The repeatability of the Visante pachy map in the standard mode was noted at 7 micron standard deviation in the center and 14 micron standard deviation in the periphery.

The Visante is also equipped with an optometer capable of changing focus from a +20 diopters to a –35 diopters. As the optometer changes focus, accommodation can be induced and as such dynamic changes of the anterior segment can be quantitatively measured.

In the Visante 2.0 software, there is an additional enhanced mode for the anterior segment mode scan and the High Res Mode scan. In the enhanced mode, four consecutive scans are performed and compressed into a single image to produce a higher density, higher contrast image. Additionally, new software tools to produce a phakic IOL template and measurement tools for endothelial clearance and lens vault distance, along with more sophisticated angle measurement tools are among the many enrichments that have been devised.

Visante anterior segment OCT images can be used in evaluation of the refractive patient, both preoperatively and postoperatively. It is capable of providing broad overview images of the anterior segment and more detailed high resolutions of specific areas. Pachymetric mapping, angle evaluations, corneal flap evaluations, and phakic IOL templates are some of the useful features that will be demonstrated in examples in the remainder of this chapter.

ATLAS CORNEAL TOPOGRAPHER AND THE VISANTE 3.0 SOFTWARE

The ATLAS Corneal Topographer (Carl Zeiss Meditech, Dublin, CA, USA) is a noncontact placido disk based system that creates anterior surface computerized topographic information. The latest 3 models, the 993, 995, and the 9000 are capable of linking data with the Visante 3.0 Software.

The ATLAS 9000, which is the latest version, is a 22 ring placido disk system (18 superiorly and 22 inferiorly) that uses nonvisible 950 nm infrared light. The information obtained is from the reflection of the rings from the corneal surface. Therefore, the data obtained as such pertains only to the anterior corneal surface.

The Visante 3.0 version is upgraded with a tracking device so that once the corneal pachymetric mapping is commenced the device will keep the sequential scans centered to the same location. Additionally, the vertex of the cornea is recognized as the point with greatest signal in a vertical scan. The vertex of the ATLAS scans and the Visante pachymetric scans are matched to represent the same location. By using the corneal thickness map (pachymetric data), with known anterior surface curvature data from the ATLAS, the posterior corneal curvature data may be calculated **(Figure 10.1)**.

LASIK PATIENTS

In evaluation of a patient for LASIK eye surgery, the Visante is able to provide preoperative pachymetric mapping of the cornea, evaluation of the angles, and any corneal pathology. In evaluation of post-LASIK surgery patients, detailed anatomical data may be obtained to further guide in clinical decision making. In combination with the ATLAS topography, the Visante 3.0 software is able to provide a more comprehensive set of data including the posterior corneal curvature both pre- and postoperatively.

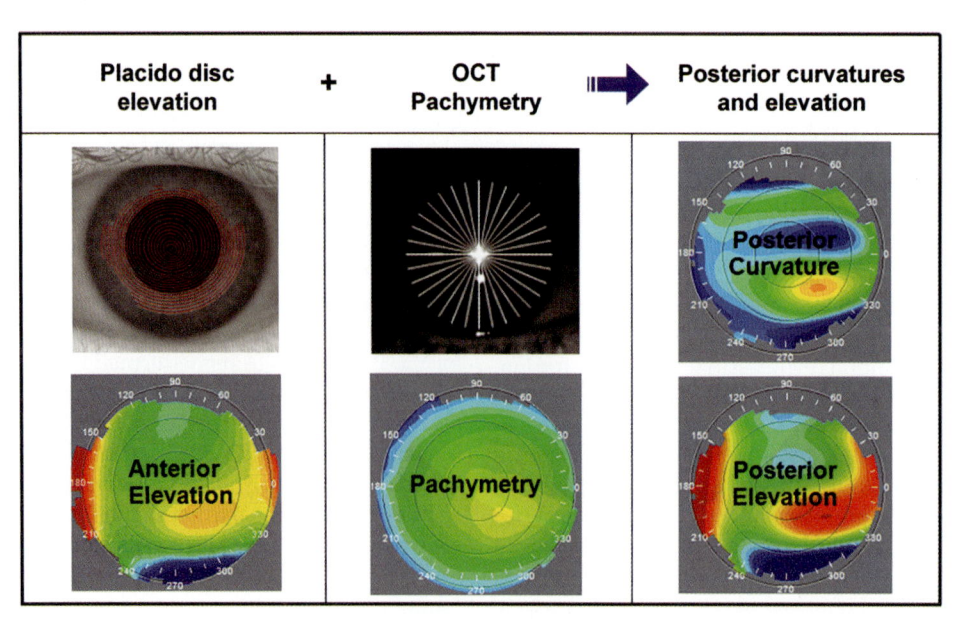

Figure 10.1 The anterior corneal elevation and curvature data from the placedo disc technology of ATLAS is added to the corneal pachymetric data of the Visante to derive the posterior corneal curvature and elevation data

Chapter 10: Evaluation of Patients for Refractive Surgery with Visante Anterior ...

Pachymetric Mapping

The pachymetric mapping of the cornea combined with the corneal topographic map provides a powerful set of information. This information may be especially important in cases where possibility of corneal ectasia is raised. A normal pachymetric map of the cornea (**Figure 10.2**) has the thinnest portion in the center with concentrically thicker tissue as it approaches the periphery. A 19 years old male presented for consideration of LASIK eye surgery with refractions of –1.75–0.25 × 111 in the right eye and –2.00 Sphere in the left eye with best corrected vision of a weak 20/20–. His corneal topographies (**Figure 10.3**)

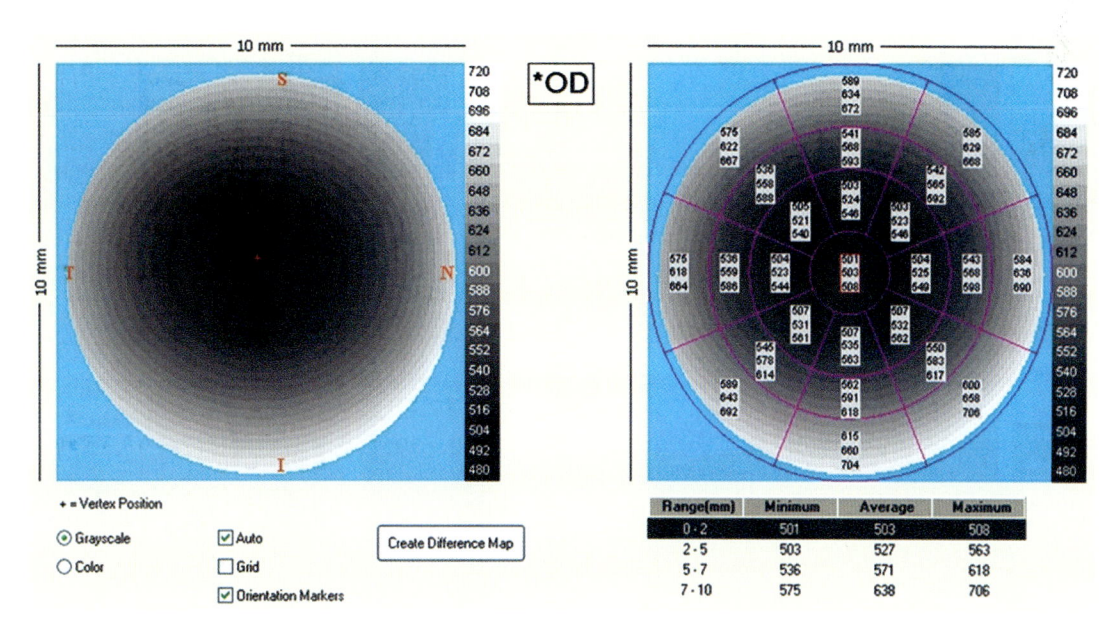

Figure 10.2 Normal pachymetric map of the cornea, demonstrating thinnest area in the center with concentric thickening of the tissue towards the periphery

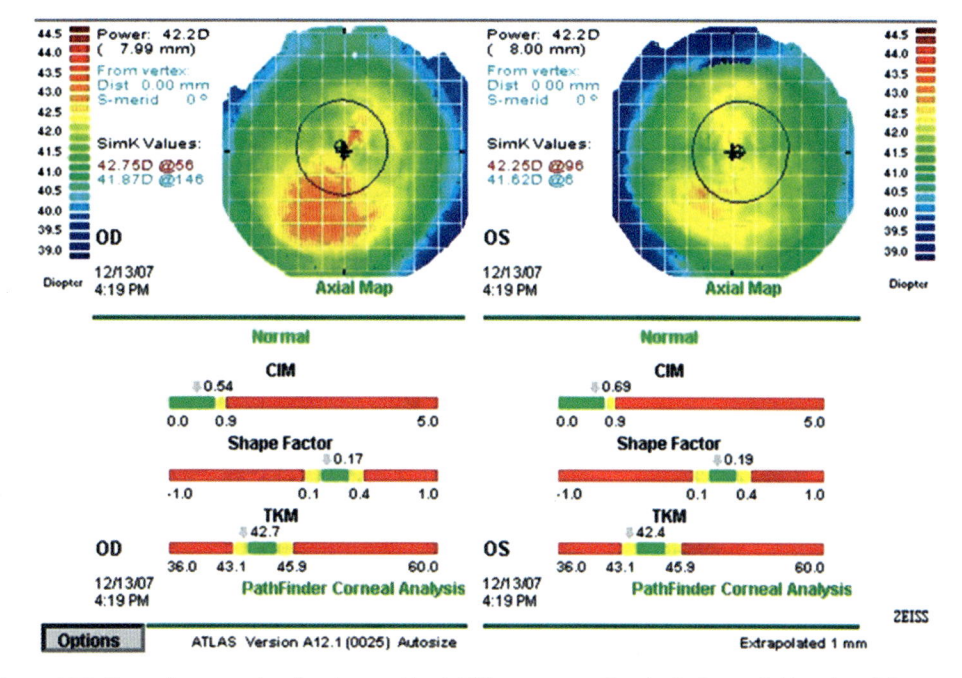

Figure 10.3 Corneal topography of patient seeking LASIK eye surgery. See the Pachymetric Mapping of the cornea in Figures 10.4 to 10.6. Figures 10.7 and 10.8 are the Holladay reports from Visante 3.0 software

were interpreted by the computer software as normal (PathFinder Corneal Analysis Software, ATLAS Topographer, Carl Zeiss Meditec, Dublin, California, USA). Slight interior steepening of the right eye prompted concerns of possible forme fruste keratoconus. A global Pachy Map of both eye **(Figures 10.4 to 10.6)** revealed an inferotemporal thinning, consistent with bilateral inferotemporal steepening on the topography. The Visante 3.0 Holladay analysis with a toric ellipsoid best corneal fit is shown in **Figures 10.7 and 10.8**. This six figured analysis starts with anterior axial curvature in top left and anterior tangential curvature in the bottom left, followed by Visante Pachymap in the center top and the relative pachymetry in the center bottom, and the anterior elevation top left and posterior elevation bottom left. This format places all pertinent data into a single printout for comprehensive review. Diagnosis of forme fruste keratoconus was entertained given the relative unusual display, 6 micron protrusion above the best-fit toric-ellipsoid curvature and the patient's age and he was encouraged to continue with his regular corrective methods and not consider excimer laser therapy at this time.

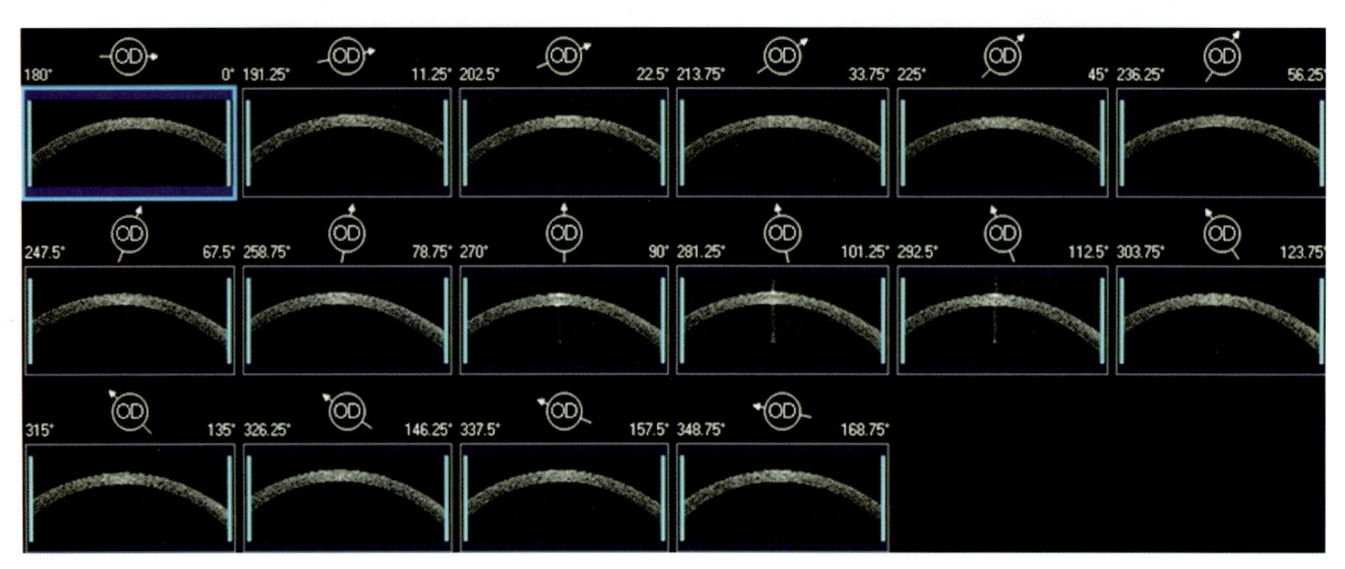

Figure 10.4 Global Pachymetric Map is created from 16 modified High Res Images as noted in this figure

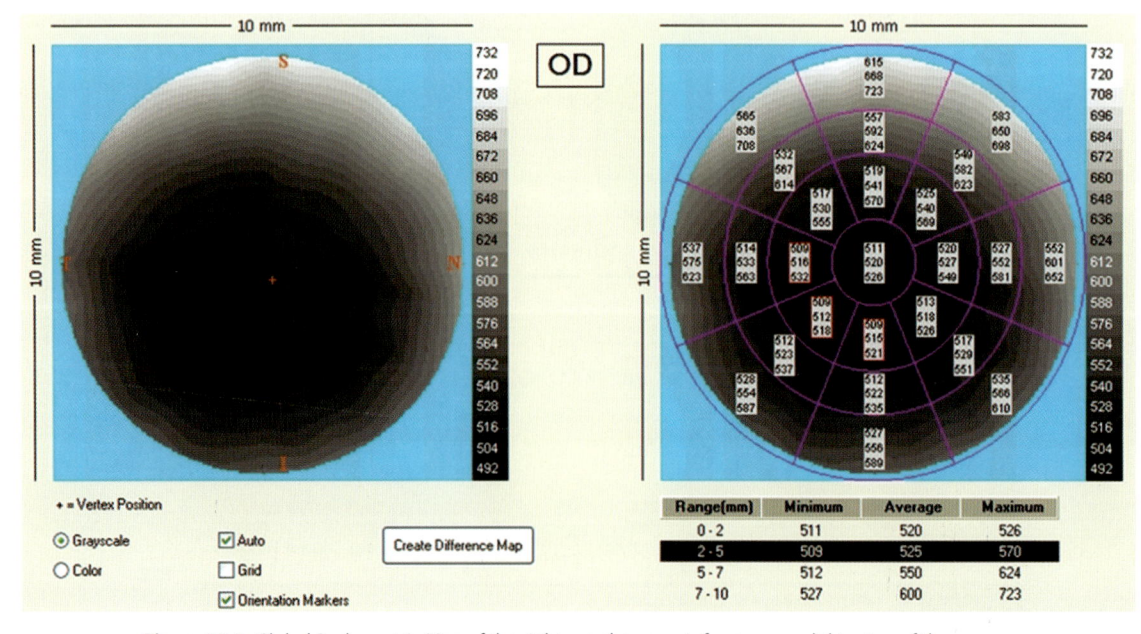

Figure 10.5 Global Pachymetric Map of the right eye shows an inferotemporal thinning of the cornea

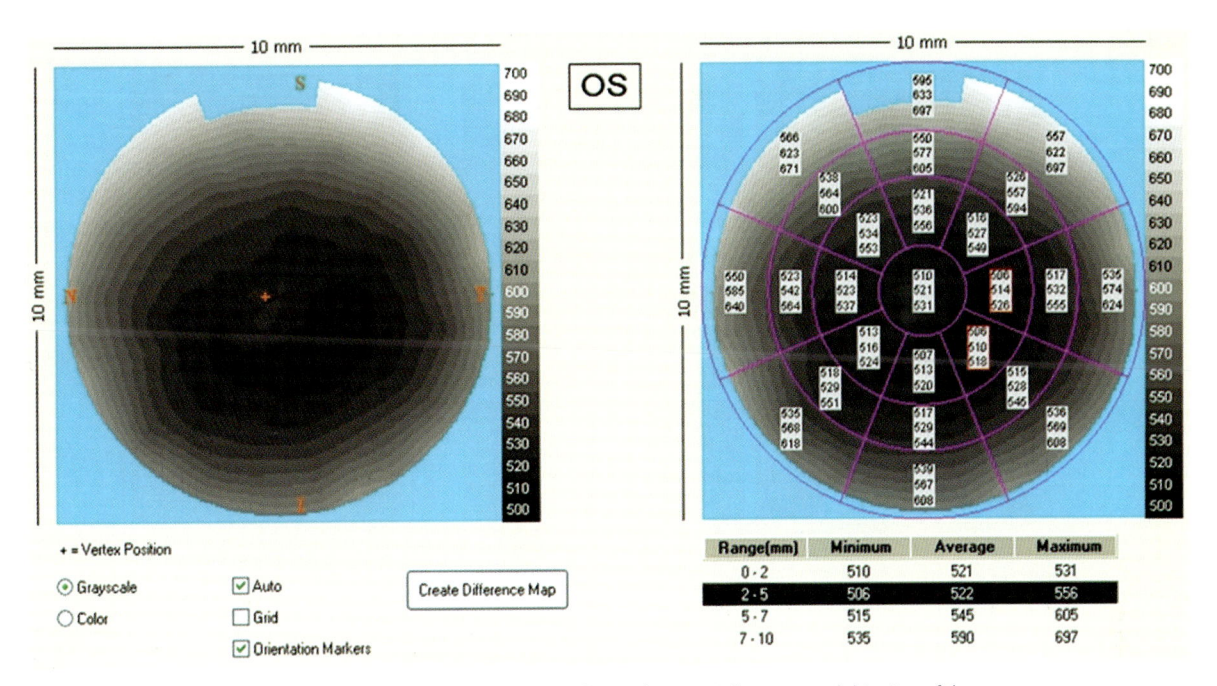

Chapter 10: Evaluation of Patients for Refractive Surgery with Visante Anterior ... 115

Figure 10.6 Global Pachymetric Map of the left eye showing inferotemporal thinning of the cornea

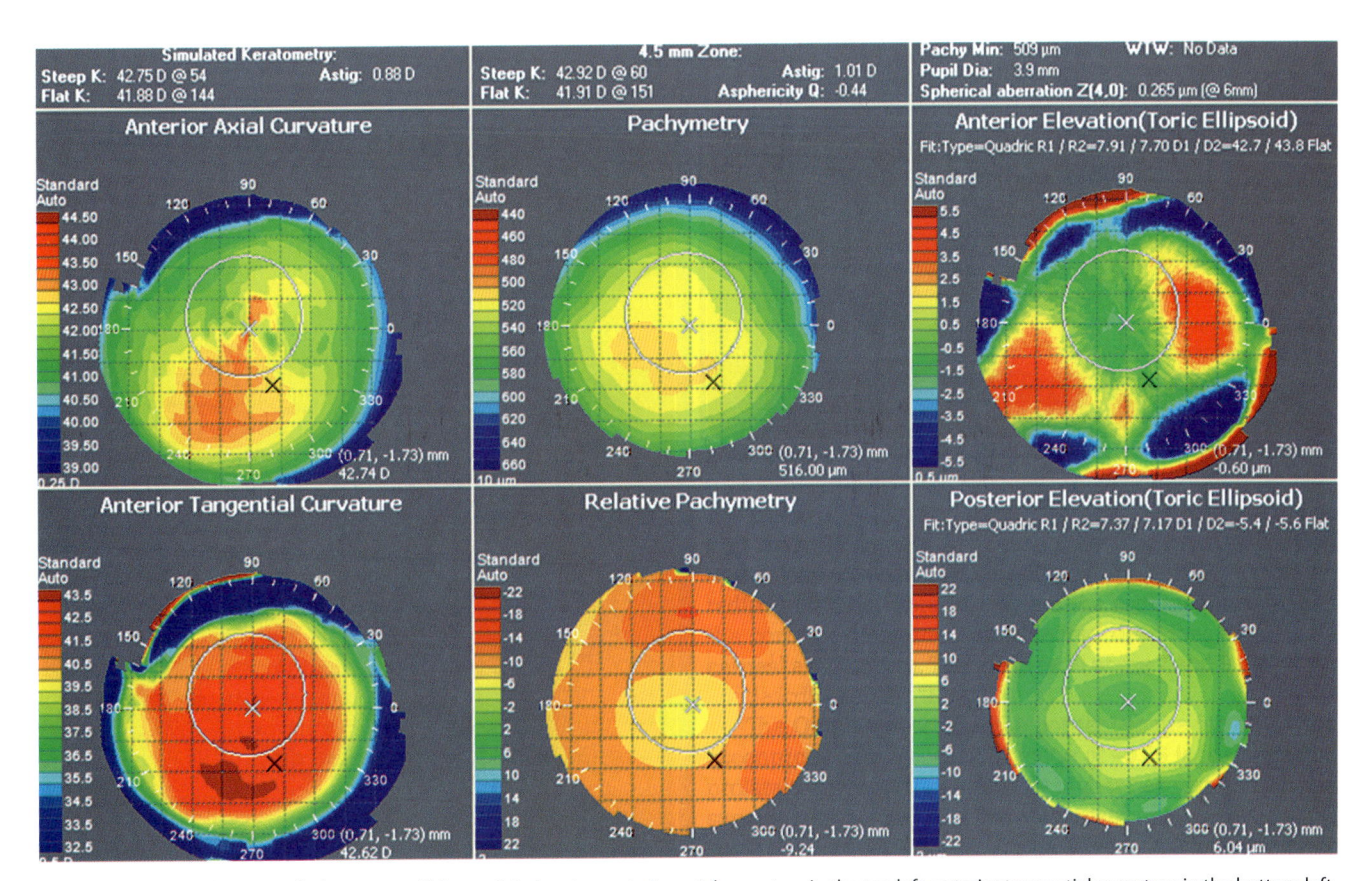

Figure 10.7 The right eye Holladay report of Visante 3.0 showing anterior axial curvature in the top left, anterior tangential curvature in the bottom left, Visante pachymetric map in the top center, relative pachymetry in the bottom center, best-fit toric ellipsoid anterior elevation curvature in the top right and best-fit toric ellipsoid posterior elevation curvature in the bottom right showing a 6 micron elevation above the sphere

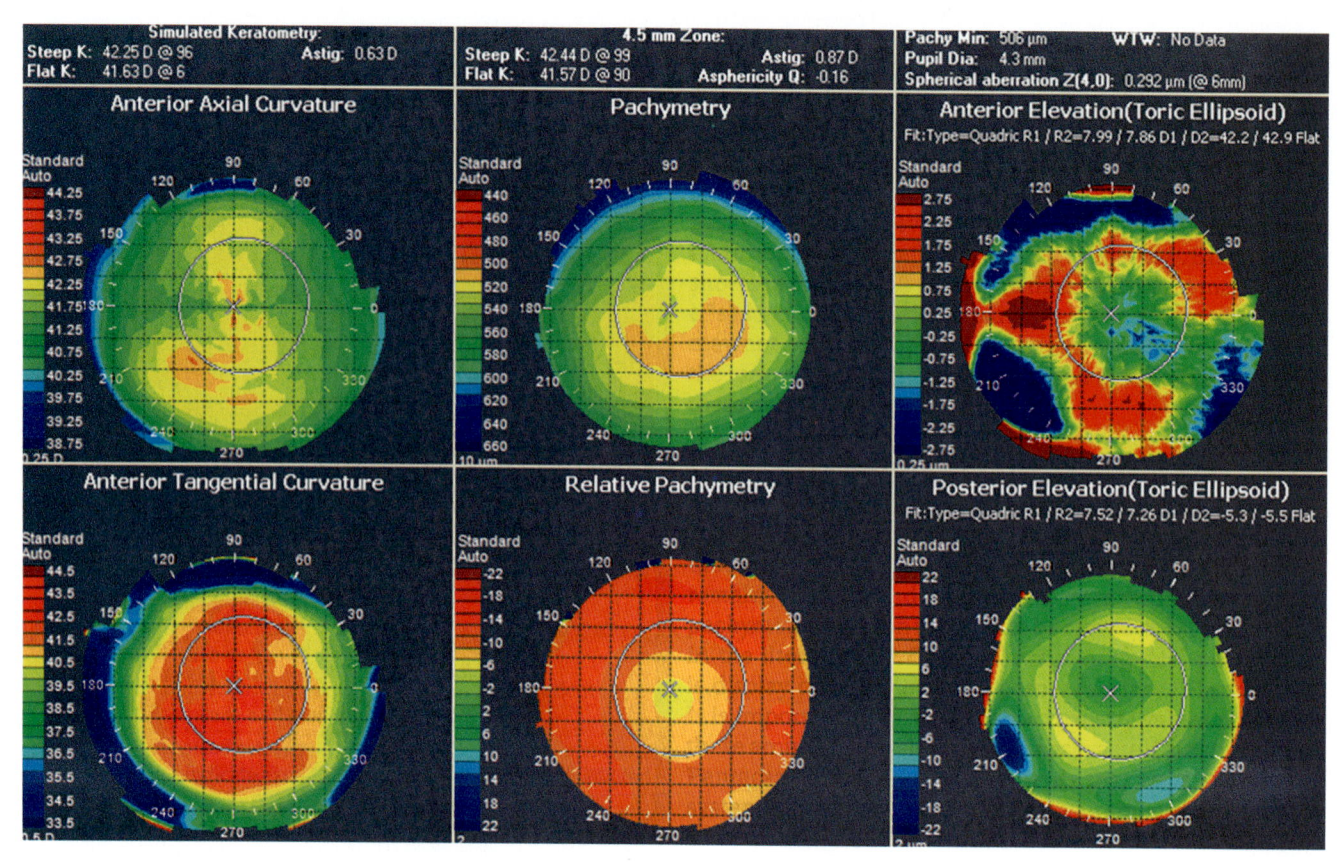

Figure 10.8 The left eye Holladay report of Visante 3.0

To counter balance the previous example, here is the case of a 13 years old male patient with rapidly progressive keratoconus. He underwent standard penetrating keratoplasty 11 months earlier in his left eye. In the span of 11 months his keratometric measurement in his fellow right eye had progressed from mean of 48 to 58 diopters. His vision had also declined from best corrected 20/20 to 20/400. In his preoperative evaluation for IntraLase Enabled Keratoplasty, the Pachy Map (**Figure 10.9**) revealed a perfectly normal pattern of pachymetric distribution, despite the clearly pathologic cornea. This case is to demonstrate that one must consider the pachymetric mapping only as an augmentation of information in consideration of LASIK surgery and may appear normal despite such advanced pathology.

The following are three examples of classic cases that may be seen in cornea and refractive clinics. A thirty years old male presented for LASIK evaluation with refractions of +3.75–5.50 × 015 OD and +3.75–5.00 × 180 OS with best corrected visual acuities of 20/15—each eye. Central ultrasound pachymetries were 502 OD and 504 OS with keratometric readings of 43.12, 48.12 D @ 096 OD and 43.37, 48.12 D @ 090 OS. **Figure 10.10** shows the Holladay report with completely normal posterior corneal maps with no protrusion (–0.25 microns) above best-fit toric ellipsoid curvature. He underwent CustomVue, IntraLase LASIK eye surgery with Iris Registration (iLASIK) (Advanced Medical Optics, Inc., Santa Ana, CA, USA) and enjoys a 20/20 uncorrected vision each eye.

A forty-four years old male with history of keratoconus and corneal transplant in the right eye has maintained a stable cornea in the left eye. A Holladay report of the left native cornea clearly shows the anterior axial curvature to be keratoconic. The posterior curvature clearly shows an inferotemporal protrusion of 53.04 microns above the best fit toric ellipsoid curvature (**Figure 10.11**).

A fifty-four years old female with history of pellucid marginal degeneration with stable refraction has the Holladay report for the left eye presented in **Figure 10.12**. The top left anterior axial curvature is a typical "crab claw" or "kissing bird beaks" display classic for pellucid marginal degeneration. Visante pachymap in the top center shows an off center corneal thinning. The bottom right image shows the inferior corneal protrusion of 86.55 microns above the best-fit toric ellipsoid sphere.

Angle Evaluation

In care of a refractive patient, one must never overlook the ophthalmic care that may be required. A fifty-five years old

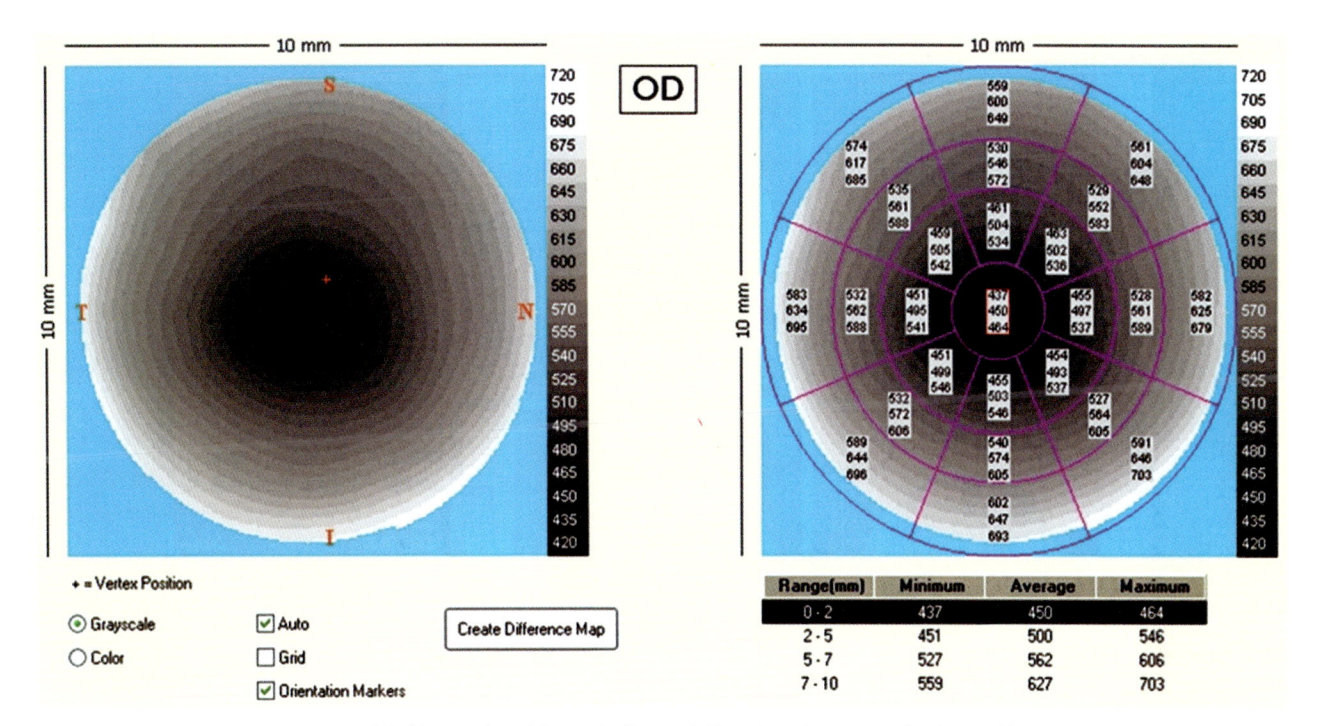

Chapter 10: Evaluation of Patients for Refractive Surgery with Visante Anterior ...   117

Figure 10.9 Pre-IntraLase enabled keratoplasty Visante Pachymetric Mapping of patient with advanced keratoconus and central keratometric readings of 58 diopters

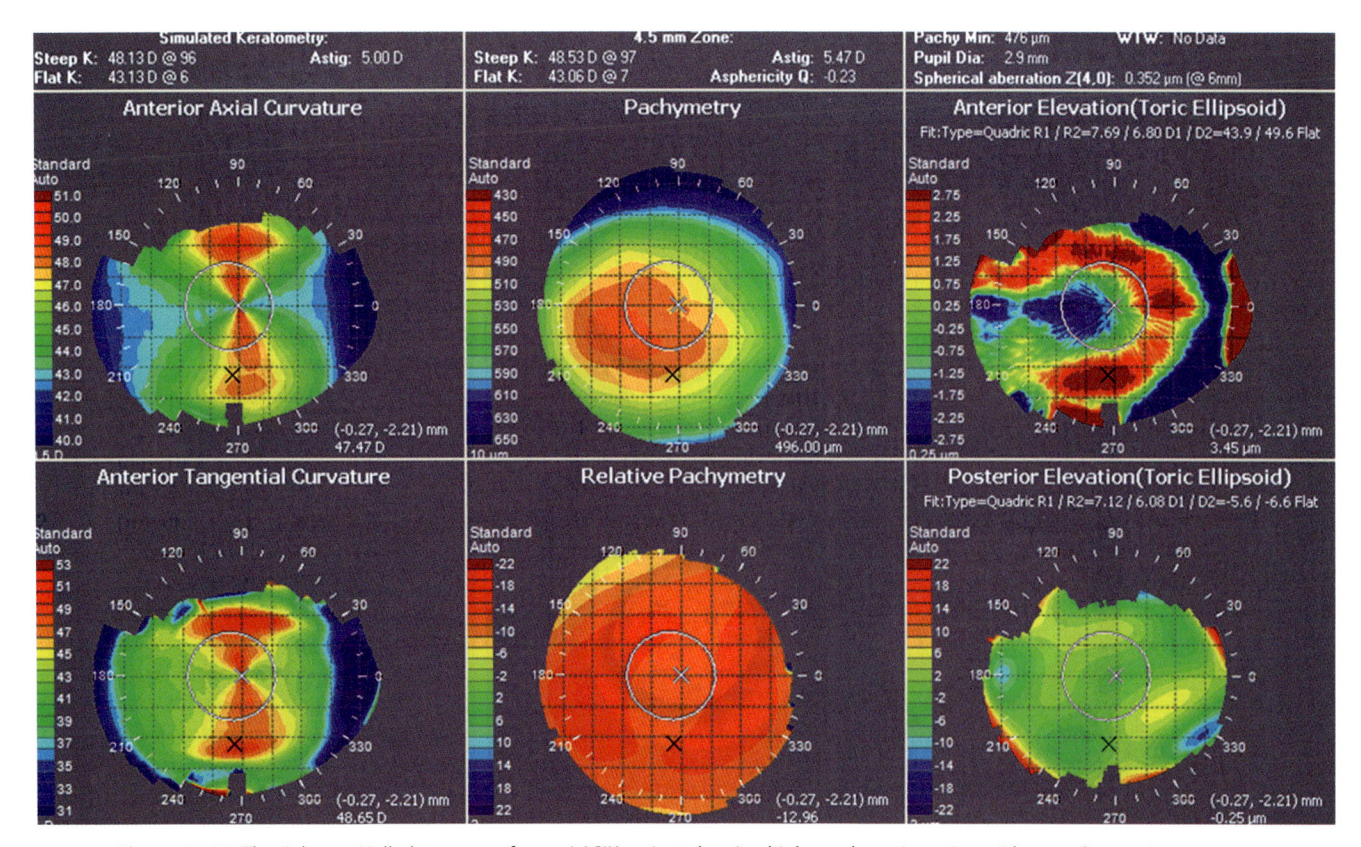

Figure 10.10 The right eye Holladay report of a pre-LASIK patient showing high regular astigmatism with normal posterior curvature

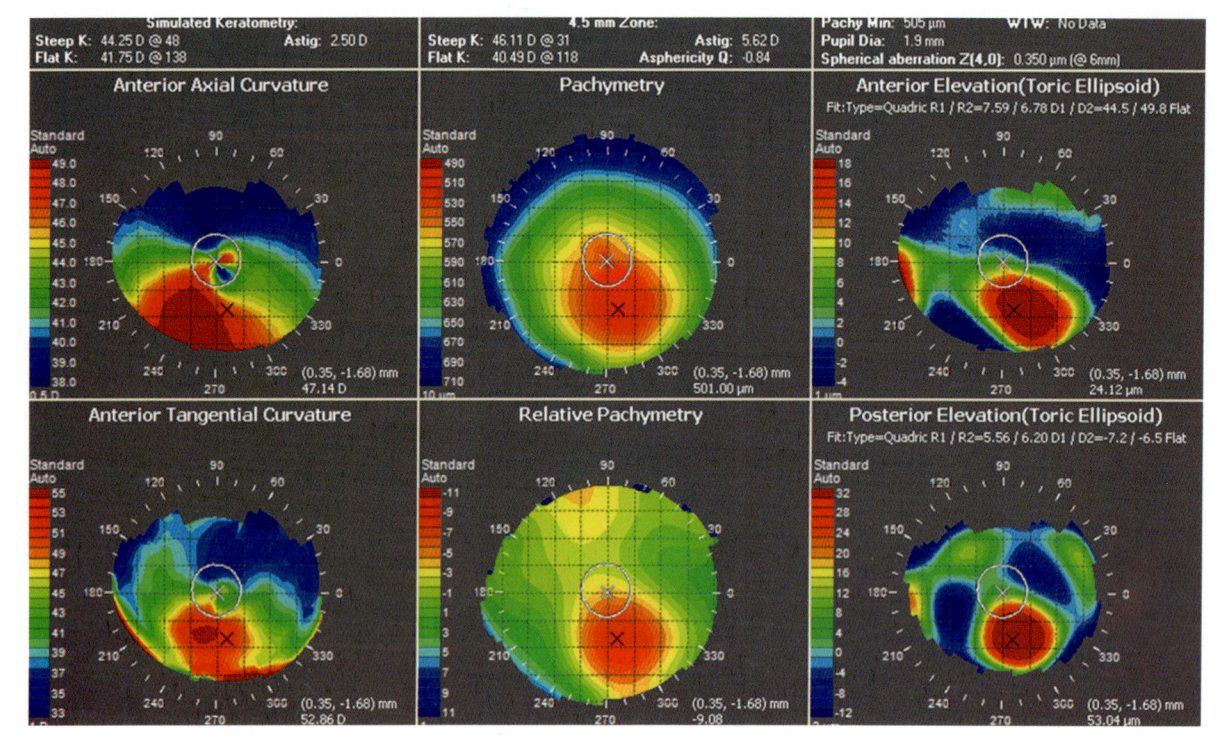

118 Section III: Pentacam and Anterior Segment Optical Coherence Tomography

Figure 10.11 The left eye Holladay report of a known stable keratoconic patient showing a 53 micron protrusion above the best-fit posterior toric-ellipsoid sphere

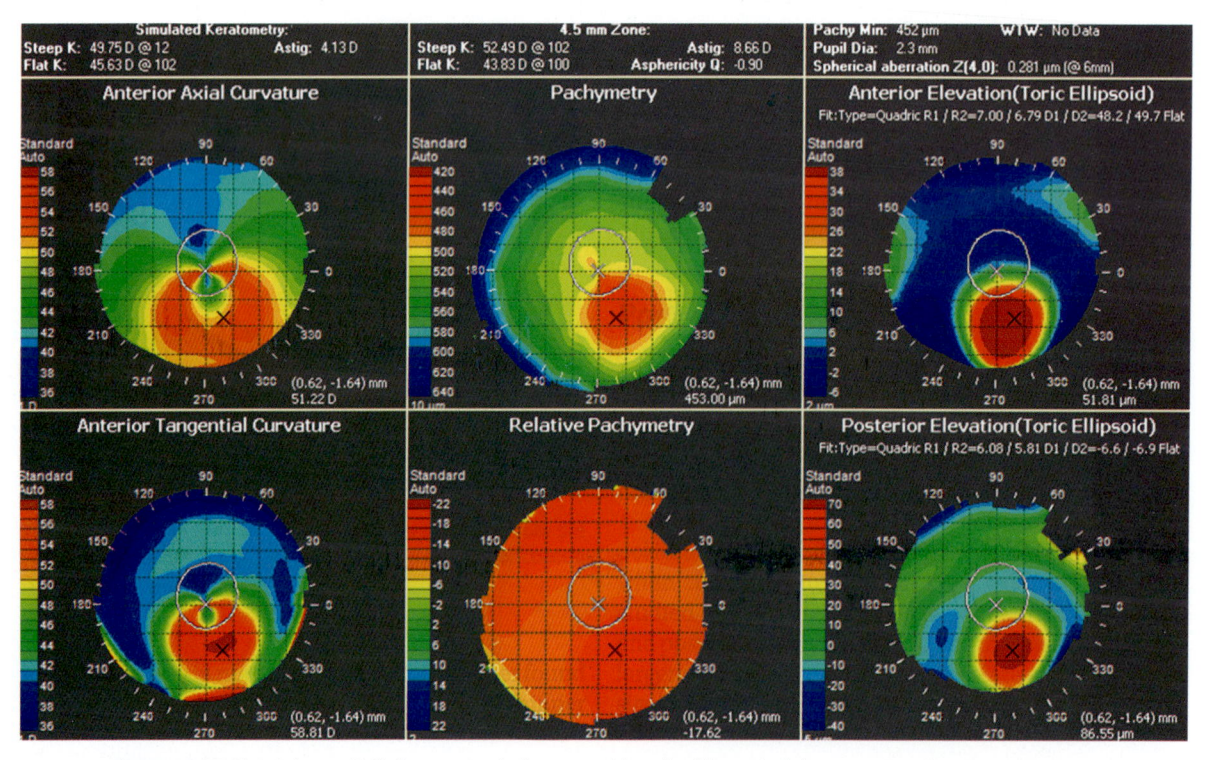

Figure 10.12 The right eye Holladay report of a known stable pellucid marginal degeneration showing a 86 micron protrusion of the cornea above the best-fit posterior toric-ellipsoid sphere

Chapter 10: Evaluation of Patients for Refractive Surgery with Visante Anterior ...   119

female patient with 2.00 diopters of hyperopia presented for LASIK eye surgery. Preoperative Visante evaluation, **Figure 10.13**, revealed narrow angles of approximately 10 degrees. Moderate anterior bowing of the posterior iris pigmented line can be noted. Peripheral iridotomies were performed weeks prior to her LASIK eye surgery. After the iridotomy, **Figure 10.14**, despite the fact that the pupil is larger compared to the preoperative image, the angles are significantly more open at approximately 25 degrees with near complete flattening of the posterior pigmented iris lines. As compared with standard slit-lamp gonioscopic examination of the eye, the angle is identified quantitatively with multiple methods of calculated angle area and distance measurements. Trabecular-iris space area (TISA) and angle opening distance (AOD) are both measured at 500 microns and 750 microns away from the scleral spur. The AOD is defined as the distance perpendicularly away from the trabecular meshwork/endothelial surface to the surface of the iris. The TISA is a trapezoidal area bordered by the AOD at 500 µm or 750 µm, and a line drawn perpendicularly from the scleral spur to the iris. The ability to acquire and present all this information in real-time to a patient represents a major advance in both diagnosis and patient education.

Corneal Pathology

A forty-four years old female contact lens user had developed a corneal ulcer in her dominant eye five years earlier with complete healing and resolution; however, best corrected visual acuity had been reduced to 20/40. The patient was seeking consultation for LASIK eye surgery. Her cornea was noted to have a paracentral scar with concordant flattening

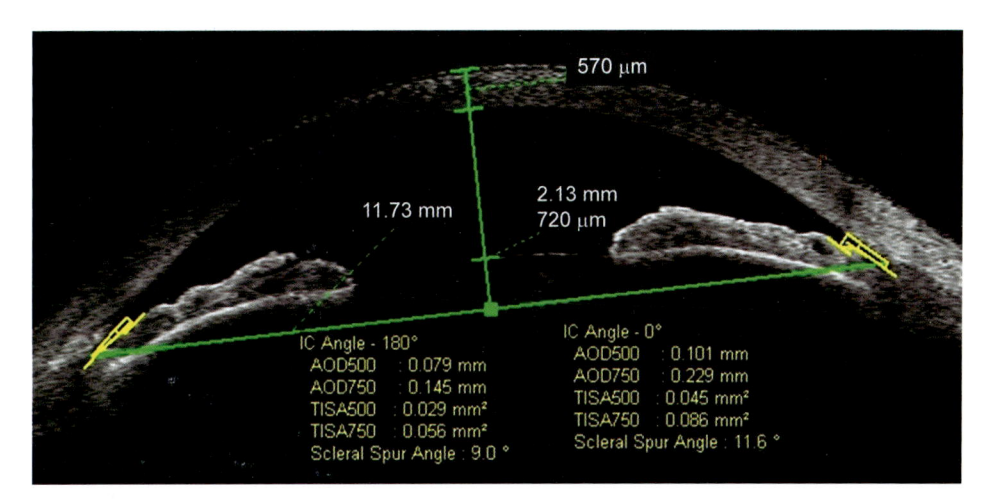

Figure 10.13 Preoperative evaluation of the anterior segment of a patient with 2 diopters of hyperopia in consideration of LASIK

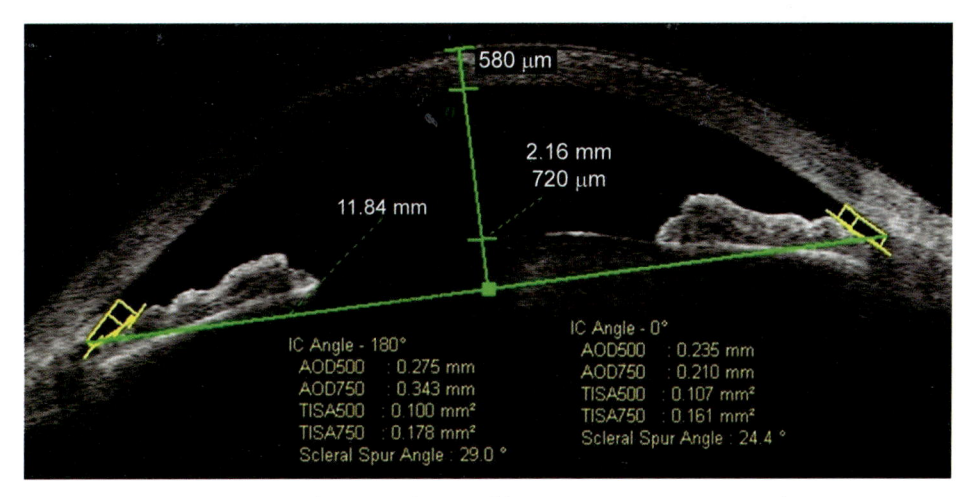

Figure 10.14 Postiridotomy evaluation of the same patient as Figure 10.1, showing greater opening of the angle and flatting of the posterior pigmented iris line

on the topographic map **(Figure 10.15)**. Her preoperative refraction was –4.00-1.50 × 110 leading to 20/40 vision. The Visante was used to measure the depth of tissue loss, epithelial filing and the corneal scar **(Figure 10.16)**. A decision was made to correct this eye conservatively with stepwise approach. As such treatment of only –2.25-1.50 × 110 was delivered via photorefractive keratectomy. Six months after the PRK, patient was elated with 20/25+ uncorrected visual acuity and correctable to 20/20 with plano –0.75 × 135. The corneal topography **(Figure 10.17)** can also be noted to have improved mire rings. The corneal scar although not obliterated by the excimer laser was reduced in thickness and opacity intensity **(Figure 10.18)**. Additionally, the epithelial pooling over the depressed scar area is also noted to be significantly less. It can

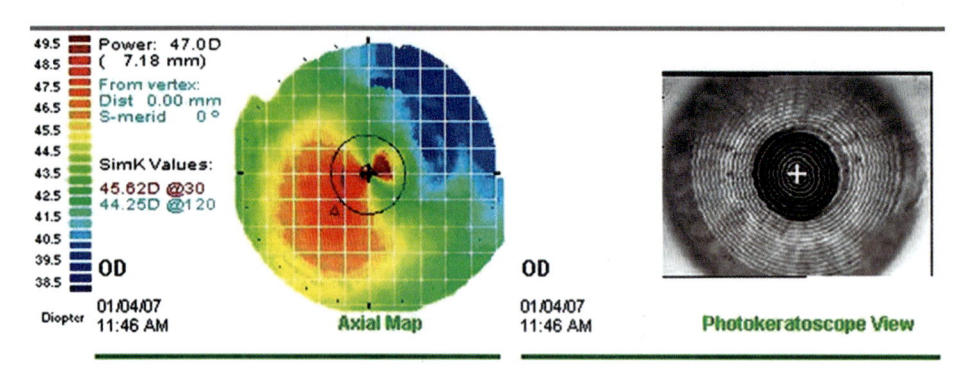

Figure 10.15 Corneal topography prior to PRK showing area of flattening associated with corneal scar at 2 o'clock paracentral position

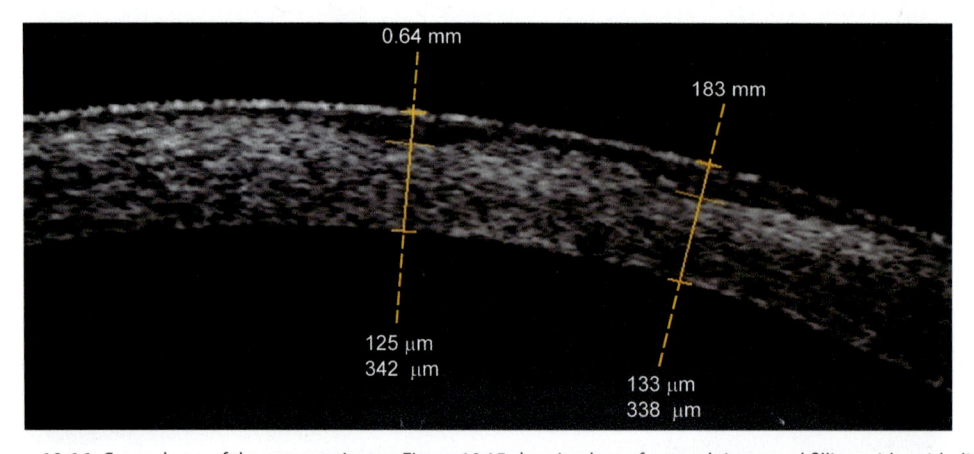

Figure 10.16 Corneal scar of the same patient as Figure 10.15 showing loss of corneal tissue and filling with epithelium

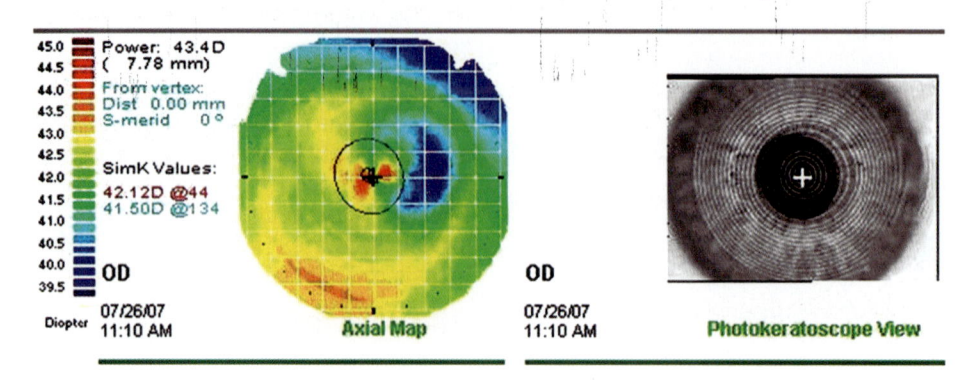

Figure 10.17 Corneal topography of the same patient as Figure 10.15 after her PRK

Chapter 10: Evaluation of Patients for Refractive Surgery with Visante Anterior ... 121

also be noted that the Bowman's membrane noted as a black line under the white epithelium in **Figure 10.16** is obliterated and nonexistent in **Figure 10.18** after PRK.

Flap Evaluation

In evaluation of postoperative LASIK patients who may be considering enhancement, the Visante can provide detailed information that would be essential to the safety of the procedure. The Visante can provide details of corneal flap shape and regularity. The LASIK flaps are created using either a mechanical microkeratome or a femtosecond laser microkeratome. An example of a mechanical microkeratome flap created using the Amadeus II (Ziemer Ophthalmic Group AG, Switzerland) **(Figure 10.19)** can be noted to have a tapered edge with thicker peripheral flap and thinner central flap. This configuration is referred to as the meniscus flap. An example of a femtosecond laser microkeratome flap created using the IntraLase (Advanced Medical Optics, Inc., Santa Ana, California, USA) shows a sharp 70 degree flap edge and an evenly thick flap throughout **(Figure 10.20)**. This flap configuration is referred to as the linear flap.

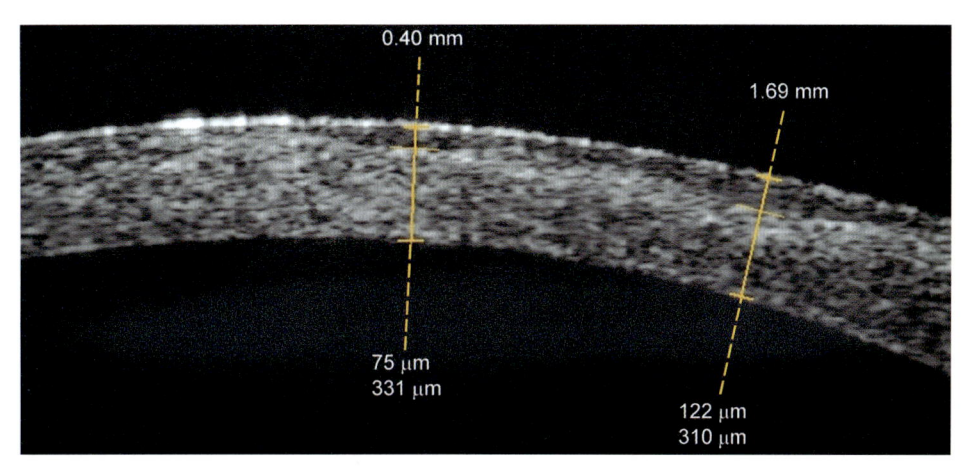

Figure 10.18 Corneal scar of the same patient as Figure 10.15 after PRK

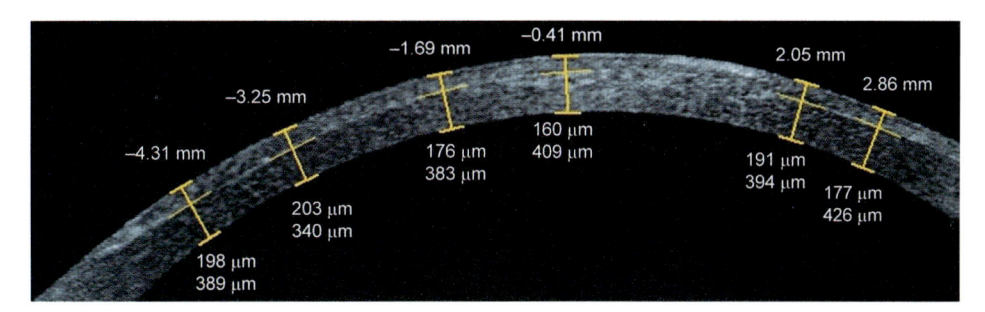

Figure 10.19 Amadeus II microkeratome created flap showing the tapered flap edge and meniscus flap configuration

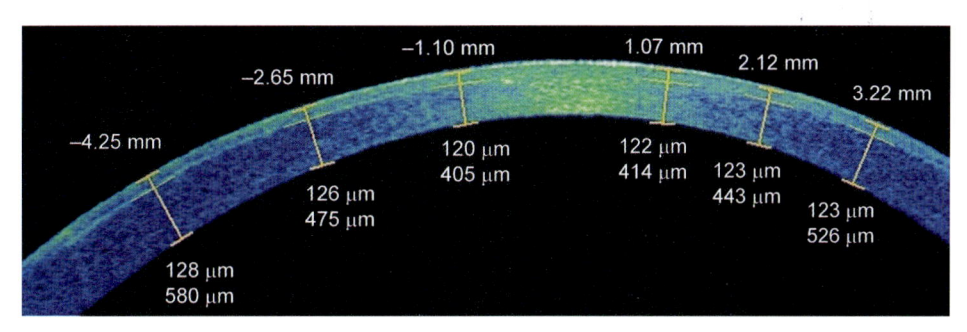

Figure 10.20 IntraLase created LASIK flap with vertical edge and linear flap configuration

A thirty-five years old male patient had LASIK eye surgery 5 years previously elsewhere and no records were available. A LASIK flap with jagged edge could be noted peripherally. The Visante was able to demonstrate presence of a very thin LASIK flap **(Figure 10.21)**. A decision was made to perform a surface ablation rather than to try to lift the previous LASIK flap. The patient obtained 20/15 vision postoperatively.

A thirty five years old female with a refraction of –8.00 –2.75 × 020 with central corneal thickness of 515 microns had CustomVue, IntraLase LASIK eye surgery with Iris Registration (iLASIK) (Advanced Medical Optics, Inc., Santa Ana, California, USA). One can note in **Figure 10.22**, the central residual stromal bed remaining after the initial iLASIK is only in the range of 280 microns. Postoperative refraction stable over 6 months is –0.25–1.75 × 010 and **Figure 10.23** provides a supportive data of regular best-fit toric ellipsoid posterior curvature. There may be as many opinions and options regarding the safety of LASIK and its enhancements in this patient as there are residual microns left, but the data provided allows the individual patient and surgeon to discuss the plan and practice the art of medicine in this case. In this iLASIK case one may note the 70° flap edge on the left side of the image and the linear flap thickness created by the IntraLase femtosecond laser. Although the range of the flap thickness is measured from 107 to 118 microns, one must also note the limitation in gradation of the flap tool in the Visante software that may be stepwise and in accordance to the resolution limits of the hardware. In specific, the axial resolution of the Visante is 18 microns and has a repeatability of +/–7 microns in measurement of the flap and +/– 11 microns in the measurement of the stromal tissue. It should also be noted that flap visibility is diminished overtime. The sensitivity at 1 day is noted at 99% and 95% at 6 months.

Complication Evaluation

A thirty-eight years old male, who had LASIK eye surgery 8 years previously elsewhere with no records available, presented for LASIK enhancement. The Visante was able to clearly demonstrate the flap and residual stromal bed thickness. Patient was assured that LASIK enhancement via lifting of the flap could be performed. The patient however, developed epithelial ingrowth postenhancement. The patient

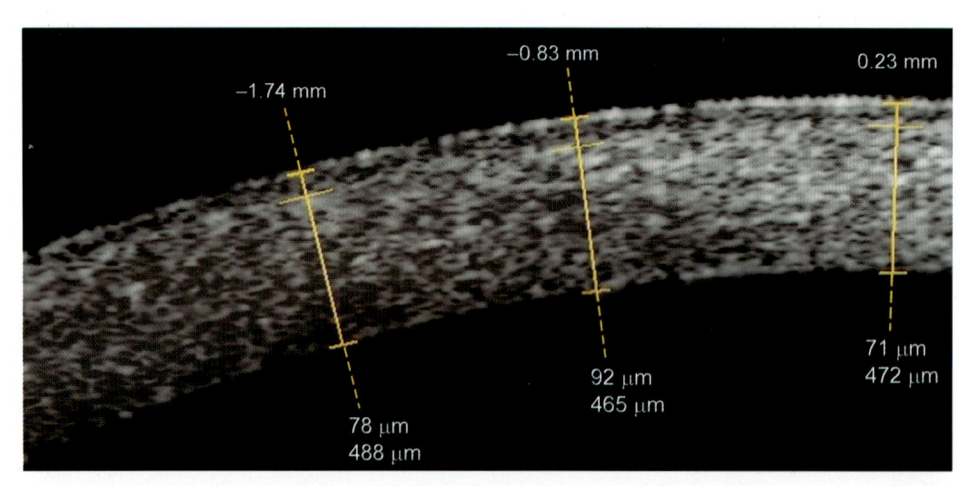

Figure 10.21 Patient asking for enhancement 5 years after initial LASIK surgery

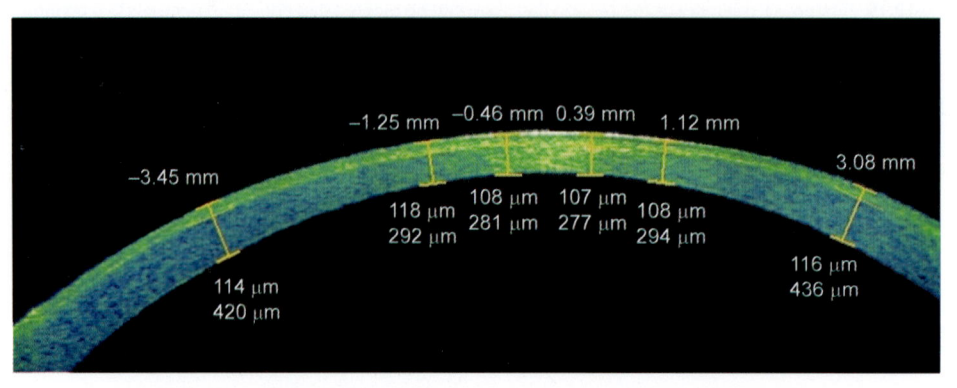

Figure 10.22 Highly myopic patient after iLASIK in need of minor enhancement

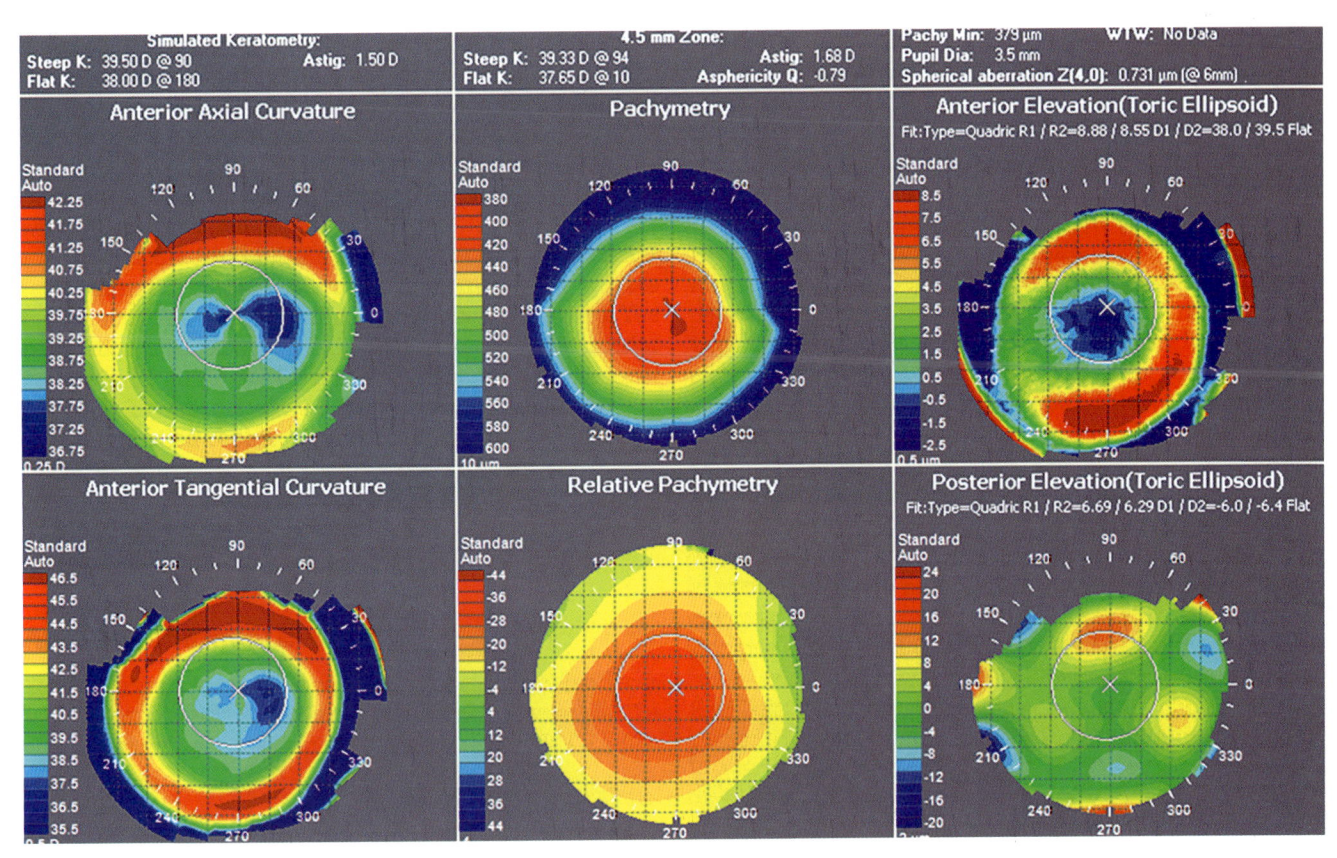

Chapter 10: Evaluation of Patients for Refractive Surgery with Visante Anterior ... 123

Figure 10.23 Holladay report of the right eye of the patient in Figure 10.22

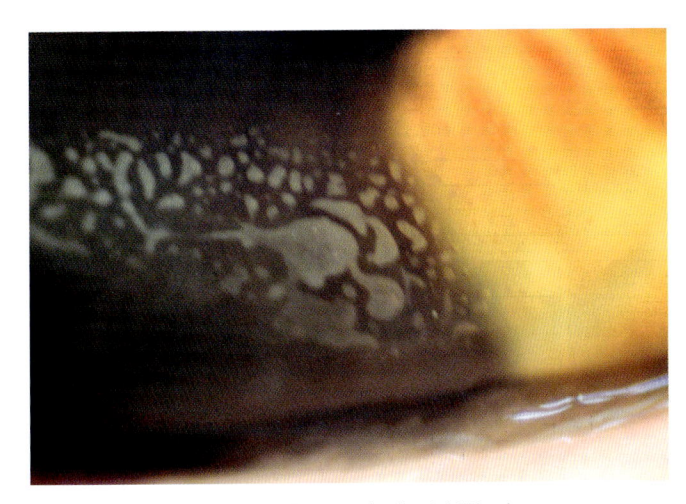

Figure 10.24 Epithelial ingrowth after LASIK enhancement

with uncorrected 20/15 vision after the enhancement chose not to have any intervention. The Visante is able to identify the leading edge of the epithelial ingrowth and allow for very precise monitoring overtime. The clinical appearance of the epithelial ingrowth at 2 months can be noted in **Figure 10.24**. The Visante Image, **Figure 10.25**, in regular High Res Mode in rainbow color scheme, performed at 2 months after the LASIK enhancement demonstrates the leading edge of the epithelial ingrowth from the flap edge. At a follow-up visit 6 months later (8 months postoperative) clinical appearance was unchanged. The Visante Image, **Figure 10.26**, was however, acquired in the enhanced High Res Mode. In this enhanced format, 4 high resolution images are composited together to provide an enhanced view with reduced graininess and increased contrast within the image. Please note that the epithelial ingrowth on the Visante has remained identical.

A sixty-three years old male patient, one year post-LASIK, acquired a new kitten. The kitten with her very sharp, narrow claws punctured the LASIK flap and seeded the interstromal space with a small infiltrate forming ulcer, **Figure 10.27**. The ulcer was treated conservatively with very close evaluation intervals, without lifting of the flap, with combined aminoglycoside (tobramycin) and fluoroquinolone (moxifloxacin) for complete resolution without any loss of visual acuity.

A fifty-six years old male patient with history of initial refractive error of $-0.50-3.00 \times 050$ right eye and $-0.75-2.25 \times 115$ left eye with pre-LASIK corneal topographies as noted in **Figure 10.28** underwent LASIK eye surgery elsewhere. The patient later underwent 2 enhancement procedures

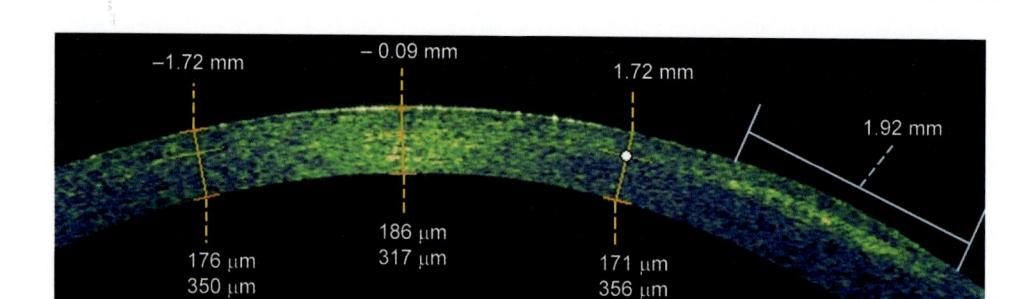

Figure 10.25 Visante (standard High Res Mode) 2 months after LASIK enhancement

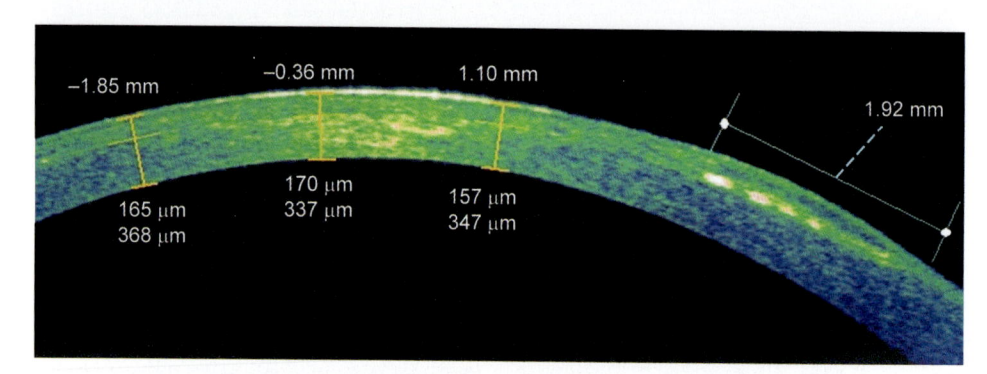

Figure 10.26 Visante (enhanced High Res Mode) 8 months after LASIK enhancement

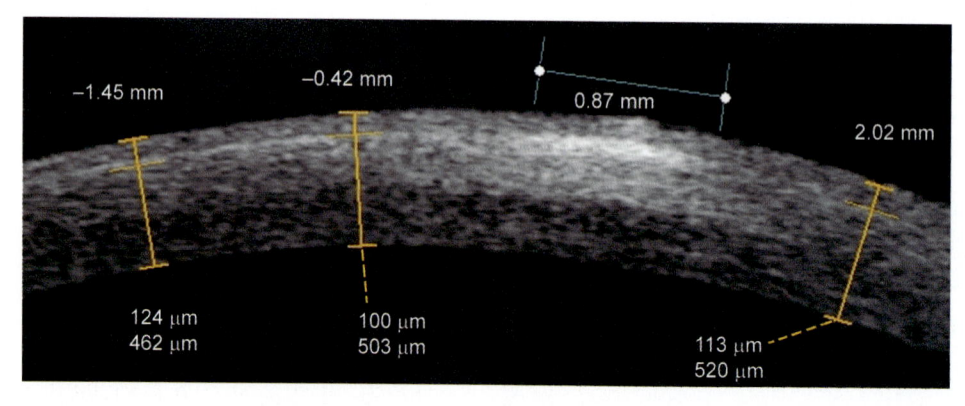

Figure 10.27 Visante image of inter-flap space ulcer

for correction of residual refraction in the right eye and one enhancement procedure in the left eye. Patient presented for second opinion in regards to his progressively declining vision. The Visante **(Figure 10.29)** was able to demonstrate that despite the residual stromal tissue of at least 300 microns, ectasia of the cornea was clearly notable. Patient underwent a corneal transplant surgery for the right eye and was fitted with hard contact lens in the left eye.

As demonstrated in the case presentations above, the Visante Anterior Segment OCT is very useful in evaluation of LASIK patients preoperatively. Evaluation of the corneal pachymetric map as an adjunct to the corneal topographic map and quantitative assessment of the angles are examples. The postoperative care is also enhanced in evaluation of patients for enhancement and also for management of complications.

PHAKIC INTRAOCULAR LENSES

Phakic intraocular lenses (phakic IOLs) are relatively new to the United States market. However, they have enjoyed much

Chapter 10: Evaluation of Patients for Refractive Surgery with Visante Anterior ... 125

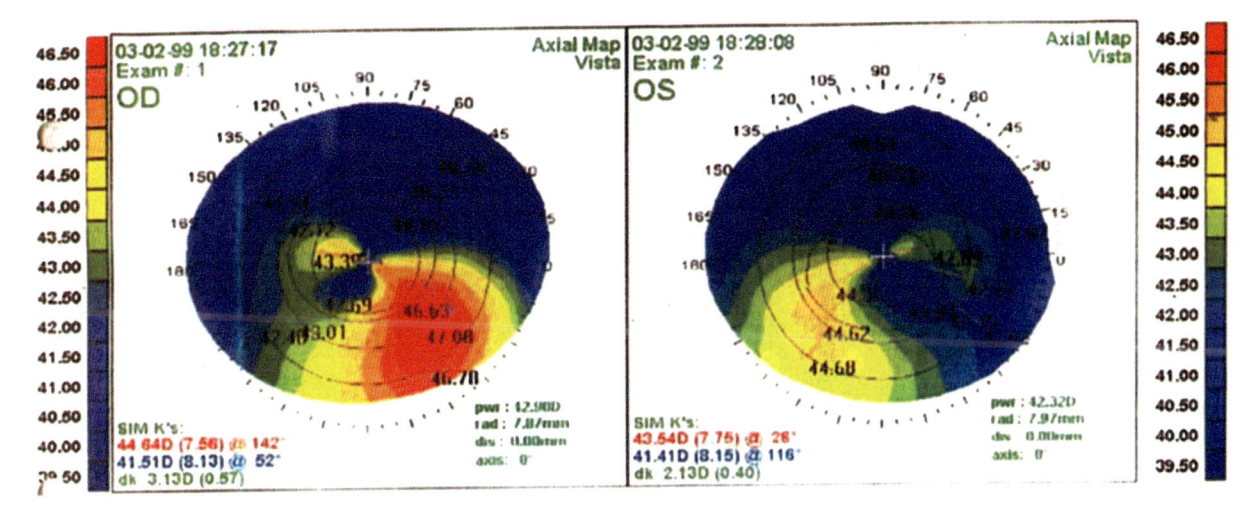

Figure 10.28 Pre-LASIK topography

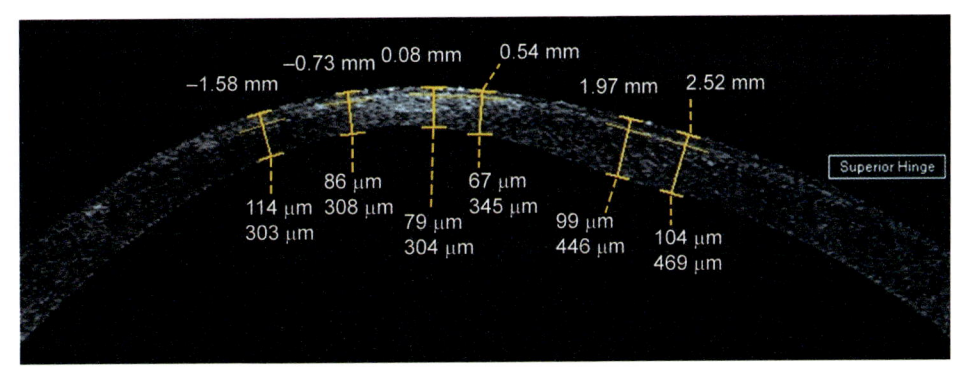

Figure 10.29 Corneal ectasia after LASIK

greater acceptance and use internationally. At the time of writing this chapter in January 2009, there are only two approved phakic IOLs that are approved by the United States Food and Drug Administration, the Verisyse (Advanced Medical Optics, Inc., Santa Ana, California, USA), and the Visian ICL (Staar Surgical, Inc., Monrovia, California, USA). Both of the phakic IOLs are only approved for correction of myopia in the USA. The Verisyse is an anterior chamber lens that is enclavated to the iris **(Figure 10.30)**. The Visian ICL is a posterior chamber lens that rests in the sulcus space anterior to the crystalline lens. There are many other lenses available in the international markets and also in clinical trials in the United States.

Endothelial Clearance

The inner lining of the cornea is populated by the corneal endothelial cells. With placement of the phakic IOLs, there is always a concern regarding the lifetime consequences that

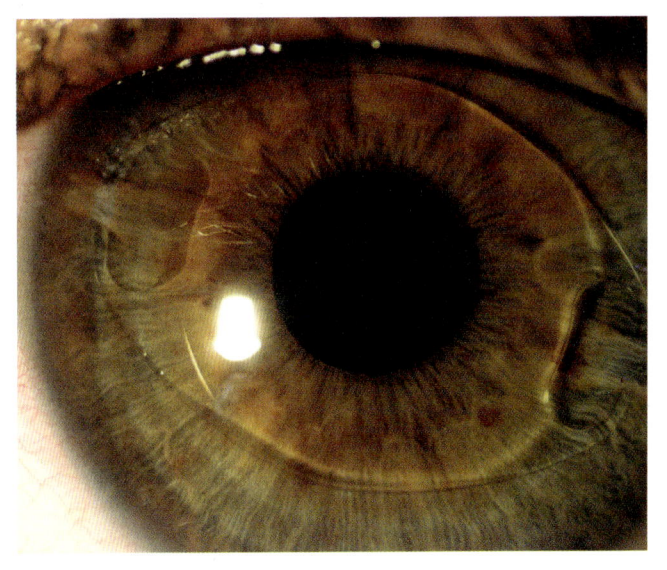

Figure 10.30 Image of an eye implanted with Verisyse

placement of these prostheses, on the population of these cells. Two of the risk factors noted and emphasized by Advanced Medical Optics, Inc., are the 1.5 mm minimal clearance of the anterior aspect of the prosthesis to the corneal endothelium and the minimum anterior chamber depth of 3.2 mm. AMO has a computer software program called the VeriCalc. This program requires the patient's prescription in sphere and cylinder, along with anterior chamber depth and the corneal keratometric measurements. Although the VeriCalc is helpful, the Visante with its new phakic IOL module may provide a much more accurate assessment of acceptable implantation requirements.

The next case is a patient that had Verisyse implantation prior to availability of the Visante and its phakic IOL module. A twenty-eight years old female with prescription of right eye −15.00−1.50 × 165, and the left eye −14.25−1.25 × 175, with the VeriCalc was estimated to have a postoperative minimal endothelial clearance of 1.56 and 1.65 in the right and left eye respectively. However, on postoperative evaluation, **(Figures 10.31 and 10.32)** the patient was noted to have significantly less endothelial—Verisyse clearance, ranging from 1.22 to 1.66 mm right eye, with average of 1.41 mm, and ranging from 1.14 to 1.53 mm left eye with average of 1.35 mm.

Crystalline Lens Rise

In the following case presentation however, the patient was evaluated with the new Phakic IOL module available with the Visante 2.0 software. A twenty years old male with right eye refraction of −14.25−2.75 × 115 leading to 20/40 vision, with slight amblyopia, was evaluated for the Verisyse implantation. In **Figure 10.33** one can evaluate the angles, anterior chamber and the gross endothelial clearance with the "rainbow" module. The anterior chamber depth (ACD) in this case equals to the anterior lens surface to endothelial distance (3.03 mm) plus the corneal thickness (590 microns = 0.59 mm). Therefore, the ACD would equal to 3.03 mm + 0.59 mm = 3.62 mm. Baikoff has described the crystalline lens rise (CLR) as measurement of lens rise above or below the horizontal line across the deepest portion of the angles. Note that although the angle measurements are done from the scleral spur, these measurements are done from the deepest angle positions. In this case, the CLR is found to be 300 microns. Baikoff describes a form of pigment dispersion syndrome (PDS) in 9 patients, 8 of whom had a CLR greater than 600 microns. This form of PDS is a direct result of iris pigment liberation from traumatized iris tissue in between the phakic IOL and the crystalline lens. As an example the patient in **Figure 10.13**, has a CLR of 720 microns and would neither have sufficient clearance of ACD nor the CLR and would not be a Verisyse candidate.

Preoperative Phakic IOL Model

After the initial quick evaluation **(Figure 10.34)**, one may proceed to a much more in depth evaluation with the Verisyse model number and power. Once the model is aligned just anterior to the posterior iris pigmented epithelium, and

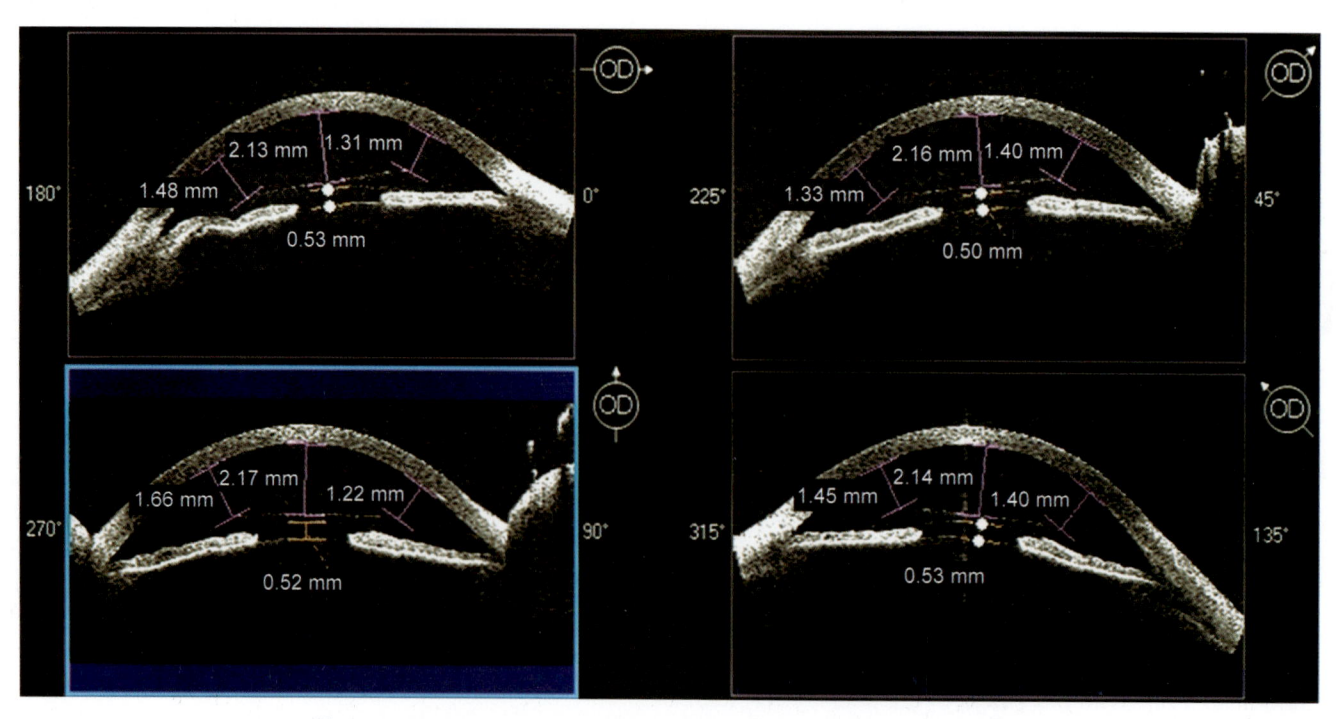

Figure 10.31 Visante images (Quad Scan) of the right eye implanted with Verisyse

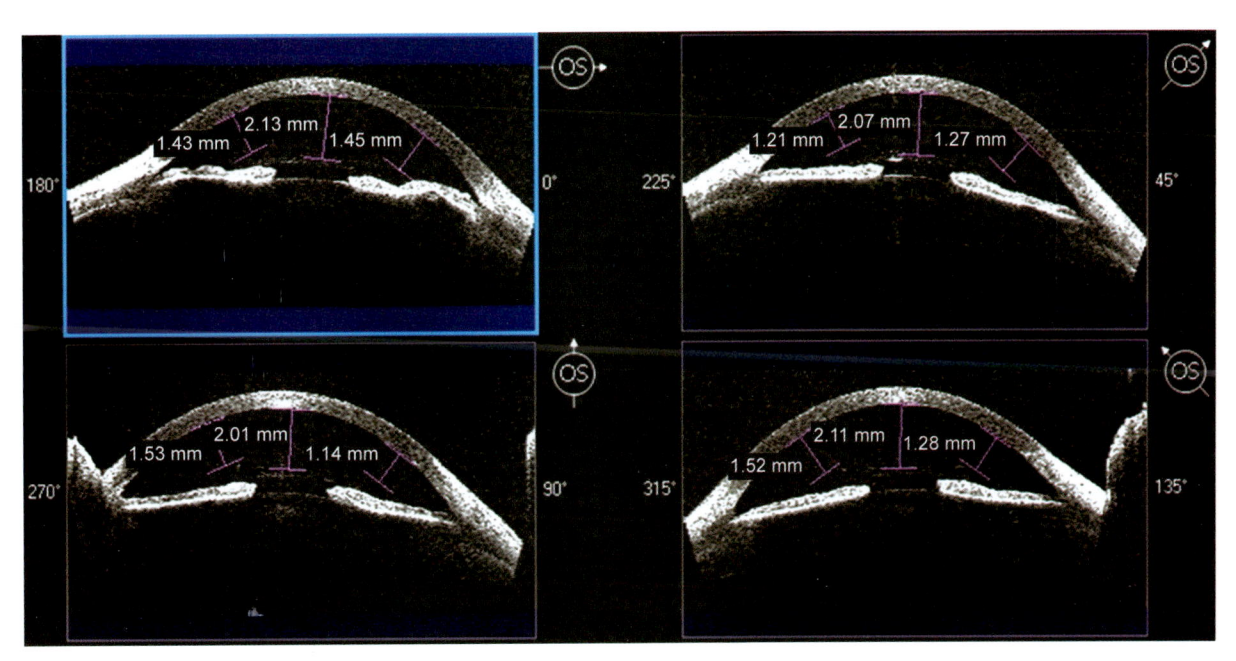

Chapter 10: Evaluation of Patients for Refractive Surgery with Visante Anterior ...   127

Figure 10.32 Visante images (Quad Scan) of the left eye implanted with Verisyse

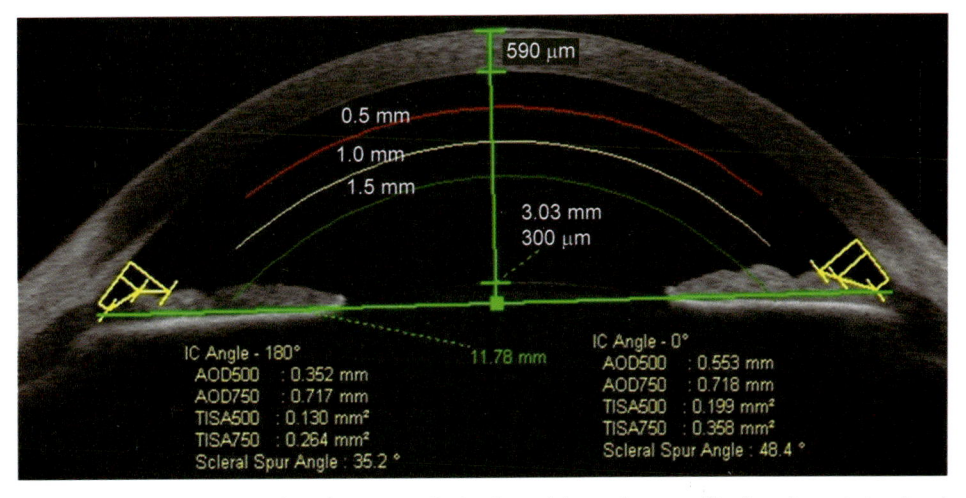

Figure 10.33 Preoperative evaluation of eye for Verisyse. Evaluations of the angles, crystalline lens rise, anterior chamber depth, and safety endothelial distance clearance are noted

centered, the measurement via the safety lines and the lens vault can be placed. The safety lines are to evaluate for the anterior surface of the phakic IOL to the posterior aspect of the cornea. The vault caliper is used to evaluate the distance from posterior aspect of the phakic IOL to the anterior crystalline lens distance.

This patient did subsequently undergo Verisyse implantation and was evaluated by the Visante (**Figure 10.35**). The VeriCalc had calculated the minimum endothelial clearance as 1.92 mm. The Visante model calculated an average of 1.59 mm phakic IOL to endothelium clearance, and a vault distance of 41.67 microns. The actual postoperative data revealed a 1.64 mm phakic IOL to endothelial clearance and a vault distance of 38.67 microns.

Dynamic Changes of the Anterior Chamber with Accommodation

Verisyse as currently available in the United States is a solid PMMA lens available in 6.0 or 5.0 mm optics, and as such must be inserted through a similar size wound. Artiflex is a foldable version of the same and may be inserted through a smaller wound. Jose Guell and colleagues published a study where they implanted Verisyse in one eye and Artiflex in the second eye. They then did an accommodative dynamic study on each eye of the 11 patients in their study. Using the optometer, accommodation was induced in the patient's eye, one diopters at a time, up to seven diopters. Their conclusion was that there were no clinical differences in how both phakic IOLs behaved relative to each other; however, with accommodation, there was a total anterior movement of the iris-lens diaphragm of up to a maximal 250 microns at the center of the phakic IOL to the endothelial distance. It must be noted that the distance of the phakic IOL edge to the endothelium is much less than the center and may prove to be more significant than the measurement of the center of the lens. Additionally, a maximal 1.5 mm pupillary constriction with accommodation was noted. Accommodation did not cause significant change in the vault distance between the crystalline lens and the posterior aspect of the phakic IOL.

In another study, Kiovula and Kugelberg studied the Phakic Refractive Lens (Medennium, Inc., Irvine, California, USA), which is not currently approved by the FDA in United States. The PRL is a posterior chamber lens that floats in the posterior chamber and rests on the zonules and freely rotates. In their study, in the hyperopic group, there were no contacts between the crystalline lens and the PRL at baseline, however with accommodation, contact was noted in 3 cases (27%) and a decrease in the distance noted in another 6 cases (55%). In the myopic group, with the lens model PRL 100, there was one case of contact (10%) at base line, 2 crystalline lenses had contact with the PRL with accommodation (20%), and 3 cases (30%) had decrease in the distance between the PRL and the crystalline lens. In the myopic PRL 101, 2 cases (6%) had baseline PRL-crystalline lens contact at baseline and another lens came in contact with accommodation for a total of 3 (10%), and 21 cases (68%) exhibited decrease in the PRL-crystalline lens distance without contact. There was a mean of 84 micron reduction in the PRL-crystalline lens distance in the PRL models 101 and 200; however, there was no reduction in the PRL model 100. The authors suggest that the smaller size of this model prevents the reduction in the PRL-crystalline lens caused by pupillary constriction and the anterior lens movement. They also suggest

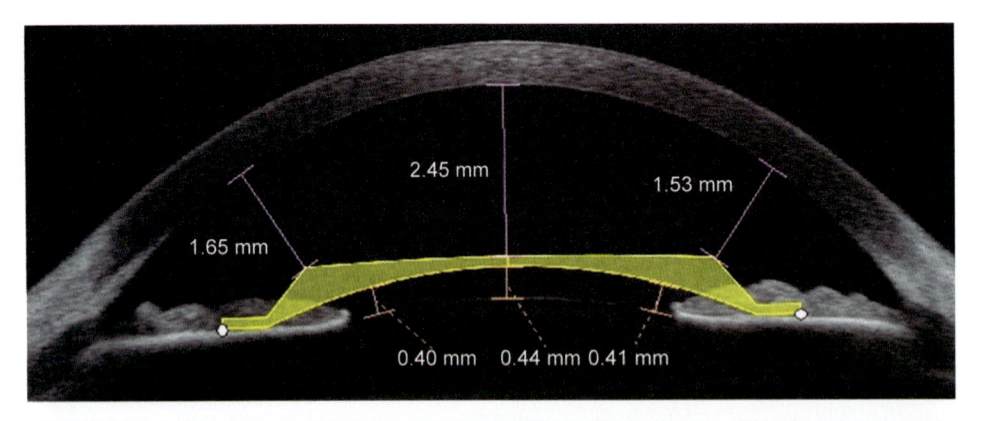

Figure 10.34 Preoperative Verisyse model placement using the Visante. The Verisyse model and power are programmed and placed properly. The lens-endothelial clearance and the vault distances are measured preoperatively

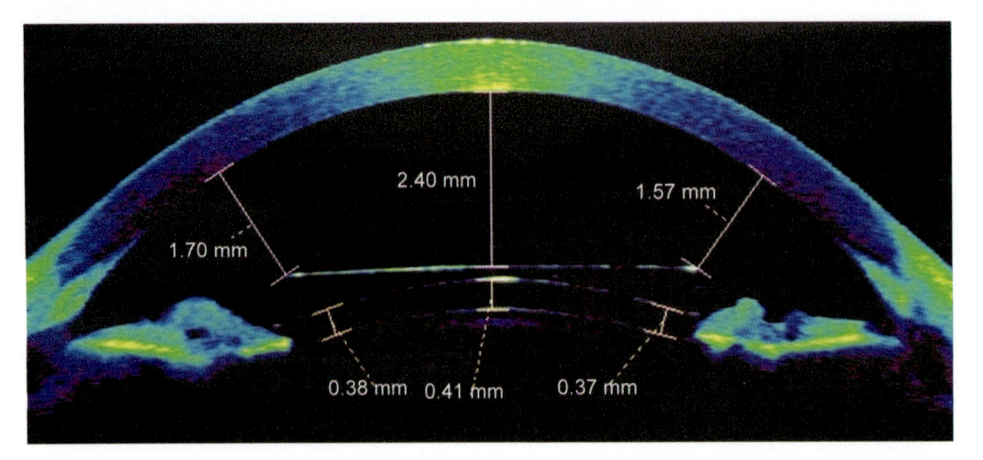

Figure 10.35 Postoperative actual Visante scan of eye implanted with Verisyse. Endothelial clearance and vault distances are measures. The iris claw hooks are noted as black spots in the iris tissue

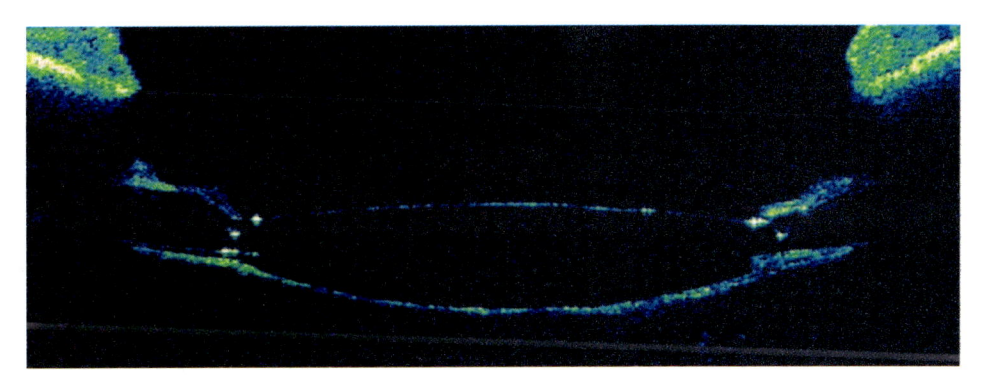

Figure 10.36 CrystaLens implanted in the eye. The optic and the hinges are clearly noted

that despite greater prosthesis—crystalline touch, the reason for fewer cataract complications of this lens compared to the sulcus fixated posterior chamber Visian ICL phakic IOL, is that the lens rotation allows for aqueous exchange.

In evaluation of the phakic IOL candidate the Visante anterior segment OCT plays a crucial role in safely evaluating the anterior chamber depth, the crystalline lens rise, the endothelial-phakic IOL distance, the phakic IOL-crystalline lens vault, and the dynamic accommodative changes of the anterior segment.

CONCLUSION

Although in this chapter we did not address one of the most commonly performed refractive surgeries, namely, cataract surgery or clear lens extraction, there is also a significant role for the Visante anterior segment OCT in those cases as well. With increasing emphasis on the premium IOL, including the accommodative lenses, the Visante becomes invaluable in demonstrating the efficacy of the lenses. Visante can be used to induce accommodation using the build-in optometer as noted under the phakic IOL section. An example of CrystaLens implanted in a patient is presented, however, no measurable movement in the lens could be noted **(Figure 10.36)**.

As demonstrated through case presentations, the Visante Anterior Segment Optical Coherence Tomography System is a powerful noncontact, real-time imaging system of the eye that shows excellent accuracy. In care of the excimer laser patients, from the preoperative stages the patients' candidacy may be enhanced with additional information such as pachymetric mapping of the cornea and posterior corneal curvature data when linked with the ATLAS topographer. The health of the eye may be assessed beyond its refraction, such as the quantitative measurement of the angle as opposed to the qualitative capabilities of the standard slit-lamp gonioscope. Corneal pathologies, such as scars, infections, flap configurations, and irregularities are quantitatively noted and are only some of the examples of the usefulness of the Visante in the care of a past, present, and future refractive patient.

REFERENCES

1. Steinert RF, Hwang D. Anterior Segment Optical Coherence Tomography; Slack, USA; 2008.
2. Baïkoff G. Anterior segment OCT and phakic intraocular lenses: A perspective. J Cataract Refract Surg. 2006;32:1827-35.
3. Güell JL, Morral M, Gris O, Gaytan J, Sisquella M, Manero F. Evaluation of Verisyse and Artiflex phakic intraocular lenses during accommodation using Visante optical coherence tomography. J Cataract Refract Surg. 2007;33:1398-404.
4. Koivula A, Kugelberg M. Optical Coherence Tomography of the Anterior Segment in Eyes with Phakic Refractive Lenses. Ophthalmology. 2007;114:2031-37.

Chapter 11

Corneal Inflammation and Optical Coherence Tomography

Dhivya Ashok Kumar (India), Amar Agarwal (India)

NORMAL CORNEAL TEXTURE

Normal cornea is seen as homogeneous structure in the optical coherence tomography (OCT). The usual corneal layers seen in conventional time domain TD-OCT are the epithelium, the stroma and the endothelial layer **(Figure 11.1)**. The epithelial layer is seen highly reflective due to the difference in the refractive indices of air and the cornea with overlying tear film. Stroma is seen below the epithelium as homogeneous structure. Bowman's layer is not routinely seen in conventional time domain OCT. However, it may be seen in patients with corneal pathologies like ectasia or keratoconus in spectral or Fourier domain OCT. Descemet membrane is seen as high reflective layer with the underlying endothelium in the posterior cornea. The high reflection is again due to the difference in the refractive indices of aqueous and endothelium.

PATHOLOGY IN CORNEAL INFLAMMATION

Keratitis may be produced by infectious organisms or by noninfectious stimuli. Microbial keratitis is a common, potentially sight threatening ocular infection that may be caused by bacteria, fungi, virus or parasites.[1] It is often assessed by the status of epithelium, type of stromal inflammation and the site of stromal inflammation. The intrinsic virulence of an organism relates to its ability to invade tissue, resist host defense mechanisms and produce tissue damage. Bacterial invasion is facilitated by proteinases that degrade basement membrane and extracellular matrix and cause cell lysis.[2] The proteases in keratitis cause degradation of basement membrane, laminin, extracellular matrix proteoglycan and collagen. The infective organism may enter the cornea after trauma or surgery (refractive surgery) easily due to the presence of break in epithelium.

ROLE OF OCT IN KERATITIS

AS OCT provides a range of qualitative and quantitative information for the assessment of microbial keratitis; serial standardized examination allows objective assessment of microbial keratitis and monitoring of the disease course.[3-6] Depending upon the clinical stage, the parameters in the OCT scan changes during the course of the disease. Serial scans can be carried out through the same area of the cornea by adhering to a scanning protocol. The common features noted in OCT are stromal thickness, epithelial integrity, infiltration dimensions, endothelial edema, Descemet changes, scar or fibrosis. Corneal high resolution mode is routinely used for corneal infiltration quantification. Time domain and FD OCT has been used widely in the recent past for prognosis of corneal infection.[3-6]

Early Stages of Inflammation

At the initial stages of microbial keratitis, even mild cases have a thickened cornea at the infiltrated area.[3] Inflammatory cells may appear to be hyper-reflective in the corneal stroma in superficial and deep keratitis **(Figure 11.2)**. In infection involving deeper cornea and anterior chamber, it may be seen as aggregates on the endothelial surface **(Figure 11.3)**.[7] Corneal ulcer prognosis can be observed by measuring the change in epithelial defect and infiltration thickness on serial OCT images. Stromal or corneal thickness (CT) is observed regularly during the course of treatment and the decrease in CT shows response to treatment and resolution of inflammation. Epithelial healing can also be assessed by the absence of heaped up layers and continuous-regular reflection from the anterior surface. AS OCT also can image and monitor the extent of stromal edema associated with the ulceration. Corneal stromal edema accompanying the ulcer can be visualized as diffuse or

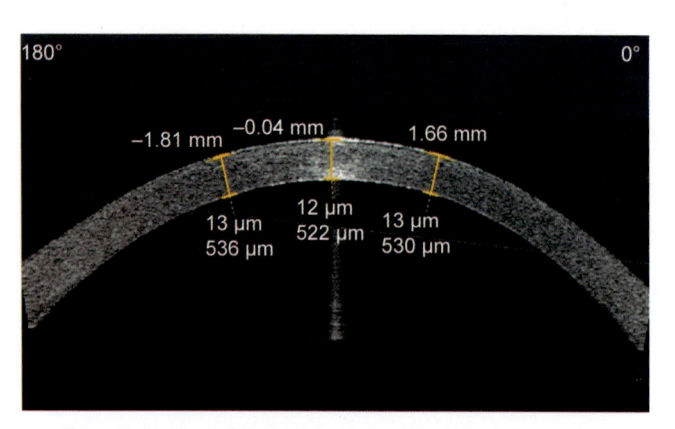

Figure 11.1 Normal cornea as seen by time domain (TD) anterior segment optical coherence tomography

Chapter 11: Corneal Inflammation and Optical Coherence Tomography

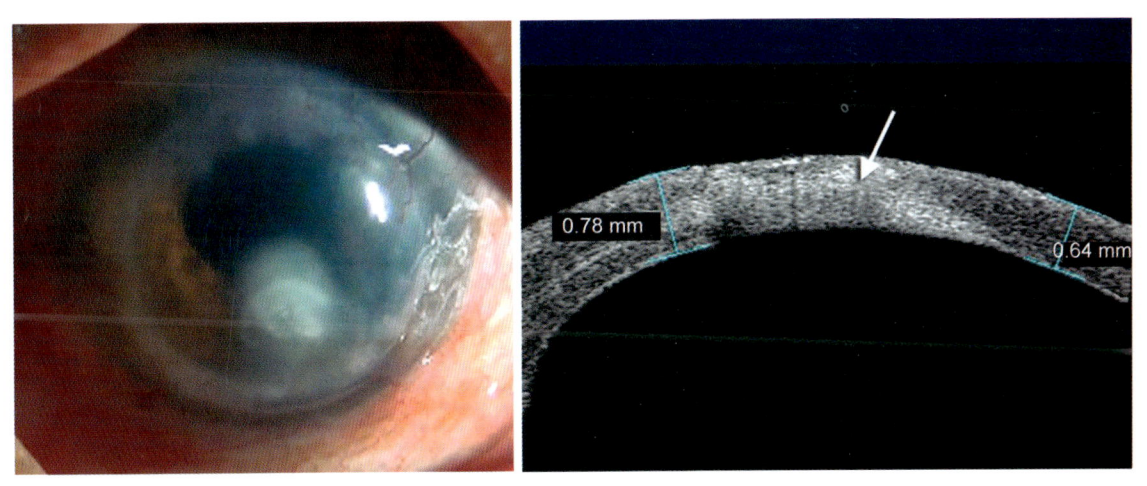

Figure 11.2 Corneal ulcer (left) and the corresponding anterior segment OCT (right) showing infiltration in stroma (arrow) with increased stromal thickness (0.78 mm)

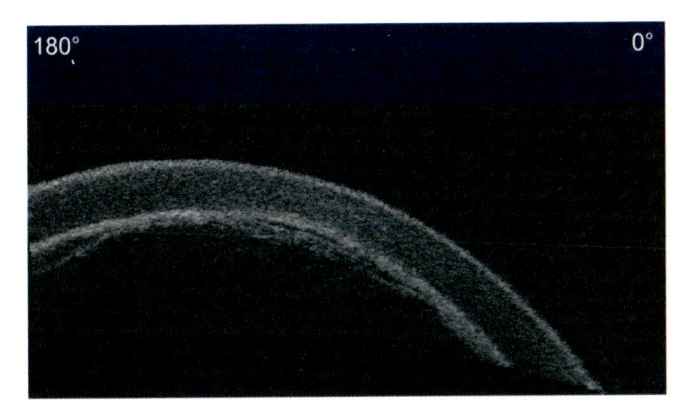

Figure 11.3 Endothelial inflammation seen as aggregates on the endothelial surface with adjacent fibrinous reaction

local thickening of stroma and increase in the convexity on the posterior surface **(Figure 11.4)**. Infiltration of microbes and underlying tissue damage is noted as hyper-reflective regions in the clear corneal surface **(Figure 11.2)**. Infiltration thickness (IT) is an important parameter which aids in post-treatment monitoring. Descemet folds can be imaged as ruffles in the normally smooth endothelial surface **(Figure 11.5)**.[3] In early corneal edema, anterior chamber can be visualized for cellular reaction clearly by OCT unlike the late stages.[7]

Advanced Inflammation

In advanced lesions, there can be stromal edema, corneal abscess and diffuse corneal involvement. Severe infection can cause necrosis and liquefaction causing thinning of the

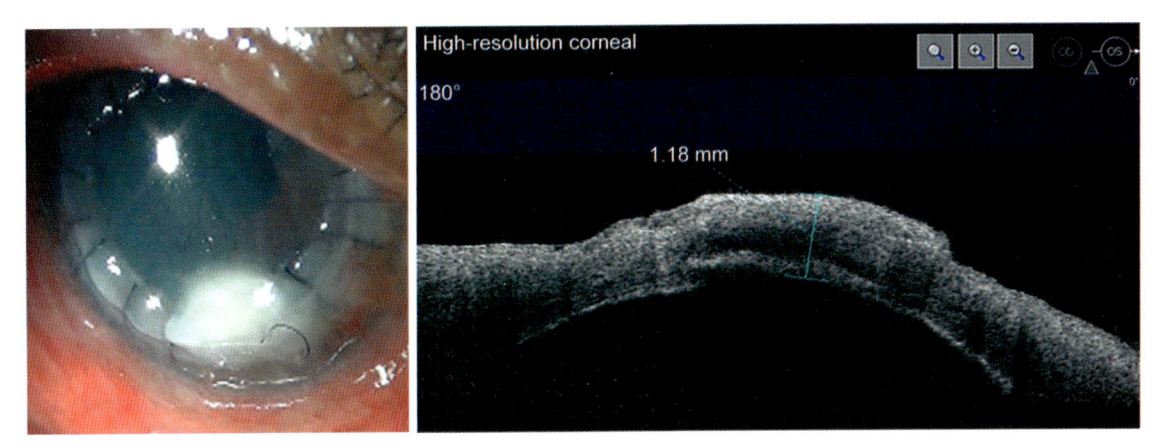

Figure 11.4 Postpenetrating keratoplasty stromal keratitis (left) and the OCT showing deep corneal infiltration with necrosis (right)

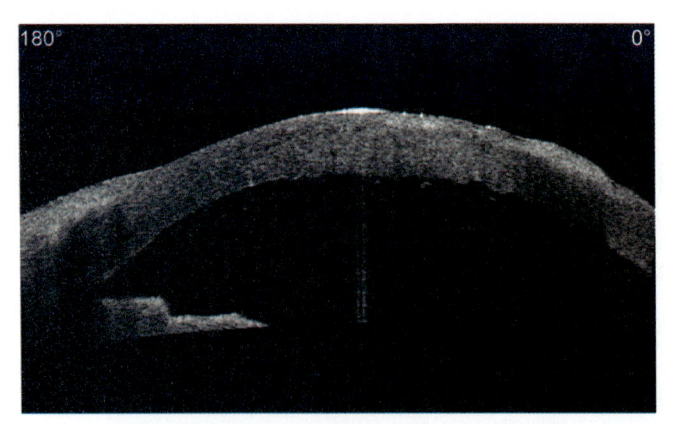

Figure 11.5 Descemet folds seen on the endothelial surface in microbial keratitis

affected cornea **(Figure 11.6)**. Risk of perforation is there in advanced fungal infections **(Figure 11.7)**. Advanced cases with endothelial inflammatory plaques can be measured using OCT. Measurement of the width of plaque or endothelial abscess **(Figure 11.8)** on serial scans allowed objective assessment of the disease course.

Healing Stage

At the later stages of the disease, scar tissue develops and the affected cornea may become thinner than adjacent healthy tissue. Scar and fibrosis can produce dense hyper-reflective zone in the corneal stroma corresponding to the region of corneal opacity as seen in the slit lamp. Sometimes there can be adherent leukoma **(Figure 11.9)** in chronic stages with synechiae. Long standing scar can lead to calcareous degeneration or plaque formation. Dense opacification or thick exudates can prevent light from entering the cornea and causes back shadowing. Cornea with blood staining due to hyphema may also hinder IR ray transmission.[7]

ADVANTAGE OF OCT IN CORNEAL INFILTRATION

The average size of the neutrophils, monocytes, and lymphocytes in inflammation usually range from 10 to 20 mm.[8] Because of the higher resolution of OCT, it may be possible to pick even early infiltration. Time domain OCT has an axial resolution of 18 microns as compared to Fourier domain which has 5 microns resolution. We have reported the use of FD-OCT in post lasik inflammation management **(Figure 11.10)**.[6] The acquisition time of FD-OCT is also lesser than TD-OCT. Number of scans taken by FD-OCT is 26,000 A-scan/s and TD-OCT is 2048 scans/s and moreover, a three dimensional image is possible in FD-OCT.[6] Therefore, it is possible to document the volume and shape of the lesion in three dimensions. AS OCT cannot replace slit-lamp examination, but it does provide information that may aid assessment. Endothelial plaque dimensions and posterior stromal infiltration dimensions can be quantified even in edematous cornea. Qualitative assessment of the infiltration also is possible, because the intensity of hyper reflectivity corresponds to the density of the infiltration on slit-lamp examination.

AS OCT FOR PROGNOSIS

Instead of single scan, serial OCT scans are recommended for assessment of response and prognosis after commencing the treatment.[3] OCT software calipers are utilized for quantification of the parameters like infiltration and corneal thicknesses in microns. In the early stages of microbial keratitis, clinical improvement is associated with reduction of IT. Decrease CT is also a necessary OCT parameter which shows the significant

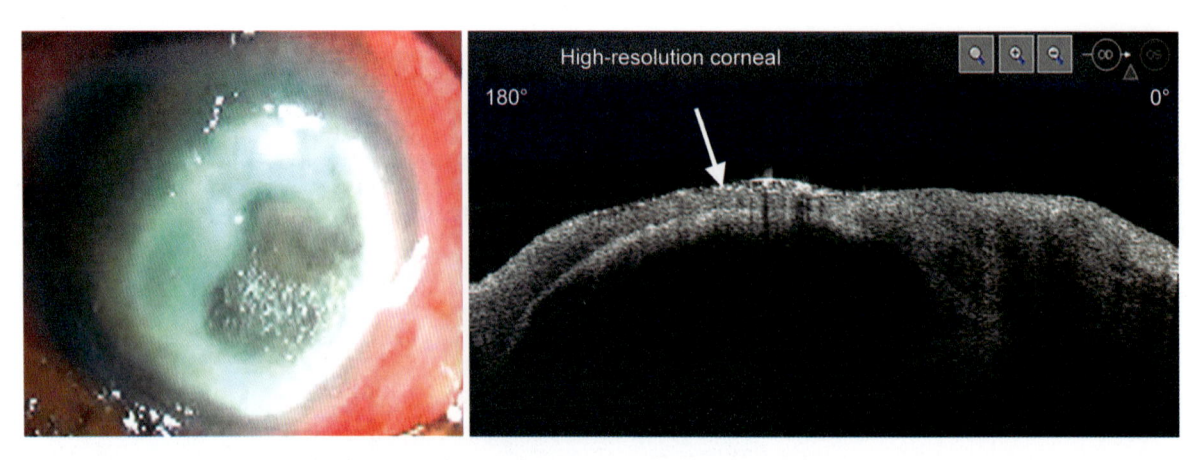

Figure 11.6 Sclerokeratitis with corneal necrosis in an female patient (left) and the corresponding thinning and stromal changes as seen in the OCT (right)

Chapter 11: Corneal Inflammation and Optical Coherence Tomography 133

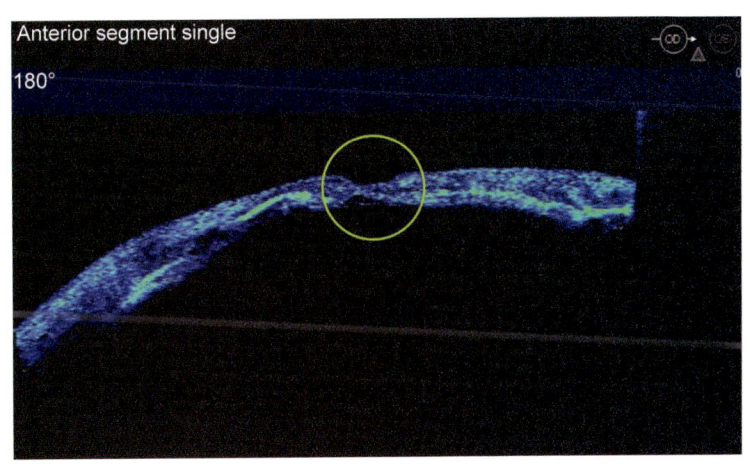

Figure 11.7 OCT showing the postcorneal infection perforation with pseudo-cornea formation (circled)

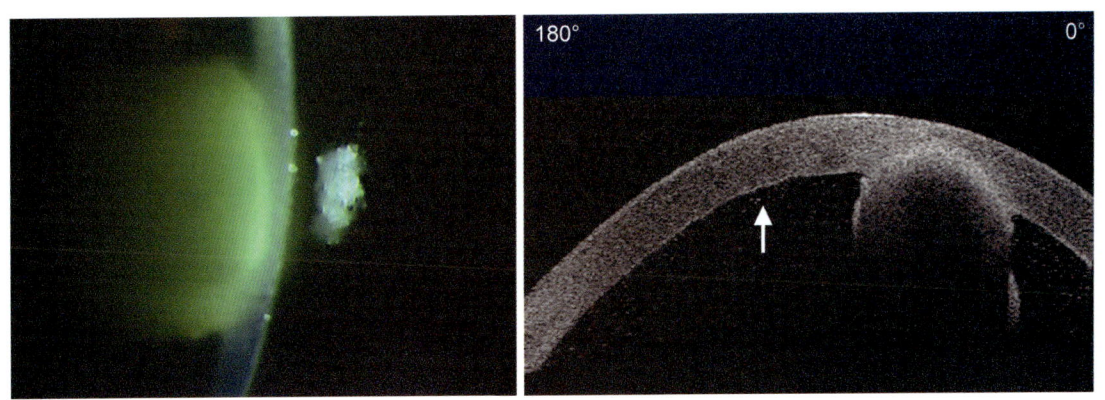

Figure 11.8 Endothelial abscess in an elderly male (left) and the corresponding OCT scan showing the abscess with infiltration in the posterior cornea and the anterior chamber (right)

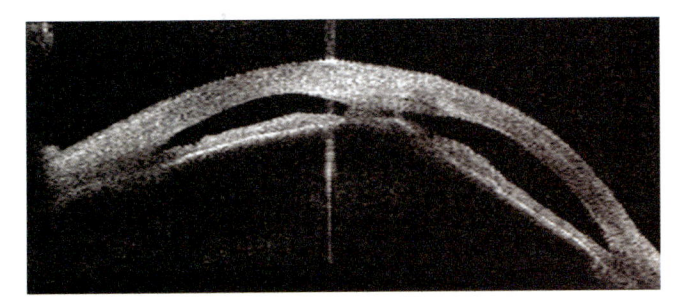

Figure 11.9 Healed corneal ulcer with adherent leukoma. Note the pulled up iris to the cornea and shallow anterior chamber

response to treatment. Increase in the IT or CT shows deterioration and no response to antimicrobials. This change may be detected on AS OCT before deterioration becomes clinically apparent. In postrefractive surgery inflammation, OCT can be used assess the sub flap infiltration thickness and prognosis to treatment (**Figure 11.10**).

AS OCT ASSESSMENT FOR SURGERY PLAN

In nonresponding microbial keratitis, the depth of involvement of cornea can be measured by OCT. This aids in elective planning for surgery like corneal debridement or therapeutic penetrating keratoplasty. Corneal abscess which is progressively increasing as seen by serial OCT scans can move into the anterior chamber and therefore it requires emergency evacuation with intracameral antibiotics (**Figure 11.8**). Eyes with localized post-infective stromal opacity involving the anterior cornea can be assessed by measuring the thickness involved and anterior lamellar keratoplasty can be planned appropriately. Eyes with localized nonhealing corneal epithelial defect with irregular

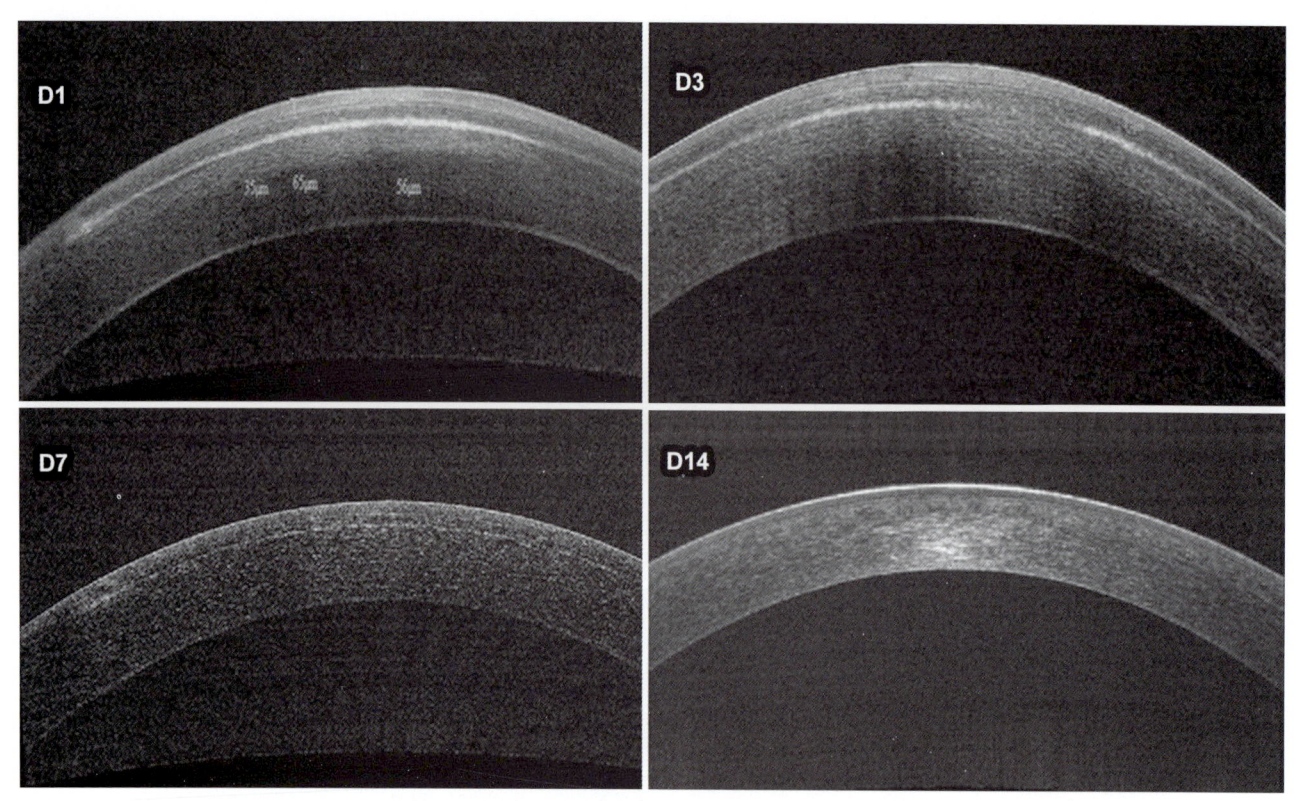

Figure 11.10 High resolution fourier domain OCT image of the cornea showing the infiltration and interface fluid on day 1 (D1), day 3 (D3), day 7 (D7) and 2 weeks (D14) of the treatment

heaped up margins may require elective amniotic membrane graft. Eyes with corneal edema hindering anterior chamber evaluation can be seen for the depth of the anterior chamber and iris configuration.

REFERENCES

1. O'Brien TP, Green WR. Keratitis. In Mandell GL, et al. (Eds). Principles and practice of infectious diseases, 4th edn, New York, Churchill Livingstone, 1995.
2. O'Brien TP. Bacterial keratitis. In Krachmer, et al. (Eds).Cornea. Cornea and external disease: Clinical diagnosis and management, 3rd edn, Missouri, Mosby, 2011.
3. Konstantopoulos A, Kuo J, Anderson D, Hossain P. Assessment of the use of anterior segment optical coherence tomography in microbial keratitis. Am J Ophthalmol. 2008;146(4):534-42.
4. Soliman W[1], Fathalla AM, El-Sebaity DM, Al-Hussaini AK. Spectral domain anterior segment optical coherence tomography in microbial keratitis. Graefes Arch Clin Exp Ophthalmol. 2013;251(2):549-53.
5. Konstantopoulos A[1], Yadegarfar G, Fievez M, Anderson DF, Hossain P. In vivo quantification of bacterial keratitis with optical coherence tomography. Invest Ophthalmol Vis Sci. 2011;52(2):1093-7.
6. Ashok Kumar D, Prakash G, Agarwal A, Jacob S, Agarwal A. Quantitative assessment of post-LASIK corneal infiltration with frequency domain anterior segment OCT: a case report. Cont Lens Anterior Eye. 2009;32(6):296-9.
7. Agarwal A, Ashok Kumar D, Jacob S, Agarwal A, Saravanan Y. High-speed optical coherence tomography for imaging anterior chamber inflammatory reaction in uveitis: clinical correlation and grading. Am J Ophthalmol. 2009;147(3):413-6.
8. Williams WJ. Clinical evaluation of patient: approach to the patient. In: Williams WJ, Beutler E, Ersler AJ, Litchman MA, (Eds). Book of hematology. 3rd edn, New York: McGraw Hill; 1983. pp. 11–9.

Chapter 12

Optical Coherence Tomography in Corneal Ectasia

Otman Sandali (France), Vincent Borderie (France), Laurent Laroche (France)

KERATOCONUS

Keratoconus is the most common primary ectatic corneal disorder. It is characterized by progressive corneal thinning, irregular astigmatism, and corneal protrusion that may eventually result in scarring and loss of vision.

This disease is associated with stromal thinning, decrease in keratocyte density, various amounts of stromal haze, Bowman's layer disruption and splitting in the region of the cone, and epithelial changes.[1]

The optical coherence tomography (OCT) provide an accurate assessment of corneal layers changes during keratoconus and should be performed systematically in association with topographic exams in the evaluation of keratoconus eyes.

OCT IN KERATOCONUS SCREENING

The diagnosis of moderate to advanced keratoconus is not difficult because of the characteristic topographic patterns. However, the identification of the forme fruste keratoconus (FFK), in patients with minimum or no clinical signs can be challenging. Preoperative accurate detection of keratoconus among refractive surgery candidates is crucial. Forme fruste keratoconus is the main cause of postoperative corneal ectasia after LASIK surgery.

Li and Huang conducted a study using a time-domain OCT system to map pachymetry for keratoconus detection.[2] They determined criteria of keratoconus diagnosis, based on the first percentile or 99th percentile cut-off points of the normal range. These criteria include:
- Asymmetric parameters SN-IT or S-I (superior-inferior) values greater than 45 µm.
- Minimum corneal thickness less than 470 µm.
- Focal thinning parameter Minimum – Maximum value less than -100 µm.

Early epithelial changes are present in subclinical cases of keratoconus. The epithelium is able to compensate fully for the sub-surface cone, topographically evident on the back surface, resulting in an apparently normal anterior surface topography.[3] The analysis of the corneal epithelial thickness profile may aid in the interpretation of corneal topography improving the detection of the FFK. In a recent study of 38 keratoconus cases, we demonstrated that the thinnest epithelial point was located inferiorly in comparison with normal cornea and corresponded to the location of the thinnest corneal point on OCT pachymetry and the maximal posterior corneal elevation zone on corneal topography. The epithelial thickness of the thinnest point was thinner in FFK in comparison with normal corneas. A pattern of thin epithelium surrounded by a zone of epithelial thickening (doughnut pattern) as described by Reinstein is suggestive of mild keratoconus **(Figures 12.1A to D)**.

OCT IN KERATOCONUS EVALUATION

Many classifications of keratoconus based on the location of the cone, slit lamp appearance, and indirect topographic patterns, have been proposed in the literature.

However, these classifications may have not taken into account direct corneal microstructure and histological changes occurring during keratoconus evolution. Indeed, a microstructural corneal analysis directly reflects corneal layers abnormalities occurring in keratoconus, and is more informative than the corneal topographic changes in the assessment of corneal architecture.

Recently, we have established an OCT keratoconus classification based on structural corneal changes occurring at the conus as follows[4] **(Figure 12.2)**:

Stage 1: Thinning of epithelial and stromal layers at the conus. Corneal layers have a normal aspect.

Stage 2: Hyper-reflective anomalies occurring at the Bowman's layer level (varying from a barely visible hyper-reflective line to a hypertrophic scar) and epithelial thickening at the conus (2a, clear stroma; 2b, stromal opacities).

Stage 3: Posterior displacement of the hyper-reflective structures occurring at the Bowman's layer level with increased epithelial thickening and stromal thinning (3a, clear stroma; 3b, stromal opacities).

Stage 4: Pan-stromal scar. In stage 4, when the residual stroma is thin, it acquires an hourglass-shaped scar with increased epithelial thickening.

Stage 5: Represents the acute form of keratoconus (hydrops): 5a, acute onset, characterized by the rupture of Descemet's

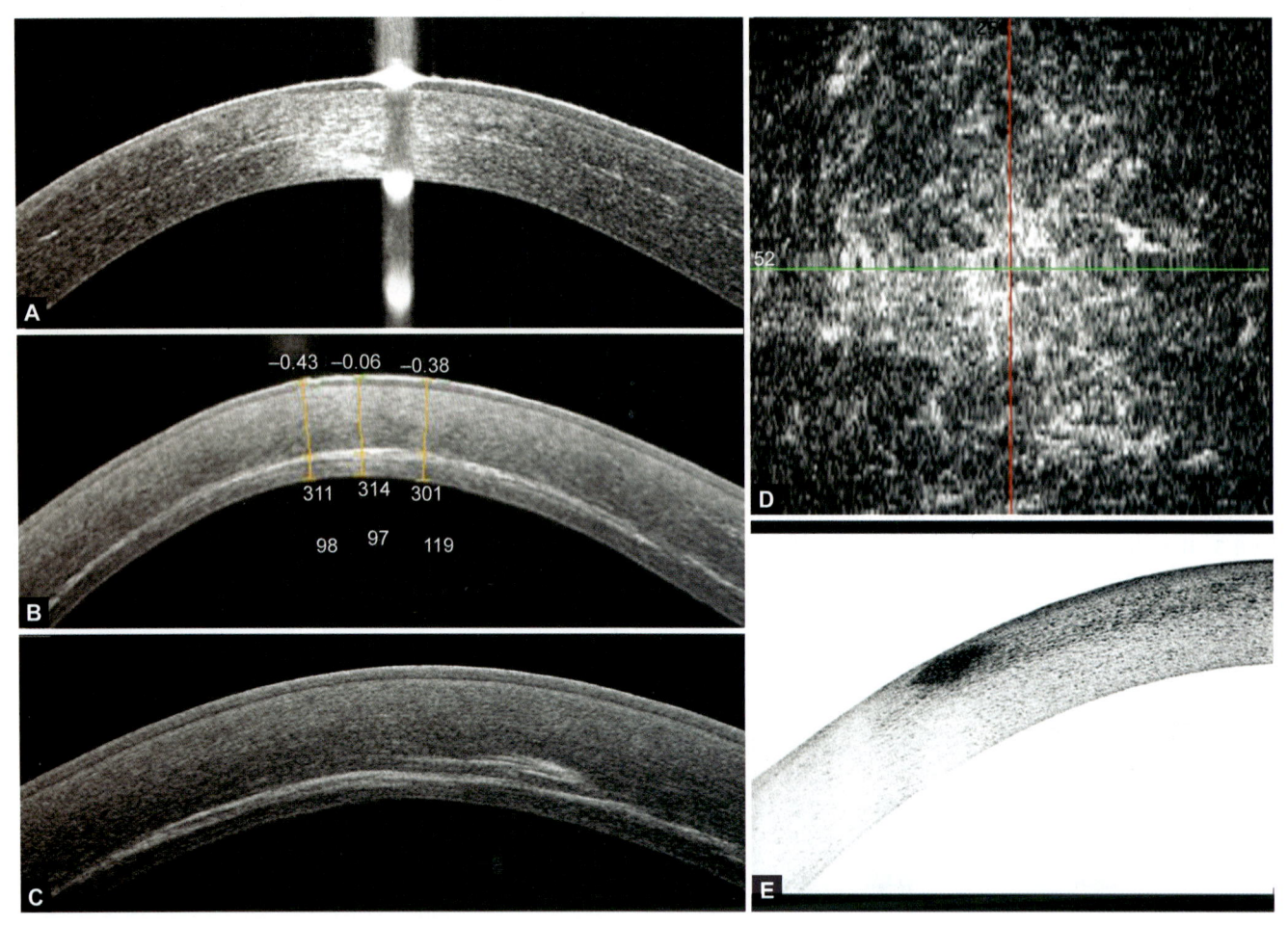

Figures 12.4A to E (A) Optical coherence tomography (OCT) in corneal cross-linking. The corneal stromal demarcation line is deeper in (B and C) cases compared with a case; (D) En-face aspect of stromal demarcation line demonstrating hyper-reflective structures; (E) A rare complication of peripheral sterile keratitis occurring after corneal cross-linking

pachymetry is performed. Indeed, we found that epithelium thickness had a negative correlation with stromal thickness in advanced keratoconus cases **(Figures 12.1A to D)**.

On optical coherence tomography (OCT) images **(Figures 12.4A to E)**, the corneal stromal demarcation line occurs 1 month after corneal cross-linking indicating probably the efficiency of the procedure and corresponds to the transition zone between the cross-linked anterior corneal stroma and the untreated posterior corneal stroma. Linear hyper-reflectivities will be present at the anterior stroma corresponding to keratocyte activation and new collagen fibers synthesis.

A temporary anterior stromal haze is frequently seen and decreases between the third and the twelve postoperative month. Peripheral sterile keratitis will occurs rarely after CXL and resolves with topical steroid therapy. Infectious keratitis is associated mainly with CXL protocols with de-epithelialization and postoperative therapeutic contact lens wear.

INTRACORNEAL RINGS IMPLANTATION

Intacs corneal inserts or implants are a minimally invasive surgical option used primarily for the treatment of keratoconus. The placement of intacs remodels and reinforces the cornea, eliminating some or all of the irregularities caused by keratoconus in order to improve vision. There are indicated in contact lens-intolerant patients who had a keratometry < 60 D and peripheral corneal thickness > 450 µm with a clear cornea.

The choice of number of implanted rings (1 or 2), their diameters and thicknesses depends on the corneal topography and the cone location.[5]

The OCT provides more accurate corneal thickness measurements at the peripheral zone of implantation (6–7 mm) in comparison with topographic pachymetry, improving the results and the safety of the procedure. The best results seem to be obtained when the rings are introduced at 60–80% stromal thickness depth. The OCT highlights the

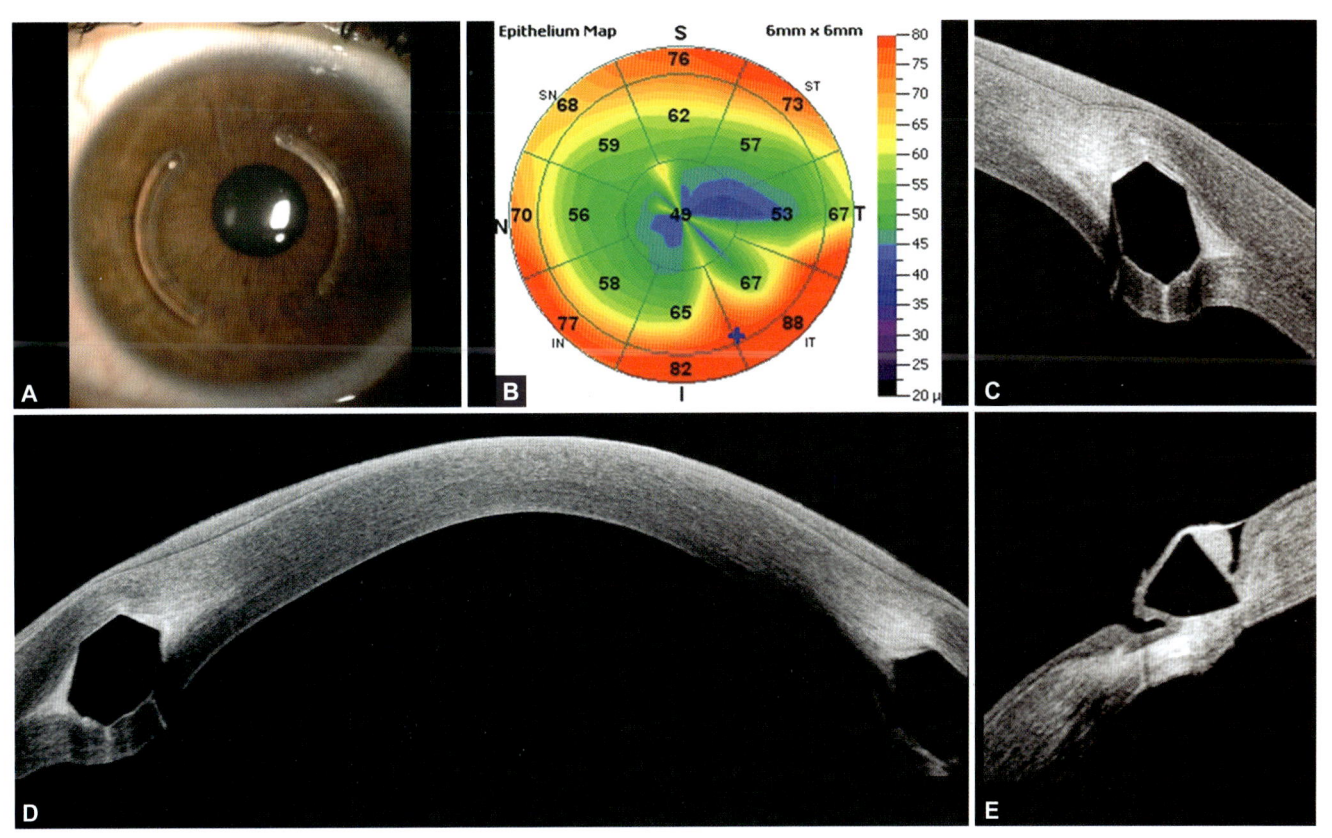

Figures 12.5A to E Intracorneal rings (A) Slit lamp examination; (B) Epithelial map showing an epithelial thickening around the ring; (C and D) Corneal remodeling after rings implantation on OCT. Next to the ring, there is a compression of stromal fibers, and the epithelium compensates the corneal irregularities maintaining the smoothness of corneal surface (epithelial thinning at the stromal protrusion and epithelial thickening around); (E) Extrusion of corneal ring segment

anatomical remodeling after rings implantation. The central portion of the cornea becomes more flat. Next to the ring, there is a compression of stromal fibers, and the epithelium compensates the corneal irregularities maintaining the smoothness of corneal surface(epithelial thinning at the stromal protrusion and epithelial thickening around) **(Figures 12.5A to E)**.

Potential complications of intrastromal rings implantation include accidental penetration through to the anterior chamber when forming the channel, postoperative corneal infection, and migration or extrusion of the segments.

CORNEAL KERATOPLASTY

In cases of contact lens intolerance and/or central corneal scars, corneal transplantation is indicated for advanced keratoconus. Deep anterior lamellar keratoplasty (DALK) is currently considered to be the first-choice operative procedure in patients with severe keratoconus. Removal of the damaged corneal stroma may be achieved by manual dissection with a surgical blade and scissors, microkeratome-assisted lamellar cut, or femtosecond laser-assisted cut. Descemet's membrane detachment from the corneal stroma can be achieved using air injection (the "big-bubble" technique).

Comparing to penetrating keratoplasty, long-term, model-predicted graft survival and endothelial densities are higher after DALK than after penetrating keratoplasty (PK). Endothelial immune reactions are prevented in DALK.

Visual recovery depends on postoperative astigmatism, stromal transparency, and the quality of the stromal interface (DALK). The big-bubble technique gives better results than manual dissection and nearly similar results in comparison with PK.[6]

OCT enables the analysis of the quality of interface and the measurement of the residual stroma in DALK (manual dissection) **(Figures 12.6A to E)**. At the recipient-graft junction, OCT shows an epithelial continuity at the corneal surface in PK and DALK. There is a better congruency at the stromal junction in DALK. The endothelium-Descemet's membrane complex is continuous at the recipient-graft junction and is discontinuous in PK.

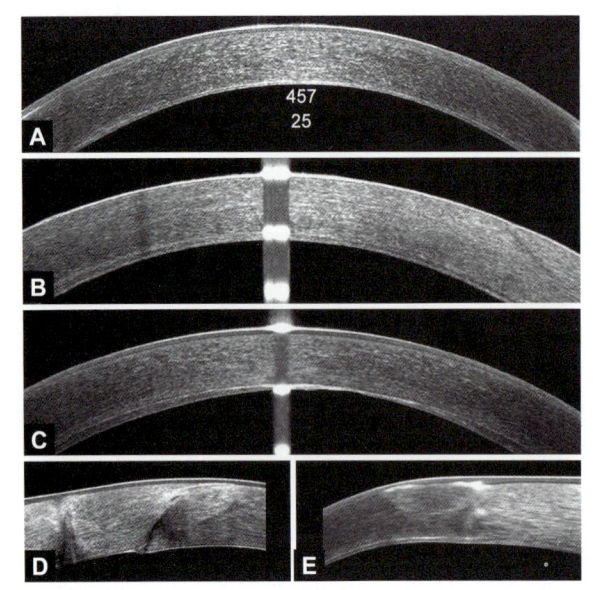

Figures 12.6A to E OCT in corneal keratoplasty (A) DALK (big-bubble technique); (B) DALK (manual dissection with regular stromal interface); (C) DALK (manual dissection with irregular stromal interface); (D) Recipient-graft junction in penetrating keratoplasty; (E) Better congruency at the recipient-graft junction in DALK. The endothelium-Descemet's membrane complex is continuous at the recipient-graft junction and is discontinuous in PK

OTHER CORNEAL ECTATIC DISORDERS

Post-LASIK Ectasia

Corneal ectasia is a serious complication of laser *in situ* keratomileusis (LASIK). The main risk factors for postoperative corneal ectasia are: undiagnosed keratoconus, family history of keratoconus, preoperative corneal thickness < 500 microns, central keratometry > 47 diopters, age < 25 years, correction of myopia > 8 diopters, reverse astigmatism > 2 diopters, residual posterior stromal bed < 250 microns.[7]

The OCT can accurately measure the corneal flap and the residual stromal bed thicknesses explaining the cause of ectasia. The presence of Bowman's layer anomalies and stromal scars on OCT in advanced cases indicate that the underlying disease is a non diagnosed keratoconus decompensated by LASIK surgery **(Figures 12.7A to D)**.

Marginal Pellucid Degeneration

Pellucid marginal degeneration (PMD) is an idiopathic, progressive, noninflammatory, ectatic corneal disorder characterized by a peripheral inferior band of corneal thinning in a crescent-shaped pattern (typically 4 o'clock to 8 o'clock). Similarities between PMD and keratoconus (KC) have led

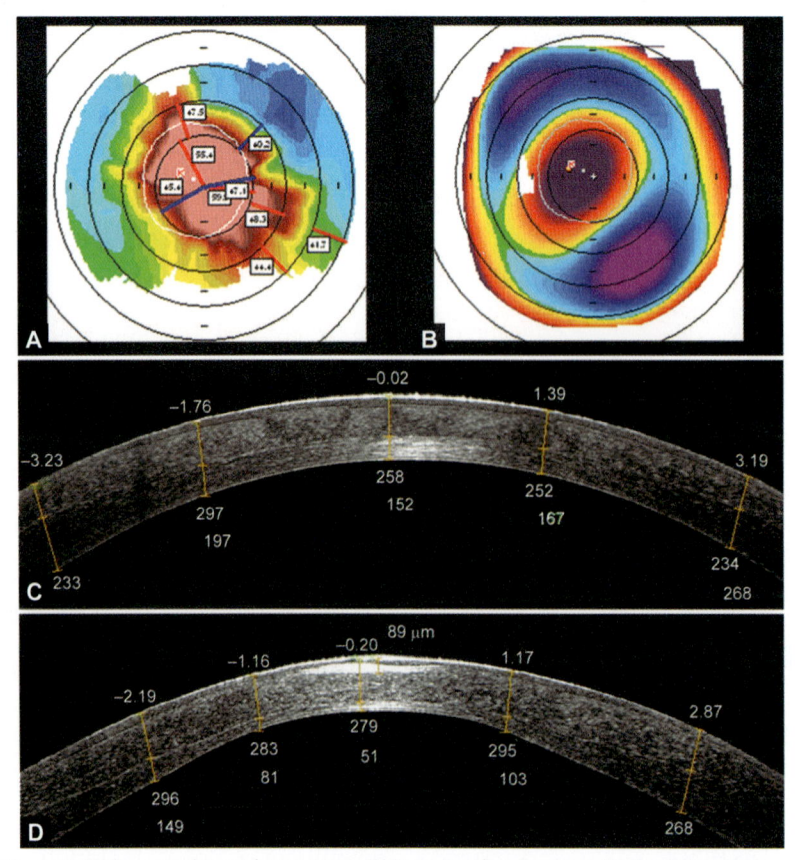

Figures 12.7A to D Post-LASIK ectasia (A) Topographic axial power map; (B) Posterior elevation map; (C) The OCT provides accurate measurements corneal flap and residual stromal bed thicknesses (152 μm); (D) Corneal scar at the Bowman's layer level and epithelial thickening at the conus in an advanced case of post-LASIK corneal ectasia

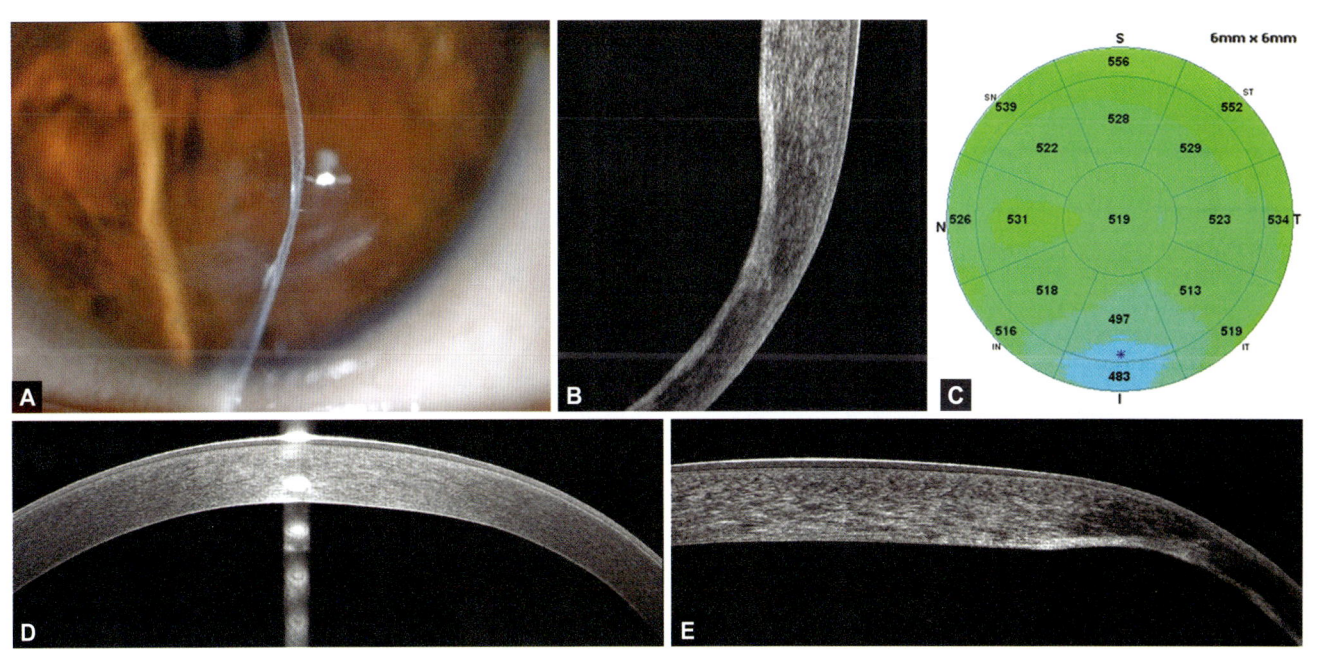

Figures 12.8A to E Pellucid marginal degeneration: (A) Slit lamp examination; (B) Corneal OCT showing a peripheral inferior band of corneal thinning in a crescent-shaped pattern; (C) Pachymetry map showing a peripheral corneal thinning in comparison with keratoconus disease; (D) Contrary to the peripheral cornea, the central cornea has a normal appearance; (E) Stromal opacities in advanced case of pellucid marginal degeneration

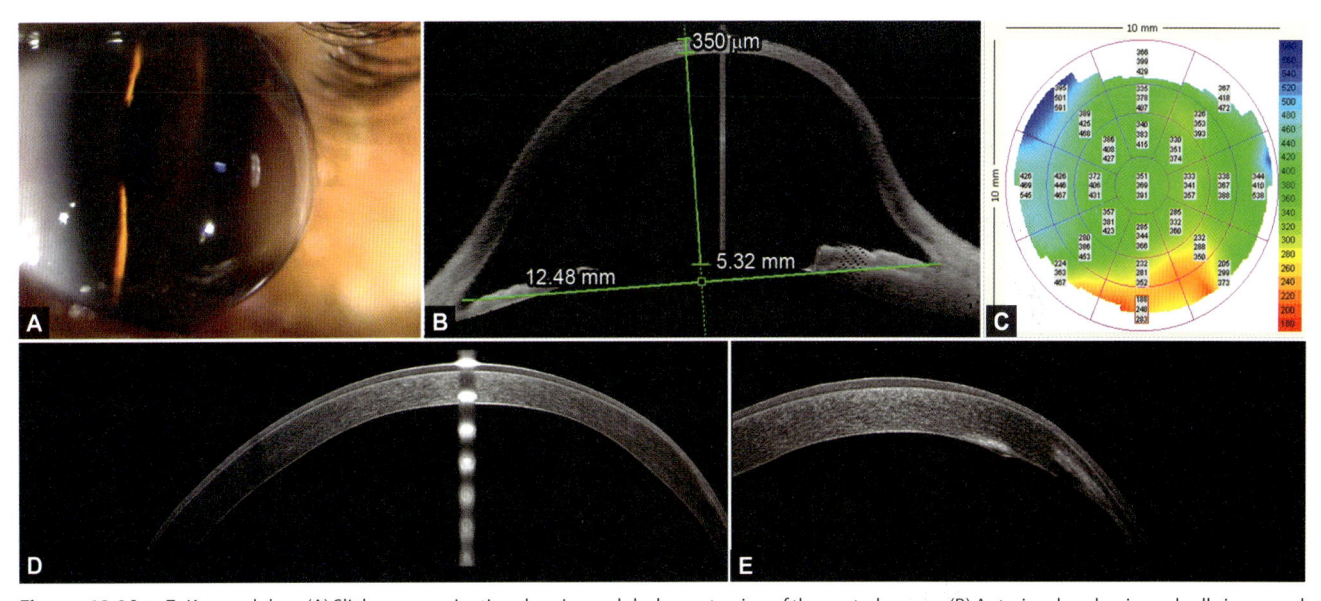

Figures 12.9A to E Keratoglobus: (A) Slit lamp examination showing a globular protrusion of the central cornea; (B) Anterior chamber is markedly increased on OCT-visante; (C) Generalized corneal thinning on visante-OCT map; (D) OCT optovue showing a thinning and protrusion of cornea; (E) Stromal and Descemetic lesions in an advanced keratoglobus case

some ophthalmologists to consider PMD to be a peripheral form of KC.

Distinguishing between the two entities is of potential clinical importance since they differ markedly in prognosis and management. The management of PMD is unique since PMD is a progressive disease despite the fact that it is encountered in the third to fifth decade of life. Accordingly, corneal cross-linking should still be one of the treatment options. When intracorneal rings (ICRs) implantation is indicated in the management of PMD, caution should be paid to the location of the inferior segment, since it passes through the inferior thinned area. Corneal thickness at the thinnest point is more accurate in the pachymetry map provided by the OCT.

In PMD, corneal tomographic analysis reveals a flattening in the vertical meridian, inducing a significant against-the-rule (ATR) astigmatism and a significant steepening around the area of maximum thinning with a classical aspect of claw pattern.

The OCT shows a peripheral and inferior stromal thinning. The central cornea has a normal appearance. Corneal pachymetry map is important to differentiate keratoconus from PMD showing a lower and more peripheral corneal thinning in PMD **(Figures 12.8A to E)**.

KERATOGLOBUS

Keratoglobus is a rare corneal disease characterized by limbus-to-limbus corneal thinning, often greatest in the periphery, with globular protrusion of the central cornea. Visual impairment in patients with keratoglobus can be profound due to severe corneal ectasia, irregular astigmatism, high myopia, and may occur secondarily to corneal scarring and rupture.

The natural course of the disease is different from keratoconus. Corneal hydrops are exceptional. However, the evolution is marked by the risk of corneal perforation or rupture.

The OCT topographic map shows a generalized thinning of the cornea (only paracentral in keratoconus). The depth of the anterior chamber is markedly increased. Stromal opacities can occur in advanced cases **(Figures 12.9A to E)**.

REFERENCES

1. Efron N, Hollingsworth JG. New perspectives on keratoconus as revealed by corneal confocal microscopy. Clin Exp Optom. 2008;91:34-55.
2. Li Y, Meisler DM, Tang M, et al. Keratoconus diagnosis with optical coherence tomography pachymetry mapping. Ophthalmology. 2008;115:2159-66.
3. Reinstein DZ, Archer TJ, Gobbe M. Corneal epithelial thickness profile in the diagnosis of keratoconus. J Refract Surg. 2009;25:604-10.
4. Sandali O, El Sanharawi M, Temset C, et al. Fourier-Domain Optical coherence tomography imaging in keratoconus: a corneal structural classification. Ophthalmology. 2013;120:2403-12.
5. Tang M, Andrade EM, Li Y, Khurana RN, Song JC, Huang D. Optical coherence tomography to assess intrastromal corneal ring segment depth in keratoconic eyes. J Cataract Refract Surg. 2006;32:1860-5.
6. Borderie VM, Sandali O, Bullet J, Gaujoux T, Touzeau O, Laroche L. Long-term Results of Deep Anterior Lamellar versus Penetrating Keratoplasty. Ophthalmology. 2012;119:249-55.
7. Randleman JB, Woodward M, Lynn MJ, Stulting RD. Risk assessment for ectasia after corneal refractive surgery. Ophthalmology. 2008;115:37-50.

Chapter 13

Spectral-domain Anterior Segment Optical Coherence Tomography in Refractive Surgery

Karolinne Maia Rocha (USA), Ronald R Krueger (USA)

Optical coherence tomography (OCT) is a promising imaging device in refractive surgery due to its real-time, high-speed and noncontact features. OCT allows for high-resolution, cross-sectional scans and two- and three-dimensional (3-D) reconstructions of the cornea, iris, anterior chamber angle and lens, as well as 3-D optical biometry.[1-8] OCT images are acquired by measuring the intensity and the time delay of wave lights diffracted from anatomical structures passing through an established reference path.[8] Spectral-domain OCT (SD OCT) systems use a charge coupled device camera to register the diffraction grating of wave lights returning from the eye structures. The time delay and intensity of the wave lights are processed using a mathematical formula (Fourier transformation). The effective acquisition speed is 26,000 axial scans per second, which is up to 100 times faster when compared to the first generation time-domain OCT systems. The system operates at 830 nm.[9] The implications of the increased speed and sensitivity offered by SD OCT are images with lower signal to noise ratio (SNR), compared to time-domain OCT (TD OCT), and high axial resolution.[8-12] A wide-angle anterior segment adaptor (CAM-L mode) for the RTVue-100 OCT (Optovue, Inc., Fremount, CA) provides denser pixel cross-sectional imaging of the cornea/anterior segment with axial resolution of 5 μm and transverse resolution of 15 μm.[10]

Most recently, a custom-developed SD OCT system, including full distortion correction (fan and optical), as well as segmentation and merging of the different volumes (cornea, iris and lens), was built to process and generate high-resolution 3-D images.[1,2,13-17] The main features of this device are: 840 nm (50 nm bandwidth) SLD is super luminescent diode illuminating source; spectrometer with a 4096-pixel line CMOS camera; axial pixel resolution of 3.4 μm and predicted axial resolution of 6.9 μm. As a result, 3-D biometrical quantification of the anterior segment can be generated.

Three-dimensional epithelial and total corneal maps can be generated by interpolating thickness profiles from multiple meridians.[18] In addition, SD OCT-based corneal tomography and visualization of all corneal layers by high-resolution cross-sectional scans are essential tools for evaluating refractive candidates, including screening and risk of ectasia assessment, progression of corneal ectasia, corneal collagen cross-linking, intrastromal corneal rings and inlays, custom ablation profiles and presbyopic treatments.

REFRACTIVE SURGERY SCREENING AND CORNEAL ECTASIA RISK SCORING SYSTEM

One of the most important screening strategies in refractive surgery is to identify risk factors for corneal ectasia and to minimize its occurrence. Several placido-based computerized videokeratoscopy indices have been described for the diagnosis of keratoconus.[19-21] The diagnosis and progression of keratoconus is based on clinical features and anterior corneal curvature data as classically seen with the Amsler-Krumeich classification.[22] Over the last few years, a comprehensive corneal analysis from the anterior and posterior corneal curvature and full pachymetric data has been used for preoperative refractive screening and early detection signs of keratoconus. New corneal tomography parameters using rotating Scheimpflug devices[23-25] and slit-scanning elevation topography[26] has shown changes on both the posterior cornea and/or corneal thickness map as earlier indicators of corneal ectasia.

Spectral-domain optical coherence tomography measures the anterior and posterior cornea curvature in addition to qualitative and quantitative analysis of the relationship of the corneal epithelium and stroma that can be expressed as topographic thickness variations. The Optovue RTVue-CAM (Optovue Inc, Fredmont, CA) pachymetry-corneal power software (Cpwr), with 1024 axial scans and 6 mm diameter scanning, measures the cornea in 8 meridians. The high resolution, cross-sectional scans are repeated 5 times and averaged to generate the pachymetry maps. The air-tear interface and the epithelial-Bowman's layer landmark were identified automatically by a computer algorithm to generate the epithelial thickness maps, as described by Lin et al.[27] The corneal pachymetry map and epithelial thickness map is divided into zones by octants and 2, 5 and 6 mm annular rings. The map is obtained in 0.32 seconds and comprises 8 meridional scans. The average of 6 mm paracentral pachymetry measurements of superior (S), inferior (I), temporal (T), nasal (N), superotemporal (ST), superonasal (SN), inferotemporal (IT) and inferonasal (IN) zones are displayed. The central measurement corresponds to the average pachymetry of the central 2 mm. The pachymetry map also includes minimum corneal thickness and location; anterior and posterior corneal power and curvature radius; and total corneal power (**Figure 13.1**). In previous studies, SD OCT pachymetry maps have shown high reproducibility in detecting eccentric

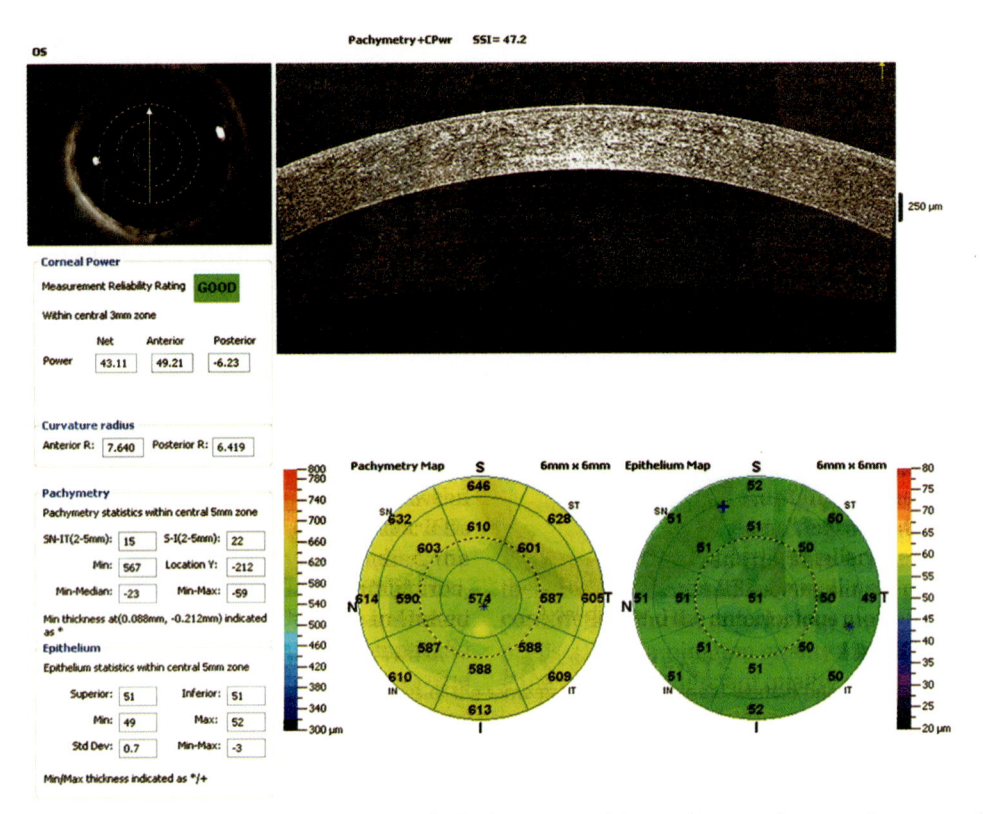

Figure 13.1 Spectral-domain optical coherence tomography CAM-L raster module scan (6-mm pachymetry+Cpwr scans - Optovue RTVue-100) display of a normal cornea including pachymetry map, epithelial thickness profile map and corneal power

and asymmetric corneal thinning in keratoconus.[27] Recently, a SD OCT pachymetry map–based keratoconus risk scoring system was developed based on these pachymetric variables.[28]

Additionally, the cross-sectional high resolution scans can show localized areas of epithelial compensation overlying areas of stromal thinning in keratoconus **(Figure 13.2)**. SD OCT high resolution cross-sectional scans demonstrated significant regional variability in corneal epithelial thickness profiles, as well as greater patterns of thickness deviation in eyes with keratoconus and postoperative corneal ectasia, compared to normal eyes.[28-30] **Figure 13.3** shows 2 patients with inferior steepening seen on placidobased corneal topography; SD OCT epithelial thickness map shows localized zone of epithelial thinning surrounded by thickened epithelium over the region of the cone in keratoconus, and thickened epithelium, corresponding to the area of inferior steepening seen on topography, in corneal warpage. The analysis of the epithelial thickness profile can be used as an adjunctive tool in refractive screening and possible early detection of keratoconus.

EPITHELIAL THICKNESS REMODELING IN REFRACTIVE SURGERY

Recently, detailed analysis of the corneal epithelial thickness profile in laser-assisted *in situ* keratomileusis (LASIK) using SD OCT has been described.[32-33] The corneal epithelium has a fast turnover and compensatory changes of the corneal epithelium helps to generate a smoother corneal surface in the setting of irregularities of the underlying stroma.[29-35]

We evaluated epithelial thickness remodeling and changes in the flap architecture after myopic LASIK using high resolution SD-OCT to correlate the anatomical findings to the preoperative spherical equivalent manifest refraction and refractive outcomes.[32] **Figure 13.4** shows the air-tear film interface and the epithelial-Bowman's layer landmark automatic segmentation and reconstruction, as described by Li et al;[36] the distance between the anterior surface of the cornea and the flap-stroma interface were manually detected to generate flap thickness maps (see *LASIK Flap Mapping by SD OCT* section).

Forty myopic eyes were included in this prospective, randomized, contralateral eye study. The preoperative manifest refraction ranged from –1.00 to –7.25 diopters (mean –3.25 ± 1.9). Flap creation was randomized between eyes, using the IntraLASE FS60 (IL, Abbott Medical Optics, Irvine, CA) in one eye and WaveLight FS200 (FS, Alcon Laboratories Inc., Ft Worth, TX) in the contralateral eye and all eyes were treated with the ALLEGRETTO®Eye-Q excimer laser (Alcon Laboratories Inc., Ft Worth, TX). SD-OCT (Optovue RTVue-100 Fremont, CA) was used to evaluate the epithelial and flap

Chapter 13: Spectral-domain Anterior Segment Optical Coherence Tomography ... 145

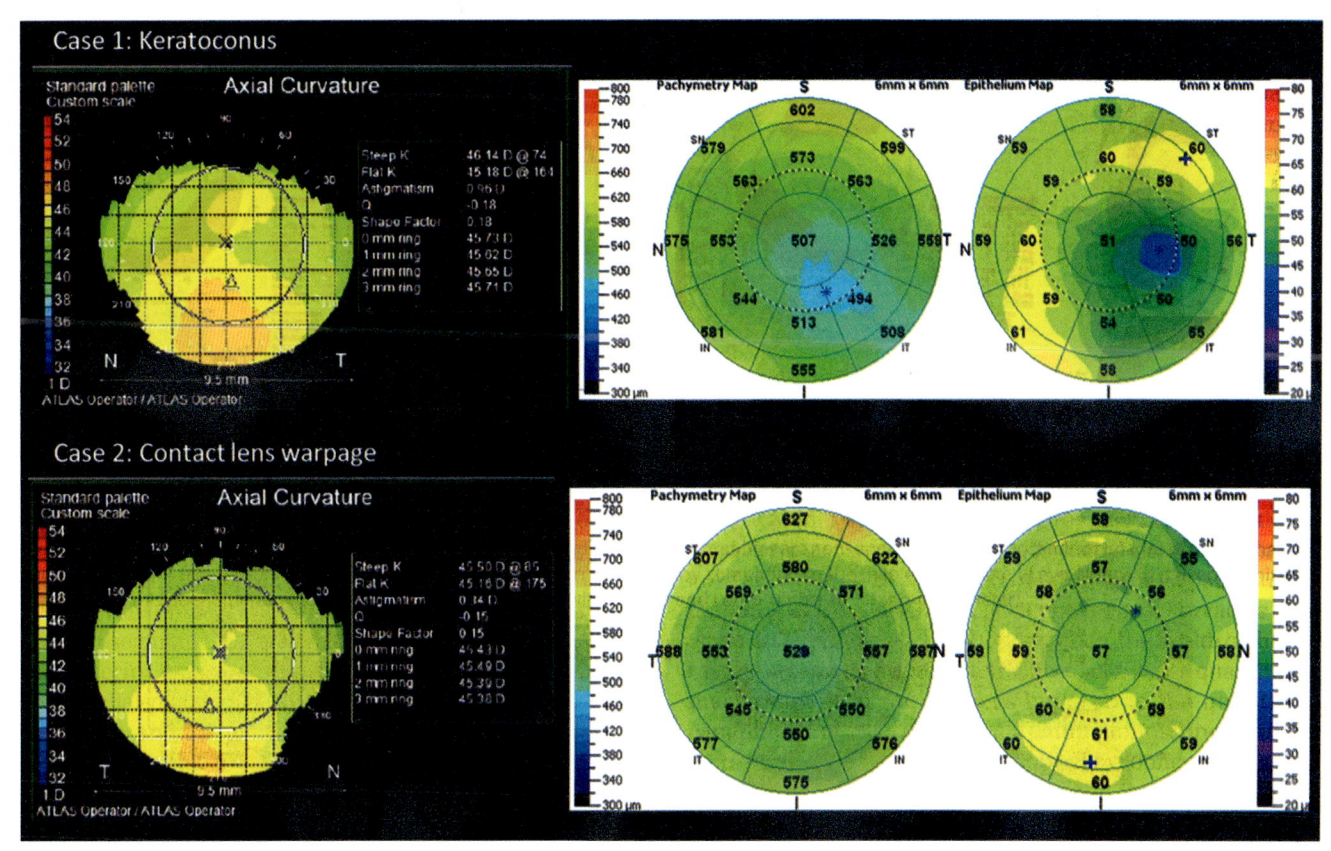

Figure 13.2 Corneal topography and spectral-domain optical coherence tomography epithelial thickness profile map in corneal warpage and keratoconus. Epithelial thickness map shows localized zone of epithelial thinning over the region of the cone in keratoconus and thickened epithelium corresponding to the area of inferior steepening seen on topography in corneal warpage

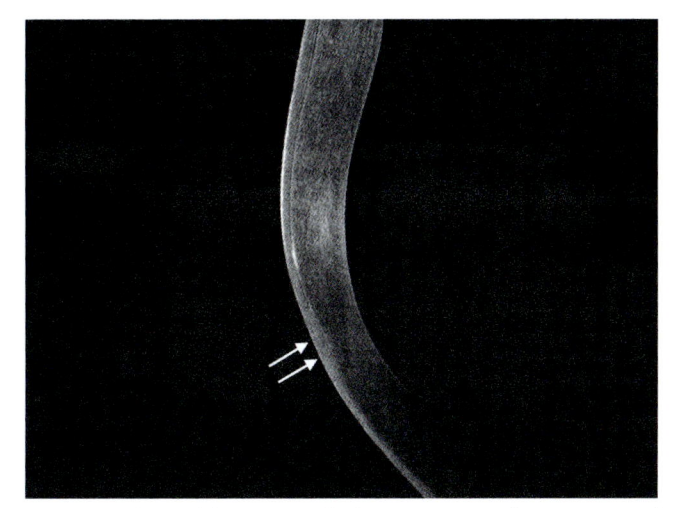

Figure 13.3 Spectral-domain optical coherence tomography cross-sectional high resolution scans across the central 6-mm of the corneal apex in the vertical meridian in keratoconus. Regional epithelial thickness profile variability, with localized areas of thickened (arrows) and thinned epithelium can be observed

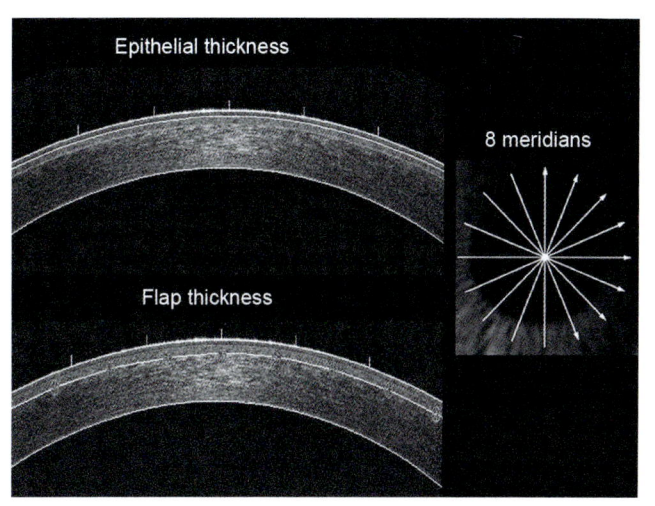

Figure 13.4 Cross-sectional spectral-domain optical coherence tomography high resolution scans reveal epithelial and flap thickness profiles, along 8 radial meridians, to generate epithelial thickness and femtosecond laser-assisted *in situ* keratomileusis flap SD OCT maps (arrows)

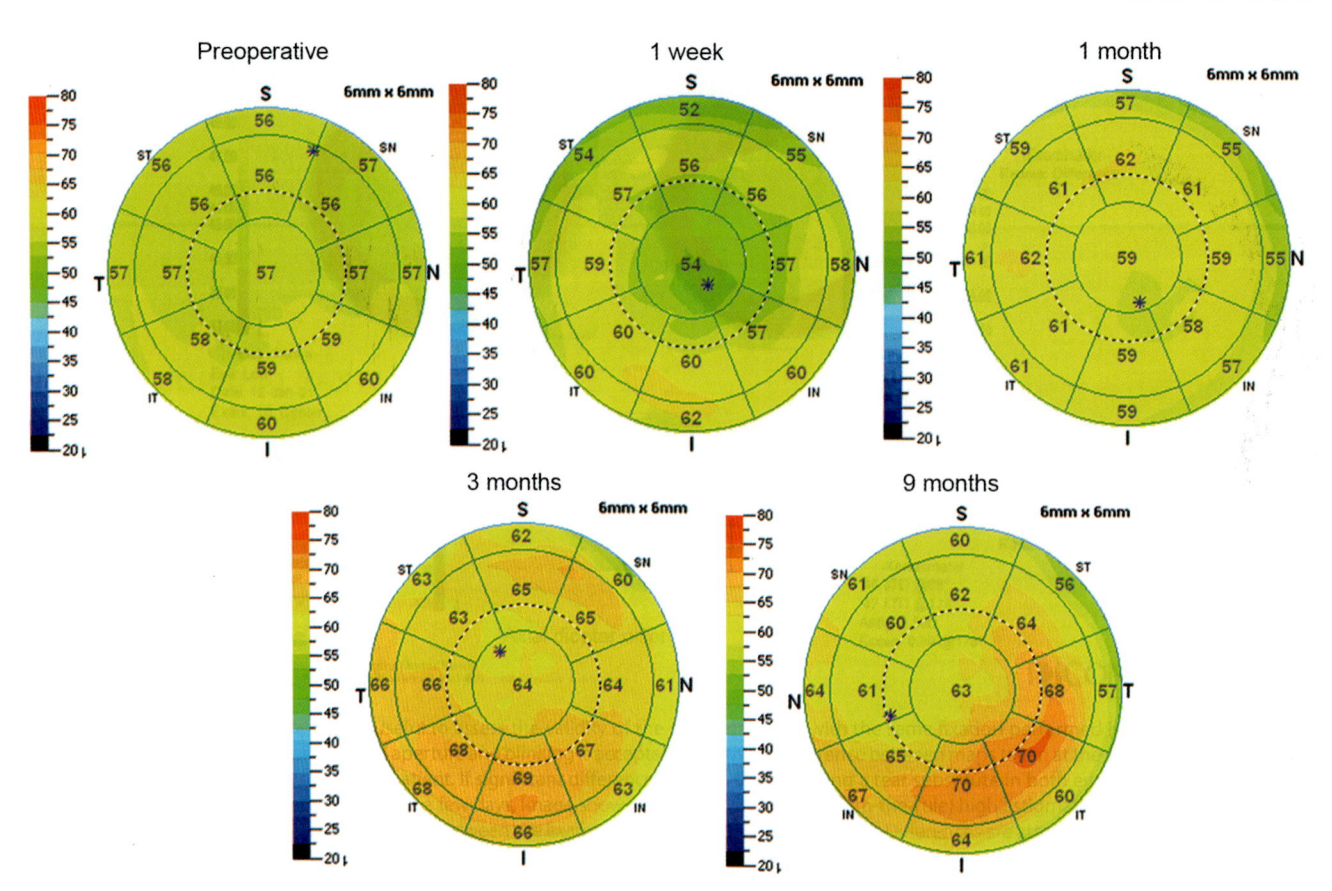

Figure 13.5 Epithelial thickness profile mapping seen preoperatively, 1 week, 1 month, 3 and 9 months post femtosecond laser-assisted *in situ* keratomileusis for myopia.

thickness profiles and corneal power preoperatively and at 1 week, 1, 3 and 9 months postoperatively. Statistically significant epithelial thickening was observed in both IL and FS groups as early as 1 month postoperatively (p = 0.033 and p = 0.042), but this stabilized between 3 (p = 0.042 and p = 0.035) and 9 months postoperatively (p = 0.043 and p = 0.041) **(Figure 13.5)**. The magnitude of epithelial and flap thickness remodeling correlated to the preoperative spherical equivalent refraction. We found a statistically significant correlation between the magnitude of preoperative myopic refraction and the central epithelial thickness at 1, 3 and 9 months (Pearson correlation coefficients 0.485, 0.587 and 0.576), (p = 0.0021, 0.0010 and 0.0011), respectively. Additionally, the corneal power change reconstructed from the SD-OCT maps showed steepening at 3 and 9 months, in correlation with both the thicker epithelium and a mild myopic shift in manifest and wavefront refraction.

The use of SD OCT in refractive surgery is important to recognize the initial instability seen after LASIK and to characterize the spatial relationship of epithelial remodeling with refractive outcomes. We believe the pattern of epithelial remodeling with different ablation profiles should be considered in the future planning of customized excimer laser ablations including topography-guided, wavefront-guided and multifocal, presbyopic excimer laser treatments.

LASIK FLAP MAPPING BY SPECTRAL DOMAIN OPTICAL COHERENCE TOMOGRAPHY

The lamellar distribution of collagen in the anterior and peripheral corneal stroma adjacent to Bowman's layer has higher cohesive tensile strength compared to the posterior stroma, presenting the sub-Bowman's region as the strongest area of the cornea.[37-39] As a result, femtosecond laser-assisted LASIK flaps that are thin and planar, and more so small incision lenticule extraction procedures, minimize biomechanical changes in the cornea.[40-43] Residual stromal bed measurements are useful when planning LASIK enhancements to avoid deeper ablations into the posterior stroma. For these reasons, advanced imaging of the predictability of refractive procedures should be incorporated into clinical practice.

Spectral-domain OCT high resolution cross-line scan of the add-on lens can easily identify the posterior edge of the LASIK flap. Traditionally, one-dimensional measurements of

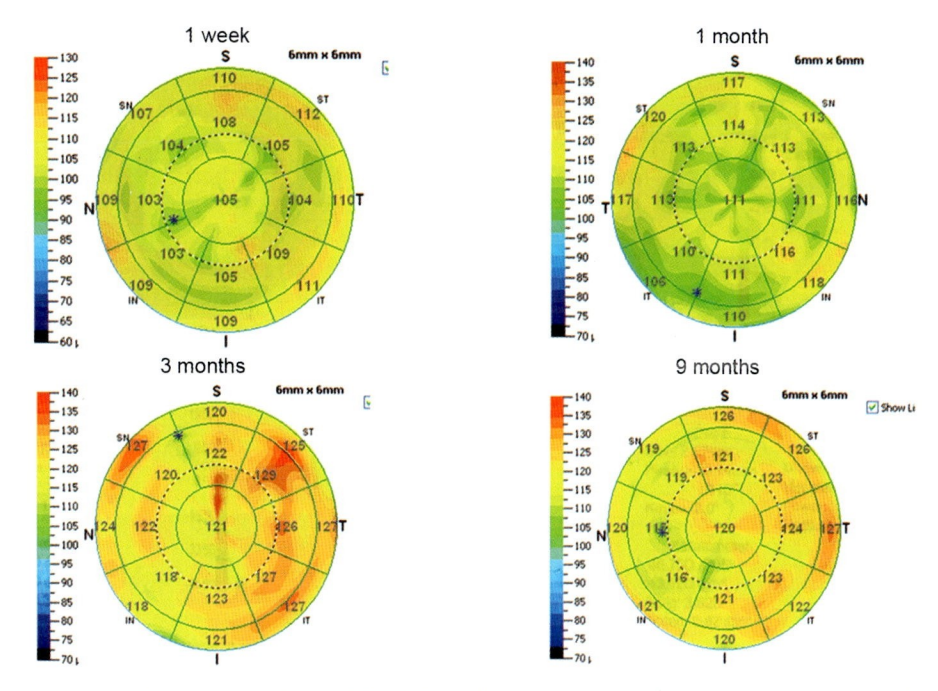

Figure 13.6 Flap thickness profile mapping at 1 week, 1, 3 and 9 months post femtosecond laser-assisted *in situ* keratomileusis for myopia

the distance between the anterior surface of the cornea and the flap-stroma interface using high resolution cross-sectional scans are used to asses flap thickness.[44-55] Pachymetric LASIK flap maps can be generated by SD OCT. In our latest study, the flap boundaries were manually detected and inspected, and 9 points were manually measured in 8 meridians to generate the flap thickness profile maps.[32] The automated algorithm built into the RTVue software was used to interpolate the high resolution scans. The color scale ranged from 20 to 80 μm for the epithelial thickness maps and from 70 to 140 μm for the flap thickness profile maps **(Figure 13.4)**.

In correlation with the change in epithelial thickness observed at 1 week, 1 month, 3 and 9 months after myopic LASIK, comparable variations in femtosecond laser flap thickness profiles were seen in both IntraLASE FS60 (IL) and WaveLight FS200 (FS) laser groups. Progressive thickening of the femtosecond LASIK flaps was observed up to 3 months after femtosecond-LASIK **(Figure 13.6)**. No statistically significant difference was found for the IL and FS lasers flaps at 1 week (p = 0.08) and 1 month postoperatively (p = 0.07). Femtosecond-LASIK flaps were thicker in the IL group in comparison to the FS group at 3 and 9 months postoperatively (p = 0.003 and p = 0.005, respectively).

ADVANCES IN ANTERIOR SEGMENT BIOMETRY AND INTRAOCULAR LENS CALCULATION

The two main sources of error in intraocular lens (IOL) power calculation after refractive surgery are measurements of the postoperative corneal power by standard keratometry and topography, and IOL formula limitations based on inaccurate estimation of the effective lens position (*ELP*).[56-65] *ELP* is the distance between the vertex of the cornea to the plane of the IOL. Keratometers and topographers do not precisely measure the central cornea power and corneal tomographers extrapolate curvature data based on elevation measurements relative to a reference shape. As a result, measurements of the cornea power (K) after refractive surgery tend to overestimate the K readings following laser corrections for myopia and under-estimate for hyperopia. Third generation formulas (e.g. SRK-T, Holladay 1, Hoffer Q) predict the *ELP* based on the axial length and keratometry. Using these formulas, a flat K power will produce a false shallow postoperative *ELP*, resulting in under-estimation of the calculated IOL power and a hyperopic error.

The measurement of both the anterior and posterior corneal surfaces and the anterior and posterior lens by SD OCT systems allows three-dimensional quantification of the cornea, anterior chamber depth, lens and effective intraocular lens position.[15,16] Additionally, SD OCT provides for the true corneal power calculation. SD OCT measurements of the central corneal power post myopic LASIK and RK are lower than conventional keratometry, therefore an OCT-based formula based on an optical vergence model of the eye (paraxial approximation of Gaussian optics) should be used.[66-68] In a pilot study, Tang, et al. showed that SD OCT-based IOL power calculation had better predictive accuracy than the Clinical History Method and was equivalent to the Haigis-L formula in post myopic LASIK eyes.[66] 3-D OCT optical biometry and 3-D anterior segment reconstruction are promising tools for ELP, IOL tilt and decentration evaluation.[16]

ADVANCED SPECTRAL-DOMAIN OPTICAL COHERENCE TOMOGRAPHY IMAGING— CASE REPORT

A 42-year-old male, right eye dominant, was referred for evaluation of epithelial ingrowth in the right eye. The patient underwent myopic LASIK in both eyes in 2000 and LASIK flap lift enhancement in the right eye in March of 2013 for mild myopic regression. At the time of presentation patient reported blurred vision at distance and near in the right eye since about 1 week after the LASIK enhancement. Best-corrected visual acuity (BDVA) was 20/30 in the right eye and 20/15 in the left eye with manifest refraction of −0.50 + 2.00 @ 58 in the right eye and plano in the left eye. **Figure 13.7** shows the anterior segment photo and cross-sectional high resolution SD OCT image. Flap lift with extensive epithelial scraping of stromal bed and posterior surface of flap and beyond edge of flap edge was performed in the right eye. At 1 week following flap lift in the right eye BDVA was 20/20 with manifest refraction of −2.00+1.00@45 (**Figure 13.8** illustrates the slit lamp photos and SD OCT). Patient returned for follow up at 1 month after flap lift and epithelial scraping in the right eye; uncorrected visual acuity was 20/20 and the manifest refraction was plano, despite recurrence of the epithelial ingrowth from 3 to 4 o'clock (**Figure 13.9**). Cross-sectional high resolution SD OCT scans and epithelial thickness mapping

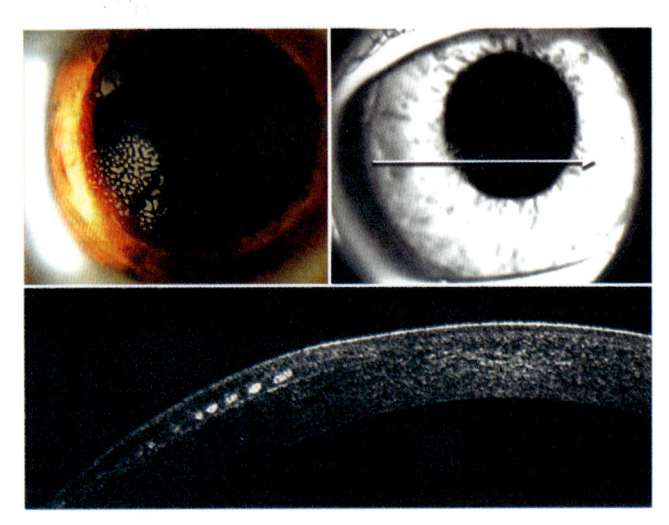

Figure 13.7 Slit lamp photo and cross-sectional spectral-domain optical coherence tomography image of postoperative epithelial ingrowth

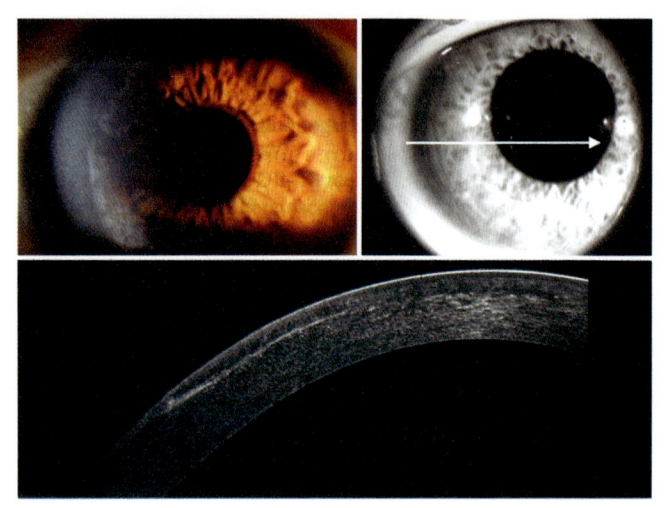

Figure 13.8 Anterior segment photo and spectral-domain optical coherence tomography image 1 week post LASIK flap lift with extensive epithelial scraping of stromal bed and posterior surface of flap and beyond edge of flap edge

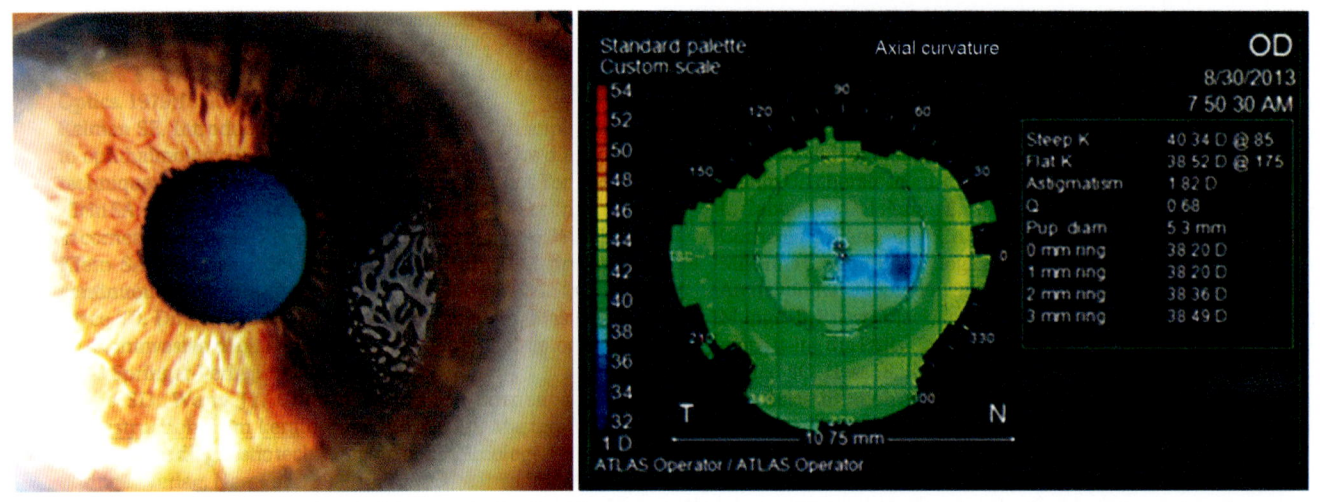

Figure 13.9 Recurrence of epithelial ingrowth after flap lift and epithelial scraping (slit lamp photo and corneal topography axial map)

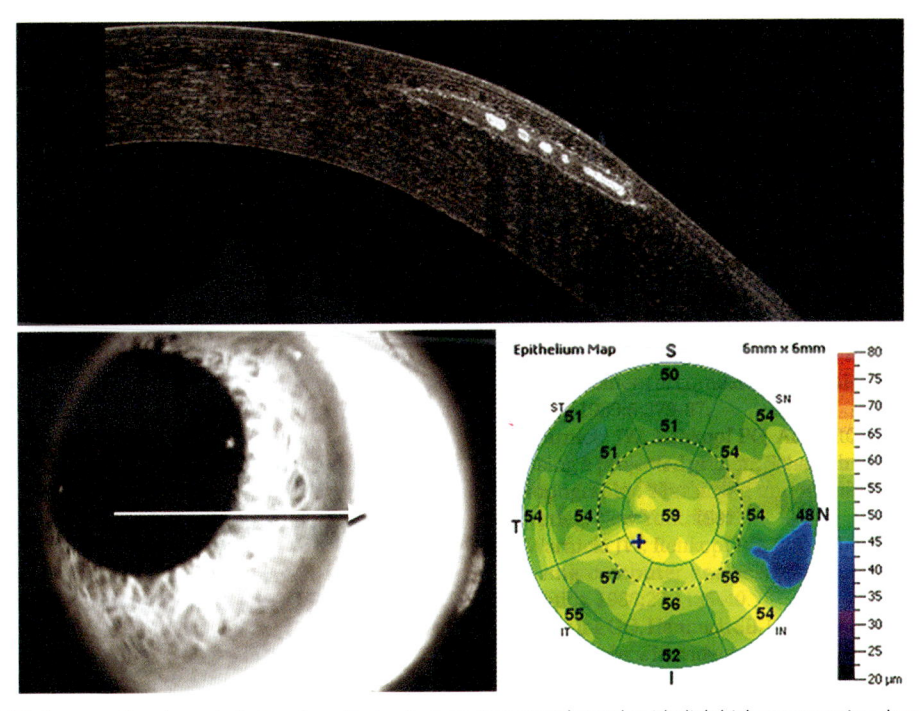

Figure 13.10 Cross-sectional spectral-domain optical coherence tomography and epithelial thickness mapping demonstrating epithelial remodeling with thinning of the corneal epithelium overlying the area of epithelial ingrowth

revealed epithelial remodeling with thinning of the epithelium overlying the area of epithelial ingrowth **(Figure 13.10)**. The treatment options were discussed with the patient. At that point the patient was asymptomatic and his visual acuity had improved. We recommended observation. This case illustrates well the epithelial compensation overlying areas of stromal irregularities producing a smooth corneal surface.

In conclusion, Spectral-domain OCT provides full assessment of all cornea layers and can be helpful in the diagnosis and management of complex refractive cases. High resolution scans, total thickness, epithelial and flap mapping add in interpretation of corneal topography and should be considered in the future planning of customized excimer laser ablation profiles. Spectral-domain OCT 3-D reconstruction of the anterior segment and measurements of the corneal power are excellent tools for complex IOL calculation cases.

REFERENCES

1. Ortiz S, Siedlecki D, Pérez-Merino P, Chia N, de Castro A, Szkulmowski M, et al. Corneal topography from spectral optical coherence tomography (sOCT). Biomed Opt Express. 2011;2(12): 3232-47.
2. Karnowski K, Kaluzny BJ, Szkulmowski M, et al. Corneal topography with high-speed swept source OCT in clinical examination. Biomed Opt Express. 2011;2(9):2709-20.
3. Radhakrishnan S, Goldsmith J, Huang D, Westphal V, Dueker DK, Rollins AM, et al. Comparison of optical coherence tomography and ultrasound biomicroscopy for detection of narrow anterior chamber angles. Arch Ophthalmol. 2005;123(8):1053-9.
4. Müller M, Dahmen G, Pörksen E, Geerling G, Laqua H, Ziegler A, et al. Anterior chamber angle measurement with optical coherence tomography: intraobserver and interobserver variability. J Cataract Refract Surg. 2006;32(11):1803-8.
5. Dada T, Sihota R, Gadia R, Aggarwal A, Mandal S, Gupta V. Comparison of anterior segment optical coherence tomography and ultrasound biomicroscopy for assessment of the anterior segment. J Cataract Refract Surg. 2007;33(5):837-40.
6. Radhakrishnan S, Rollins AM, Roth JE, Yazdanfar S, Westphal V, Bardenstein DS, et al. Real-time optical coherence tomography of the anterior segment at 1310 nm. Arch Ophthalmol. 2001;119(8): 1179-85.
7. Gambra E, Ortiz S, Perez-Merino P, Gora M, Wojtkowski M, Marcos S. Static and dynamic crystalline lens accommodation evaluated using quantitative 3-D OCT. Biomed Opt Express. 2013; 8;4(9):1595-609.
8. Huang D, Swanson EA, Lin CP, Schuman JS, Stinson WG, Chang W, et al. Optical coherence tomography. Science. 1991; 254(5035):1178-81.
9. Keane PA, Bhatti RA, Brubaker JW, Liakopoulos S, Sadda SR, Walsh AC. Comparison of Clinically Relevant Findings from High-Speed Fourier-Domain and Conventional Time-Domain Optical Coherence Tomography. Am J Ophthalmol. 2009;148(2):242-8.e1.
10. Sarunic MV, Asrani S, Izatt JA. Imaging the ocular anterior segment with real-time, full-range Fourier-domain optical coherence tomography. Arch Ophthalmol. 2008;126:537-42.
11. Prakash G, Agarwal A, Jacob S, et al. Comparison of Fourier-Domain and Time-Domain Optical Coherence Tomography for

Assessment of Corneal Thickness and Intersession Repeatability. Am J Ophthalmol. 2009;148(2):282-90.
12. Wojtkowski M, Srinivasan V, Ko T, et al. Ultrahigh-resolution, high-speed, fourier domain optical coherence tomography and methods for dispersion compensation. Optics Express. 2004;12(11):2404-22.
13. Ortiz S, Siedlecki D, Grulkowski I, Remon L, Pascual D, Wojtkowski M, et al. Optical distortion correction in optical coherence tomography for quantitative ocular anterior segment by three-dimensional imaging. Opt Express. 2010;18(3):2782-96.
14. Zhao M, Kuo AN, Izatt JA. 3D refraction correction and extraction of clinical parameters from spectral domain optical coherence tomography of the cornea. Opt Express. 2010;18(9):8923-36.
15. Ortiz S, Siedlecki D, Remon L, et al. Three-dimensional ray tracing on Delaunay-based reconstructed surfaces. Appl Opt. 2009;48(20):3886-93.
16. Ortiz S, Pérez-Merino P, Durán S, Velasco-Ocana M, Birkenfeld J, de Castro A, et al. Full OCT anterior segment biometry: an application in cataract surgery. Biomed Opt Express. 2013;4(3):387-96.
17. Ruggeri M, Uhlhorn SR, De Freitas C, Ho A, Manns F, Parel JM. Imaging and full-length biometry of the eye during accommodation using spectral domain OCT with an optical switch. Biomed Opt Express. 2012;3(7):1506-20.
18. Haque S, Jones L, Simpson T. Thickness mapping of the cornea and epithelium using optical coherence tomography. Optom Vis Sci. 2008;85(10):963-76.
19. Rabinowitz YS. Videokeratographic indices to aid in screening for keratoconus. J Refract Surg. 1995;11:371-9.
20. Rabinowitz YS, Rasheed K. KISA% index: a quantitative videokeratography algorithm embodying minimal topographic criteria for diagnosing keratoconus. J Cataract Refract Surg. 1999;25:1327-35.
21. Schwiegerling J, Greivenkamp JE. Keratoconus detection based on videokeratoscopic height data. Optom Vis Sci. 1996;73:721-8.
22. Kamiya K, Ishii R, Shimizu K, et al. Evaluation of corneal elevation, pachymetry and keratometry in keratoconic eyes with respect to the stage of Amsler-Krumeich classification. Br J Ophthalmol. 2014;98(4):459-63.
23. Smadja D, Touboul D, Cohen A, Doveh E, Santhiago MR, Mello GR, et al. Detection of subclinical keratoconus using an automated decision tree classification. Am J Ophthalmol. 2013;156(2):237-46.
24. Ambrosio R, Jr, Caiado AL, Guerra FP, Lousada R, Roy AS, Luz A, et al. Novel pachymetric parameters based on corneal tomography for diagnosing keratoconus. J Refract Surg. 2011;27:753-8.
25. Michael W Belin, Renato Ambrósio, Jr. Scheimpflug imaging for keratoconus and ectatic disease. Indian J Ophthalmol. 2013; 61(8):401-6.
26. Saad A, Gatinel D. Topographic and tomographic properties of forme fruste keratoconus corneas. Invest Ophthalmol Vis Sci. 2010;51(11):5546-55.
27. Li Y, Meisler DM, Tang M, Lu AT, Thakrar V, Reiser BJ, et al. Keratoconus diagnosis with optical coherence tomography pachymetry mapping. Ophthalmology. 2008;115(12):2159-66.
28. Qin B, Chen S, Brass R, Li Y, Tang M, Zhang X, et al. Keratoconus diagnosis with optical coherence tomography-based pachymetric scoring system. J Cataract Refract Surg. 2013;39(12):1864-71.
29. Rocha KM, Perez-Straziota CE, Randleman JB, et al. Spectral-domain OCT analysis of regional epithelial thickness profiles in keratoconus, postoperative corneal ectasia, and normal eyes. J Refract Surg. 2013;29(3):173-9.
30. Rocha KM, Perez-Straziota CE, Randleman JB, et al. Epithelial and stromal remodeling after corneal collagen cross-linking evaluated by Spectral-domain OCT. J Refract Surg. 2014;30(2):122-7.
31. Sandali O, El Sanharawi M, Temstet C, Hamiche T, Galan A, Ghouali W, et al. Fourier-domain optical coherence tomography imaging in keratoconus: a corneal structural classification. Ophthalmology. 2013;120(12):2403-12.
32. Rocha KM, Krueger RR. Spectral-domain optical coherence tomography epithelial and flap thickness mapping in femtosecond laser-assisted in situ keratomileusis. Am J Ophthalmol. 2014, in press.
33. Kanellopoulos AJ, Asimellis G. Longitudinal postoperative LASIK epithelial thickness profile changes in correlation with degree of myopia correction. J Refract Surg. 2014;30(3):166-71.
34. Reinstein DZ, Archer TJ, Gobbe M. Change in epithelial thickness profile 24 hours and longitudinally for 1 year after myopic LASIK: three-dimensional display with Artemis very high-frequency digital ultrasound. J Refract Surg. 2012;28(3):195-201.
35. Reinstein DZ, Silverman RH, Raevsky T, et al. Arc-scanning very high-frequency digital ultrasound for 3D pachymetric mapping of the corneal epithelium and stroma in laser in situ keratomileusis. J Refract Surg. 2000;16(4):414-30.
36. Li Y, Tan O, Brass R, et al. Corneal epithelial thickness mapping by Fourier-domain optical coherence tomography in normal and keratoconic eyes. Ophthalmology. 2012;119(12):2425-33.
37. Dawson DG, Grossniklaus HE, McCarey BE, Edelhauser HF. Biomechanical and wound healing characteristics of corneas after excimer laser keratorefractive surgery: is there a difference between advanced surface ablation and sub-Bowman's keratomileusis? J Refract Surg. 2008;24(1):S90-6.
38. Dupps WJ, Jr., Roberts C. Effect of acute biomechanical changes on corneal curvature after photokeratectomy. J Refract Surg. 2001;17(6):658-69.
39. Randleman JB, Dawson DG, Grossniklaus HE, et al. Depth-dependent cohesive tensile strength in human donor corneas: implications for refractive surgery. J Refract Surg. 2008;24(1):S85-9.
40. Yao P, Zhao J, Li M, Shen Y, Dong Z, Zhou X. Microdistortions in Bowman's Layer Following Femtosecond Laser Small Incision Lenticule Extraction Observed by Fourier-Domain OCT. J Refract Surg. 2013;6:1-7.
41. Zhao J, Yao P, Li M, Chen Z, Shen Y, Zhao Z, et al. The morphology of corneal cap and its relation to refractive outcomes in femtosecond laser small incision lenticule extraction (SMILE) with anterior segment optical coherence tomography observation. PLoS One. 2013;5;8(8):e702-08.
42. Reinstein DZ, Archer TJ, Randleman JB. Mathematical model to compare the relative tensile strength of the cornea after PRK, LASIK, and small incision lenticule extraction. J Refract Surg. 2013;29(7):454-60.
43. Agca A, Ozgurhan EB, Demirok A, Bozkurt E, Celik U, Ozkaya A, et al. Comparison of corneal hysteresis and corneal resistance factor after small incision lenticule extraction and femtosecond laser-assisted LASIK: a prospective fellow eye study. Cont Lens Anterior Eye. 2014;37(2):77-80.
44. Stahl JE, Durrie DS, Schwendeman FJ, Boghossian AJ. Anterior segment OCT analysis of thin IntraLase femtosecond flaps. J Refract Surg. 2007;23:555-8.

45. Wylegała E, Teper S, Nowińska AK, et al. Anterior segment imaging: Fourier-domain optical coherence tomography versus time-domain optical coherence tomography. J Cataract Refract Surg. 2009;35(8):1410-14.
46. von Jagow B, Kohnen T. Corneal architecture of femtosecond laser and microkeratome flaps imaged by anterior segment optical coherence tomography. J Cataract Refract Surg. 2009;35(1):35-41.
47. Duffey RJ. Thin flap laser in situ keratomileusis: flap dimensions with the Moria LSK-One manual microkeratome using the 100-microm head. J Cataract Refract Surg. 2005;31(6):1159-62.
48. Kymionis GD, Portaliou DM, Tsiklis NS, et al. Thin LASIK flap creation using the SCHWIND Carriazo-Pendular microkeratome. J Refract Surg. 2009;25(1):33-6.
49. Kim JH, Lee D, Rhee KI. Flap thickness reproducibility in laser in situ keratomileusis with a femtosecond laser: optical coherence tomography measurement. J Cataract Refract Surg. 2008;34:132-6.
50. Miranda D, Smith SD, Krueger RR. Comparison of flap thickness reproducibility using microkeratomes with a second motor for advancement. Ophthalmology. 2003;110(10):1931-4.
51. Krueger RR, Dupps WJ Jr. Biomechanical effects of femtosecond and microkeratome-based flap creation: prospective contralateral examination of two patients. J Refract Surg. 2007;23(8):800-7.
52. Li Y, Netto MV, Shekhar R, et al. A longitudinal study of LASIK flap and stromal thickness with high-speed optical coherence tomography. Ophthalmology. 2007;114(6):1124-32.
53. Hood CT, Krueger RR, Wilson SE. The association between femtosecond laser flap parameters and ocular aberrations after uncomplicated custom myopic LASIK. Graefes Arch Clin Exp Ophthalmol. 2013;251(9):2155-62.
54. Rocha KM, Kagan R, Smith SD, et al. Thresholds for interface haze formation after thin-flap femtosecond laser in situ keratomileusis for myopia. Am J Ophthalmol. 2009;147(6):966-72.
55. Rocha KM, Randleman JB, Stulting RD. Analysis of Microkeratome Thin Flap Architecture Using Fourier-domain Optical Coherence Tomography. J Refract Surg. 2011;27(10):759-63.
56. Aramberri J. Intraocular lens power calculation after corneal refractive surgery: double-K method. J Cataract Refract Surg. 2003;29:2063-8.
57. Arce CG, Soriano ES, Weisenthal RW, Hamilton SM, Rocha KM, Alzamora JB, et al. Calculation of intraocular lens power using Orbscan II quantitative area topography after corneal refractive surgery. J Refract Surg. 2009;25(12):1061-74.
58. Yang R, Yeh A, George MR, Rahman M, Boerman H, Wang M. Comparison of intraocular lens power calculation methods after myopic laser refractive surgery without previous refractive surgery data. J Cataract Refract Surg. 2013;39(9):1327-35.
59. Awwad ST, Kilby A, Bowman RW, Verity SM, Cavanagh HD, Pessach Y, et al. The accuracy of the double-K adjustment for third-generation intraocular lens calculation formulas in previous keratorefractive surgery eyes. Eye Contact Lens. 2013;39(3):220-7.
60. Saiki M, Negishi K, Kato N, Arai H, Toda I, Torii H, et al. A new central-peripheral corneal curvature method for intraocular lens power calculation after excimer laser refractive surgery. Acta Ophthalmol. 2013;91(2):e133-9.
61. Javadi MA, Feizi S, Malekifar P. Intraocular lens power calculation after corneal refractive surgery. J Ophthalmic Vis Res. 2012;7(1):10-6.
62. Kwitko S, Marinho DR, Rymer S, et al. Orbscan II and double-K method for IOL calculation after refractive surgery. Graefes Arch Clin Exp Ophthalmol. 2012;250(7):1029-34.
63. Awwad ST, Kelley PS, Bowman RW, et al. Corneal refractive power estimation and intraocular lens calculation after hyperopic LASIK. Ophthalmology. 2009;116(3):393-400.
64. Awwad ST, Manasseh C, Bowman RW, Cavanagh HD, Verity S, Mootha V, et al. Intraocular lens power calculation after myopic laser in situ keratomileusis: Estimating the corneal refractive power. J Cataract Refract Surg. 2008;34(7):1070-6.
65. Gimbel HV, Sun R. Accuracy and predictability of intraocular lens power calculation after laser in situ keratomileusis. J Cataract Refract Surg. 2001;27(4):571-6.
66. Tang M, Wang L, Koch DD, et al. Intraocular lens power calculation after previous myopic laser vision correction based on corneal power measured by Fourier-domain optical coherence tomography. J Cataract Refract Surg. 2012;38(4):589-94.
67. Tang M, Li Y, Huang D. An intraocular lens power calculation formula based on optical coherence tomography: a pilot study. J Refract Surg. 2010;26(6):430-7.
68. Huang D, Tang M, Wang L, Zhang X, Armour RL, Gattey DM, et al. Optical coherence tomography-based corneal power measurement and intraocular lens power calculation following laser vision correction (an American Ophthalmological Society thesis). Trans Am Ophthalmol Soc. 2013;111:34-45.

Section IV

Aberropia, Aberrations and Topography

CHAPTERS

14. Corneal Topographers and Wavefront Aberrometers: Complementary Tools
15. Aberrometry and Topography in the Vector Analysis of Refractive Laser Surgery
16. Aberropia: A New Refractive Entity
17. Differences Between Various Aberrometer Systems
18. Corneal Wavefront Guided Excimer Laser Surgery for the Correction of Eye Aberrations
19. Ocular Higher Order Aberration Induced Decrease in Vision (Aberropia): Characteristics and Classification
20. Topographic and Aberrometer Guided Laser
21. NAVWave: Nidek Technique for Customized Ablation

Chapter 14

Corneal Topographers and Wavefront Aberrometers: Complementary Tools

Tracy Schroeder Swartz (USA), Ming Wang (USA), Arun C Gulani (USA)

INTRODUCTION

The accessibility of the cornea and the non-intraocular designation of its anatomical status makes it the focus of refractive surgery. The cornea has therewith enjoyed this privilege for decades of refractive surgery. These very advantages also have us refractive surgeons constantly vying to make this delicately transparent yet inherently elastic tissue more predictable.

Thus began our search for that perfect tool which could study and analyze the cornea and also determine our consistency for cornea-based refractive surgery. Corneal topographers have been the gold standard for understanding corneal shape which is the basis of laser refractive surgery. Recently with the advent of aberrometers, the bar has been raised. We have a new technology as well as a new language to address the cornea with and thereby translate the same into effective and accurate surgical outcomes.

This bridge from topography to wavefront technology is actually an adjunct and not about the past or future. These are complementary technologies as of now and this chapter therewith addresses the application of the two.

With the advent of complex topographic systems and wavefront aberrometers, opthalmologists now benefit from a deeper understanding of the optics of the cornea and their effect on vision.

KERATOMETERS

The first instrument to measure the surface of the cornea was the ophthalmometer. This device measured the curvature of the cornea using reflected rings. It is important to remember the following assumptions related to keratometry:[1]

- The formula used is based on spherical geometry. The cornea, however, is not spherical but is a prolate (flattened) ellipsoid. Thus, the central radius is slightly steeper than actually measured.
- Keratometry is based on four data points within the central 3 mm of the cornea. It provides no insight into the area inside or outside of the 3 mm ring.
- Keratometry theory assumes paraxial optics. While the approximation may be clinically acceptable for fitting contacts or estimating corneal astigmatism, it may not be when measuring peripheral curvature.
- Keratometers assume alignment of the corneal apex, line of sight and instrument axis. However, this rarely occurs during actual measurement.
- The formula used to calculate the radius (r) approximates the distance to the convex focal point, which in the case of the Reichert keratometer, may introduce up to 0.12D of error. This error may increase, if the instrument is not correctly focused or the operator accommodates during measurement.
- Since the indexes may differ between manufacturers, one must be careful comparing the readings in diopters between different instruments.

CORNEAL TOPOGRAPHY

Such assumptions result in significant errors when considering the peripheral cornea, especially in eyes with irregular surfaces such as in keratoconus or S/P keratorefractive surgery. With the growth of computers came the corneal topography systems widely used today to evaluate the shape characteristics of the cornea.

Early videokeratoscopes used axial power maps to illustrate the information from captured raw data. The power at each point was calculated according to the Javal ophthalmometer convention, and suffered many of keratometry's assumptions.

The axial map is a traditional but poor descriptor of corneal refraction because it does not take into account spherical aberration.[2,3] Despite its limits, the axial map became known as "the corneal topography map". With the development of arc-step algorithms, placido systems could not only approximate axial power, but also measure corneal shape. Elevation maps became available. An example of an axial and elevation map of an eye with with-the-rule astigmatism is shown in **Figure 14.1**.

In the early to the mid 1990s, the explosion of excimer laser refractive surgery necessitated more accurate optical instruments to create more detailed representation of the corneal surface. At this point, the path divided as two parallel paths emerged. Some believed the answers to problems encountered in refractive surgery could be answered using

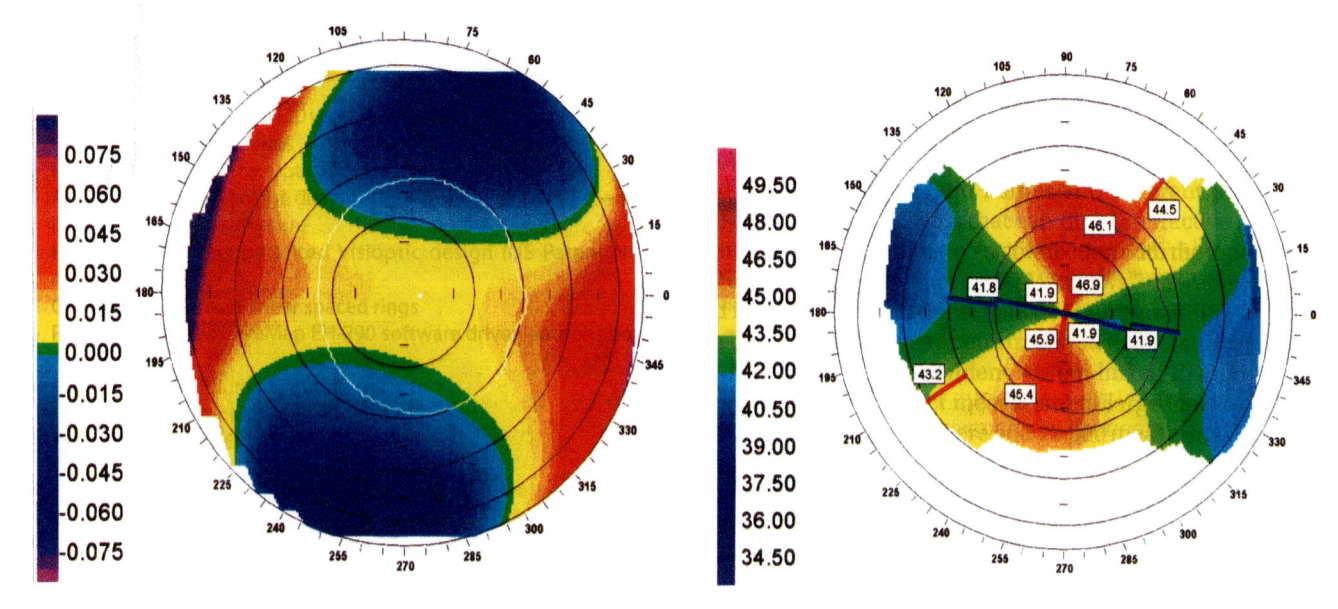

Figure 14.1 An axial (Right) and elevation (Left) map of an eye showing with-the-rule astigmatism

elevation-based topography, while others supported wavefront aberrometry-based platforms.

ELEVATION BASED TOPOGRAPHY

Placido disc imaging systems are limited to evaluation of the anterior cornea only, and calculate rather than directly measure elevation data. Systems emerged which directly measured corneal elevation, and evaluated anatomy posterior to the anterior cornea. The PAR Corneal topography system (PAR-CTS) was the first system to directly measure anterior elevation topography, using principles of triangulation. The distortion of a grid projected on to the cornea was mathematically compared to the true grid in a reference plane. Because the geometry of the reference surface and the grid projection is known, rays can be intersected in three dimensional space to compute the X, Y and Z coordinates of the surface.[4] This system was generally accepted to be more accurate when measuring complex bicurve and multicurve test surfaces, but poor reproducibility was reported.

Slit-scanning technology addressed both the need for direct measurement of elevation as well as evaluation of the posterior structures within the eye. The Orbscan II (Bausch & Lomb, Roschester, New York) combined a placido disc to measure curvature and slit scanning to measure both surfaces of the cornea. The most commonly used display for this system is the Quad map, shown in **Figure 14.2**. A placido image is captured to evaluate curvature data. Then, over 1.5 seconds, two scanning slit lamps project a total of 40 images each at 45 degrees of the video axis. A proprietary tracking system reduced eye movements. It produced pachymetry and anterior chamber depth information for the first time. This system remains the only type capable of evaluation of the posterior surface. Thus, there is no way to validate the information found in the posterior map.

Another technology was developed to address two problems associated with currently used topographic technology: assumptions inherent to power calculation and paracentral measurement of the cornea. The Pentacam (Oculus) addressed these deficiencies. It is a rotating Scheimpflug camera which provides a complete picture from the anterior surface of the cornea to the posterior surface of the lens, as shown in **Figure 14.3**.

As topographic systems advanced, understanding of the optics resulting from changes in shape induced by disease or refractive surgery, and the need to correct optical problems grew. Unfortunately, significantly irregular corneas, dry eyes, and scarring may cause topographic systems to fail.

Programs such as the Custom Corneal Ablation Planner (Custom CAP) utilized elevation data and computer analysis to create custom ablation profiles in an attempt to correct decentered ablations and relieve patients of visual distortion. An example is shown in **Figure 14.4**. Topography-driven programs fail to address the refractive error, however, and refractive changes induced by such treatments were somewhat unpredictable.

WAVEFRONT: ANOTHER VIEW OF CORNEAL OPTICS

Just as topographic analysis was facilitated by computers, so was measurement of optical aberrations. This advance in technology occurred slightly later and parallel to the growth of topography. The most common types of aberrometers are

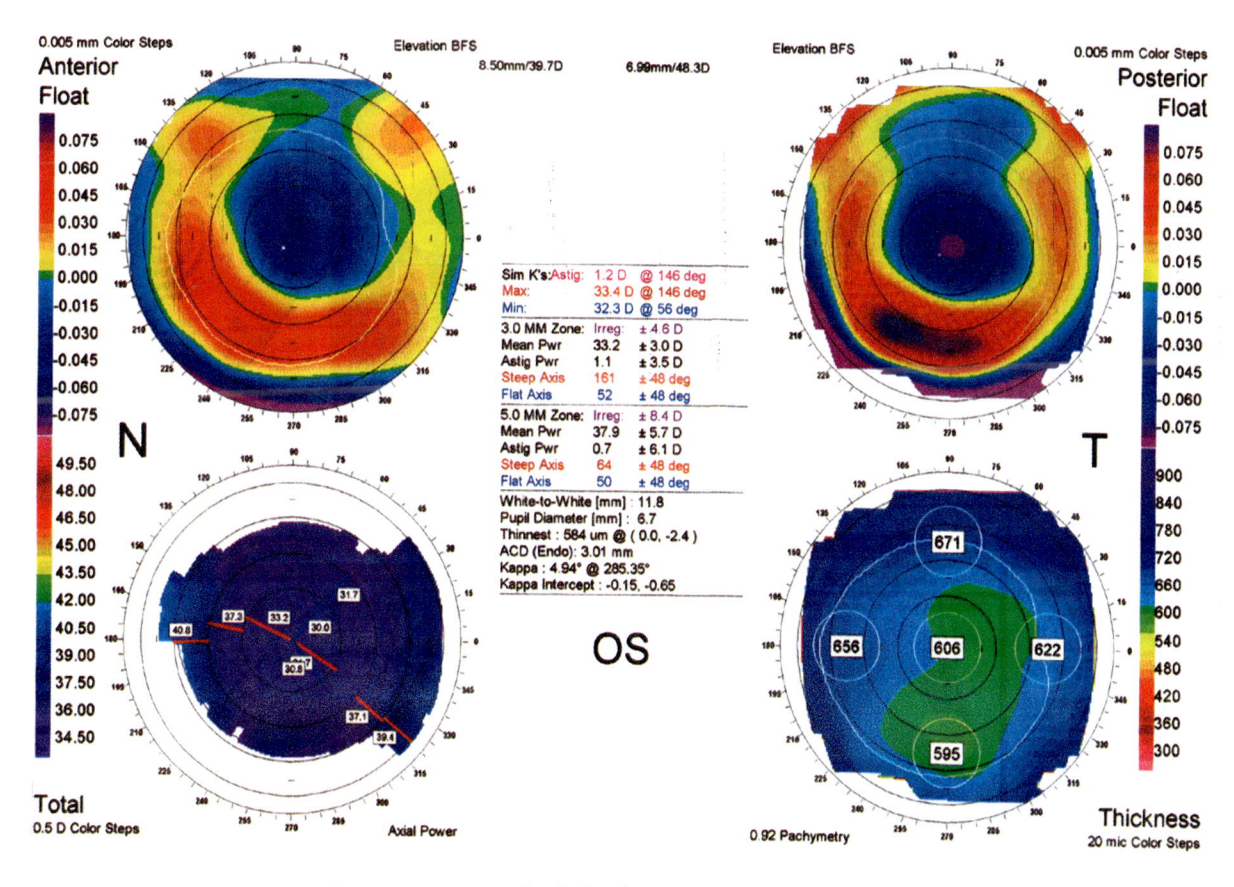

Chapter 14: Corneal Topographers and Wavefront Aberrometers: . . . 157

Figure 14.2 An example of a Quad map in a patient S/P myopic LASIK

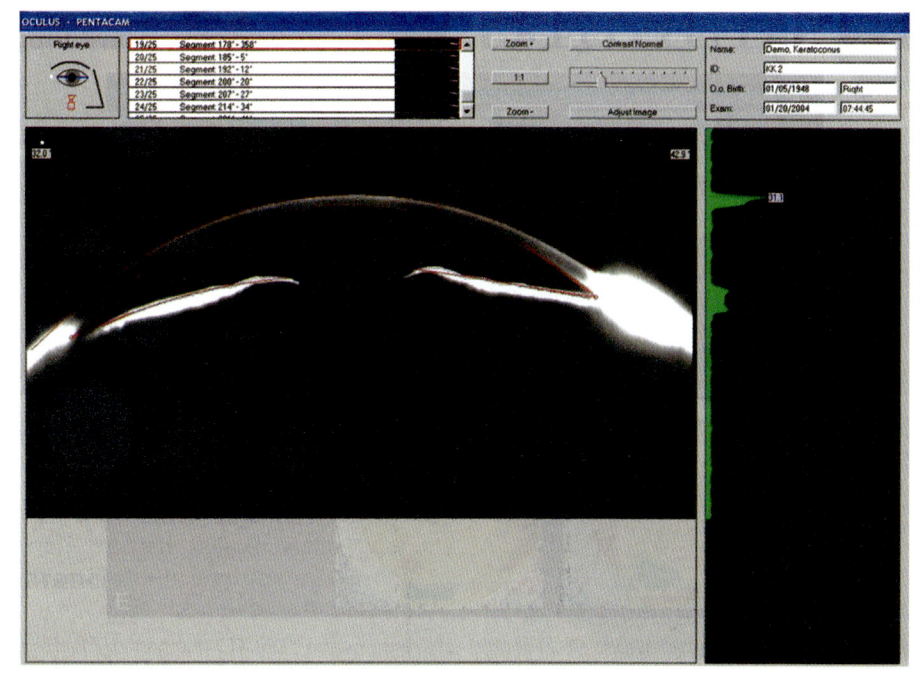

Figure 14.3 Scheimpflug image

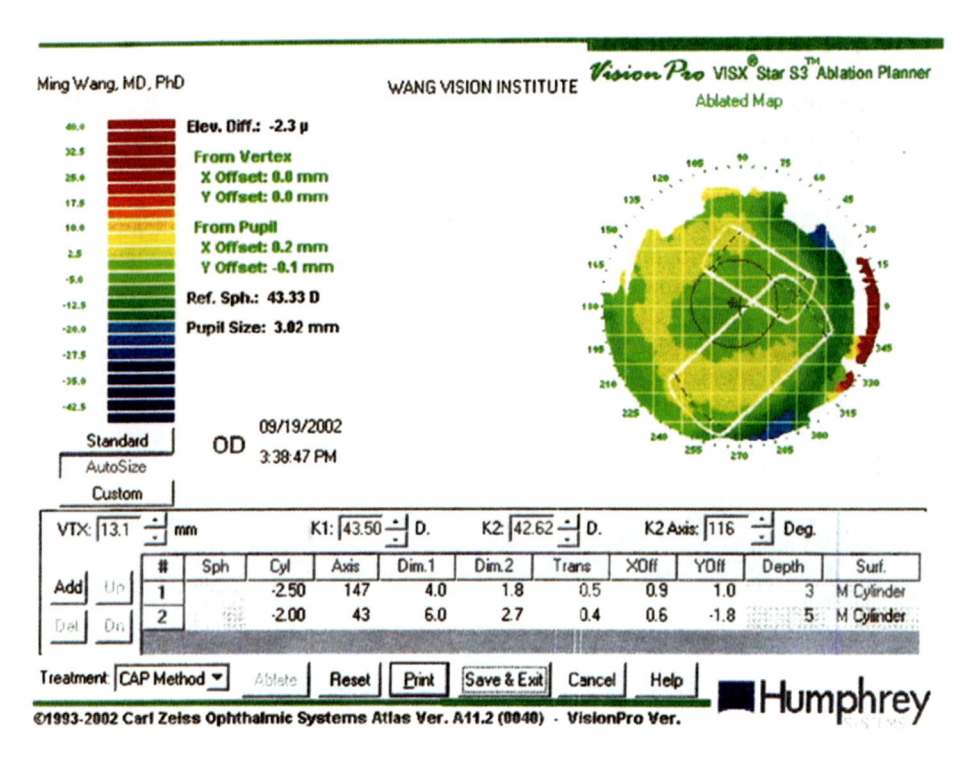

Figure 14.4 Custom CAP case

the Hartmann-Shack and the ray tracing models. Hartmann-Shack models utilize several hundred lenslets to measure the wavefront. Ray tracing models utilize individual rays of light to measure the wavefront. Both models measure aberrations as a deviation from the plane wave in microns, and measurements are limited by pupil size. This is problematic in eyes with smaller pupils.

The shape of the wavefront is then mathematically described, most commonly using Zernicke polynomials.[5] **Figure 14.5** shows this polynomial pyramid. Zernicke polynomials are a combination of radial trignometric functions which describe the wavefront mathematically. While second order terms of defocus and astigmatism are addressed by the manifest refraction, the irregular astigmatism primarily attributed to the cornea can be described by higher order terms such as coma, spherical aberration, and trefoil.

Just as topographers exhibit difficulty capturing irregular corneal surfaces, aberrometers falter on irregular wavefronts (typically due to irregular astigmatism). This is especially true for diseased eyes and those S/P keratorefractive procedures. Smolek and Klyce studied Zernicke fitting methods for corneal elevation and reported 4th order Zernicke polynomials may not be adequate in their description of corneal aberrations in significantly aberrant eyes.[6]

Because topography failed to address lower order aberrations, and aberrometry failed to address focal topography irregularities, advanced methods were needed. Several case examples later in this chapter demonstrate how using several systems to gain information about the topography and aberrometry combined is beneficial in determination of the etiology of the visual complaint. It is also beneficial in creating a management plan for surgery.

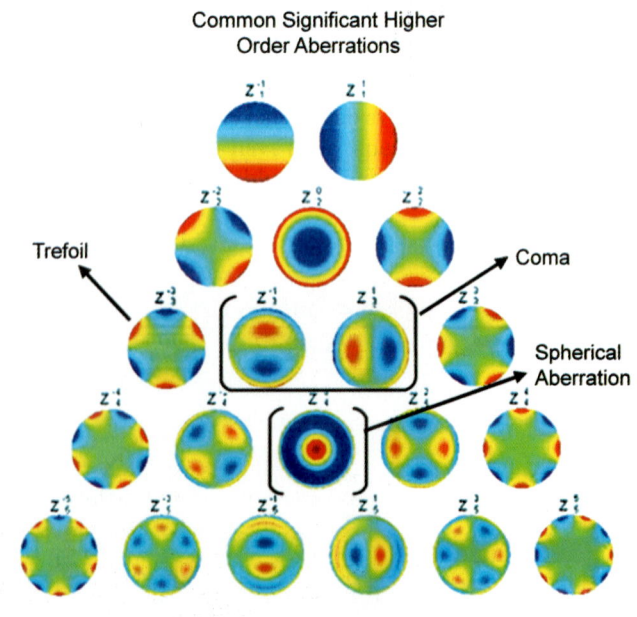

Figure 14.5 Zernicke polynomial pyramid

Chapter 14: Corneal Topographers and Wavefront Aberrometers: ... 159

As the limitations of wavefront became apparent, interest turned to corneal wavefront measurements—the ability to measure the amount of aberration attributable to the cornea alone. Systems which subtracted the corneal wavefront from the total ocular wavefront emerged. The EyeSys system is capable of using wavefront aberrometry and corneal topography to develop a corneal wavefront map. **Figures 14.6A and B** illustrate the aberrations found in a keratoconic patient with a 4 mm pupil (A) as well as the topography (B). **Figure 14.7** illustrates the corneal and internal aberrations of the same eye.

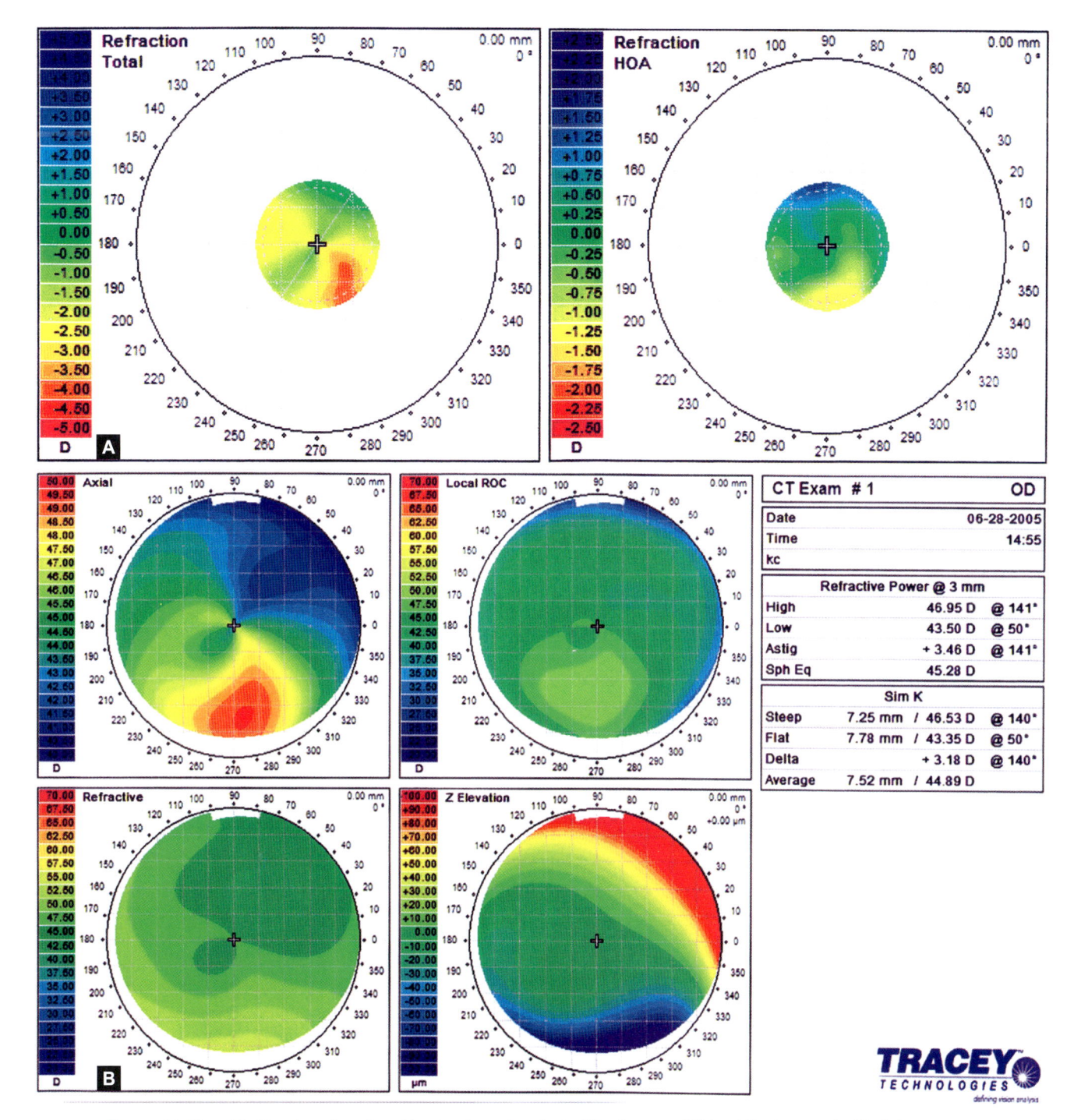

Figures 14.6A and B The aberrations found in a keratoconic patient with a 4 mm pupil (A) and the topography (B) of the same eye

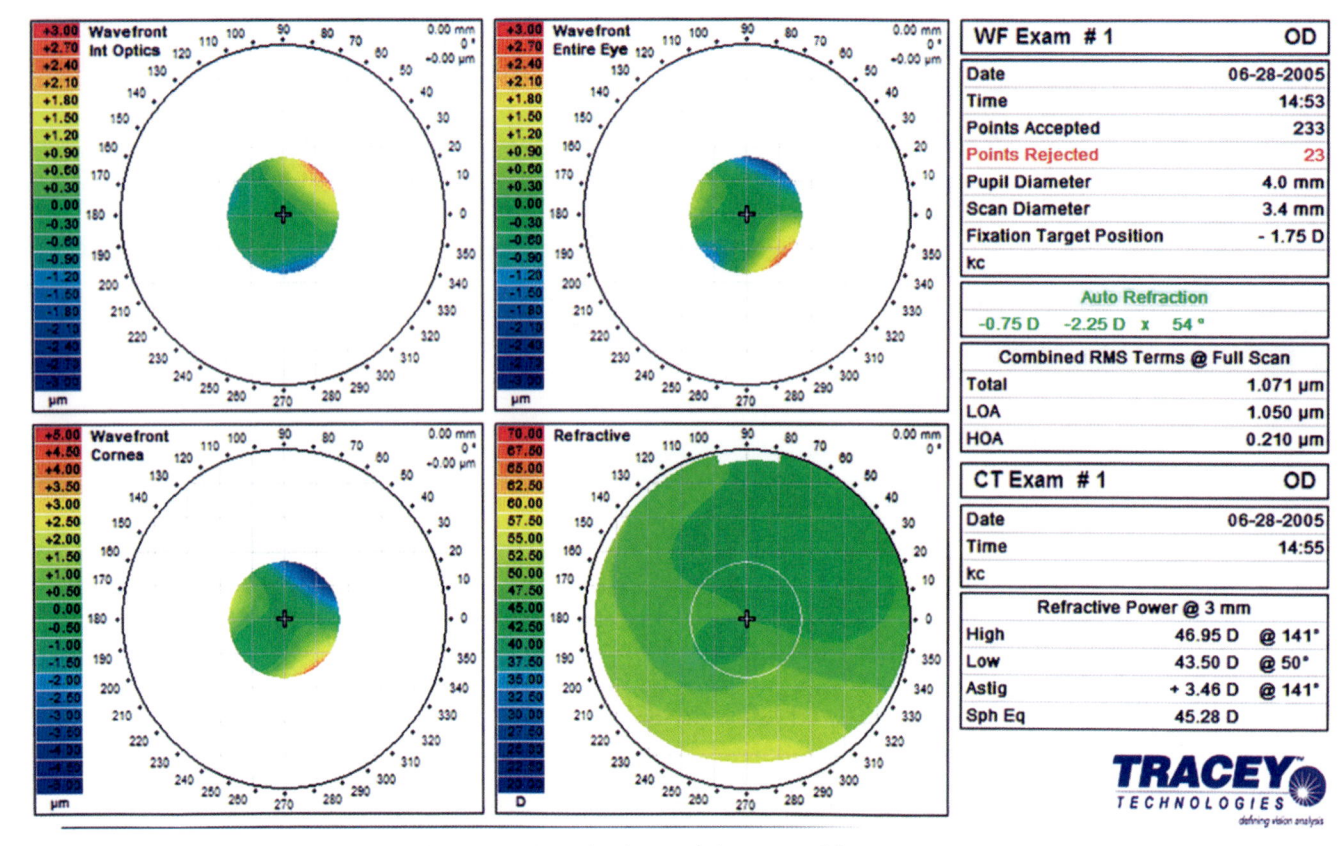

Figure 14.7 Corneal and internal aberrations of the same eye

It has been suggested that surgeons consider the rule of three when considering corneal surgery: for every 3 microns of distortion from the ideal shape of the cornea, about +1 micron difference in the OPD map and −1 micron difference in the wavefront error map. It should be noted, however, that the precision of both excimer lasers and wavefront aberrometers far surpasses that of human healing.

CASES

As previously suggested, rather than look at the technologies as separate, it is advantageous to consider them in conjunction with each other. Using both topography and wavefront measurements to determine the etiology of a visual complaint can be advantageous in the clinical setting. This is illustrated by the following case discussions.

Case I: Double Vision Complaints S/P Lasik

Patient WR presented complaining of "terrible night vision OS after LASIK. Preoperatively, he was significantly nearsighted, and correctable to 20/20. Postoperatively, he refracted to −2.75+1.75 × 160, with a BVA of 20/30. An RGP improved his vision to 20/20 with a significant reduction in monocular diplopia. His preoperative Wavescan map is shown in **Figure 14.8A**, with the preoperative topography in the upper right corner of the difference map shown in **Figure 14.8B**. Elevation mapping revealed a decentered ablation. Significant coma is evident in the aberrometry map, as expected with decentered ablations. We performed a Custom-CAP treatment, which treats the decentered ablation directly without taking the refractive error into account, and the visual distortion improved significantly, indicated by the drop in the RMS value shown in **Figure 14.9**.

Case II: Night Vision Complaints S/P LASIK

Patient WR presented with complaints of "terrible night vision, starbursts and halos" after LASIK in 2000. Preoperatively, she was −2.50 DS. Postoperatively, she refracted to −1.00+0.25 × 160, with a BVA of 20/30 OD, her dominant eye. **Figure 14.10A** shows her topography, revealing central irregularities. Wavescan, found in **Figure 14.10B**, revealed coma and trefoil. We suspected the central irregularities were exaggerated by her dry eye, and treated her aggressively with punctual occlusion, Restasis BID, and Liqugel nightly. Her symptoms improved slightly, and she is waiting for more advanced custom treatment.

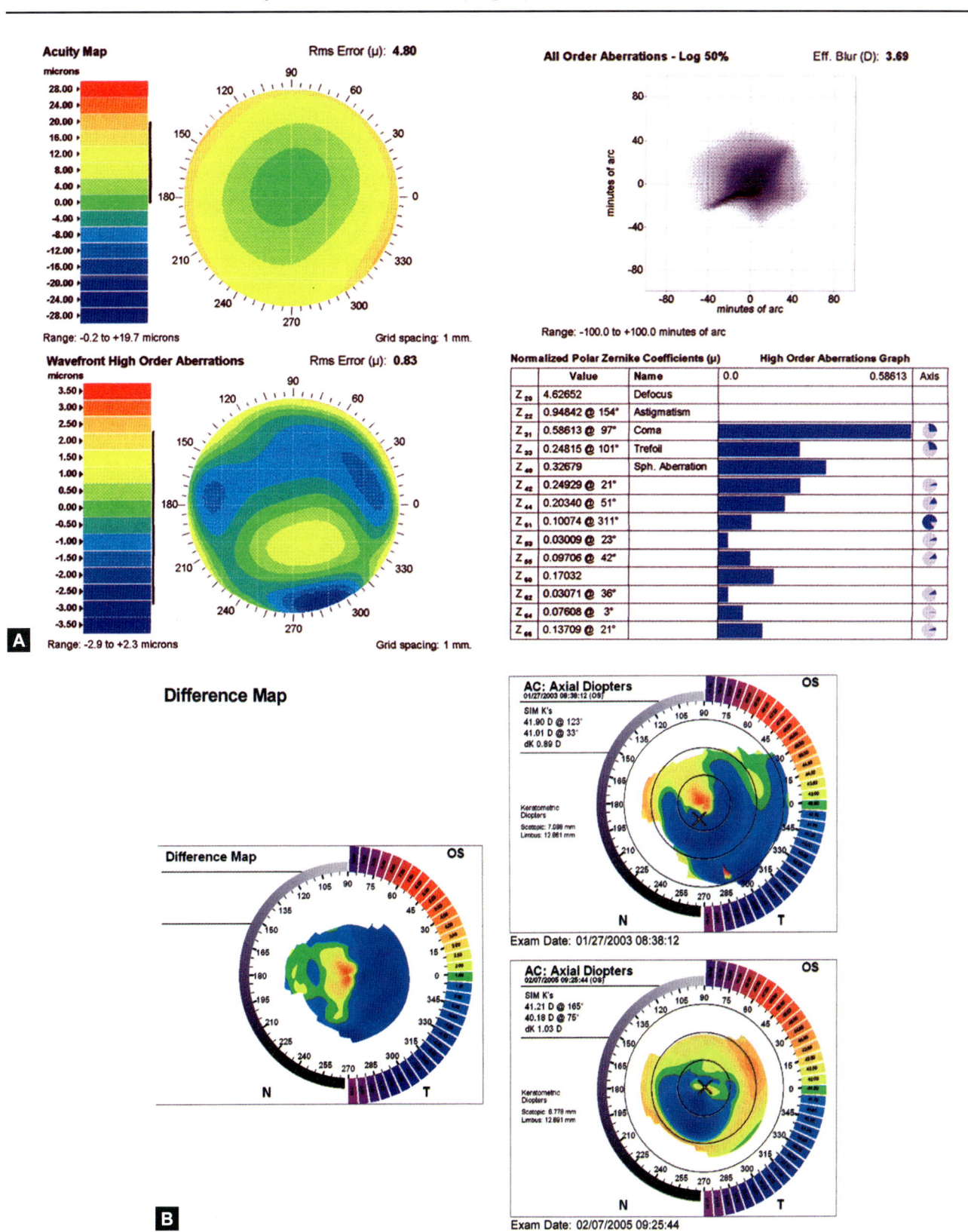

Figures 14.8A and B Preoperative Wavescan map, and topography difference map showing the change in topography following a custom CAP treatment

162 Section IV: Aberropia, Aberrations and Topography

Acuity Map — Rms Error (μ): **1.64**

All Order Aberrations - Log 50% — Eff. Blur (D): **2.85**

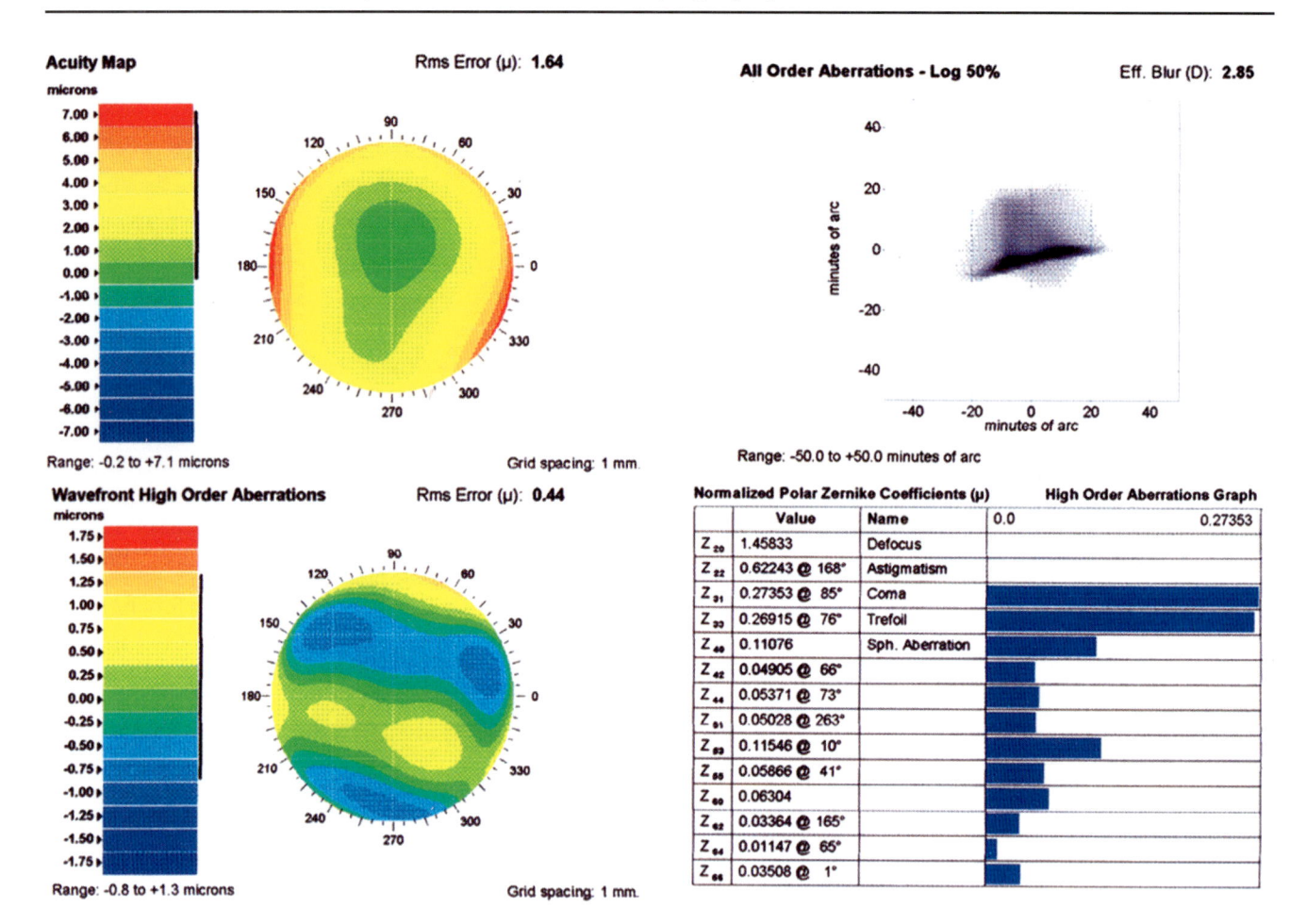

Range: -0.2 to +7.1 microns — Grid spacing: 1 mm

Range: -50.0 to +50.0 minutes of arc

Wavefront High Order Aberrations — Rms Error (μ): **0.44**

Range: -0.8 to +1.3 microns — Grid spacing: 1 mm

Normalized Polar Zernike Coefficients (μ) — **High Order Aberrations Graph**

	Value	Name	0.0	0.27353
Z_{20}	1.45833	Defocus		
Z_{22}	0.62243 @ 168°	Astigmatism		
Z_{31}	0.27353 @ 85°	Coma		
Z_{33}	0.26915 @ 76°	Trefoil		
Z_{40}	0.11076	Sph. Aberration		
Z_{42}	0.04905 @ 66°			
Z_{44}	0.05371 @ 73°			
Z_{51}	0.05028 @ 263°			
Z_{53}	0.11546 @ 10°			
Z_{55}	0.05866 @ 41°			
Z_{60}	0.06304			
Z_{62}	0.03364 @ 165°			
Z_{64}	0.01147 @ 65°			
Z_{66}	0.03508 @ 1°			

Figure 14.9 Wavescan S/P custom cap treatment

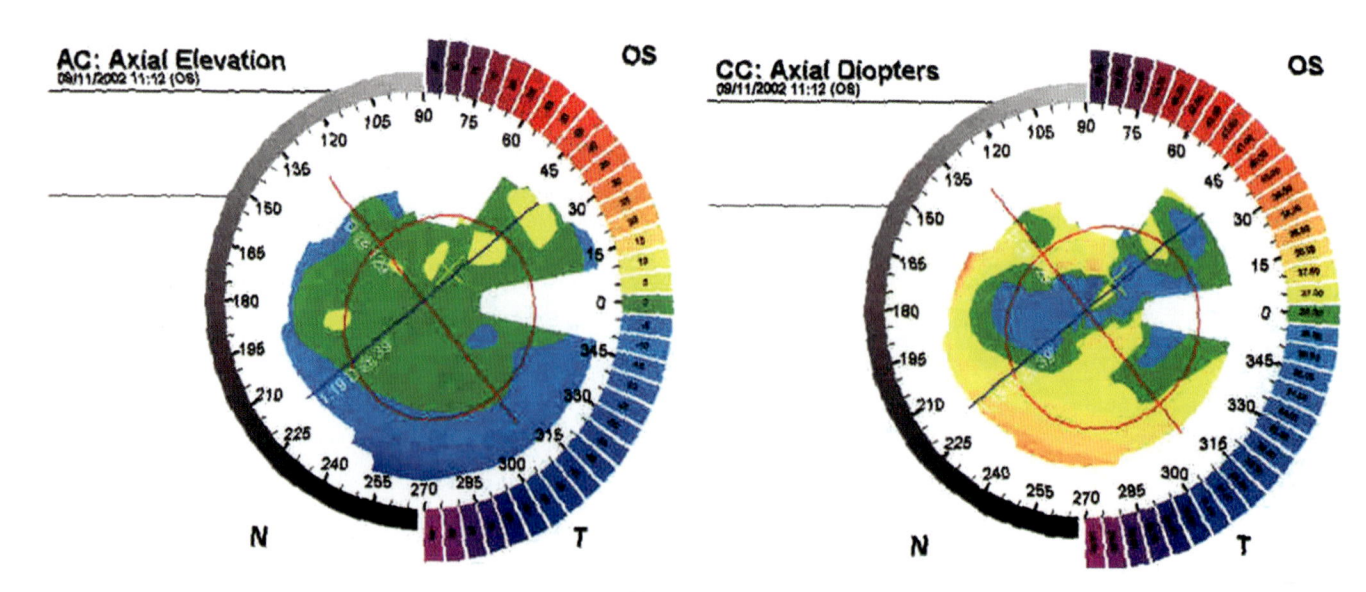

Figure 14.10A

Figure 14.10B

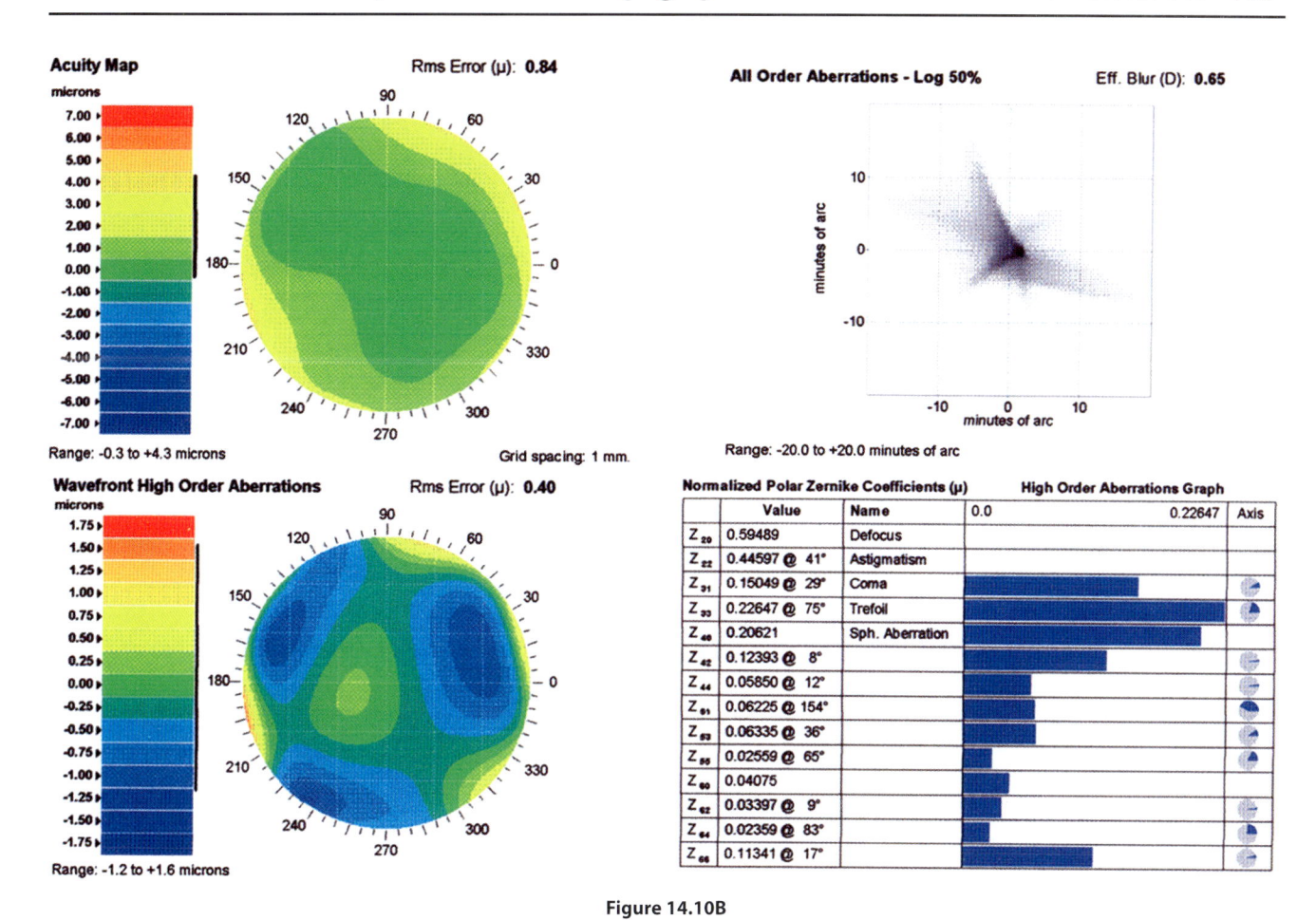

Figures 14.10A and B Central irregularities were revealed with topography, while aberrometry found coma and trefoil. Dry eye treatment only partially resolved this patient's complaints

Case III: Complaint of Multiple Images after Hyperopic LASIK

Patient TD presented complaining of light sensitivity, ghosting, halos and starbursts at night. Preoperatively she was +4.50D OU. Postoperatively, she refracted to PL, 20/25+ OD, +0.25+0.50 × 150, 20/25+ OS. Despite her unaided 20/20- Snellen acuity, she complained bitterly about her quality of vision. Topography found a smaller optical zone OS with greater steepening in the dominant left eye, as shown on the axial map in **Figure 14.11A**. Wavescan found significant spherical aberration (**Figure 14.11B**). Note the spherical aberration is negative due to the hyperopic treatment. We have prescribed Alphagan P in an attempt to decrease the pupil size and minimize the night vision issues, and fit the patient with gas permeable lenses.

Case IV: Double Vision with Loss of Best Correction S/P LASIK

Patient RD presented for evaluation of double vision S/P LASIK, even with glasses. Preoperatively, he was −4.75+0.75 × 105, with a BVA of 20/20. After his original surgery, he underwent two enhancements and AK in the affected eye, leaving him with −2.00 DS. He was fit with an RGP, which he reported did not resolve the diplopia, so he rarely wore the lens. Clinical notes from the fitting doctor report BCCLVA of 20/25. The topography was surprisingly regular in the pupillary zone despite the repeated corneal surgery. Wavefront analysis found significant COMA and trefoil, and can be seen in **Figure 14.12**. We attribute this to early lenticular changes, and elected to monitor rather than proceed with corrective ablation.

Case V: Hyperopic Keratorefractive Surgery Results in Steep Cornea

A 19-year-old female presented for LASIK evaluation. Manifest refraction was +1.75+05.0 × 25 OD (20/40) and +0.75 OS (20/25). Cycloplegic found latent hyperopia: +4.25 OD (20/50) and +1.50 (20/40) OS. Her preoperative topography was normal, and is shown in **Figure 14.13A**. After considerable discussion, she elected to undergo LASIK in both eyes. The latent hyperopia OD was partially addressed, and the goal was a correction of

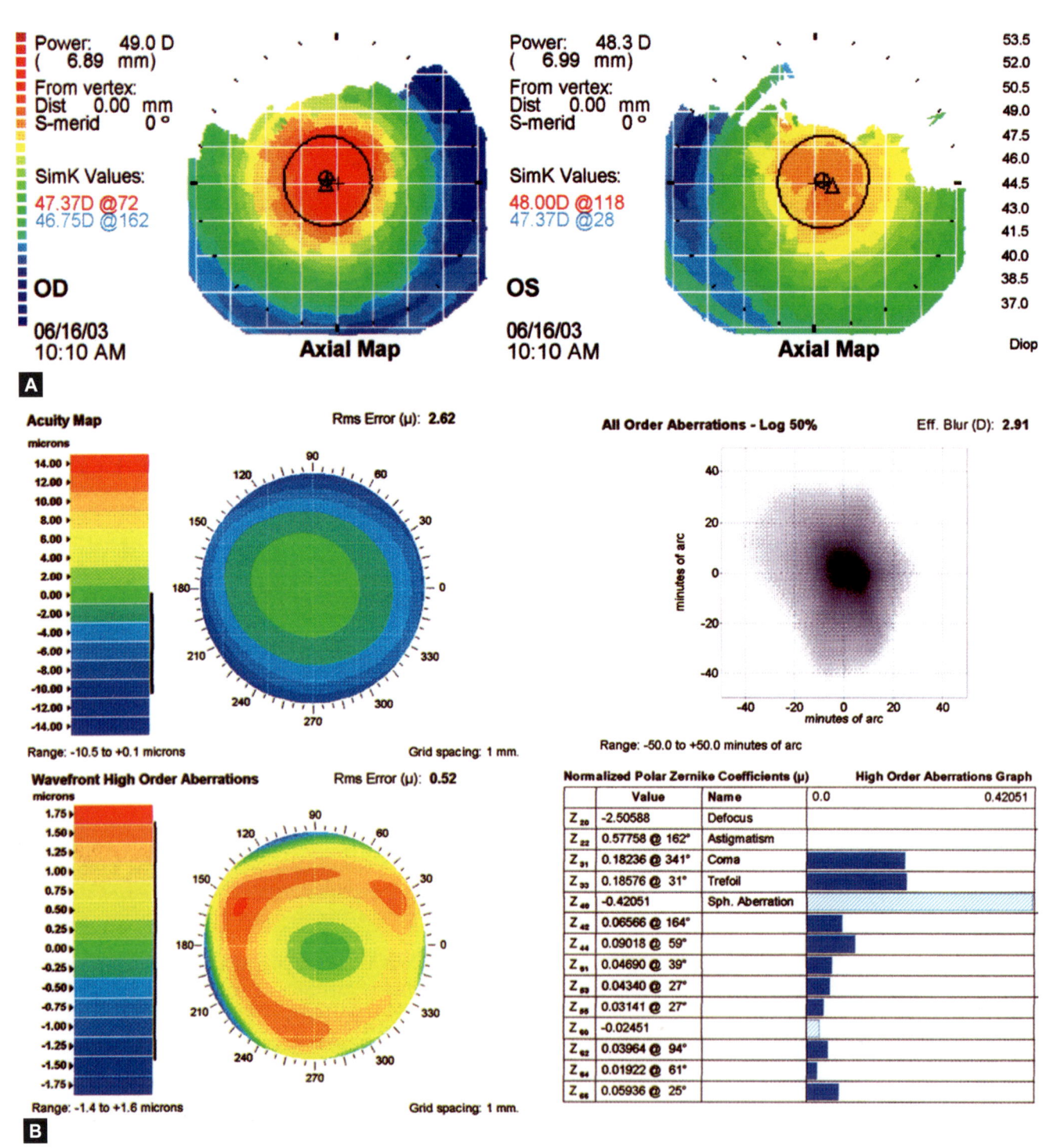

164   Section IV: Aberropia, Aberrations and Topography

Figures 14.11A and B Patient's complaint of glare and night vision disturbances secondary to the HOA caused by the small area of central steepening OS

+2.75 OD, +1.00 OS. She underwent bilateral femtosecond laser-assisted keratomileusis using a VISX Star 4 laser.

S/P LASIK, the patient complained of blurred vision OD, and the UCVA dropped to 20/50. Manifest refraction found +1.50+1.25 × 180 while the cycloplegic again revealed the latent hyperopia: +3.00+1.25 × 180, yielding a VA of 20/30. Her visual complaint was relieved with simple hyperopic correction, and the patient underwent an enhancement by relift of +1.50+1.25 × 180.

At one month, she presented complaining of decreased vision OD, multiple images, and "an unbalanced feeling". Manifest refraction found −1.50+0.75 × 75, and corrected

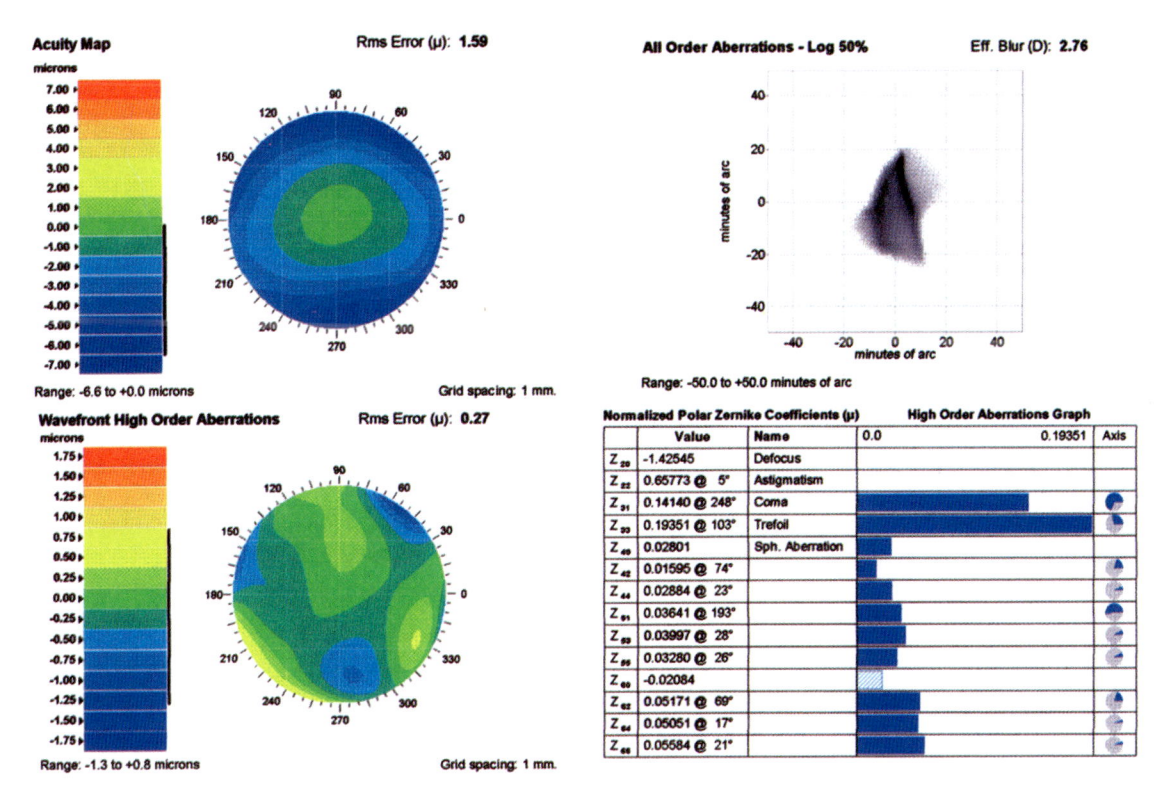

Chapter 14: Corneal Topographers and Wavefront Aberrometers: ... 165

Figure 14.12 Aberrometry revealed the cause of the patient's complaint when topography found a relatively normal shape: early cataracts

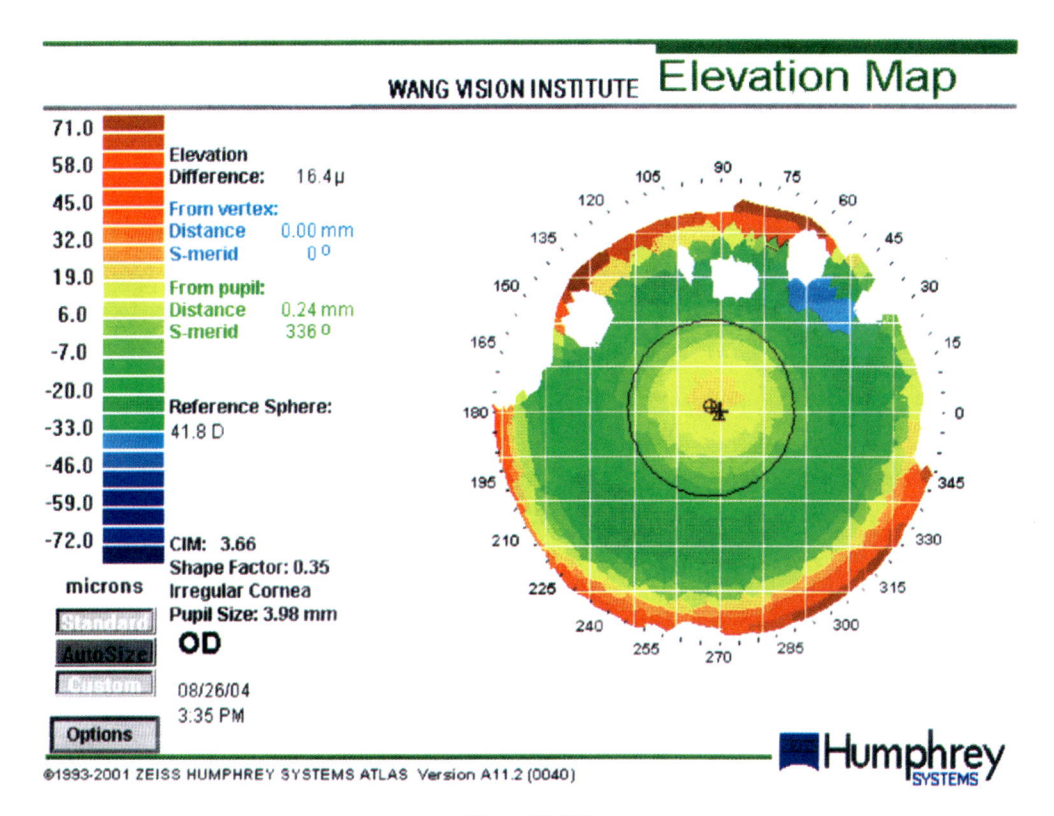

Figure 14.13A

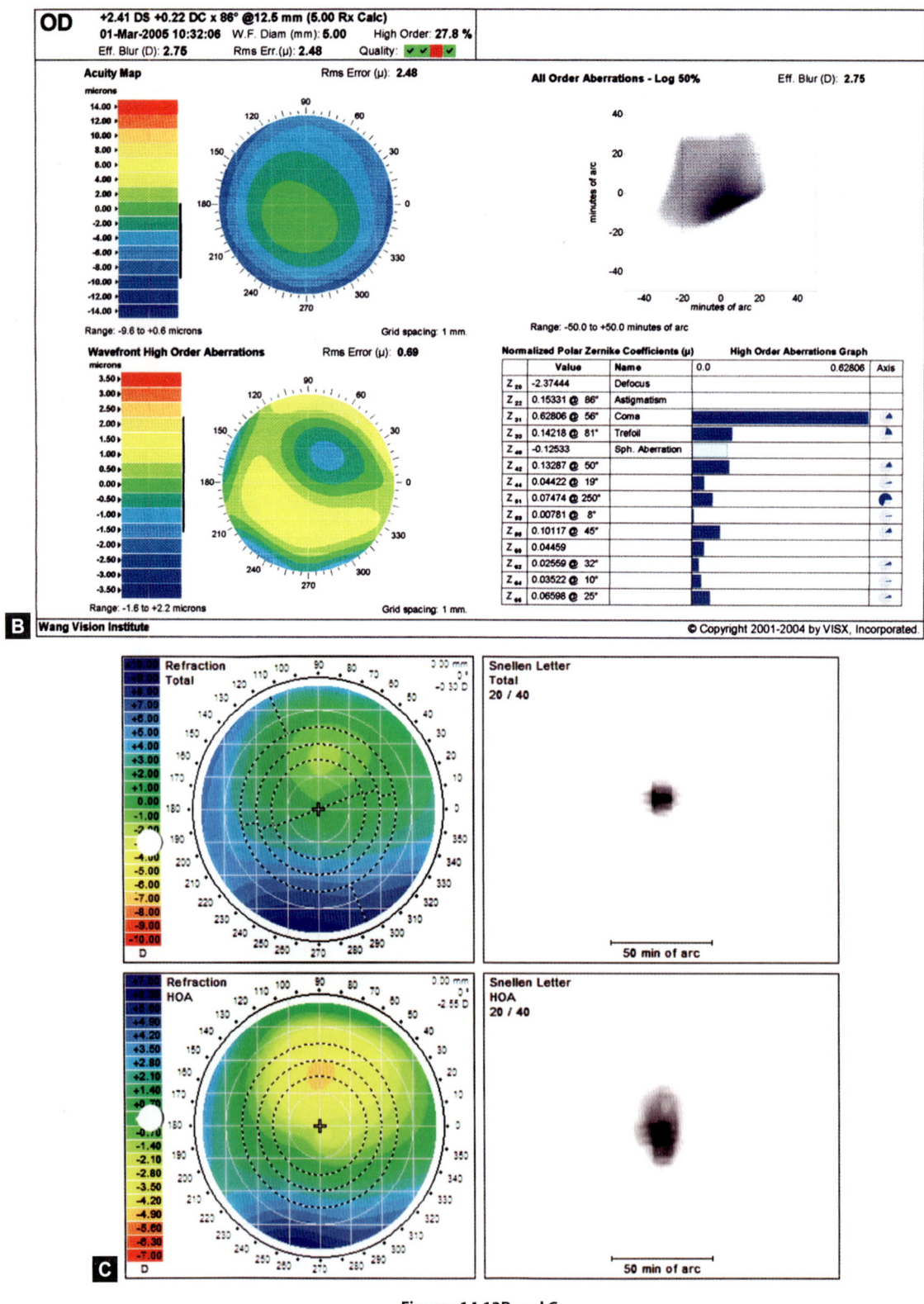

Figures 14.13B and C

Figures 14.13A to C Elevation maps reveal marked central steepening OD S/P hyperopic LASIK with hyperopic enhancement, as seen on the elevation map in (A). Her Wavescan map (B) and Itrace map (C) revealed coma, and reported hyperopic refractions despite a manifest of −1.50DS

her to only 20/50. Her elevation maps reveal marked central steepening OD as seen on the elevation map in **Figure 14.13A**. Her wavefront aberrometry measurements revealed coma OD, shown in **Figure 14.13B and C**. Interestingly, the Wavescan and I-Trace both found hyperopic refractions. The coma suggested a decentered apex, and topography revealed a significant steepening just above the geographical center.

Neither correction of the manifest refraction with a soft lens nor Alphagan-P to change the pupil size corrected the patient's complaint. While a gas permeable lens did restore functional vision, the patient is not able to tolerate the lens. It appears that the patient only uses the tip of the cornea for vision, resulting in the preferred myopia refraction. As time progresses and the natural smoothing of the cornea occurs, her symptoms lessening, and we may perform a custom treatment in the future.

CONCLUSION

While topographers and aberrometers may work well in virgin eyes, for surgeons striving for technology to address irregular astigmatism, current systems fall short. Improved understanding of the relationship between aberrometry, topography and corneal optics must be gained with continued advancement of the current technology.

Several generalizations can be made regarding the relationship between topography and wavefront aberrometry. The loss of the prolate cornea results in an increase in spherical aberration. Irregular astigmatism may be associated with an increase in coma and trefoil. Decentered ablations have been linked to increased coma. The irregular surface associated with dry eyes has been found to be improved with punctual occlusion and accompanied by a secondary reduction in HO aberrations.[7]

For patients with visual complaints S/P keratorefractive surgery, it is advantageous to obtain information from various sources about the etiology of the visual complaint. Using wavefront aberrometry and corneal topography to investigate the source of the patient's problem, and better understand the visual system as a whole, will better enable us to manage our patient's. Systems such as the Advanced Corneal Ablation Pattern (VISX), which combine topographic and wavefront information to create computerized simulations for surgery, may enable correction of irregular surfaces as well as refractive errors.

REFERENCES

1. Horner DG, Salmon TO, Soni PS. Chapter 17, Corneal Topography. In Benjamin WJ (Ed): Borish's Clinical Refraction, WB Saunders Company, Philadelphia, 1998.
2. Klein SA. A corneal topography algorithm that produces continuous curvature. Optom Vis Sci. 1992;69:829-34.
3. Roberts C. The Accuracy of "Power" maps to display curvature data in corneal topography systems. Invest Ophtalmol Vis Sci. 1994;35:3524-32.
4. Belin MW, Cambier JL, Nabors JR, Ratliff CD. PAR Corneal Topography System (PAR CTS): the clinical application of close-range photogrammetry. Optom Vis Sci. 1995;72:828-37.
5. Campbell C. A new method for describing the aberrations of the eye using zernike polynomials. Optometry and Vision Science. 2003;80(1):79-93.
6. Smolek MK, Kyce SD. Zernicke polynomial fitting fials to represent all visual signficant corneal aberrations. Invest Ophthalmol Vis Sci. 2003;44:4676-81.
7. Pepose J, Huang B, Mirza A, Quazi M. Effect of punctal occlusion on wavefront aberrations in dry eyes after LASIK. Invest Ophthalmol Vis Sci. 2003;44: E-Abstract 26-28.

Chapter 15

Aberrometry and Topography in the Vector Analysis of Refractive Laser Surgery

Noel A Alpins (Australia), Gemma Walsh (Australia)

INTRODUCTION

Refractive laser surgery techniques such as laser *in situ* keratomileusis (LASIK) and photorefractive keratectomy (PRK) are effective methods of treating spherical myopic errors up to 12 D and hyperopic errors up to 6 D, with good visual outcomes. However, generally more than half of the people who are suitable candidates for refractive surgery have enough astigmatism to warrant its inclusion in the surgical correction. As astigmatism has both direction and magnitude, its incorporation into the treatment makes planning more complex. It has been shown that vector analysis can improve the visual outcome of spherocylindrical treatments by combining the topographic and refractive astigmatic components to target a reduced level of corneal astigmatism compared to using refractive parameters alone.[1-9]

MEASUREMENT OF ASTIGMATISM

There are three differing categories of astigmatism; naturally occurring regular astigmatism, naturally occurring irregular astigmatism and secondary irregular astigmatism associated with ocular trauma, disease, infection or previous ocular surgery.[1] There are many different ways to measure astigmatism, some assessing corneal astigmatism only, and the others measuring refractive astigmatism including the internal optics of the eye. It is important in routine clinical practice to utilize more than one method in the preoperative examination.

The manifest subjective refraction is a measure of the spherocylindrical correction required for the patient's perception of their best vision. The principal contribution to the cylindrical error is the corneal astigmatism, but also includes astigmatism from the internal optics of the eye (such as the crystalline lens) as well as the interpretation of the image by the cerebral cortex. The measured result depends on many variables such as chart illumination and contrast, test distance and room lighting.

The technology of wavefront analysis provides a spatially oriented refractive map of the pathway of light through the eye, which provides a greater amount of information on the refractive system than the manifest refraction data alone. It too includes the internal optics of the eye, but unlike subjective responses does not include the conscious perception of the cerebral cortex, thus giving no information regarding the nonoptical interpretation of astigmatic images on the retina and visual cortex. This subjective value conventionally forms part of the ablative treatment and is an important component for patient satisfaction. The application of wavefront analysis in the treatment plan is discussed further on.

Keratometry is a useful objective test to measure average corneal curvature at the paracentral region of the cornea. However, as it requires the manual alignment of optical mires to identify the steepest and flattest corneal axes, there is a potential problem with reproducing reliable results due to variability between different observers. Corneal topography, or computer assisted videokeratography (CAVK), provides a more detailed quantified view of the corneal astigmatism displayed as a map based on the measurement of refractive power of thousands of separate points over the entire cornea. Average topographical astigmatism can be represented by a simulated keratometry value, which is a mean value derived from a number of constant reference points. It is a best fit compromise, and determined in various ways by the different types of topographers.

SURGICAL PLANNING ~ REFRACTION, TOPOGRAPHY, OR BOTH?

In an ideal world the goal of astigmatic refractive surgery is to completely eliminate astigmatism from the eye and its optical correction. However, it has since been recognized that this is not possible in the majority of cases due to the inherent differences between corneal astigmatism (represented by the simulated keratometry value from topography) and refractive astigmatism (represented by lower [second] order aberrations from aberrometry).[6,7] Most surgeons traditionally treat the refractive value alone based on the principle that treating what the patient perceives to give their best corrected vision will provide a superior visual outcome.

However, this is not necessarily the case. Disregarding the shape of the cornea while changing it flies in the face of the fundamental principles of corneal surgery. In fact, simple arithmetic analysis shows that an excessive amount of corneal astigmatism may be left if treatment is applied exclusively based on the parameters derived from the refractive cylinder magnitude and axis.[2,5] This occurs because failing to align the maximum ablation closer to the flattest corneal meridia results in off-axis loss of effect when reducing corneal astigmatism. Consequently, lower (second) order astigmatic aberrations and (third order) coma would not be minimized, with more remaining than otherwise necessary.[1] This may result in post-surgical symptoms such as reduced visual acuity and contrast sensitivity, creating difficulty with night driving and thus actually diminishing satisfaction in a proportion of patients.

It becomes particularly important to consider this in patients with form fruste or mild keratoconus as there is usually a large discrepancy between the refractive and corneal astigmatism in these cases. It has been shown that optimizing the PRK treatment by combining the refractive parameters with the corneal topography can improve the total astigmatic and visual outcomes for these patients.[3]

As it becomes more widely recognized that a zero overall astigmatism is mostly unattainable, effective contemporary treatment methods target astigmatism outcomes that combine both the refractive and topographic measurements in the analytical planning process. This should ensure the distribution of the remaining astigmatism to achieve the optimal outcome. That is, choosing a maximal treatment that leaves the minimum amount of astigmatism in the most favorable orientation. With-the-rule astigmatism is more prevalent in the younger population undergoing laser vision correction, and is thought to be more visually tolerable to refractive perception than against-the-rule astigmatism (Javals rule).[5,7,10]

VECTOR ANALYSIS BY THE ALPINS METHOD

The surgical planning and analysis process is expedited by the implementation of computer and software technology. Calculations performed for the publication of this chapter utilized the ASSORT® program developed by the first author (the Alpins Statistical System for Ophthalmic Refractive surgery Techniques). It employs the principles of vector planning and analysis[1-8] and utilizes a paradigm that favors with-the-rule astigmatism while minimizing measurable postoperative refractive astigmatism quantified as second order aberrations.

The amount and axis of astigmatic change that the surgeon *intends* to induce is called the target induced astigmatism vector (TIA). This is determined by using an optimal combination of refractive and topographic data, as seen in the example later on. The surgically induced astigmatism vector (SIA) is the astigmatic change *actually* induced by the surgery. It is possible to determine whether the treatment was on-axis or off-axis, and also whether too much or too little treatment was applied by examining the various relationships between the SIA and TIA. The Correction index (CI) is the ratio of the SIA to TIA and ideally is 1.0. An overcorrection occurs if the CI is greater than 1.0 and less than 1.0 for an undercorrection. The magnitude of error (ME) is the arithmetic difference between the magnitudes of the SIA and TIA. This is positive for overcorrections and negative for undercorrections. The angle of error (AE) is the angle contained by the SIA and TIA vectors. If the achieved correction is oriented counterclockwise (CCW) to where it was intended then the AE is positive. If the achieved correction is clockwise (CW) to the intended axis then the AE is negative.

An absolute measure of success of the surgery is described by the difference vector (DV). This is the induced astigmatic change that would enable the initial surgery to achieve its intended target, and is ideally zero. The DV is a useful dioptric measure of uncorrected astigmatism. A relative measure of success is the Index of success (IOS) which is calculated by dividing the DV by the intended change, the TIA. This is also preferably zero.

As previously mentioned, the corneal and refractive astigmatism are rarely equivalent. This difference may be represented vectorially by the ocular residual astigmatism (ORA).[11] In other words, the ORA is the noncorneal component of total refractive astigmatism, and quantifies by magnitude and axis orientation the minimum intraocular second order astigmatism aberrations. It is also the amount of corneal astigmatism expected to remain after treatment guided by refractive values alone, to neutralize this intraocular astigmatism.

ABERROMETRY AND WAVEFRONT GUIDED TREATMENT

Wavefront technology offers theoretical guidance to reduce spherical aberrations by achieving the most effective prolate aspheric profile. However, wavefront-assisted LASIK does not address the amount of resultant corneal astigmatism, and therefore is similar to LASIK based on manifest refraction. In addition, as aberrometry includes the internal optics of the eye in its calculations, any changes over time to the crystalline lens may undermine any benefit gained from the wavefront ablation.[1,9]

Furthermore, if wavefront guided ablation corrects all ocular aberrations at the corneal surface, it would produce an uneven corneal treatment resulting in induced corneal irregularities. This might be an undesirable result when it is widely recognized that a regular cornea with orthogonal and symmetrical astigmatism gives a superior visual result.[1,8] Permanently changing regional corneal shape in this manner is also complicated by the fact that this form of treatment may in fact be neutralized by epithelial healing.[9] Despite these potential limitations wavefront technology does provide useful refractive information. Rather than employing wavefront data exclusively, it can be combined with the vector planning method described in this chapter to produce an optimal treatment with reduced postsurgical aberrations.

Combining Wavefront Analysis and Topography with Vector Planning

A typical wavefront analysis is depicted in **Figure 15.1**. The spherocylindrical refraction as measured by the wavefront device at the spectacle plane is +0.52/−1.83 × 3. The two dimensional illustration of the wavefront analysis on the left shows a moderate level of mixed astigmatism with a typical saddle appearance. The higher order spherical aberrations

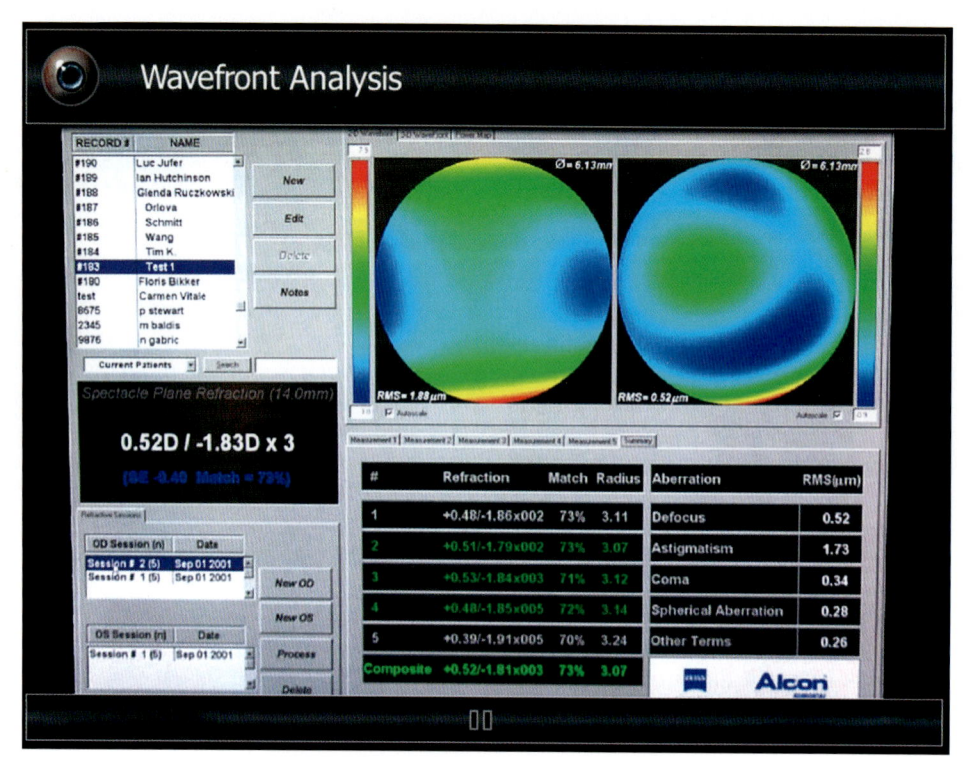

Figure 15.1 A typical wavefront analysis display

are quantified as root-mean-square values in the lower right hand corner of the display. The spherical component of the correction (+0.52) is shown as the defocus. The cylindrical component is displayed beneath this. Third order aberrations (coma and trefoil) are listed separately, with 4th order spherical aberrations. 'Other terms' indicates 5th order and higher order aberrations.

Figure 15.2 displays a topographical map of the matching astigmatic eye. The typical bow-tie appearance of the regular corneal astigmatism is evident. In this example, the astigmatism measures 2.62 D at the steepest meridian of 96 degrees as quantified by the simulated keratometry values. These parameters can then be examined together with those from the wavefront analysis spherocylindrical (second order) values to produce an optimal treatment by using the Alpins method contained in the ASSORT® program. This is shown in the treatment planning screen in **Figure 15.3**. In this diagram the treatment has been set to a base of 100% emphasis for correction of refractive astigmatism parameters.

This treatment screen in **Figure 15.3** has been disassembled further for ease of understanding the various components. **Figure 15.4** is the top central section on the ASSORT® treatment screen, displaying the preoperative spherocylindrical refractive values taken from the wavefront analysis and also the corneal plane conversion. The cylindrical component here is 1.81 D of astigmatism at axis 3. This figure also displays the spherocylindrical target for the treatment, which in this case is zero.

The treatment vector being employed is shown in the polar diagram in **Figure 15.5**. Here the TIA is 1.81 D at axis 3. The pre- and postoperative target astigmatism values are shown in **Figure 15.6**. The postoperative refractive target value is zero with the target corneal astigmatism value (obtained from **Figure 15.7**) displayed in blue.

The simulated keratometry values from the preoperative topographical map are shown in **Figure 15.7**. Also displayed here are the ORA and the target for the corneal postoperative astigmatism. A vectorial calculation is used to determine the ORA, which in this case is 0.84 D. That is, there is a calculated amount of 0.84 D of intraocular astigmatism that cannot be eliminated from this eye. As the spherocylindrical refractive target has already been guided to zero, this can only leave the whole of the remaining astigmatism on the cornea at a near vertical meridian of 103 degrees to neutralize the ORA 90 degrees away, as seen in the target value of **Figure 15.7**.

However, as the emphasis is shifted towards the left, the treatment is more closely aligned to the principal corneal meridian. **Figure 15.8** shows the optimal treatment for this eye, with the emphasis placed at 33% topography and 67% refraction. The ORA is still 0.84 D, but now it is apportioned

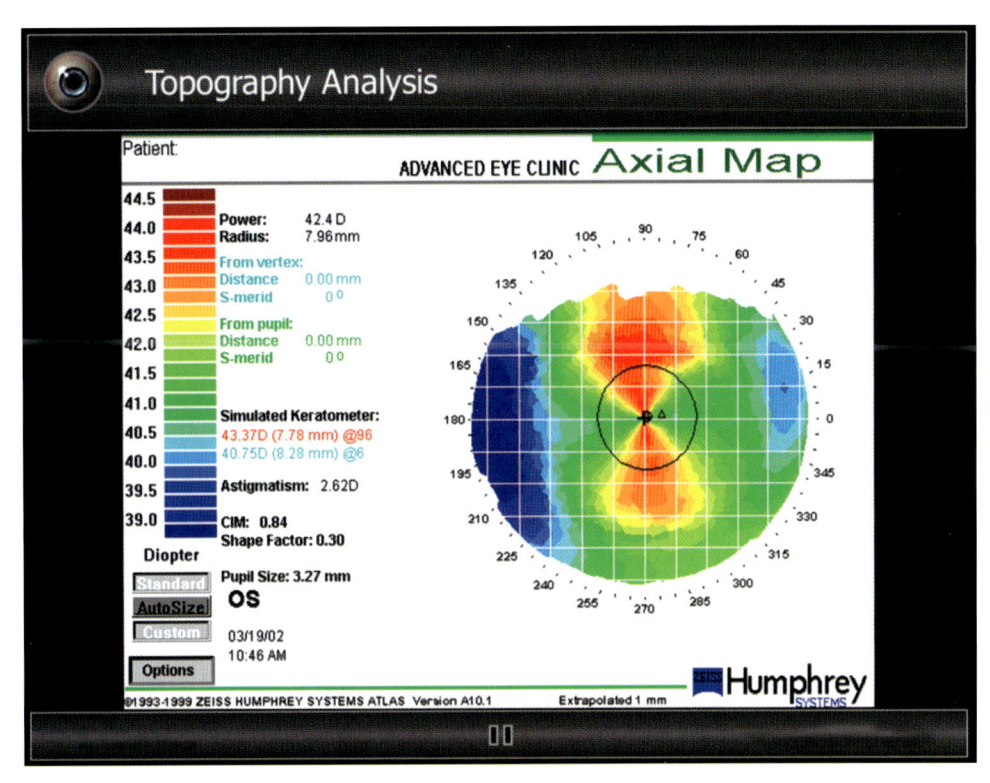

Chapter 15: Aberrometry and Topography in the Vector Analysis of Refractive... 171

Figure 15.2 Topographical analysis of the same eye

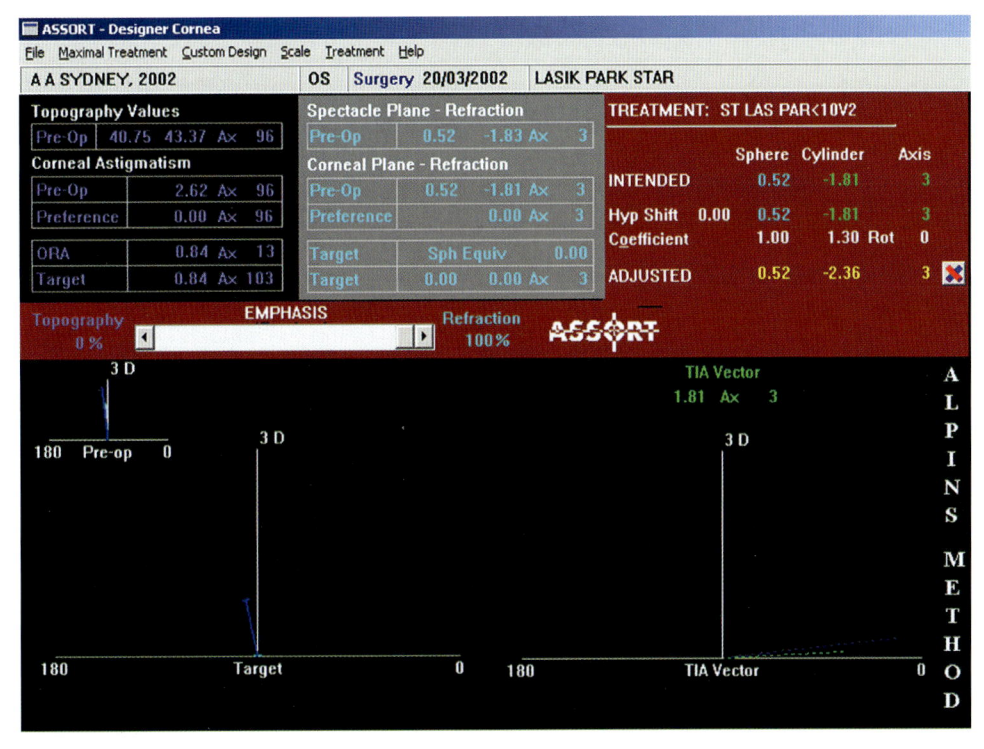

Figure 15.3 The ASSORT surgical planning module for this eye

Spectacle Plane—Refraction			
Preoperative	0.52	−1.83 Ax	3
Corneal Plane—Refraction			
Preoperative	0.52	−1.81 Ax	3
Preference		0.00 Ax	3
Target	Sph Equiv		0.00
Target	0.00	0.00 Ax	3

Figure 15.4 The top central section of the ASSORT screen displaying the preoperative refractive data obtained from the wavefront analysis (both spectacle and corneal plane values) and the chosen refractive spherocylindrical target

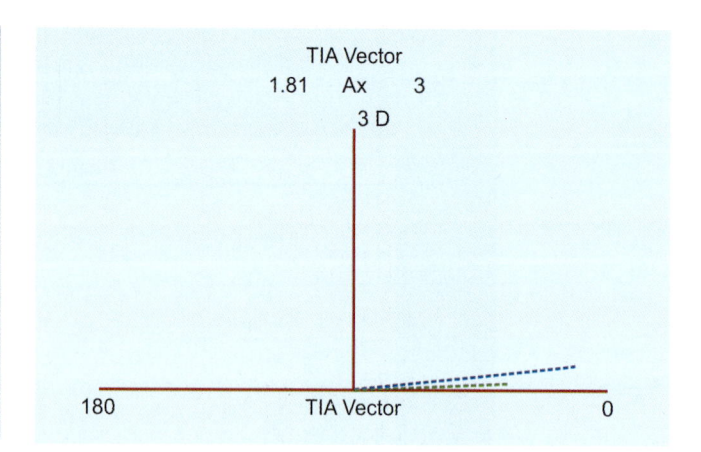

Figure 15.5 The lower right hand graph on the ASSORT screen with a polar display of the TIA vector

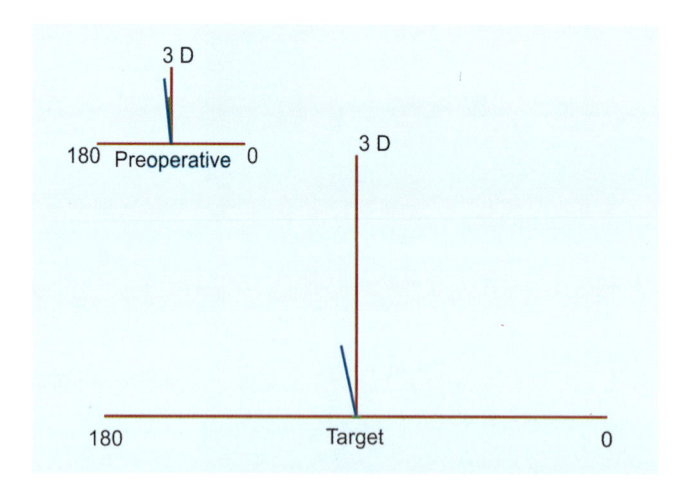

Figure 15.6 Preoperative and postoperative target astigmatism vectors. The postoperative refractive target value is zero with the target corneal astigmatism vector displayed in green

Topography Values			
Preoperative	40.75	43.37 Ax	96
Corneal Astigmatism			
Preoperative		2.62 Ax	96
Preference		0.00 Ax	96
ORA		0.84 Ax	13
Target		0.84 Ax	103

Figure 15.7 The top left hand box of the ASSORT screen displaying the corneal topographical preoperative values and the targeted corneal postoperative value. The minimum amount of astigmatism is displayed as the ORA, which in this case matches the magnitude target for the corneal astigmatism and is 90 degrees away

between the refraction and the cornea. Here less corneal astigmatism is targeted and has been reduced to 0.56 D at an unchanged meridian 103 (**Figure 15.9**). The remaining 0.28 D which is included in the spherocylindrical target of a spherical equivalent of zero, is not necessarily detected by the perceptive system at these levels, particularly as it is oriented favorably towards with-the-rule. Thus, with this method of vectorial planning, although the targeted spherocylindrical outcome is not zero, but 0.14/−0.28 × 103 as displayed in **Figure 15.10**, the measured postoperative refractive and wavefront astigmatism is likely to be negligible.

Despite not targeting a zero spherocylindrical outcome, by directing the remaining astigmatism away from the cornea the overall astigmatism is also less, and there are fewer aberrations remaining. This treatment results in an overall higher patient satisfaction.

TREATMENT OF IRREGULAR ASTIGMATISM

Differences in the two opposite superior and inferior hemi-divisions of the corneal topographical contour map are widely prevalent. This is known as irregular astigmatism and occurs if the two sides of the bow-tie representation differ in magnitude (asymmetrical) or are not aligned at 180 degrees to each other (nonorthogonal), or most commonly a combination of the two.[1,8] Irregular astigmatism may also be identified optically using wavefront devices. Unlike other

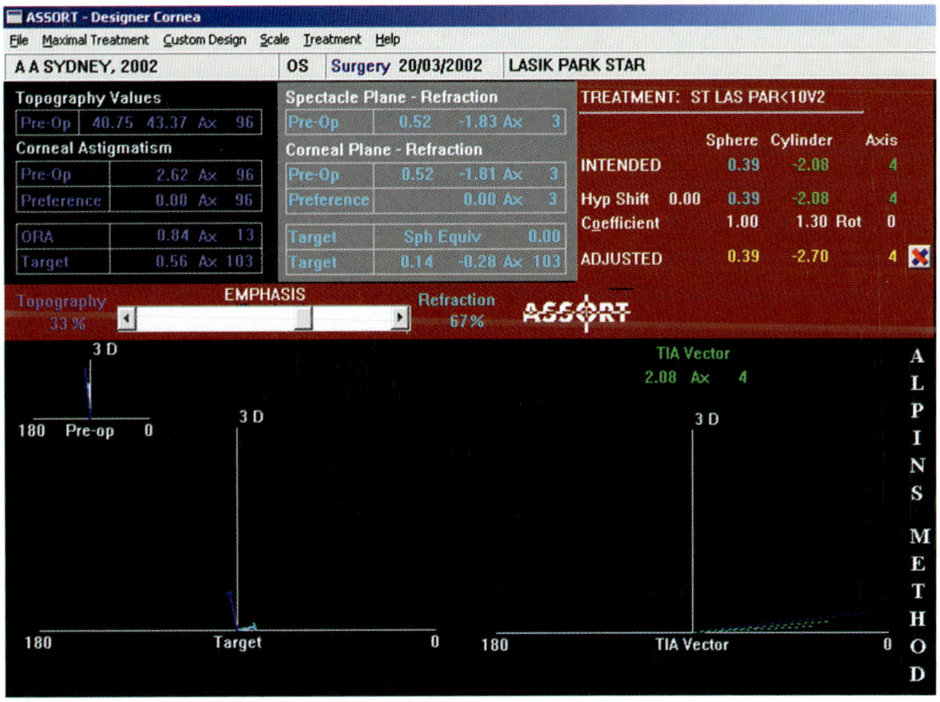

Chapter 15: Aberrometry and Topography in the Vector Analysis of Refractive... 173

Figure 15.8 The ASSORT treatment screen displaying the optimal treatment for the same eye. Here the emphasis bar has been shifted 33% towards the left so that not all of the surgical emphasis is placed on complete refractive astigmatism correction

Topography Values			
Preoperative	40.75	43.37 Ax	96

Corneal Astigmatism			
Preoperative		2.62 Ax	96
Preference		0.00 Ax	96

ORA		0.84 Ax	13
Target		0.56 Ax	103

Figure 15.9 The optimal treatment for the same eye. Here the amount of corneal astigmatism remaining after treatment has been reduced by one third to 0.56 D, though the total ORA remains unchanged at 0.84 D

Spectacle Plane—Refraction			
Preoperative	0.52	−1.83 Ax	3

Corneal Plane—Refraction			
Preoperative	0.52	−1.81 Ax	3
Preference		0.00 Ax	3

Target	Sph Equiv		0.00
Target	0.14	−0.28 Ax	103

Figure 15.10 The new spherocylindrical target for this eye is not zero, but 0.14/-0.28x103. This distributes the ORA between the postoperative refractive and corneal modes to produce a more favorable corneal shape and therefore less second order aberrations following surgery. The favorably oriented and minimal refractive target is not likely to be perceived by the patient

methods of astigmatism analysis, the method described in this chapter may theoretically also be applied independently to each hemidivision in a cornea displaying pre-existing idiopathic irregularity. This would theoretically allow analysis and treatment of this irregular astigmatism to produce an orthogonal, symmetrical cornea.

The target refractive and corneal astigmatism values must be considered separately for each hemimeridian, with individual treatment plans required for both the superior and inferior topographic magnitudes and meridian values with the common refractive astigmatism value. From this, minimum target astigmatism values may be calculated for each part of the cornea, and their orientations are used to guide the choice for the optimal TIA for that side.[8]

The vectorial difference between the two opposite semimeridian values for magnitude and axis in each corneal part is called the topographic disparity (TD). When displayed on a 720 degree double-angle vector diagram, the TD quantifies the irregular astigmatism of the cornea in diopters, and the treatment required to reduce or eliminate the irregular astigmatism can be determined from this.[8]

The information gained from computerized topography regarding the corneal height (either directly such as the Z dimension on the Orbscan device, or indirectly inferred from slope measurement) may be translated into planned tissue ablation patterns using the Munnerlyn formula. This ablative pattern may then be applied at specific points on the corneal surface to reduce the irregularity.[1] There are various methods to link topographical information with tailored ablation, though a real time preoperative link is yet to be achieved.

In this way, the corneal shape may be manipulated by asymmetrical surgical treatment to the irregular hemidivisions of the cornea, allowing the achievement of any corneal shape (thus producing regular astigmatism where selected). In cases of irregular astigmatism a rearrangement rather than a reduction of the corneal astigmatism may be of benefit, as regularizing the cornea may improve best corrected visual acuity to better approach the goal of supernormal vision.

SUMMARY

Due to natural differences in the vast majority of eyes between total astigmatism as measured by refraction and corneal techniques, it is impossible to completely eliminate astigmatism from the eye's optical system and its correction. It can therefore be beneficial to combine both these elements when considering the plan for refractive laser surgery to produce an optimal, individualized outcome. If the treatment plan utilizes manifest refraction data alone, it may actually increase the postoperative aberrations, thereby reducing the final visual result.

The Alpins method of vector planning utilizes information from both corneal topography and manifest refraction/wavefront data to target less postoperative corneal astigmatism and minimize postoperative aberrations. Though this often means that the postoperative refractive astigmatism target is not zero, this minor refractive error (with a spherical equivalent of zero) that remains postoperatively in a favorable orientation may not be significant enough for patient perception. In fact, overall the patient satisfaction is potentially higher due to the lesser amount of lower order aberrations.

This method of vector planning and analysis may also be used to optimize treatment for each separate hemimeridian of the cornea in cases of irregular astigmatism. This would enable the surgeon to rearrange the corneal astigmatism and regularize the cornea, thus producing a potential increase in the best corrected visual acuity. Though a real time preoperative link to the topographical and wavefront information for this specialized ablation is yet to be formed, this integration of these diagnostic modalities utilizing vector planning may be a reality in the future.

REFERENCES

1. Goggin M, Alpins N, Schmid, L, Management of irregular astigmatism. Current Opinion in Ophthalmology. 2000;11:260-6.
2. Alpins NA. Astigmatism by the Alpins Method. J Cataract Refract Surg. 2001;27:31-49.
3. Alpins NA, Stamatelatos G. Customized photoastigmatic refractive keratectomy using combined topographic and refractive data for myopia and astigmatism in eyes with form fruste and mild keratoconus. J Cataract Refract Surg. 2007;33:591-602.
4. Alpins NA, Stamatelatos G.* Clinical outcomes of LASIK using combined topography and refractive wavefront treatments for myopic astigmatism. J Cataract Refract Surg. 2008; (in print).
5. Croes KJ. The Alpins Method: A breakthrough in astigmatism analysis. Medical Electronics, September 1998.
6. Alpins NA. A new method of analyzing vectors for changes in astigmatism. J Cataract Refract Surg. 1993;19:524-33.
7. Alpins NA. New method of targeting vectors to treat astigmatism. J Cataract Refract Surg. 1997;23:65-75.
8. Alpins NA. Treatment of irregular astigmatism. J Cataract Refract Surg. 1998;24:634-46.
9. Alpins NA.* Wavefront technology: A new advance that fails to answer old questions on corneal vs refractive astigmatism correction. J of Refractive Surg; 2002. pp. 737-9.
10. Javal E. Memoirs d'Ophthalmometrie. 1890, G Masson, Paris.
11. Duke-Elder S, (Ed). System of Ophthalmology. Vol 5: Ophthalmic optics and refraction. St Louis, Mosby; 1970. pp. 275-8.

*of special interest

Chapter 16

Aberropia: A New Refractive Entity

Amar Agarwal (India), Athiya Agarwal (India)

INTRODUCTION

The next evolution to come on to the visual science scene in refractive ocular imaging is the aberrometer, the Orbscan and wavefront analysis. This technology is based on astrophysical principles, which astronomers use to perfect the images impinging on their telescopes. Dr Bille, the Director of the Institute of Applied Physics at the University of Heidelberg first began work in this field while developing this specific technology for astronomy applications in the mid-1970s. For perfect imaging, astrophysicists have to be able to measure and correct the imperfect higher-order aberrations or wavefront distortions that enter their telescopic lens system from the galaxy. To achieve this purpose, adaptive optics are used wherein deformable mirrors reform the distorted wavefront to allow clear visualization of celestial objects. Extrapolating these same principles to the human eye, it was thought that removal of the wavefront aberrations of the eye might finally yield the long awaited and much desired ultimate goal of "super vision".

So far, the only parameters that could be modified to obtain the optical correction for a given patients refractive error were the sphere, cylinder and axis even though this does not give the ideal optical correction many a times. This is because the current modes for correcting the optical aberrations of the eye do not reduce the higher order aberrations. The ideal optical system should be able to correct the optical aberrations in such a way that the spatial resolving ability of the eye is limited only by the limits imposed by the neural retina, i.e. receptor diameter and receptor packing.

Thus, there may be a large group of patients whose best corrected visual acuity (BCVA) may actually improve significantly on removal of the optical aberrations. These optical aberrations are contributed to by the eye's entire optical system, i.e. the cornea, the lens, the vitreous and the retina. This study was conducted to determine the existence of a hitherto unidentified entity which we label as "aberropia" wherein patients with best corrected visual acuity of ≤ 6/9 (0.63), corneal topography not accounting for the lack of improvement in BCVA and with no other known cause for decreased vision improved by ≥ two Snellen lines after refractive correction of their wavefront aberration.

MATERIALS AND METHODS

Sixteen eyes of 10 patients were included in this retrospective study carried out at the Dr Agarwal's Eye Institute, India between May to December 2002. Only patients who had visual acuity less than 6/9 (0.63) prior to the procedure and whose visual acuity improved by more than or equal to two lines after the procedure were included in the study. None of these patients had any other known cause for decreased vision and their corneal topography did not account for the lack of improvement in BCVA. The routine patient evaluation including uncorrected (UCVA) and best corrected (BCVA), slit lamp examination, applanation tonometry, manifest and cycloplegic refractions, Orbscan, aberrometry, corneal pachymetry, corneal diameter, Schirmer test and indirect ophthalmoscopy had been performed for all the patients. Patients wearing contact lenses had been asked to discontinue soft lenses for a minimum of 1 week and rigid gas permeable lenses for a minimum of 2 weeks before the preoperative examination and surgery. Informed consent was obtained from all patients after a thorough explanation of the procedure and its potential benefits and risks.

The Zyoptix procedure was then performed using the Bausch and Lomb Technolas 217 Z machine. The parameters used were: wavelength 193 nm, fluence 130 mJ/cm^2 and ablation zone diameters between 4.8 mm and 6 mm. The Hansatome (Bausch and Lomb) was used in all the eyes. Either the 180 μm or the 160 μm plate was used in all the eyes. The aberrometer and the Orbscan, which checks the corneal topography, are linked and a zylink created. An appropriate software file is created which is then used to generate the laser treatment file.

Postoperatively, the patients underwent complete examination including UCVA, BCVA, slit lamp examination, Orbscan and aberrometry. The mean follow-up was 37.5 days.

For statistical analysis, the Snellen acuity was converted to the decimal notation. Continuous variables were described with mean, standard deviation, minimum and maximum values.

Results: 16 eyes of 10 patients satisfied the inclusion criteria. The mean age of the patients was 29.43 years (range 22-35 years). Six patients were females and four were males. The mean preoperative pupil diameter measured on aberrometer was 4.69 mm and mean postoperative pupil diameter measured on aberrometer was 4.53 mm.

The mean preoperative spherical equivalent was – 4.94 D (range –12.50 to –1.5 D). The mean spherical equivalent at 1 month postoperative period was –0.16 ± 0.68 D (range –1.0 to 1.5). Mean preoperative sphere was –4.95 D (range –12.50 to –0.75 D) and the mean postoperative sphere was –0.13 ± 0.68 D (range –1 to 1.5) at 1 month. The mean preoperative cylinder was –1.34 D (range 0 to –3.50). The mean postoperative cylinder was –0.08 ± 0.24 D (range 0 to –0.75 D) at one month. Postoperatively, at the end of first month, 70% of the patients were within ± 0.5D and 90% were within ± 1 D of emmetropia **(Figure 16.1)**. Preoperatively mean RMS (root mean square) values **(Figure 16.2)** were: Z 200 Defocus –9.22, Z 221 Astigmatism 0.12, Z 220 Astigmatism 1.02, Z 311 Coma –0.041, Z 310 Coma –0.04, Z 331 Trefoil 0.23, Z 330 Trefoil 0.016, Z 400 Spherical aberration –0.054, Z 420 Secondary astigmatism 0.103, Z 421 Secondary astigmatism 0.029, Z 440 Quadrafoil –0.103, Z 441 Quadrafoil –0.021, Z 510 Secondary coma 0.025, Z 511 Secondary coma –0.015, Z 530 Secondary trefoil 0.0049, Z 531 Secondary trefoil –0.00219, Z 550 Pentafoil 0.023, Z 551 Pentafoil 0.046. Postoperative mean RMS values were: Z 200 Defocus –0.429, Z 221 Astigmatism 0.07, Z 220 Astigmatism –0.07, Z 311 Coma 0.149, Z 310 Coma –0.079, Z 331 Trefoil –0.102, Z 330 Trefoil –0.004, Z 400 Spherical aberration –0.179, Z 420 Secondary astigmatism 0.015, Z 421 Secondary astigmatism 0.031, Z 440 Quadrafoil 0.019, Z 441 Quadrafoil –0.069, Z 510 Secondary coma –0.008, Z 511 Secondary coma 0.008, Z 530 Secondary Trefoil –0.002, Z 531 Secondary Trefoil –0.014, Z 550 Pentafoil 0.006, Z 551 Pentafoil 0.026.

Root mean square (RMS) pre and postlaser showed a reduction in the higher order aberrations **(Tables 16.1 and 16.2)**. 6.25% patients achieved 6/9, 31.25% patients achieved ≥ 6/6 (1.00), 37.50% achieved a BCVA of 6/5 (1.25) and 25% achieved a BCVA of 6/4 (1.6) **(Figure 16.3)**. **Figure 16.4** shows the preoperative Orbscan picture of a patient showing no abnormality. **Figures 16.5A and B** shows the aberrometer maps of the right eye and left eye of a patient in which we can see the aberrations reduced postlaser.

DISCUSSION

Zyoptix is the new generation of excimer laser used for the treatment of refractive disorders. Until recently, refractive disorders were treated with standard techniques, which took into consideration only the subjective refraction. Zyoptix technique on the other hand, takes into account the patient's subjective refraction, ocular optical aberrations and corneal topography, with the latter not only for the diagnosis, but also for the therapeutic treatment, in order to design a personalized

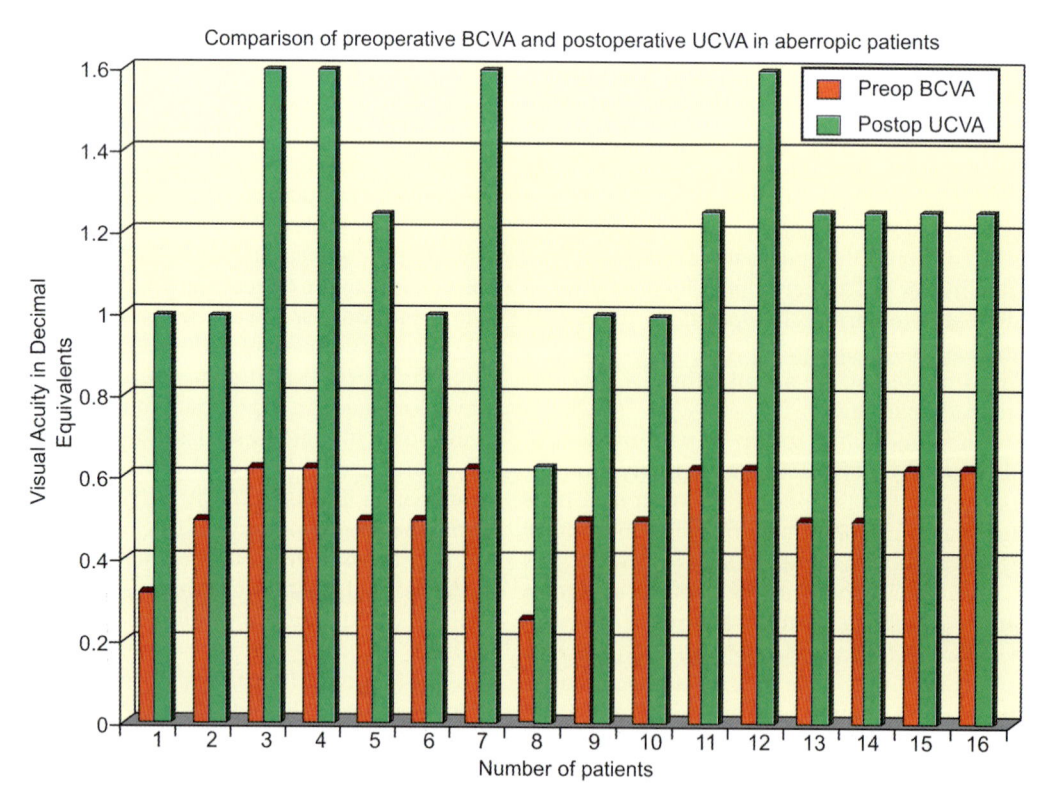

Figure 16.1 Preoperative BCVA versus postoperative UCVA

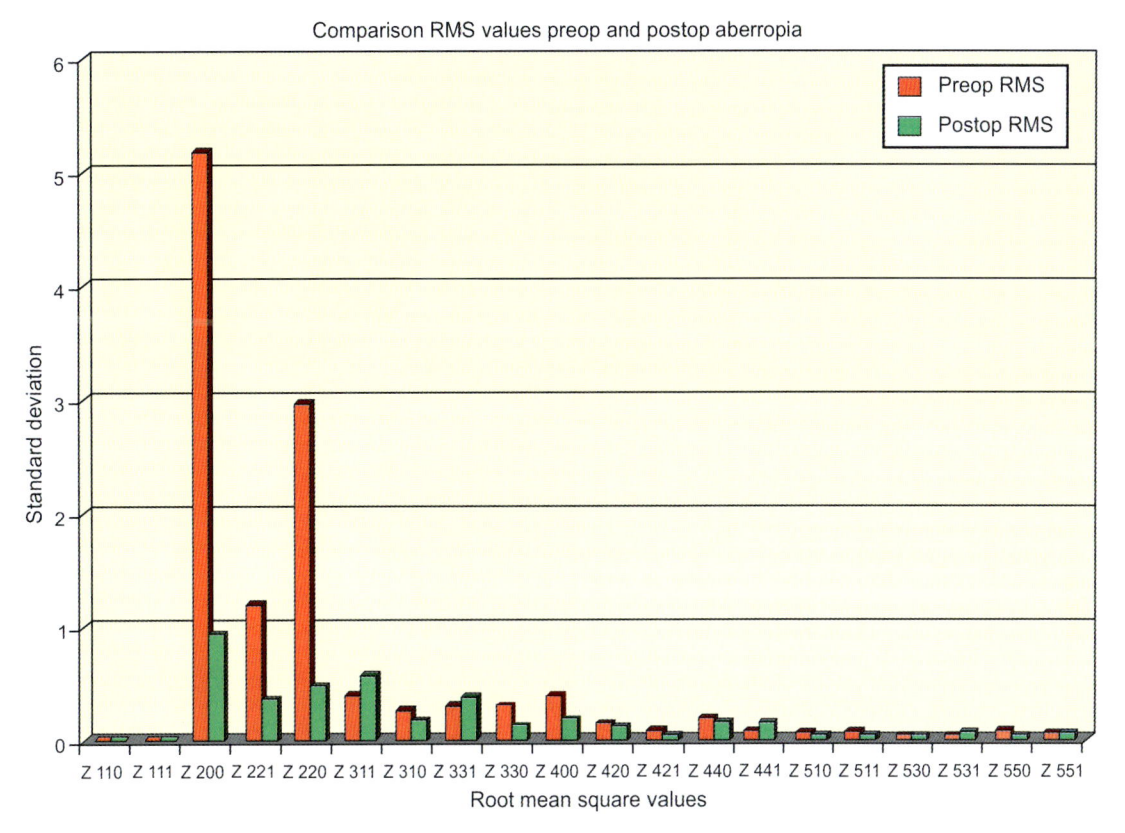

Figure 16.2 Root mean square (RMS) values preoperative and postoperative

treatment based on the total structure of the eye. The wavefront technology in Zyoptix uses the Hartmann Shack aberrometer based on the Hartmann-Shack principle[1] demonstrated by Liang et al[2] to measure the eye's wave aberration. This wavefront sensor has been improved by increasing the density of samples taken of the wavefront slope in the pupil.[3] All Hartmann-Shack devices are outgoing testing devices in that they evaluate the light being bounced back out through the optical system. A narrow laser beam is focused onto the retina to generate a point source. The outcoming light rays which experience all the aberrations of the eye pass through an array of lenses which detects their deviation. The wavefront deformation is calculated by analyzing the direction of the light rays using this lenslet array. Parallel light beams indicate a good wavefront and nonparallel light beams indicate a wavefront with aberrations, which does not give equidistant focal points. This image is then captured onto a charge-coupled device (CCD) camera and the wavefront is reconstructed. The data is explained mathematically in three dimensions with polynomial functions. Most investigators have chosen the Zernike method for this analysis although Taylor series can also be used for the same purpose.[4] Data from the wavefront map is presented as a sum of Zernike polynomials each describing a certain deformation. At any point in the pupil, the wavefront aberration is the optical path difference between the actual image wavefront and the ideal spherical wavefront centered at the image point.[5]

Any refractive error which cannot be corrected by spherocylindrical lens combinations is referred to by physicists as higher order aberrations, i.e. coma, spherical aberration, chromatic aberration. The Zernike polynomials, which describe ray points, are used to obtain a best fit toric to correct for the refractive error of the eye. The points are described in the X and Y coordinates and the third dimension, height is described in the Z-axis. The local refractive correction of each area of the entrance pupil can be determined by calculating from the wavefront polynomial the corresponding local radii of curvature and hence the required spherocylindrical correction.[6] Thus, each small region of the entrance pupil has its own three parameters that characterize the local refractive correction: sphere, cylinder and axis.[6] The global aberrations of the entire optical system including the cornea, lens, vitreous and the retina are thus measured. The great advantage of wavefront analysis is that it can describe these other aberrations.

The first order polynomial describes the spherical error or power of the eye. The second order polynomial describes the

Table 16.1 Root mean square (RMS) preoperative of 16 eyes

RMS Values Prelaser

Patient No	Z110	Z111	Z200	Z221	Z220	Z311	Z310	Z331	Z330	Z400	Z420	Z421	Z440	Z441	Z510	Z511	Z530	Z531	Z550	Z551	Z6
1	0	0	-5.77	4.055.	-6.131	0.299	-0.113	0.725	-0.44	0.009	-0.03	0.102	-0.233	0.109	0.131	0.027	-0.048	-0.041	0.052	0.039	-9999
2	0	0	-4.323	-1.719	6.005	-0.273	0.022	-0.353	0.275	0.092	0.092	-0.145	0.199	-0.013	-0.006	0.011	0.034	-0.039	0.042	0.042	-9999
3	0	0	-11.8	-0.088	0.116	0.435	-0.658	-0.444	-0.567	-0.779	-0.089	0.043	-0.202	-0.053	-0.052	-0.057	-0.04	-0.001	0.13	0.111	-9999
4	0	0	-12.46	0.514	-0.155	0.29	-0.006	0.016	0.529	-0.91	0.124	0.124	-0.431	-0.222	0.074	-0.04	0.001	-0.063	-0.141	0.119	-9999
5	0	0	-6.535	-0.123	-0.886	0.156	-0.09	0.094	-0.128	-0.084	-0.072	0.035	-0.009	-0.044	0.001	-0.031	0.01	-0.005	0.001	-0.041	-9999
6	0	0	-7.867	0.185	1.704	-0.02	0.414	0.441	0.197	0.365	0.197	0.107	-0.155	-0.002	0.123	0.026	-0.001	0.049	0.048	0.032	-9999
7	0	0	-4.28	0.167	2.571	0.007	-0.089	0.356	0.125	0.585	0.101	-0.002	-0.17	-0.062	-0.077	0.198	0.001	-0.104	-0.022	0.029	-9999
8	0	0	-10.4	0.502	-0.587	-0.007	-0.331	0.165	-0.126	-0.054	-0.071	0.036	-0.118	-0.128	0.009	0.017	-0.007	-0.026	0.063	-0.052	-9999
9	0	0	-17.15	-0.414	-1.217	0.093	-0.106	0.343	-0.18	-0.254	0.009	0.002	0.001	-0.025	0.007	-0.022	-0.007	-0.042	0.037	0.04	-9999
10	0	0	-16.78	-0.162	-0.637	0.122	-0.159	0.279	0.2	-0.181	0.115	0.007	-0.002	0.042	-0.034	-0.028	0.021	-0.043	-0.006	-0.017	-9999
11	0	0	-4.513	2.916	4.661	-0.634	-0.205	0.477	0.44	0.094	0.377	0.058	-0.201	0.101	0.133	-0.147	0.009	0.011	-0.055	0.118	-9999
12	0	0	-5.736	-1.501	5.195	-1.126	0.32	0.665	-0.254	0.218	0.479	0.122	-0.253	-0.045	0.099	-0.025	0.012	-0.006	-0.05	0.11	-9999
13	0	0	-15.46	1.605	2.754	0.378	0.443	0.208	0.458	0.643	-0.083	0.09	0.407	-0.006	-0.021	0.09	0.033	0.032	0.239	0.149	-9999
14	0	0	-15.26	-0.557	2.865	-0.26	-0.059	0.107	0.122	0.168	0.025	-0.256	-0.003	0.257	0.007	0.051	0.136	-0.061	-0.114	0.124	-9999
15	0	0	-4.955	0.735	0.383	-0.401	0.003	0.62	-0.494	-0.676	0.391	0.163	-0.421	-0.264	0.039	-0.261	-0.079	0.241	0.103	-0.067	-9999
16	0	0	-4.367	-0.195	-0.238	0.28	-0.04	0.021	0.11	-0.112	0.084	-0.022	-0.061	0.013	-0.018	-0.063	0.004	0.063	0.044	0	-9999

Chapter 16: Aberropia: A New Refractive Entity

Table 16.2 Root mean square (RMS) postoperative of 16 eyes

RMS Values Postlaser

Patient No	Z 110	Z 111	Z 200	Z 221	Z 220	Z 311	Z 310	Z 331	Z 330	Z 400	Z 420	Z 421	Z 440	Z 441	Z 510	Z 511	Z 530	Z 531	Z 550	Z 551	Z 6
1	0	0	-0.022	0.74	-1.294	0.117	-0.067	0.141	0.052	-0.063	-0.076	0.1	0.054	-0.037	-0.028	0.001	0.008	0.007	0.013	0.006	-9999
2	0	0	-0.508	0.12	0.194	-0.085	0.039	-0.12	-0.018	-9999	-9999	-9999	-9999	-9999	-9999	-9999	-9999	-9999	-9999	-9999	-9999
3	0	0	-1.398	-0.606	0.697	-0.558	-0.351	0.841	0.345	-0.39	0.392	0.038	-0.303	-0.038	-0.001	0.103	-0.066	-0.105	-0.021	0.137	-9999
4	0	0	-2.05	-0.499	-0.375	-0.027	-0.269	-0.534	-0.289	-0.58	0.114	0.058	0.236	-0.161	0.034	-0.083	0.004	0.039	0.01	-0.077	-9999
5	0	0	0.229	0.1	-0.123	-9999	-9999	-9999	-9999	-9999	-9999	-9999	-9999	-9999	-9999	-9999	-9999	-9999	-9999	-9999	-9999
6	0	0	-0.036	-0.17	0.425	-0.002	0.069	-0.045	-0.042	-0.342	-0.032	0.094	0.075	-0.05	0.068	0.03	0.064	-0.014	0.012	0.002	-9999
7	0	0	0.687	0.128	-0.028	-0.117	-0.043	0.062	0.088	-0.178	0.179	0.024	-0.045	0.055	0.013	0.016	-0.034	-0.013	-0.013	0.059	-9999
8	0	0	-2.164	0.279	-0.696	-0.25	-0.398	-0.147	-0.128	-0.581	-0.238	0.02	0.032	-0.088	-0.129	0.028	-0.029	0.007	0.089	0.059	-9999
9	0	0	-0.298	0.002	-0.311	0.158	-0.206	0.129	-0.116	-0.105	-0.045	-0.043	-0.1	-0.1	-9999	-9999	-9999	-9999	-9999	-9999	-9999
10	0	0	0.109	0.241	-0.503	0.233	-0.119	-0.16	-0.204	-9999	-9999	-9999	-9999	-9999	-9999	-9999	-9999	-9999	-9999	-9999	-9999
11	0	0	0.034	-0.092	0.076	0.013	-0.03	-0.067	0.003	-9999	-9999	-9999	-9999	-9999	-9999	-9999	-9999	-9999	-9999	-9999	-9999
12	0	0	0.187	0.061	0.004	-0.097	0.015	0.067	0.035	-0.428	-0.013	0.204	0.258	-0.636	-0.082	0.113	0.069	-0.239	0.062	0.059	-9999
13	0	0	-0.701	0.291	0.598	2.161	0.349	-1.062	-0.201	-0.118	-0.077	0.003	0.157	0.034	-0.006	-0.025	0.004	0.018	-0.066	-9999	-9999
14	0	0	-0.638	0.094	0.391	0.517	-0.328	-0.336	0.188	-0.111	0.053	0.07	-0.019	-0.084	-0.007	-0.051	-0.052	0.063	0.011	-9999	-9999
15	0	0	-0.148	0.493	0.017	0.261	0.017	-0.354	0.302	0.025	-0.008	-0.059	-0.028	-9999	-9999	-9999	-9999	-9999	-9999	-9999	-9999
16	0	0	-0.161	-0.038	-0.331	0.072	0.049	-0.05	-0.086	0.025	-0.008	-0.059	-0.028	-9999	-9999	-9999	-9999	-9999	-9999	-9999	-9999

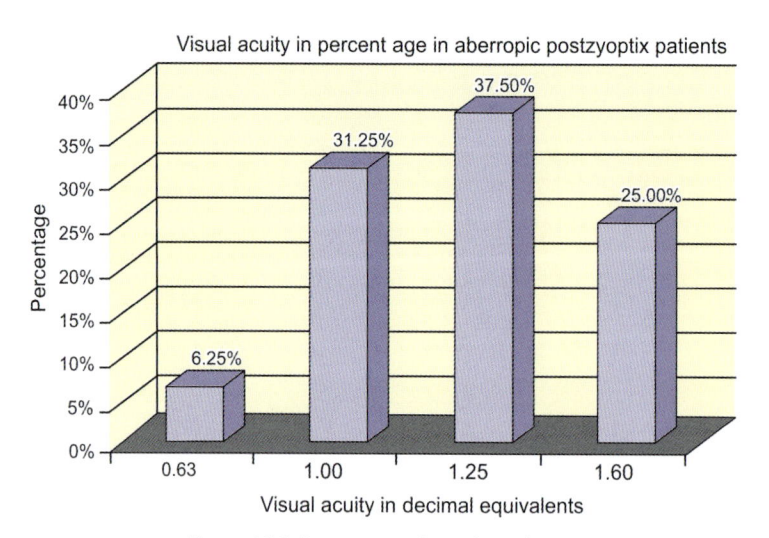

Figure 16.3 Percentage values of visual acuity

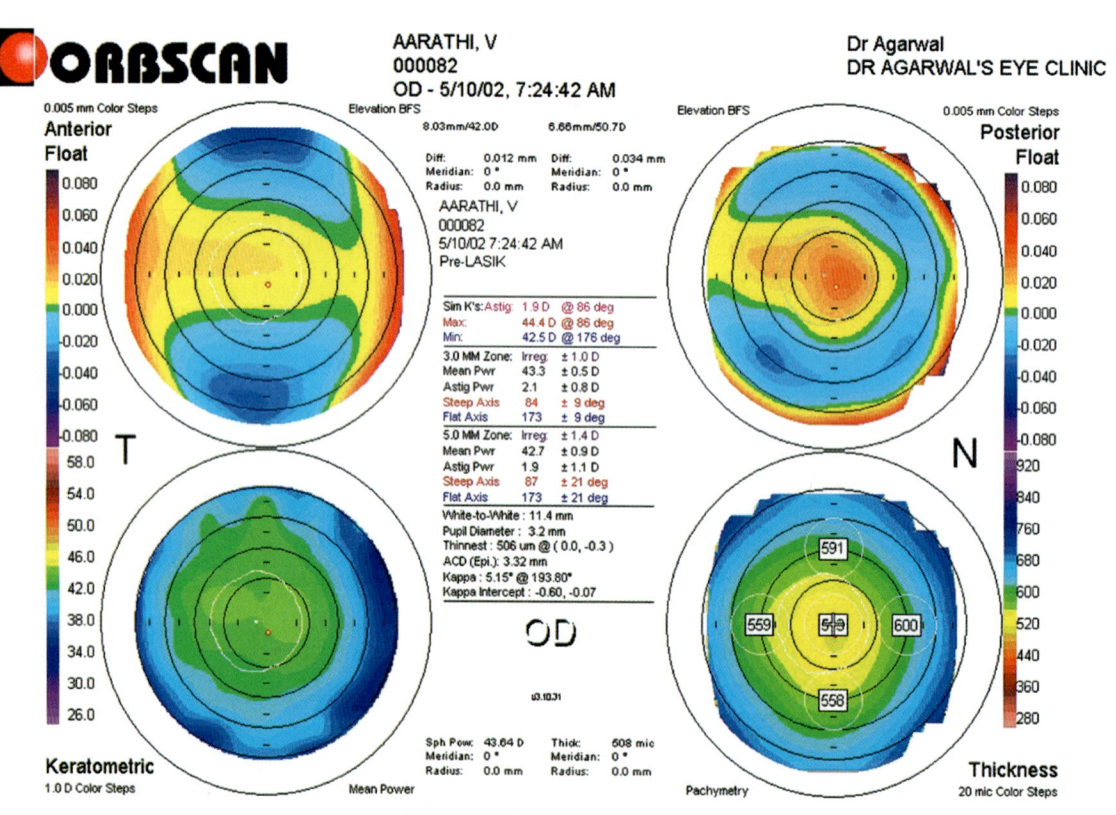

Figure 16.4 Preoperative Orbscan

regular astigmatic component and its orientation or axis. Third order aberrations are considered to be coma and fourth order aberrations are considered to be spherical aberration. Zernike polynomial descriptions for wavefront analysis typically go up to the tenth order of expression. The first and second orders describe the morphology of a normal straight curve. More local maximum and minimum points require higher orders of the polynomial series to describe the surface. Normal eyes exhibit spherical[7,8] and coma[9,10] aberrations in addition to exhibiting defocus and astigmatism.

Ideally, the difference in the magnitude of the local refractive correction of each area of the entrance pupil should not exceed 0.25 D. Lower spherocylindrical corrections are generally associated with lower wavefront aberrations.[6] These

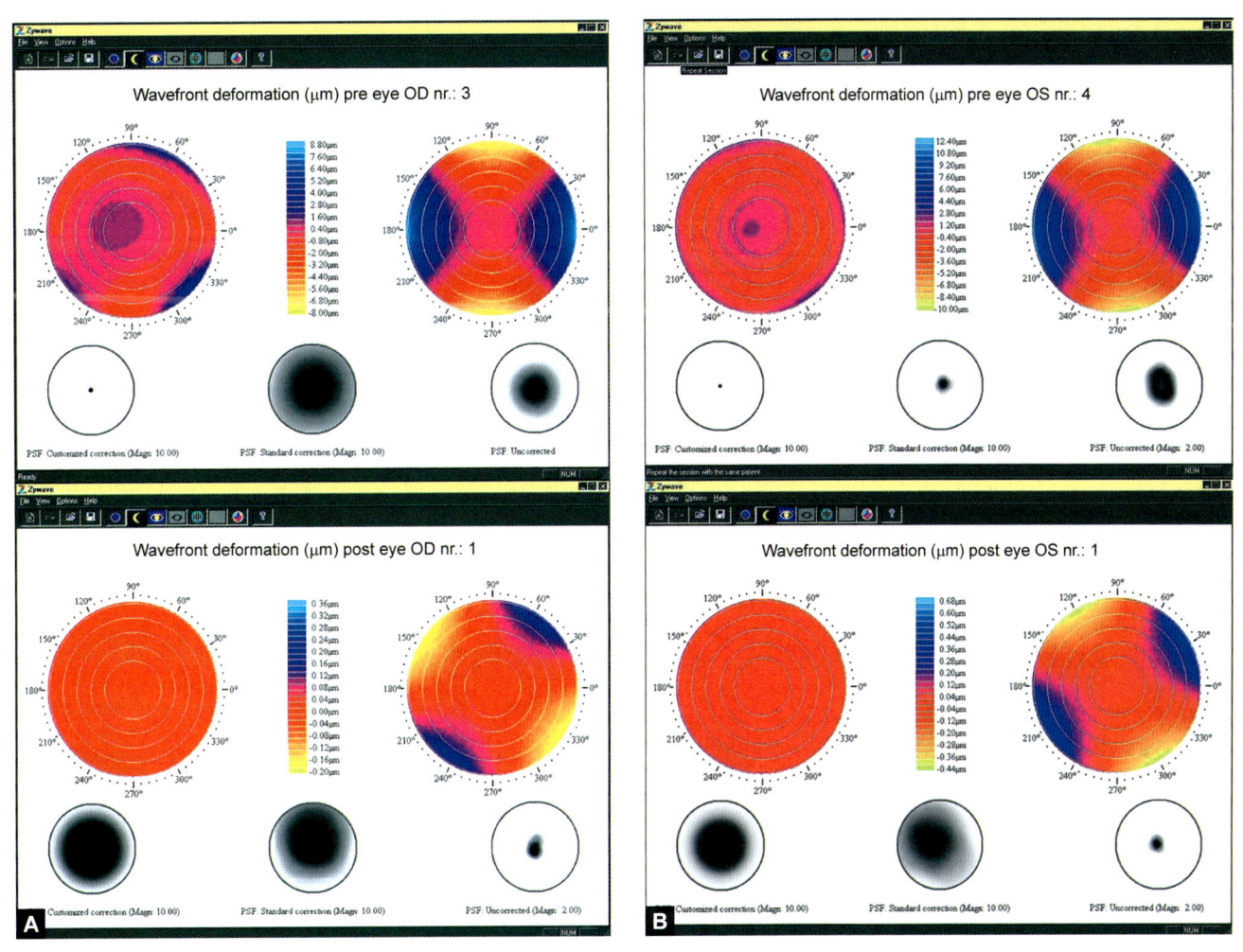

Figures 16.5A and B Pre- and postoperative aberrometry of the right and left eye of the same patient showing removal of higher order aberrations

observations regarding variation in local ocular refraction along different meridians are also confirmed by Ivanoff[11] and Jenkins.[12] Van den Brink[13] also commented on the change in refraction across the pupil. Clinically significant changes of at least 0.25 D in one or both components of the spherocylindrical correction might normally be expected for decentrations of about 1 mm. Rayleigh's quarter wavelength rule states that if the wavefront aberration exceeds a quarter of a wavelength, the quality of the retinal image will be impaired significantly.[14] Thus, the aberration in eyes starts to become significant when the pupil diameter exceeds 1–2 mm.[6] Thus, it is not possible to correct the entire wavefront aberration with a single spherocylindrical lens. As conventional refractive procedures such as LASIK also reduce only the second order aberrations, the visual acuity will still be limited by aberrations of third and higher order aberrations. These patients are likely to undergo tremendous improvement in their BCVA after correction of their aberrations by Zyoptix.

In the Zyoptix system, the aberrometer and the Orbscan, which checks the corneal topography, are linked and a zylink created. An appropriate software file is created which is then used to generate the laser treatment file. The truncated gaussian beam shape used in Zyoptix combines the advantages of the common beam shapes, i.e. flat top beam and the gaussian beam, creating a maximized smoothness and minimized thermal effect. Thus, Zyoptix gives a smoother corneal surface, reducing glare and increasing visual acuity. The larger optical zones reduce haloes. Zyoptix also causes a reduction of the ablation depth by 15–20% and a reduced enhancement rate.

In a patient with higher order aberrations, LASIK does not remove the higher order aberrations and the point-spread function is a large blur. Zyoptix on the other hand, performs customized ablation and removes the higher order aberrations thus minimizing the wavefront deformation. The point-spread function is therefore a small spot of light.

In our study, the mean preoperative spherical equivalent improved from –4.78 D to –0.16 D ± 0.68 and the mean preoperative cylinder improved from –1.34 D to –0.08 D ± 0.24. The aberrations were reduced drastically in all the eyes and the BCVA improved in all cases by more than and equal to two lines. Reduction of the aberrations of the eye can thus result in an improved BCVA postoperatively.

Improving the optics of the eye by removing aberrations increases the contrast and spatial detail of the retinal image. Reduction of higher order aberrations may not improve high contrast acuity much more in eyes where spherocylindrical lenses alone improve the BCVA to 6/3 (2.00) or better. In contrast, in otherwise normal eyes where the BCVA is limited to 6/9 (0.50) or 6/6 (1.00) due to optical aberrations, reduction of higher order aberrations should improve visual acuity.

Realization of the best possible unaided visual acuity may be limited at the cortical, retinal and the spectacle, corneal, or implant level. All maculae may not be able to support 6/3 (2.00) vision. Insufficient cone density or suboptimal orientation of cone receptors or a suboptimal Stiles-Crawford profile of the macula may make 6/3 (2.00) vision impossible. Clinical or subclinical amblyopia may make achievement of super vision impossible. But, in spite of this, there may be a certain patient population who have the potential for an improved BCVA on removal of their wavefront aberrations. The corneal topography does not account for the decreased preoperative visual acuity in these patients, neither do they have any other identifiable cause for the decrease in acuity except for an abnormal wavefront. It is important that this subgroup of patients are identified and their optical aberrations neutralized so that they are not deprived of the opportunity to gain in their BCVA.

Wavefront sensing technology, at present, does not in most cases define the exact locale of the pathology causing the aberration. Hence, clinical examination and other refractive tools, such as corneal topographic mapping, along with sound clinical judgment is required for proper understanding of the eye and its individual refractive status. Also, wavefront aberrations may not remain static. Numerous authors,[15-18] have shown that ocular optical aberrations probably remain constant between 20 and 40 years of age but increase after that. Aberrations also change during accommodation [19,20] and may be affected by mydriatics.[21] Thus, the patient should be informed about these possibilities while taking the consent for the procedure. Long-term studies are required to determine the stability of the postoperative refraction, residual aberrations and changes in BCVA if any.

The question of magnification factor improving visual acuity does not arise as these patients preoperatively did not improve with contact lenses. Further the refractive error in some of these patients was not very large.

CONCLUSION

In conclusion, removal of the wavefront aberration may extend the benefit of an improved BCVA to patients with an abnormal wavefront. The subgroup of patients with higher order aberrations, normal corneal topography and no other known cause for decreased vision may thus benefit immensely with wavefront-guided refractive surgery. Customized refractive surgery tailor-made for these individual patients, aimed at neutralizing the wavefront aberrations of the eye is safer, more predictable, provides better visual acuities and reduces the incidence of unsatisfactory outcomes. Further studies are required to assess the long-term outcomes.

Till now, when we discuss refractive errors we discuss about spherical and a cylindrical correction. But in todays world we have to think of a third parameter which is the aberrations present in the eye which can be anywhere in the optical media. These can be corrected in the corneal level by the laser treatment.

REFERENCES

1. Platt B, Shack RV. "Lenticular Hartmann screen," Opt Sci Center News (University of Arizona) 5,1971:5-16.
2. Liang J, Grimm B, Goelz S, Bille J. Objective measurement of the wave aberrations of the human eye with the use of a Hartmann-Shack wavefront sensor. J Opt Soc Am. 1994;11:1949-57.
3. Liang J, Williams DR, et al. Aberrations and retinal image quality of the normal human eye. J Opt Soc Am A. 1997;14(11):2873-83.
4. Oshika T, Klyce SD, Applegate RA, et al. Comparison of corneal wavefront aberrations after photorefractive keratectomy and laser in situ keratomileusis. Am J Ophthalmol. 1999;127:1-7.
5. Fincham WHA, Freeman MH. Optics, 9th edn. London: Butterworths, 1980.
6. Charman WN, Walsh G. Variations in the local refractive correction of the eye across its entrance pupil. Optometry and Vision Science. 1989;66(1):34-40.
7. Rosenblum WM, Christensen JL. "Objective and subjective spherical aberration measurement of the human eye," in Progress in Optics, e Wolf, ed. (North-Holland, Amsterdam) 1976;13:69-91.
8. Campbell MC, Harrison EM, Simonet P. Psychophysical measurement of the blur on the retina due to optical aberrations of the eye: Vision Res. 1990;30:1587-1602.
9. Howland HC, Howland B. A subjective method for the measurement of monochromatic aberrations of the eye. J Opt Soc Am. 1977;67:1508-18.
10. Walsh G, Charman WN, Howland HC. Objective technique for the determination of monochromatic aberrations of the human eye. J Opt Soc Am A1; 1984. pp. 1987-92.
11. Ivanoff A. About the spherical aberration of the eye. J Opt Soc Am. 1956:46:901-03.
12. Jenkins TCA. Aberrations of the eye and their effects on vision. Part 1. Br J Physiol Opt. 1963;20:59-91.
13. Van den Brink G. Measurements of the geometric aberrations of the eye. Vision Res. 1962;2:233-44.

14. Born M, Wolf E. Principles of Optics, 2nd edn. New York: Macmillan 1964:203-32.
15. Kaemmerer M, Mrochen M, Mierdel P, et al. Optical aberrations of the human eye. Nature Medicine (in press).
16. Oshika T, Klyce SD, Applegate RA, et al. Changes in corneal wavefront aberration with aging. Invest Ophthalmol Vis Sci. 1999; 40:1351-55.
17. Calver RI, Cox MJ, Elliot DB. Effect of aging on the monochromatic aberrations of the human eye. J Opt Soc Am A. 1999;16:2069-78.
18. Guirao A, Gonzalez C, Redondo M, et al. Average optical performance of the human eye as a function of age in a normal population. Invest Ophthalmol Vis Sci. 1999;40:203-13.
19. Krueger R, Kaemerrer M, Mrochen M, et al. Understanding refraction and accommodation through "ingoing optics" aberrometry: A case report. Ophthalmology (in press).
20. He JC, Burns SA, Marcos S. Monochromatic aberrations in the accommodated human eye. Vis Res. 2000;40:41-8.
21. Fankhauser F, Kaemerrer M, Mrochen M, et al. The effect of accommodation, mydriasis, and cycloplegia on aberrometry. ARVO abstract 2248. Invest Ophthalmol Vis Sci. 2000;41;S461.

Chapter 17

Differences Between Various Aberrometer Systems

Ronald R Krueger (USA)

INTRODUCTION

Custom ablation is a very broad term. It can refer to treatment of the cornea that does not depend on recent technological advances: Surgeon-oriented customization occurs, for instance, if the surgeon decides to treat a small zone for a central island that has developed following laser vision correction.

The implied meaning of custom ablation today does involve recent advances. Custom ablation can be guided by topography, and more recently by wavefront mapping. Wavefront guided customization will be the most successful method of corneal ablation in the future. Most companies in the ophthalmic vision correction industry are focusing their resources on this technology because it promises to yield all the information needed for doing customized laser treatment.

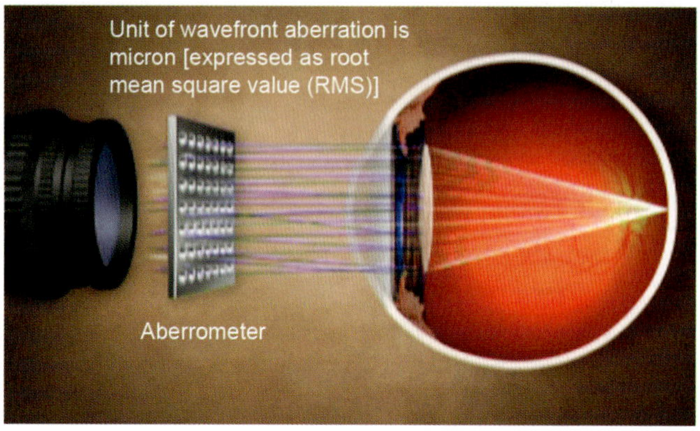

MAPPING A PROFILE OF THE WHOLE EYE

The wavefront sensing device provides a new and objective way of mapping the profile of refraction and of higher order defects in the eye such as coma and spherical aberrations. Whereas corneal topography allows us to map a profile of the corneal surface, wavefront mapping makes it possible to map a profile of the whole eye.

Wavefront analysis is a more sophisticated method of defining aberrations that the surgeon is trying to correct through refractive surgery. Until the present time the basis for diagnosis has essentially been corneal topography.

DIFFERENT METHODS AVAILABLE

Wavefront technology originated from two main sources more than 100 years ago. A physicist named Hartmann developed principles of subjectively measuring optical aberrations in a reproducible way. This system was later developed into what is called the Hartmann-Shack wavefront analyzing device, which is used by most manufacturers today **(Figure 17.1)**. Tscherning, an ophthalmologist working in the late 1800s, devised another method of doing wavefront mapping. Tscherning's method was further developed by Howland and Howland in the 1970's and more recently, Theo Seiler modified this method for clinical use, as adopted by two German manufacturers. The Tscherning's

Figure 17.1 Hartmann Shack aberrometer
(*Courtesy:* Dr Agarwal's Eye Hospital, India)

principle is also utilized in a retinal tracing method applied with the Tracey technology.

A third method is used by the group at Emory University in Atlanta, Georgia. Their method involves a spatially resolved refractometer which evaluates the wavefront profile by soliciting the patient's subjective response to a series of light rays entering the eye. Still another method of wavefront analysis, which Nidek is using, operates more by retinoscopic principles.

The Mechanisms of Wavefront Devices

Light passing in and out of the eye has to go through multiple structures like the vitreous, lens and the back and front surfaces of the cornea. Aberrations inside the eye can affect the passage of the light **(Figures 17.2 to 17.5)**. Ultimately, seeing where the light is emitted from the eye in relation to the cornea allows the ophthalmologist to predict the change in corneal shape needed to give the patient perfect focus.

Wavefront devices can be categorized into four groups. With "outgoing" wavefront analysis, the wavefront is defined by the foveally reflected laser light going out of the eye. The Hartmann-Shack devices represented by Alcon, Visx, Bausch and Lomb, Meditec and Topcon are all based on this form of wavefront analysis. The Tscherning device, named after a

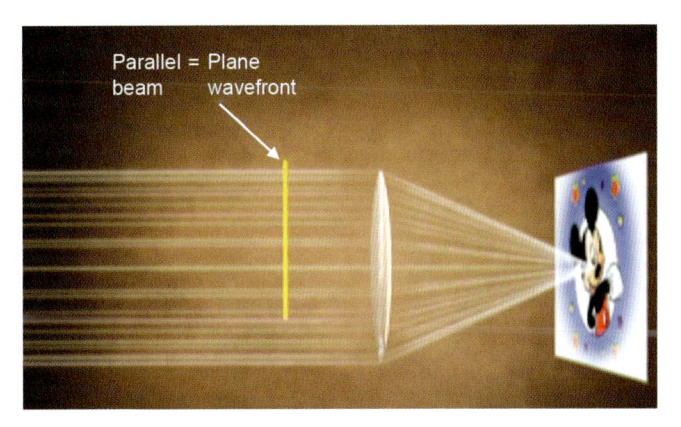

Chapter 17: Differences Between Various Aberrometer Systems

Figure 17.2 Plane wavefront (*Courtesy*: Dr Agarwal's Eye Hospital, India)

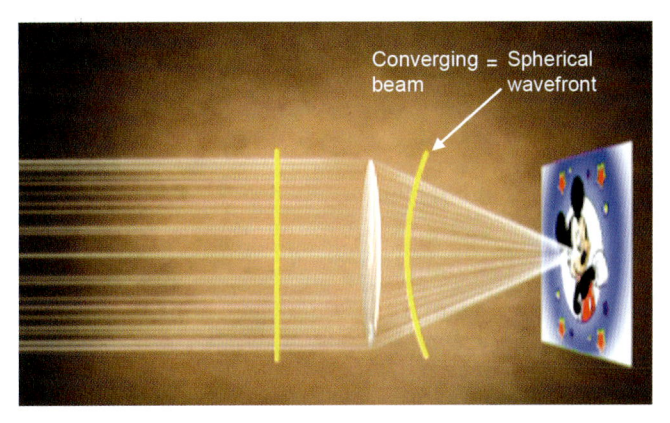

Figure 17.3 Spherical wavefront (*Courtesy*: Dr Agarwal's Eye Hospital, India)

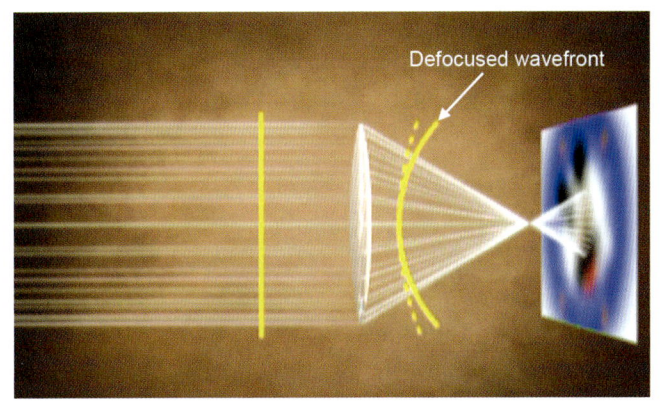

Figure 17.4 Defocused wavefront (*Courtesy*: Dr Agarwal's Eye Hospital, India)

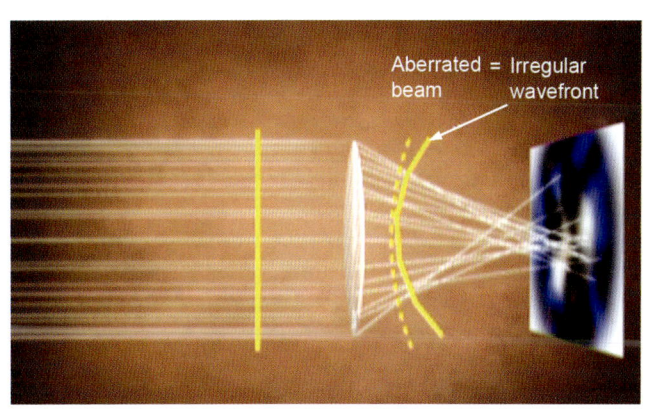

Figure 17.5 Irregular wavefront (*Courtesy*: Dr Agarwal's Eye Hospital, India)

prominent ophthalmologist from the late 1800s, is based on "retinal imaging" wavefront analysis. The Tscherning device involves a grid of laser energy shone into the eye. The way the grid deviates as it enters the eye and is imaged on the retina defines the wavefront pattern. This device uses the retina to obtain the wavefront pattern. It has been popularized through the efforts of Dr Theo Seiler, who introduced the technology to two German companies, Wavelight, and Schwind. The Tracey retinal ray tracing method sequentially delivers one ray at a time which is imaged on the retina in a rapid (<10 msec) fashion. The third method is an ingoing adjustable way of determining the wavefront pattern. It measures the light rays coming in, being manually adjusted by the patient to a central retinal focus. The Spatially Resolved Refractometer use this mechanism. The final method uses a double pass (in and out) method of analyzing the wavefront by slit skioloscopy, using retinoscopic principles. The Nidek OPD scan uses this mechanism.

Benefits of Wavefront Analysis

Probably the best analogy to the development of wavefront technology relates to the early days of radial keratotomy in refractive surgery. At that point, before the age of corneal topography, all the surgeon needed to know was the keratometry value and certain other numbers about the shape of the cornea. The advent of corneal topography allowed us to map a whole profile of the shape of the cornea, giving us much more information for diagnosis.

Approaching patients with spherocylindrical refraction, we base the laser treatment on the refractive error with sphere, cylinder and axis. But those are only three numbers, just as keratometry is defined with only a few numbers. Our goal is to get the whole profile of refraction, with an equivalent value at every point within the pupillary aperture. Once this information is obtained, the ophthalmologist can use the laser to create the perfect optical surface.

Linking Diagnostic Information from Wavefront Mapping to Laser Treatment

It is already possible to link diagnostic information obtained from wavefront analysis to the excimer laser treatment. Several companies are actively doing this form of customized treatment in studies performed in non-US countries. Alcon is using the technology as part of clinical trials in cooperation with the US Food and Drug Administration (FDA). Autonomous Technologies Corp, which had a very effective scanning spot laser, was purchased by Summit Technologies, which owns many patents in the US. Now Summit has been acquired by Alcon. Alcon is now refining their LADARVision excimer laser to be used with the custom cornea wavefront device. The specific aberrations can be used to obtain diagnostic information. Then, with the laser, that diagnostic information can be directly applied to the treatment. This custom cornea platform of Alcon was recently approved in the US for the correction of myopia.

All the companies that have excimer lasers are developing their own unique wavefront devices. Alcon has the LADAR Wave Wavefront Device. Visx has the WaveScan device, Bausch and Lomb has the Zywave device and Zeiss-Meditec has the Wavefront Sciences Device as part of their WASCA program. Each of these modified Hartmann-Shack devices uses "outgoing optics" to define the wavefront pattern. Wave Light and Schwind have their own wavefront devices based on Tscherning's design of "retinal imaging" optics. Nidek has the OPD scan, which is a special device based on slit skioloscopy, using a modification of retinoscopic principles.

Because there is variation among all these types, it would not be wise to obtain a device from Alcon and a laser from Nidek, because the two may not correspond to allow for custom ablation. At this point in the development of the technology no one really knows which is the best device, and comparative studies are yet to be done. The best approach is to examine the technology, consider the manufacturers behind the various devices, and try to predict which are likely to be successful.

WAVEFRONT ANALYSIS IN CONJUNCTION WITH CORNEAL TOPOGRAPHY

Ophthalmologists have learned to depend on corneal topography devices to help screen for disease before surgery and to monitor patients after surgery. More and more we will use the wavefront device for diagnostic testing before and after surgery. Wavefront mapping in conjunction with corneal topography will provide the most complete picture. Although it is uncertain whether corneal topography will continue to be used a decade from now as technology continues to advance, there is definitely a place for it now. Meanwhile, the wavefront device provides even more detailed information about what the patient is likely to see because it measures the light passage into the eye focusing on the retina. Whereas the shape of the cornea is important, it is more important to ensure that the focus on the retina is perfectly sharp.

PERSONALIZED LASIK NOMOGRAMS

At present there is considerable interest in developing a commercial database system for nomograms. A number of researchers and companies are working on programs tailor-made for collecting data and determining individual nomograms. There may be several ways to achieve this goal. You can obtain your own Excel file. Using this file you can compare the attempted correction to what is achieved, and then assess the difference. Through regression analysis according to different variables, a nomogram can be derived.

In the future wavefront mapping may be used to refine some of these measures. However, at present with custom cornea wavefront guided treatment, a nomogram is not necessary, but rather simply an offset feature which can be adjusted according to a particular surgeon, climate and environment.

Chapter 18

Corneal Wavefront Guided Excimer Laser Surgery for the Correction of Eye Aberrations

Jorge L Alió (Spain), David P Piñero (Spain), Mohamad Rosman (Spain)

INTRODUCTION

Higher-order corneal aberrations (HOAs) can result in significant visual symptoms and visual impairment, especially in some patients who have undergone corneal refractive surgery. Advancements in excimer laser refractive surgery have led to the introduction of wavefront guided excimer laser refractive surgery. Wavefront guided excimer laser refractive surgery, based on correcting global (or total) aberrations of the eye, has been shown to reduce the induction of higher-order aberrations during PRK and LASIK of normal eyes and has also been shown to reduce the amount of higher-order aberrations in highly aberrated eyes. However, as 80% of the refractive power of the eye is attributed to the first corneal surface, higher-order aberrations from the corneal surface will have a greater impact on visual quality. Hence, the correction of corneal higher-order aberrations, as opposed to the correction of total higher-order aberrations, may have a greater impact on visual quality in the long-term. This chapter will illustrate the rationale and clinical results of corneal wavefront guided excimer laser surgery for the correction of eye aberrations.

IMPACT OF HIGHER-ORDER ABERRATIONS

Higher-order aberrations in significant amount may cause symptomatic visual impairment, especially among patients who have undergone corneal refractive surgery. Symptoms of glare, haloes and starburst are associated with spherical, coma and other types of aberrations.[1,2] Coma-like aberration of the eye has been shown to significantly affect contrast sensitivity function,[3] cause haloes[2] and may also cause monocular diplopia.[1,4] While the effect of these higher-order aberrations may not be significant when the pupil is small (3 mm), they play a substantial role in degrading visual performance when the pupil is large, i.e. in scotopic light conditions,[5,6] hence, resulting in significant night vision symptoms.

The normal cornea has a positive 4th order spherical aberration that changes with age, with mirror symmetry between the right and left eyes.[7,8] The amount of higher-order aberrations measured in normal eyes vary among subjects and increases with age.[7-9] Wang et al reported that there is a wide range of individual variability among normal individuals in aberrations with ranges of individual Zernike terms from −0.579 to +0.572 μm. The mean coefficient of the 4th-order spherical aberration (SA) (Z_4^0) was 0.280 +/− 0.086 μm and was positive in all corneas. The mean root-mean-square (RMS) values were 0.479 +/− 0.124 μm for HOA, 0.281 +/− 0.086 μm for SA (Z_4^0) and (Z_6^0), and 0.248 +/− 0.135 μm for coma (Z_3^{-1}), (Z_3^1), (Z_5^{-1}), and (Z_5^1).[7] Changes on the cornea due to surgery and disease can result in changes of higher-order aberrations which may be visually significant. Laser refractive surgery, in particular, is well-known to induce higher-order aberrations.[6] Myopic laser refractive surgery induces a positive spherical aberration while hyperopic corrections induce a negative spherical aberration.[10-12] These induced aberrations are increased when higher corrections are attempted. PRK and LASIK have also been noted to increase ocular higher-order aberrations differently. The difference between the two types of surgery may be correlated with the change of the corneal shape, the conversion of biodynamics, the healing of the corneal cut, and re-structured corneal epithelium and/or the stroma.[13] Studies have also shown that significant higher-order aberrations are induced in eyes which have undergone LASIK with a microkeratome-created flap compared to eyes which have undergone LASIK with an Intralase-created flap.[14-16] The induction of higher-order aberrations is further exaggerated in eyes with complications during laser refractive surgery.[17] On average, eyes with central islands had the most vertical coma while eyes with central islands and decentered ablations had elevated amounts of spherical aberration compared with successful postoperative LASIK eyes.[18]

Of all the aberrometric components, the primary spherical aberration and coma aberration are the most symptomatic and the most frequent after refractive surgery. As mentioned, the most frequent aberration after an uncomplicated refractive surgery is spherical aberration. The primary spherical aberration is a higher order aberration corresponding to the fourth order of the Zernike decomposition. Basically, this error is due to the difference of refractive power between the central and the peripheral area of the optical ocular system (between the ablated and the nonablated area). As a result, all the light rays passing through the system do not focus at the same point. Several light rays will be focused in front of the retinal plane, whereas others will be focused behind it.

188 Section IV: Aberropia, Aberrations and Topography

This phenomenon generates a concentric circle of blurred light around the focused point or halo. The higher the aperture of the system (the pupil diameter), the halo generated is more significant, because the aberrated peripheral area has a greater impact on the retinal image. Thus, this optical situation induces significant disturbances and discomfort in the patient under scotopic conditions **(Figures 18.1A and B)**.

Coma aberrations are commonly associated with decentered treatments **(Figures 18.2A and B)** which results in asymmetry in the cornea. This produces an enlargement of the image light distribution along an axis, generating a comet-like image of a point source light object.

To a certain extent, newer aspheric ablation profiles may have reduced the induction of spherical aberrations in uncomplicated laser refractive surgery,[19] while more advanced eye-tracking systems have reduced the risk of decentered ablations and thereby reduced the risk of coma aberrations. However, the risk of visually significant higher-order aberration after laser refractive surgery and other causes, like cornea surgery or diseases, still persists. The challenge to all refractive

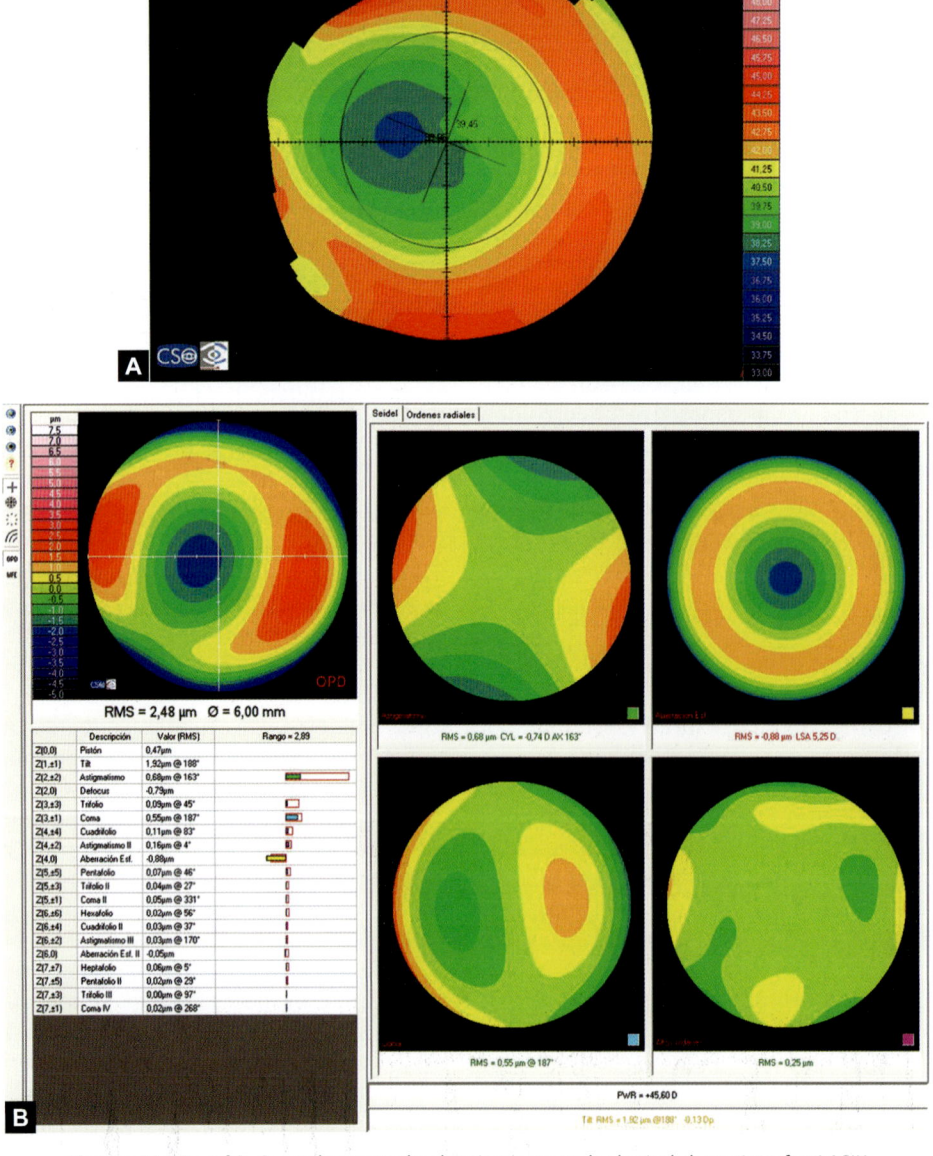

Figures 18.1A and B Corneal topography showing increased spherical aberration after LASIK

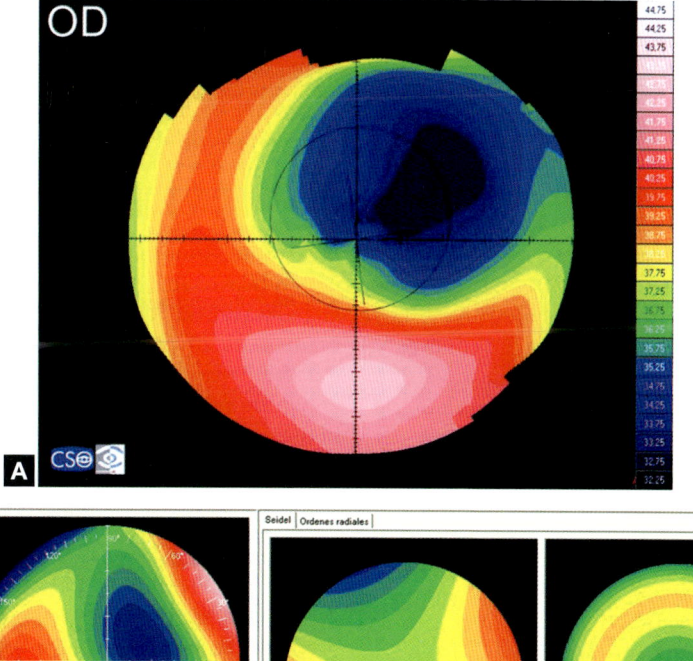

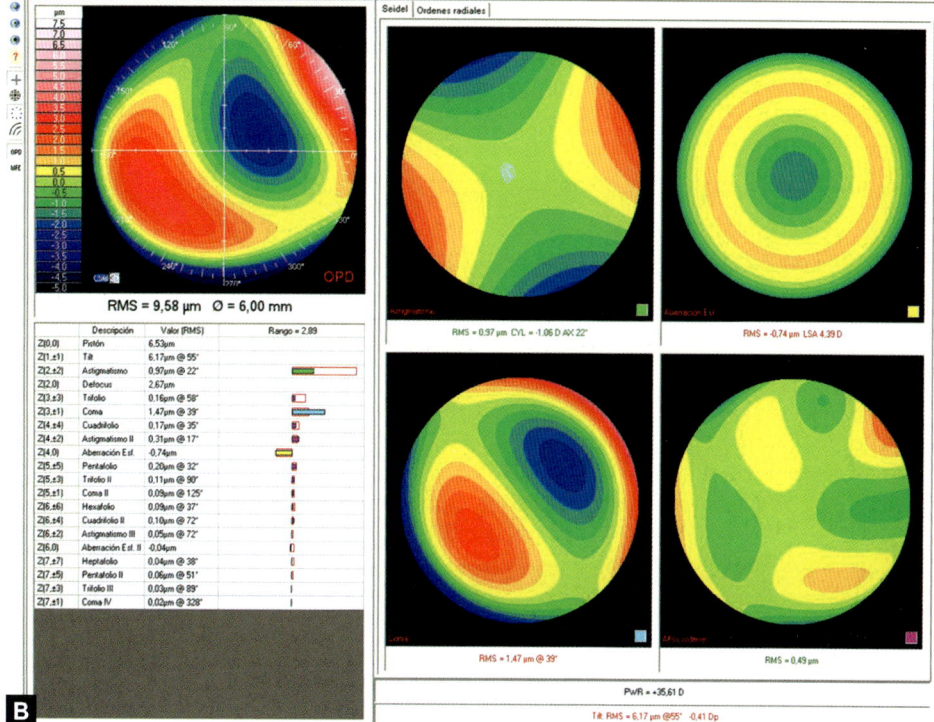

Figures 18.2A and B Corneal topography showing increased coma aberrations due to decentered ablation

surgeons is how to treat such patients and to reduce the amount of higher-order aberrations which are present.

WAVEFRONT GUIDED REFRACTIVE SURGERY

The concept of wavefront guided ablations in excimer laser refractive surgery was introduced in 2000.[20,21] The aim of wavefront guided excimer laser refractive surgery was to correct pre-existing individual optical aberrations while correcting the refractive error during excimer laser refractive surgery. Thus, it has the potential advantage of reducing post-LASIK night-vision problems and may even result in improved post-LASIK vision.

The basic concept of wavefront guided LASIK involves the measurement of the wavefront aberrations with a wavefront analyzer such as the Hartmann-Shack aberrometer and to transfer the aberrations into an appropriate ablation pattern to be performed by a scanning-spot excimer laser. However, the results of wavefront guided LASIK are influenced by other variables in the LASIK procedure, which includes accurate centration of the laser spot, creation and replacement of the corneal flap and wound healing. Cyclotorsion in the supine position may also influence the spot position as related to the aberrometer data.

Studies have shown wavefront guided LASIK to be as safe and efficacious as conventional LASIK.[22-25] Wavefront guided LASIK has also been shown to reduce the amount of induced higher-order aberrations compared to conventional LASIK.[26] But other studies have shown that wavefront guided LASIK only reduced higher-order aberrations in less than 50% of eyes.[27] Furthermore, the clinical benefits of performing wavefront guided LASIK compared to conventional LASIK in a normal eye may not be apparent.[28]

Perhaps the value of wavefront guided excimer laser treatment lies in correcting aberrated eyes with significant visual symptoms and the retreatment of LASIK for residual refractive errors. Wavefront guided LASIK appears to be superior to conventional LASIK when used to correct residual refractive errors after excimer laser refractive surgery as it induces less high-order aberrations and is less likely to cause a reduction in contrast sensitivity.[29,30]

Patients who are more likely to benefit from wavefront guided excimer laser treatment include those with significant aberrations after uneventful conventional refractive surgery, patients with complications during refractive surgeries and patients with aberrated corneas due to cornea surgery or diseases. In general, the treatment of aberrated cornea with wavefront guided LASIK results in significant reduction in higher-order aberrations. Patients also noticed a reduction in their pre-existing visual symptoms and reported improvement in quality of vision.[31-37] Wavefront guided PRK has also been reported to be effective in treating a patient with visual symptoms secondary to coma and a loss of best corrected visual acuity due to a LASIK flap button hole.[38]

CORNEAL WAVEFRONT GUIDED REFRACTIVE SURGERY

Having established the efficacy of wavefront guided excimer laser treatment for cases of retreatment and the treatment of aberrated corneas, the debate now lies between the efficacy of wavefront guided (total wavefront) treatments versus corneal wavefront guided treatments. Current technology enables the measurement of both corneal and total ocular aberrations. Global (or total) aberrations are analyzed by wavefront sensors such as the Hartmann-Shack aberrometer, while corneal aberrations are obtained by a mathematical transformation from corneal topography.

In the normal eye, 90% of the total aberrations are caused by the corneal optics; this proportion is largely the majority of the global aberration pattern of the eye when the cornea shows some degree of irregularity. Thus, targeting the corneal aberrations instead of the global aberration may be more efficacious in the treatment of highly aberrated corneas.

Global wavefront sensors available today only analyze up to 1452 points.[39] It is usually ineffective to register data of highly irregular corneas, and its information is limited to the pupil size area and by accomodation. The data is also affected by intraocular optics. With topographical systems, more than 6000 points can be studied and an exhaustive analysis performed. About 90% of the corneal surface can be analyzed with a higher resolution of 1 μm (compared to 210 μm for global wavefront aberrometry). Thus, corneal aberrometry, as mathematically transformed from corneal topography, offers data from nearly the whole cornea, providing a larger quantity and more specific information about the optical performance of the anterior corneal surface. Moreover, this measurement is not influenced by intraocular optics and accommodation.

The terms *topography guided* and *corneal wavefront guided* can be confusing. Systems that try to reduce corneal irregularity by changing the corneal shape without considering corneal wavefront analysis are called topography guided. These systems are less accurate and thus were improved by the introduction of corneal wavefront data derived from corneal elevation data in the calculation of the ablation profile.

In summary, the justifications for the use of corneal wavefront guided treatment for the treatment of highly aberrated corneas are:

1. The first refractive interface corresponding to air-cornea is the most important contributor to the total power of the eye because the greatest difference in refractive indices between media in the eye is found at that point.
2. In highly aberrated corneas with previous keratorefractive procedures, the contribution of the aberrations in the cornea generated by the surgery will be the most significant source of optical errors.
3. The sampling provided by most ocular wavefront sensors or aberrometers is more limited than that obtained with corneal topographers.
4. Ocular wavefront sensors or aberrometers have limitations in the analysis of highly aberrated eyes. These include the crowding or superimposition of the light spots or the assumption of a flat slope for each analyzed portion of the wavefront (Hartmann-Shack devices).

Computerized Corneal Topography and Corneal Wavefront Analysis

In our center, corneal aberrations were derived from the CSO corneal topography system (CSO, Florence Italy). The CSO topography system is a corneal topographer that is capable of evaluating the optical function of the anterior corneal surface, in addition to the topography. The CSO topography system measures 6144 points on the anterior corneal surface enclosed in a circular annulus defined by an inner radius of 0.33 and an outer radius of 10 mm respective to the cornea vertex. This is performed by projecting 24 placido rings into the cornea and then capturing the images of these rings using a high-resolution camera. The software of the CSO, Eye Top/Eye Image V.6.4, analyzes the perceived placido rings and then constructs different topographic maps, which also provide the wavefront error or corneal aberration demonstrated in a wavefront map.

The CSO corneal topographer/aberrometer makes the conversion of the corneal elevation profile into corneal wavefront data using the Zernike polynomials, taking into account that deviations in the topography are directly proportional to wavefront deviations of the anterior surface of the cornea. Higher order aberrations values are expressed as root-mean-square (RMS) values in micrometers. Eye alignment and the tear film stability are of extreme importance during topography acquisition. Pupil position and its size in low mesopic conditions also are provided.

Ablation Design

Data obtained from the CSO topographer are then transferred to the Optimized Refractive Keratectomy software (ORK-W or ORK-CAM; Schwind, Kleinostheim, Germany), which transforms the wavefront data into a three-dimensional ablation profile. These softwares allow the surgeon to modify and select the corneal aberrations to be treated by the laser, and modify the size of the optical and transition zones in the treatment profile. The ORK-CAM software is an upgraded version of the ORK-W software and is currently in use at our center. Data from ORK-W or ORK-CAM Schwind softwares are then transferred and used by the ESIRIS/Schwind Laser platform (Schwind Eye-Tech Solutions) to ablate the cornea.

Surgical Technique and Ablation Profile

The ESIRIS/Schwind excimer laser (Schwind Eye-Tech Solutions) has a flying-spot technology with a repetition rate of 200 Hz and a para-Gaussian profile spot diameter of 0.8 mm. The ESIRIS eye-tracker has 330 Hz and 6 to 8 milliseconds mean response time.

The ablation profile used was generated by the ORK-W or the ORK-CAM software based on the data obtained from the CSO topographer. In general, the main intention of the customized corneal wavefront guided ablation was to reduce higher-order aberrations which were considered significant, in particular spherical-like and coma-like aberrations.

In most cases of previous LASIK, the original flaps were re-lifted where possible. However, PRK was performed in eyes with previous PRK or with inadequate residual stromal bed.

RESULTS OF CORNEAL WAVEFRONT GUIDED REFRACTIVE SURGERY

Several studies have reported the results of corneal wavefront guided technology in highly aberrated corneas,[40-46] such as after complicated refractive surgery, keratoplasty, or corneal penetrating injuries. The results confirm the applicability of these excimer laser profiles.

We will now highlight our experience in the treatment of highly aberrated corneas with corneal wavefront guided excimer laser surgery.

Corneal Wavefront Guided Retreatments for Significant Night Vision Symptoms after Myopic Laser Refractive Surgery[47]

We evaluated the safety and efficacy of corneal wavefront guided retreatments with aspheric profiles for patients with significant night vision disturbances and high positive corneal spherical aberrations (SA) induced by conventional myopic laser refractive surgery. Previous studies of conventional and wavefront guided laser refractive surgery found a factor of between 2.2 and 9.4 for SA induction after myopic ablation.[11,24,27,48,49] Clinically, patients with night vision symptoms (glare, haloes and starbursts) after myopic laser refractive surgery had significantly higher SA than asymptomatic patients.[18,50] Although determination of a cut-off level is not always possible, it was postulated that SA (Z_4^0) higher than 0.5 µm can lead to significant night vision symptoms.[51] Based on these facts, we treated eyes with significant night vision disturbances and more than 0.5 µm of positive corneal SA (Z_4^0) induced by previous myopic ablation.

METHODS

We performed corneal wavefront guided retreatments for 28 eyes (14 right and 14 left) of 20 patients (16 men, 12 women) with significant postoperative night vision symptoms that did not improve after a trial of corrective lenses for at least three months. Mean patient age was 41.0 +/- 14.6 years (range, 24 to 63 years).

Inclusion criteria were:
1. Availability of preoperative and six-month postoperative visual symptom evaluation.
2. Topography maps with no missing data points within the central 7.0 mm zone.
3. No intraoperative or postoperative complications.
4. SA (Z_4^0) higher than 0.5 µm.
5. No contact lens wear for two weeks before the baseline retreatment examination.
6. Stable refractive error for at least two months before surgery.
7. Stable refraction achieved at least three months after the procedure.

Exclusion criteria were:
1. Ectasia.
2. Keratoconus suspect.

3. Decentration as evidenced by corneal topography.
4. Active ocular or systemic disease likely to affect corneal wound healing.
5. Pregnant or nursing.
6. Inability to comply with postoperative follow-up regimen.

The main outcome measures were visual symptoms, change in corneal SA (Z_4^0), and corneal asphericity (Q-value).

Evaluation of Subjective Symptoms

Before and after the retreatment, patients underwent a grading of night vision symptoms that was recorded using a subjective scale **(Table 18.1)**. All patients underwent a full ophthalmologic examination including manifest and cycloplegic refraction, determination of uncorrected visual acuity (UCVA), best-corrected visual acuity, computerized videokeratography with the CSO topographer (CSO, Firenze, Italy), slit-lamp biomicroscopy, Goldmann applanation tonometry, binocular indirect ophthalmoscopy, and ultrasonic pachymetry before and after retreatment. Before surgery, pupil diameter was measured using the Procyon P2000D pupillometer (Procyon Instruments, Ltd, London, United Kingdom) under low mesopic condition (3 cd/m^2). Postoperative assessments were performed routinely at one day, one month, three months, and six months after surgery. An independent survey was made regarding the night vision symptoms of the patients recorded from different examinations.

Analysis of Corneal Aberrations

Corneal aberrations were derived from the CSO corneal topography system. The software of this topography system, the EyeTop2005 (CSO, Firenze, Italy), performed the conversion of the corneal elevation profile into corneal wavefront data. Taking into account specific coefficients of the Zernike decomposition of the corneal wavefront, different root mean square (RMS) values were calculated. Specifically, the RMS for total wavefront aberration (TWA), coma-like aberration ($Z_3^{+/-1}$, $Z_5^{+/-1}$), spherical-like aberration (Z_4^0, Z_6^0), spherical Seidel aberration (Z_4^0), coma Seidel aberration ($Z_3^{+/-1}$), and Strehl ratio were compared before and after surgery. In all cases, the aberrometric study was performed for a 7 mm zone.

Ablation Algorithm

Enhancement surgery was planned to remove residual refractive error and corneal SA (Z_4^0) in all (n = 28) eyes. Using custom ablation manager software (ORK-CAM; Schwind Eye-Tech Solutions, Kleinostham, Germany) and data derived from the CSO corneal topographer, specific ablation profiles for treating corneal aberrations were created. The main intention of customized ablation was to reduce SA (Z_4^0), but accompanying high coma and other HOAs also were treated when they were significant considering the physiologic level of each kind of Zernike error. Customized ablation for the correction of SA (Z_4^0) and coma ($Z_3^{+/-1}$) was performed in 18 of 28 eyes, for the correction of only SA (Z_4^0) in five eyes, all HOA in three eyes, and all third- and fourth-order aberration in two eyes. The age of the patient, subjective spherocylindrical refraction, central corneal thickness, and flap thickness also must be introduced for the calculation of the ablations with this software. Using all these data, an ablation profile was generated and modified until the more appropriate profile (regarding the corneal asphericity) was obtained for the specific case. The software automatically calculates the optical and transition zones, taking into account the low mesopic pupil diameter, corneal thickness, and specific targeted Zernike terms.

The designed algorithms of the ORK-CAM software had an adjustment of the sphere correction depending on the level of SA corrected. This adjustment factor depended on the features of each specific case. The potential change in corneal aberrations was always calculated according to the ORK-CAM eye model, always having, as an objective a postoperative asphericity, –0.25 μm (approximately the mean value of the corneal asphericity in the normal population).

Primary Refractive Surgery

All eyes had myopia or compound myopic astigmatism before primary refractive surgery. All eyes underwent refractive surgery for myopia using the Planoscan algorithm with the Technolas 217-Z (Bausch & Lomb, Rochester, New York, USA). Twenty-three (82%) of 28 eyes underwent LASIK and five (18%) of 28 eyes underwent PRK as primary surgery. Of the 23 eyes that underwent LASIK as primary surgery, a flap was created using a femtosecond laser (Intralase, Inc,

Table 18.1 Grading of the night vision symptoms[47]

Grade	Symptoms
0 (None)	No symptoms
1 (Mild)	Halos, starburst, or acuity distortion noted to affect light sources at night but not interfering with functions
2 (Moderate)	Halos or starburst noted to affect usual activities; especially while driving or looking at light sources at night
3 (Disturbing)	Halos or starburst forcing the patient to refrain from certain activities at night, such as driving or looking at light sources
4 (Incapacitating)	Patients cannot drive at night at all

Irvine, California, USA) in 14 eyes and using a mechanical microkeratome in nine eyes (Moria M2 [Moria, Antony, France], eight eyes; Hansatome [Bausch & Lomb], one eye).

Surgical Technique

The enhancement procedure was performed after a minimum follow-up of six months after the initial surgery. Retreatments were performed under topical anesthesia. The original LASIK flap was relifted in 21 (75%) of 28 eyes, whereas the remaining seven (25%) eyes underwent PRK because of previous PRK (five eyes) or inadequate residual stromal bed (two eyes). Patients underwent corneal wavefront guided laser refractive surgery retreatment with the ESIRIS/SCHWIND excimer laser system (Schwind Eye-Tech Solutions).The ablation was centered on the pupil center in all eyes. The mean optical zone was 6.50 +/- 0.27 mm (range, 6.00 to 7.00 mm), and the treatment zone was 7.54 +/- 0.34 mm (range, 6.88 to 8.39 mm). No intraoperative complications occurred. All eyes had one retreatment, and no additional retreatment was performed in any eye.

RESULTS

Night Vision Symptoms

Before surgery, all patients reported symptoms of significant night vision disability (moderate [grade 2] or disturbing [grade 3]). After surgery, night time glare and halo symptoms subjectively improved to none or mild (grade 1) in all patients at the six-month follow-up. The mean preoperative pupil diameter under low mesopic condition was 6.68 +/- 0.62 mm (range, 5.69 to 7.68 mm). Eight (28.5%) of 28 eyes had pupil diameters of more than 7 mm under low mesopic conditions.

Aberrations

The mean preoperative corneal TWA significantly decreased from 3.03 +/- 1.33 µm to 2.44 +/- 1.55 µm after surgery ($P = 0.002$). Of the 28 eyes treated, 22 (79%) had a decrease in corneal TWA, 24 (86%) had a decrease in spherical-like aberrations, 19 (68%) had a decrease in coma-like aberrations, 25 (89%) had a decrease in SA (Z_4^0), and 22 (79%) had a decrease in coma ($Z_3^{+/-1}$) after enhancement.

We observed an increase in SA (Z_4^0) in three (11%) of 28 eyes after the retreatment, but the average magnitude of increase was low (mean, 0.09 µm; range, 0.002 to 0.16 µm). These three eyes had a mean myopic correction of -1.71 diopters.

Asphericity

The mean asphericity (Q-value) under the 4.5-mm zone decreased significantly after enhancement, whereas it did not change significantly under the 8.0 mm zone.

DISCUSSION

Treatment of eyes with significant night vision disturbances and more than 0.5 µm of positive corneal SA (Z_4^0) induced by previous myopic ablation using a topographic corneal WF-guided customization with aspheric profile resulted in a significant improvement in night vision symptoms and a decrease in corneal SA. Although we targeted SA in all eyes, treatment of corneal aberrations other than SA might have contributed to the improvement in the night vision in our patients.

Corneal Wavefront guided LASIK Retreatments for Correction of Highly Aberrated Corneas Following Refractive Surgery[52]

We evaluated the use of customized anterior surface corneal wavefront guided excimer laser surgery in improving visual quality, best spectacle-corrected visual acuity (BSCVA), and refractive outcome in symptomatic patients with elevated higher order aberrations following LASIK.

METHODS

Seventy-five consecutive eyes of 59 patients (27 men and 32 women) were included in this prospective consecutive, observational nonrandomized, noncomparative study. The eyes had previously undergone LASIK procedures for myopia or hyperopia (diopteric range: -8.00 to +4.00) between 2001 and 2004 and were referred with significant visual symptoms. Mean patient age was 31.5 +/- 4.8 years.

The eyes included in this study were divided into two groups for analysis of results. The night symptoms group included 37 (49.3%) eyes that suffered from significant night vision disability in the form of halos and glare under low illumination in the presence of uneventful primary LASIK surgery. The corneal complications group included 38 (50.7%) eyes that had corneal complications following the primary surgery; these complications included flap complications, decentration, and an irregular ablation profile evidenced by topography in the form of micro- and macro-irregularities.

Inclusion criteria were patients with:

1. No other eye disease or corneal problem that could be related to the visual symptoms.
2. Significant symptoms affecting visual performance in at least one activity of daily living, associated with a decrease in at least one line of BSCVA.
3. An interval of at least 6 months following the LASIK procedure.
4. Presence of an abnormal increase in the normal limits of global (if measurable) and corneal higher-order aberrations following the first surgery.

In addition, eyes were required to have at least a total higher-order aberration >0.50 μm for the night symptoms group and 0.80 μm for the corneal complications group. No eye was excluded because of an excessive corneal irregularity.

Exclusion criteria were:
1. Moderate or severe dry eye syndrome
2. Detectable slit lamp changes in crystalline lens
3. Cornea thickness <400 μm at any location in the cornea.

All patients underwent a complete ophthalmologic examination that included manifest and cycloplegic refraction, predilatation computerized corneal topography (CSO, Florence, Italy), and postdilatation corneal wavefront measurement using the 7.5 mm central corneal area (CSO). For all eyes, data concerning corneal point spread function (PSF) was measured as obtained from the corneal topography at each visit. The examinations were performed preoperatively and at 1, 3, and 6 months postoperatively. Patients were also asked about the presence of visual symptoms (e.g. halos, glare, and double vision) for each eye, whether the symptoms were significant enough to limit their normal day or night activities, and whether these symptoms were eliminated by the surgery.

Analysis of Corneal Aberrations and Surgical Technique

Corneal wavefront measurements were performed using the CSO topography system. Data from the CSO topographer were then transferred to the Optimized Refractive Keratectomy software (ORK-W, Schwind Eye-Tech Solutions) which transforms the wavefront data into a three-dimensional ablation profile. In this study, a large optical zone of 6 to 6.5 mm with a standard transition zone of 1 to 1.5 mm was used in all cases. Data from the ORK-W Schwind software were then transferred and used by the ESIRIS/Schwind Laser platform to ablate the cornea.

The surgical technique performed in this study was similar in all the eyes. Flap elevation was performed followed by laser ablation on the corneal stroma.

RESULTS

Visual Outcome

Uncorrected visual acuity In the night symptoms group, mean preoperative UCVA was 20/32 (0.6 +/- 0.2 decimal value) and 6 months postoperative UCVA was 20/25 (0.8 +/- 0.2 decimal value). In the corneal complications group, mean preoperative UCVA was 20/40 (0.5 +/- 0.2 decimal value) and 6 months postoperative UCVA was 20/30 (0.7 +/- 0.2 decimal value). The difference between preoperative and postoperative UCVA was statistically significant in both groups ($P < 0.001$).

Best spectacle-corrected visual acuity In both groups, mean preoperative and 6-month postoperative BSCVA were 20/25 (0.8 +/- 0.2 decimal value). The difference between preoperative and postoperative BSCVA in both groups was not statistically significant ($P = 0.219$ for the night symptoms and $P = 0.149$ for the corneal complications group).

Safety and efficacy indices The safety index was 1.1 in both groups, and the efficacy index was 0.93 in the night symptoms group and 0.92 in the corneal complications group.

Refractive Outcome

Sphere In the night symptoms group, mean sphere was –0.20 +/– 0.90 D preoperatively and –0.20 +/– 0.40 D at 6 months postoperatively; this difference was statistically significant ($P = 0.005$). In the corneal complications group, mean sphere was 0.80 +/– 1.60 D preoperatively and 0.30 +/– 0.70 D at 6 months postoperatively; this difference was not statistically significant ($P = 0.100$).

Cylinder In the night symptoms group, mean cylinder was –0.70 +/– 0.40 D preoperatively and –0.50 +/– 0.50 D at 6 months postoperatively; this difference was not statistically significant ($P = 0.122$). In the corneal complications group, mean cylinder was –1.20 +/– 0.80 D preoperatively and –0.70 +/– 0.70 D at 6 months postoperatively; this difference was statistically significant ($P < 0.001$).

Spherical equivalent refraction In the night symptoms group, mean spherical equivalent refraction was –0.50 +/– 0.80 D preoperatively and –0.01 +/– 0.50 D at 6 months postoperatively; this difference was not statistically significant ($P = 0.006$). In the corneal complications group, mean spherical equivalent refraction was 0.12 +/– 1.60 D preoperatively and –0.04 +/– 0.70 D at 6 months postoperatively; this difference was not statistically significant ($P = 0.639$).

Corneal Aberrations

Total higher-order aberrations In the night symptoms group, mean total higher-order aberrations decreased from 1.25 +/– 0.39 μm preoperatively to 0.92 +/– 0.31 μm at 6 months postoperatively. In the corneal complications group, mean total higher-order aberrations decreased from 1.64 +/– 0.55 μm preoperatively to 1.25 +/– 0.43 μm at 6 months postoperatively.

Tilt In the night symptoms group, mean tilt decreased from 1.38 +/–0.88 μm preoperatively to 1.03 +/–0.52 μm at 6 months postoperatively. In the corneal complications group, mean tilt decreased from 2.38 +/–1.35 μm preoperatively to 1.65 +/–0.95 μm at 6 months postoperatively.

Spherical aberrations In the night symptoms group, mean spherical aberrations decreased from 0.89 +/– 0.35 μm preoperatively to 0.69 +/–0.29 μm at 6 months postoperatively. In the corneal complications group, mean spherical aberrations decreased from 1.03 +/–0.55 μm preoperatively to 0.86 +/– 0.46 μm at 6 months postoperatively.

Coma. In the night symptoms group, mean coma decreased from 0.76 +/– 0.32 μm preoperatively to 0.58 +/–0.21 μm at

6 months postoperatively. In the corneal complications group, mean coma decreased from 1.18 +/−0.47 μm preoperatively to 0.87 +/−0.36 μm at 6 months postoperatively. The differences between the preoperative and postoperative values for corneal aberrations were statistically significant in both groups.

Point Spread Function

The PSF percentage represents the relation in percentage between the light intensity peak obtained in our cases and that corresponding to the theoretical perfect eye (only diffraction-limited eye). In the night symptoms group, mean PSF percentage increased from 11.60 +/−7.17 preoperatively to 19.22 +/− 10.90 at 6 months postoperatively. In the corneal complications group, mean PSF percentage increased from 7.66 +/− 5.33 preoperatively to 10.75 +/− 6.786 at 6 months postoperatively. The differences between preoperative and postoperative PSF were statistically significant in both groups.

DISCUSSION

In this study, the corneal aberrations were measured and used as a base for the treatment performed by the excimer laser. Approximately 50% of patients in the night symptoms group did not complain of decreased visual acuity but had significant complaints regarding night vision disability such as halos and glare. Eyes in the corneal complications group were more complicated cases because of previous corneal refractive surgery. Marked improvement occurred in both groups with regard to total aberrations, tilt, and improvement of spherical aberrations and coma, as well as in PSF, UCVA, and BSCVA.

The eyes in both groups had a mean improvement in UCVA of 2 lines. In the night symptoms group, 30 (81.1%) of the eyes retained their BSCVA or gained at least 1 line of BSCVA compared with 34 (89.5%) eyes in the corneal complications group. All patients experienced improvement of their visual acuity, double vision problem, and night vision capabilities, which could be explained by the improvement in their PSF values.

The stability of the spherical equivalent refraction was another factor that added to the success of the surgery. The difference between mean preoperative and postoperative spherical equivalent refraction was +0.50 +/− 0.99 D in the night symptoms group and −0.12 +/− 1.50 D in the corneal complications group. This means the ablation performed by the laser during customized retreatment caused a shift within +/− 0.50 D from the original refraction. This result means the software used in the ablation profile (ORK-W ablation for ESIRIS excimer laser) played an important role in compensating the ablation performed by the laser maintaining the curvature of the cornea within the pretreatment range.

The treatment of LASIK-induced symptoms associated with significant higher-order aberrations using corneal wavefront guided technology is safe and effective in this select group of patients whose corneas were of adequate thickness and who had no additional lenticular or corneal pathology.

Corneal Wavefront Guided Retreatments for Corneas with High Levels of Corneal Coma Aberration after LASIK[53]

We evaluated the improvement in visual and optical performance after corneal wavefront guided LASIK enhancement with the ORK-CAM system (Schwind eye-tech solutions) in patients with high levels of corneal coma aberration and complaints about their quality of vision resulting from decentered primary LASIK procedures.

METHODS

We studied 34 consecutive symptomatic eyes of 29 patients with a hyperopic or myopic spherical equivalent (SE) who had unsuccessful primary LASIK.

Inclusion criteria were previous LASIK surgery with residual symptomatic myopia, hyperopia, or astigmatism and a significant level of primary corneal coma aberration. Thus, corneas with relevant asymmetry after surgery caused by improper centration were selected. The level of corneal coma was considered significant when the associated root mean square (RMS) for the corneal primary coma (measured over a pupil of 6.0 mm) was higher than 0.5 μm.[7,51] This criterion was chosen based on previously reported physiologic levels of corneal HOAs. The 0.5 μm cutoff point was selected because the associated probability of it being a normal value was less than 1%.[7,51]

Exclusion criteria were:
1. Corneas with flap-related problems at the time of surgery.
2. Postoperative inflammation at the interface.
3. Epithelial ingrowth under the flap.
4. Corneal opacity.
5. A formal contraindication to LASIK.

In all cases, primary LASIK had been performed at least 6 months before the evaluation for enhancement. No treatment was performed if the refraction was not stable at 2 consecutive examinations performed at least 3 weeks apart. The target postoperative refraction was emmetropia in all cases. The postoperative follow-up was 6 months.

Preoperative Examination

The preoperative examination included uncorrected decimal visual acuity (UCVA); best spectacle-corrected decimal visual acuity (BSCVA); manifest and cycloplegic refractions;

slit-lamp biomicroscopy; applanation tonometry; ultrasonic pachymetry (DHG500 US pachymeter, DHG Technology, Inc.); scotopic, low, and high mesopic pupillometry (Procyon Pupillometer P2000SA, Procyon Instruments Ltd.); corneal topography (CSO system, Costruzione Strumenti Oftalmici); and fundus evaluation. Corneal aberrations were derived from corneal topography following the protocol described below in Corneal Aberrations. In addition, patients were asked to evaluate the levels of halos and glare they perceived at night using the following qualitative scale: none, low, moderate, high, or severe.

Corneal Aberrations and Ablation Profile

Corneal aberrations were derived from the data of the anterior surface of the cornea obtained with the CSO topography system. The corneal elevation profiles were converted into corneal wavefront data with the system's software (EyeTop 2005).

The corneal wavefront guided customized ablation was designed and calculated using commercially available ORK-CAM software. The main goal of the designed ablation in all cases was to minimize the primary coma ($Z_3^{+/-1}$). The spherical aberration (Z_4^0) was treated if it was significant (55.9% of cases). The aim was to create a corneal surface with an elevation profile that would generate a minimally distorted wavefront. In addition, all treatments were designed to leave an expected residual stromal bed thicker than 250 mm in the central cornea.

Surgical Technique

All LASIK procedures were performed by the same surgeon (J.L.A.) at Vissum Instituto Oftalmologico de Alicante using the Esiris excimer laser (Schwind eye-tech solutions).

The optical zone of the treatment was selected according to the preoperative scotopic pupil size. Depending on the pachymetry, optical zones with a diameter at least as large as the scotopic pupil were targeted to prevent unwanted optical phenomena.

RESULTS

The mean age of the 29 patients was 40.82 +/- 9.79 years (range 26 to 64 years). The mean preoperative SE was +0.47 +/- 1.16 diopters (D) (range -1.75 to +3.00 D) **(Table 18.2)**.

Thirteen eyes (38.2%) had a myopic SE and 21 eyes (61.8%), a hyperopic SE. The mean preoperative scotopic pupil size was 6.43 +/- 0.76 mm and the mean optical zone, 6.56 +/- 0.28 mm (range 6.00 to 7.00 mm). The mean total ablation zone designed with ORK-CAM software was 7.71 +/- 0.40 mm (range 6.88 to 8.50 mm).

Refractive Outcomes (Table 18.2)

Statistically significant reductions were observed in sphere and cylinder at 1 month (both $P < 0.01$). At 6 months, the mean efficacy index was 0.88 +/- 0.12 (range 0.67 to 1.06) and the mean safety index was 1.03 +/- 0.16 (range 0.78 to 1.50). The improvement in both parameters at 1 month was statistically significant. ($P = 0.01$ for efficacy and $P < 0.01$ for safety). After that, there were no statistically significant changes.

Six months postoperatively, the UCVA was statistically significant better ($P = 0.01$). The loss of 2 lines in 1 eye (2.94%) was due to the proliferation of a superior epithelial ingrowth, which was responsible for an unpredictable irregularity. In addition, in 2 eyes with a loss of 1 line of BSCVA, corneal alterations (significant punctuate keratitis in 1 eye and proliferation of epithelial ingrowth in the other) were found at the 6 month examinations.

Table 18.2 Comparison of preoperative and postoperative refractive outcome

	Mean + SD (Range)			
		Postoperative		
Parameter	Preoperative	1 month	3 months	6 months
UCVA (decimal)	0.63 + 0.19 (0.20 to 1.00)	0.62 + 0.25 (0.20 to 1.00)	0.72 ± 0.20 (0.30 to 1.00)	0.75 ± 0.20 (0.20 to 1.00)
Sphere (D)	+1.13 + 1.30 (–1.00 to +5.00)	+0.35 ± 0.52 (–0.75 to +1.50)	+0.41 ± 0.50 (–0.50 to +1.50)	+0.31 ± 0.66 (–0.75 to +1.50)
Cylinder (D)	–1.32 + 0.74 (–4.50 to –0.50)	–0.84 + 0.65 (–2.50 to +0.00)	–0.83 ± 0.70 (–3.00 to 0.00)	–0.76 ± 0.61 (–2.25 to +0.00)
SE (D)	+0.47 + 1.16 (–1.75 to +3.00)	–0.06 ± 0.57 (–1.50 to +1.25)	–0.01 ± 0.50 (–1.00 to +0.88)	–0.02 ± 0.58 (–1.25 to +0.88)
BSCVA (decimal)	0.85 + 0.18 (0.30 to 1.20)	0.76 ± 0.23 (0.30 to 1.00)	0.86 ± 0.15 (0.50 to 1.00)	0.86 ± 0.18 (0.35 to 1.20)
Efficacy	–	0.73 + 0.23 (0.20 to 1.00)	0.83 ± 0.16 (0.43 to 1.19)	0.88 + 0.12 (0.67 to 1.06)
Safety	–	0.91 + 0.22 (0.44 to 1.42)	1.00 + 0.13 (0.83 to 1.50)	1.03 + 0.16 (0.78 to +1.50)

Abbreviations: BSCVA = Best spectacle corrected visual acuity, SE = Spherical equivalent, UCVA = Uncorrected visual acuity

Corneal Aberrations

At 1 month, there was a statistically significant reduction in total RMS ($P = 0.01$), astigmatic RMS ($P = 0.01$), and primary coma RMS ($P < 0.01$). The (Z_4^0) coefficient changed significantly to negative values ($P < 0.01$). There were no significant changes in these aberrometric parameters at 3 months and 6 months.

Subjective Symptoms

Complications

The existing flaps were lifted without complications in all cases, and all procedures were centered at the pupillary center. No eye required retreatment during the postoperative follow-up.

DISCUSSION

Corneal wavefront guided LASIK enhancement using the ORK-CAM software was useful in treating cases of high levels of primary coma caused by a previous decentered refractive surgery procedure. It provided excellent safety and efficacy for correction of 2nd-order components. In addition, primary coma was significantly reduced and night-vision symptoms were decreased. Spherical aberration can also be corrected using this technique.

The improvement observed in corneal aberrations after the corneal wavefront guided enhancement was related to a reduction in the bothersome symptoms perceived by patients preoperatively. Specifically, the presence of night halos and glare was studied because patients with highly aberrated corneas often report these symptoms and they are easy to describe and understand. An increase in HOAs increases the incidence of night-vision complaints, especially after refractive surgery. These optical errors significantly increase image distortion, especially when the pupil dilates because the most aberrated part of the ocular optical system takes part in the generation of the retinal image. We did not report other symptoms associated with aberrated vision, such as double vision or ghost images.

LIMITATIONS OF CORNEAL WAVEFRONT GUIDED REFRACTIVE SURGERY

Currently, one limitation of customized refractive surgery is the size of the laser spot. The ideal spot for complete correction of HOAs is 0.5 mm or smaller.[54] This will allow a smoother and more precise ablation profile. The Esiris laser has a spot size of 0.8 mm, which could be responsible for the partial correction of some HOAs. However, with the advent of newer excimer lasers with laser spot size of 0.5 mm or smaller, for example, the Amaris excimer laser (Schwind Eye-tech solutions); the results of customized laser ablations are likely to improve.

Another limitation of customized refractive surgery is the wound-healing response of the cornea. The cornea is made of complex structural composite material that undergoes biomechanical changes and healing responses after damage or injury.[55] The ablation of tissue with the excimer laser could generate subtle unexpected modifications that could limit the effect of a customized ablation.[56] Therefore, although the ablation profile was planned to achieve a more regular corneal surface, biomechanical changes and wound-healing responses could reduce the effectiveness of the customized ablation.

CONCLUSION

Higher-order aberrations are correlated with bothersome visual symptoms and night-vision disturbances. These aberrations are usually seen in postrefractive surgery patients, especially in eyes with complications. Corneal wavefront guided excimer laser retreatments in such eyes have been shown to reduce the amount of higher-order aberrations with resulting improvement in visual quality and reduction in visual symptoms.

REFERENCES

1. Chalita MR, Xu M, Krueger RR. Correlation of aberrations with visual symptoms using wavefront analysis in eyes after laser in situ keratomileusis. J Refract Surg. 2003;19:S682-6.
2. Villa C, Gutierrez R, Jimenez JR, Gonzalez-Meijome JM. Night vision disturbances after successful LASIK surgery. Br J Ophthalmol. 2007;91:1031-7.
3. Oshika T, Okamoto C, Samejima T, et al. Contrast sensitivity function and ocular higher-order wavefront aberrations in normal human eyes. Ophthalmology. 2006;113:1807-12.
4. Melamud A, Chalita MR, Krueger RR, Lee MS. Comatic aberration as a cause of monocular diplopia. J Cataract Refract Surg. 2006;32:529-32.
5. Liang J, Williams DR. Aberrations and retinal image quality of the normal human eye. J Opt Soc Am A Opt Image Sci Vis. 1997;14:2873-83.
6. Joslin CE, Wu SM, McMahon TT, Shahidi M. Higher-order wavefront aberrations in corneal refractive therapy. Optom Vis Sci. 2003;80:805-11.
7. Wang L, Dai E, Koch DD, Nathoo A. Optical aberrations of the human anterior cornea. J Cataract Refract Surg. 2003;29:1514-21.
8. Wang L, Koch DD. Ocular higher-order aberrations in individuals screened for refractive surgery. J Cataract Refract Surg. 2003;29:1896-903.
9. Netto MV, Ambrosio R, Jr., Shen TT, Wilson SE. Wavefront analysis in normal refractive surgery candidates. J Refract Surg. 2005;21:332-8.
10. Yoon G, MacRae S, Williams DR, Cox IG. Causes of spherical aberration induced by laser refractive surgery. J Cataract Refract Surg. 2005;31:127-35.
11. Wang L, Koch DD. Anterior corneal optical aberrations induced by laser in situ keratomileusis for hyperopia. J Cataract Refract Surg. 2003;29:1702-8.

12. Kohnen T, Mahmoud K, Buhren J. Comparison of corneal higher-order aberrations induced by myopic and hyperopic LASIK. Ophthalmology. 2005;112:1692.
13. Wang Y, Zhao KX, He JC, et al. Ocular higher-order aberrations features analysis after corneal refractive surgery. Chin Med J (Engl). 2007;120:269-73.
14. Tran DB, Sarayba MA, Bor Z, et al. Randomized prospective clinical study comparing induced aberrations with IntraLase and Hansatome flap creation in fellow eyes: potential impact on wavefront guided laser in situ keratomileusis. J Cataract Refract Surg. 2005;31:97-105.
15. Medeiros FW, Stapleton WM, Hammel J, et al. Wavefront analysis comparison of LASIK outcomes with the femtosecond laser and mechanical microkeratomes. J Refract Surg. 2007;23:880-7.
16. Lim T, Yang S, Kim M, Tchah H. Comparison of the IntraLase femtosecond laser and mechanical microkeratome for laser in situ keratomileusis. Am J Ophthalmol. 2006;141:833-9.
17. Tanabe T, Miyata K, Samejima T, et al. Influence of wavefront aberration and corneal subepithelial haze on low-contrast visual acuity after photorefractive keratectomy. Am J Ophthalmol. 2004;138:620-4.
18. McCormick GJ, Porter J, Cox IG, MacRae S. Higher-order aberrations in eyes with irregular corneas after laser refractive surgery. Ophthalmology. 2005;112:1699-709.
19. Zhou C, Chai X, Yuan L, et al. Corneal higher-order aberrations after customized aspheric ablation and conventional ablation for myopic correction. Curr Eye Res. 2007;32:431-8.
20. Mrochen M, Kaemmerer M, Seiler T. Wavefront guided laser in situ keratomileusis: early results in three eyes. J Refract Surg. 2000;16:116-21.
21. Mrochen M, Kaemmerer M, Seiler T. Clinical results of wavefront guided laser in situ keratomileusis 3 months after surgery. J Cataract Refract Surg. 2001;27:201-7.
22. Caster AI, Hoff JL, Ruiz R. Conventional vs wavefront guided LASIK using the LADARVision4000 excimer laser. J Refract Surg. 2005;21:S786-91.
23. Bahar I, Levinger S, Kremer I. Wavefront guided LASIK for myopia with the Technolas 217z: results at 3 years. J Refract Surg. 2007;23:586-90, discussion.
24. Aizawa D, Shimizu K, Komatsu M, et al. Clinical outcomes of wavefront guided laser in situ keratomileusis: 6-month follow-up. J Cataract Refract Surg. 2003;29:1507-13.
25. Nuijts RM, Nabar VA, Hament WJ, Eggink FA. Wavefront guided versus standard laser in situ keratomileusis to correct low to moderate myopia. J Cataract Refract Surg. 2002;28:1907-13.
26. He R, Qu M, Yu S. Comparison of NIDEK CATz wavefront guided LASIK to traditional LASIK with the NIDEK CXII excimer laser in myopia. J Refract Surg. 2005;21:S646-S649.
27. Kohnen T, Buhren J, Kuhne C, Mirshahi A. Wavefront guided LASIK with the Zyoptix 3.1 system for the correction of myopia and compound myopic astigmatism with 1-year follow-up: clinical outcome and change in higher order aberrations. Ophthalmology. 2004;111:2175-85.
28. Phusitphoykai N, Tungsiripat T, Siriboonkoom J, Vongthongsri A. Comparison of conventional versus wavefront guided laser in situ keratomileusis in the same patient. J Refract Surg. 2003;19:S217-S220.
29. Schwartz GS, Park DH, Lane SS. CustomCornea wavefront retreatment after conventional laser in situ keratomileusis. J Cataract Refract Surg. 2005;31:1502-5.
30. Alio JL, Montes-Mico R. Wavefront guided versus standard LASIK enhancement for residual refractive errors. Ophthalmology. 2006;113:191-7.
31. Kanellopoulos AJ, Pe LH. Wavefront guided enhancements using the wavelight excimer laser in symptomatic eyes previously treated with LASIK. J Refract Surg. 2006;22:345-9.
32. Hiatt JA, Grant CN, Wachler BS. Complex wavefront guided retreatments with the Alcon CustomCornea platform after prior LASIK. J Refract Surg. 2006;22:48-53.
33. Durrie DS, Stahl JE, Schwendeman F. Alcon LADARWave custom cornea retreatments. J Refract Surg. 2005;21:S804-S807.
34. Carones F, Vigo L, Scandola E. Wavefront guided treatment of abnormal eyes using the LADARVision platform. J Refract Surg. 2003;19:S703-S708.
35. Montague AA, Manche EE. CustomVue laser in situ keratomileusis treatment after previous keratorefractive surgery. J Cataract Refract Surg. 2006;32:795-8.
36. Mrochen M, Krueger RR, Bueeler M, Seiler T. Aberration-sensing and wavefront guided laser in situ keratomileusis: management of decentered ablation. J Refract Surg. 2002;18:418-29.
37. Salz JJ. Wavefront guided treatment for previous laser in situ keratomileusis and photorefractive keratectomy: case reports. J Refract Surg. 2003;19:S697-S702.
38. Chalita MR, Roth AS, Krueger RR. Wavefront guided surface ablation with prophylactic use of mitomycin C after a buttonhole laser in situ keratomileusis flap. J Refract Surg. 2004;20:176-81.
39. Rozema JJ, Van Dyck DE, Tassignon MJ. Clinical comparison of 6 aberrometers. Part 1: Technical specifications. J Cataract Refract Surg. 2005;31:1114-27.
40. Alio JL, Belda JI, Osman AA, Shalaby AM. Topography-guided laser in situ keratomileusis (TOPOLINK) to correct irregular astigmatism after previous refractive surgery. J Refract Surg. 2003;19:516-27.
41. Cosar CB, Acar S. Topography-guided LASIK with the wavelight laser after penetrating keratoplasty. J Refract Surg. 2006;22:716-9.
42. Kanellopoulos AJ. Topography-guided custom retreatments in 27 symptomatic eyes. J Refract Surg. 2005;21:S513-S518.
43. Koller T, Iseli HP, Donitzky C, et al. Topography-guided surface ablation for forme fruste keratoconus. Ophthalmology. 2006;113:2198-202.
44. Lee DH, Seo SJ, Shin SC. Topography-guided excimer laser ablation of irregular cornea resulting from penetrating injury. J Cataract Refract Surg. 2002;28:186-8.
45. Rajan MS, O'Brart DP, Patel P, et al. Topography-guided customized laser-assisted subepithelial keratectomy for the treatment of postkeratoplasty astigmatism. J Cataract Refract Surg. 2006;32:949-57.
46. Toda I, Yamamoto T, Ito M, et al. Topography-guided ablation for treatment of patients with irregular astigmatism. J Refract Surg. 2007;23:118-25.
47. Alio JL, Pinero D, Muftuoglu O. Corneal wavefront guided retreatments for significant night vision symptoms after myopic laser refractive surgery. Am J Ophthalmol. 2008;145:65-74.

48. Erdem U, Muftuoglu O. Optical factors in increased best spectacle-corrected visual acuity after LASIK. J Refract Surg. 2006; 22:S1056-S1068.
49. Kim TI, Yang SJ, Tchah H. Bilateral comparison of wavefront guided versus conventional laser in situ keratomileusis with Bausch and Lomb Zyoptix. J Refract Surg. 2004;20:432-8.
50. Chalita MR, Chavala S, Xu M, Krueger RR. Wavefront analysis in post-LASIK eyes and its correlation with visual symptoms, refraction, and topography. Ophthalmology. 2004;111:447-53.
51. Vinciguerra P, Camesasca FI, Calossi A. Statistical analysis of physiological aberrations of the cornea. J Refract Surg. 2003;19: S265-9.
52. Alio J, Galal A, Montalban R, Pinero D. Corneal wavefront guided LASIK retreatments for correction of highly aberrated corneas following refractive surgery. J Refract Surg. 2007;23:760-73.
53. Alio JL, Pinero DP, Plaza Puche AB. Corneal wavefront guided enhancement for high levels of corneal coma aberration after laser in situ keratomileusis. J Cataract Refract Surg. 2008;34:222-31.
54. Krueger RR. Technological requirements for customized corneal ablation. In: McRae SM, Krueger RR, Applegate RA, (Eds). Customized Corneal Ablation; the Quest for SuperVision. Thorofare, NJ: Slack; 2001. pp. 133-48.
55. Dupps WJ, Jr., Wilson SE. Biomechanics and wound healing in the cornea. Exp Eye Res. 2006;83:709-20.
56. Roberts C. Biomechanics of the cornea and wavefront guided laser refractive surgery. J Refract Surg. 2002;18:S589-92.

Chapter 19

Ocular Higher Order Aberration Induced Decrease in Vision (Aberropia): Characteristics and Classification

Amar Agarwal (India), Soosan Jacob (India), Dhivya Ashok Kumar (India), Athiya Agarwal (India)

ABERROPIA

We describe two patients who had been diagnosed to have amblyopia and underwent wavefront guided refractive surgery (Zyoptix) for correction of co-existing myopia. Both patients had a significant increase in their best corrected high contrast visual acuity (HCVA) and low contrast visual acuity (LCVA) over preoperative levels. An analysis of their pre- and postoperative higher order aberrations (HOA) lead to the conclusion that this increase in HCVA and LCVA must have been due to an alteration in their HOA.

We propose and classify a new refractive error—aberropia which we define as a refractive error which results in a decrease in the visual acuity or quality due to HOA and which is not correctable by standard spherocylindrical correction. This is due to a net detrimental HOA, postinteraction between different types of aberrations so that there is deterioration in the visual performance of the patients. We also propose that selected cases of so called "amblyopia" may actually be aberropia and these patients have the potential to gain significantly in their visual acuity on correction of aberropia.

INTRODUCTION

Astrophysicists have to be able to measure and correct the imperfect higher-order aberrations (HOA) or wavefront distortions that enter their telescopic lens system from the galaxy for perfect imaging. To achieve this purpose, adaptive optics are used wherein deformable mirrors reform the distorted wavefront to allow clear visualization of celestial objects. Extrapolating these same principles to the human eye raises the question of whether removal or alteration of the wavefront aberrations of the eye might result in a significant improvement in the preoperative best corrected visual acuity.

Prior to the advent of wavefront guided LASIK, the only parameters that could be modified to obtain optical correction for a given patients refractive error were the sphere and cylinder. This would often not give the ideal optical correction, many a times resulting in poor visual quality in an otherwise 20/20 postrefractive surgery patient and in some patients, even resulting in a decrease in best spectacle corrected visual acuity (BSCVA). This situation is usually because of either the persistence or induction of significant amounts of higher order aberrations after LASIK.

There may therefore be a large group of patients, either with virgin eyes or postrefractive surgery, whose best corrected visual acuity (BCVA) or visual quality may actually improve significantly over preoperative levels on altering their optical aberrations. These optical aberrations are contributed to by the eye's entire optical system, i.e. the cornea, lens, vitreous and the retina.

We report two patients with subnormal visual acuity throughout their lives in the eye that underwent wavefront guided LASIK, both of whom had a significant improvement in their best corrected visual acuity to better than normal levels postwavefront guided refractive surgery. They had both been diagnosed as being amblyopic preoperatively.

CASE REPORT

Both patients underwent routine preoperative patient evaluation including uncorrected and best corrected high and low contrast visual acuity, slit lamp examination, applanation tonometry, manifest and cycloplegic refractions, Orbscan, aberrometry, corneal pachymetry, corneal diameter, Schirmer test and indirect ophthalmoscopy. Patients wearing contact lenses had been asked to discontinue soft lenses for a minimum of 1 week and rigid gas permeable lenses for a minimum of 2 weeks before the preoperative examination and surgery.

The Zywave machine has a real time pupillometer setting, which can be used for measuring exact pupil size. We examined the visual acuity and aberrometry at the same mesopic pupil size. The Matlab 7.1 version software was used to generate wavefront maps **(Figures 19.1A and B)**, the modulation transfer function (MTF) **(Figure 19.2A)**, phase transfer function (PTF) **(Figure 19.2B)**, point spread function (PSF) **(Figures 19.3A and B)**, and the individual polynomial RMS from the preoperative and postoperative file of zernicke coefficients (Zerfiles) at mesopic pupil size and at 6 mm pupil. Zernicke polynomial ordering was done based on OSA/VSIA standards. Strehls ratio was also calculated for preoperative and postoperative higher order aberrations. Equivalent defocus was calculated for both mesopic pupil size and 6 mm.

Chapter 19: Ocular Higher Order Aberration Induced Decrease in Vision... 201

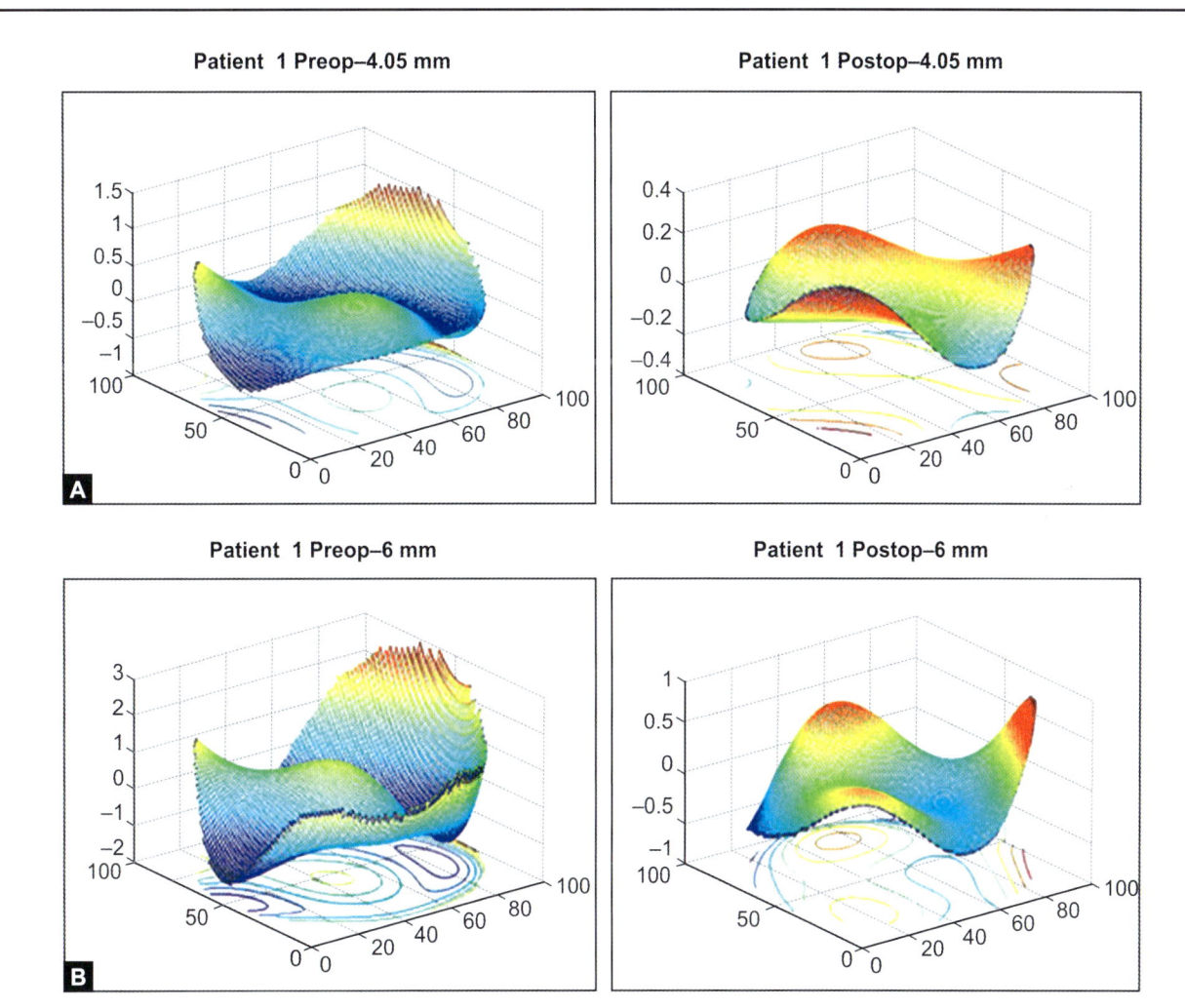

Figures 19.1A and B Pre- and postoperative 3 D wavefront maps for patient 1 for mesopic (4.05 mm) and 6 mm pupils

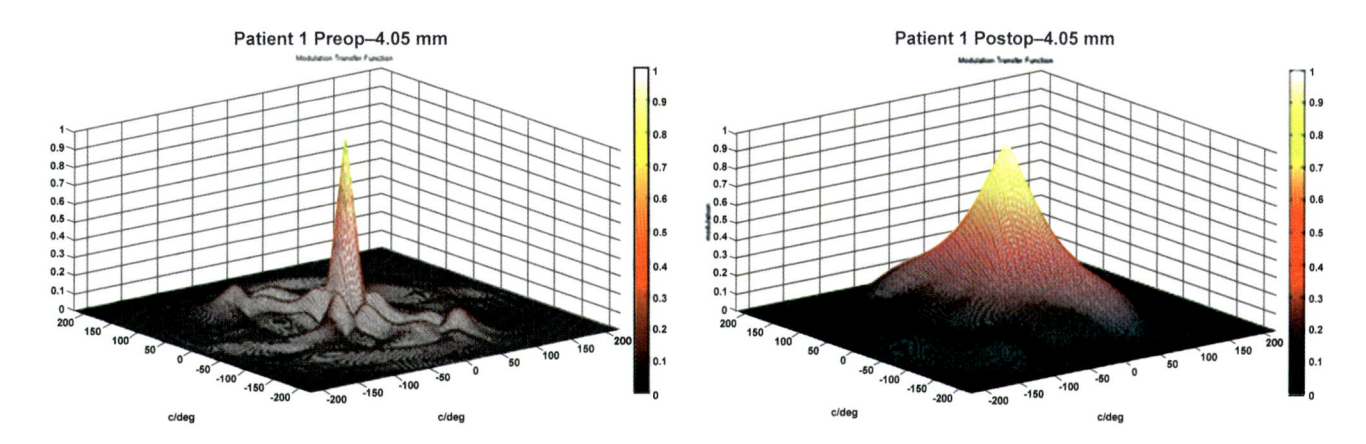

Figure 19.2A Pre- and postoperative modular transfer function with mesopic pupil for patient 1 showing improvement

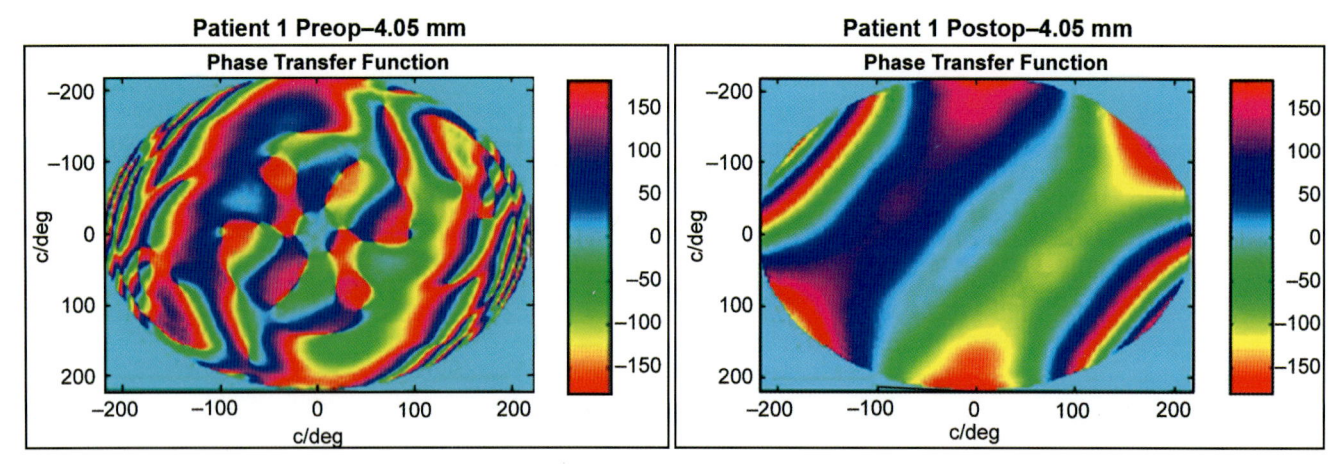

Figure 19.2B Pre- and postoperative phase transfer function with mesopic pupil for patient 1 showing improvement

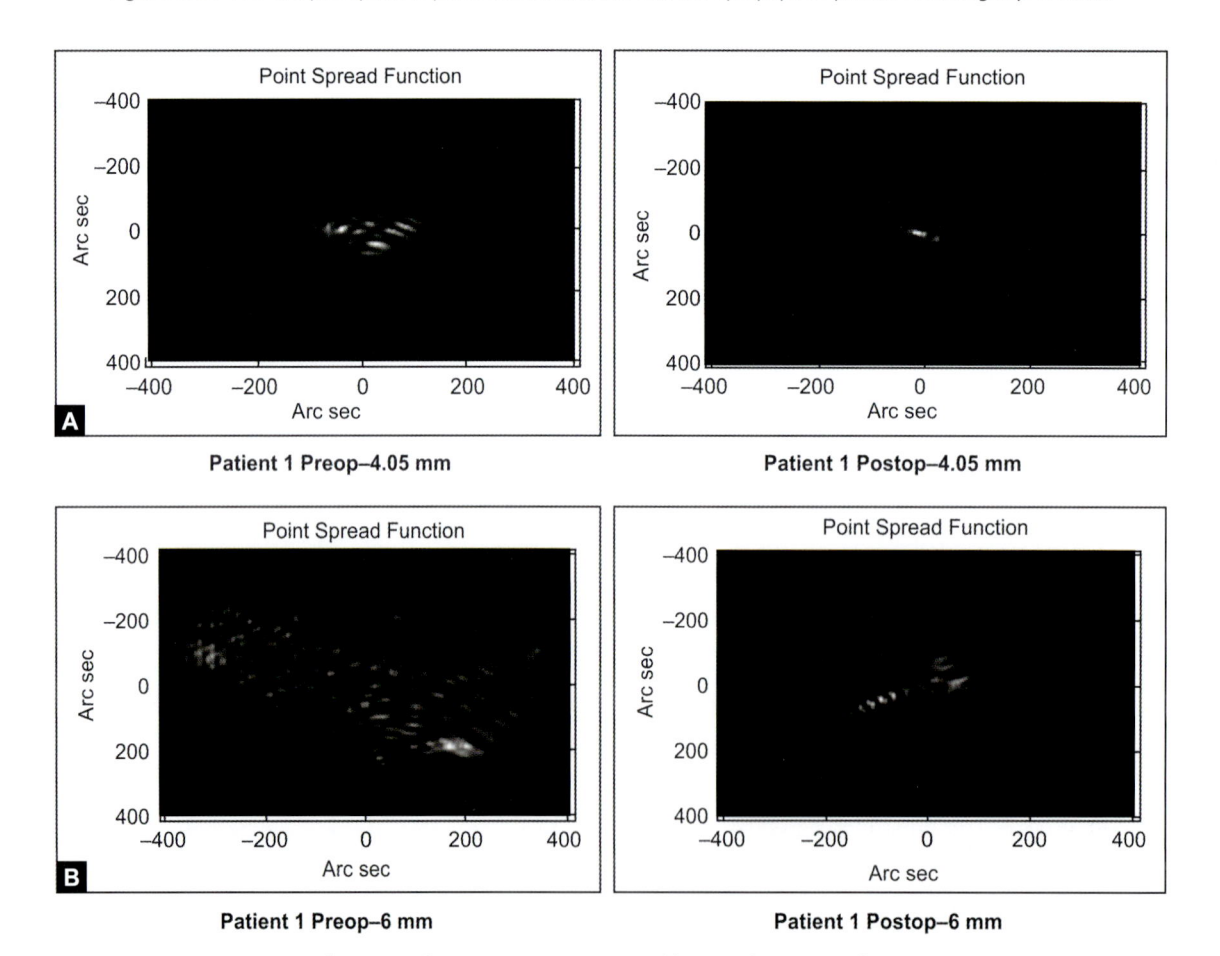

Figures 19.3A and B Pre- and postoperative point spread function for patient 1 for mesopic (4.05 mm) and 6 mm pupils showing decrease in size

Patient 1

The first patient was a 23-year-old female patient with history of decreased vision in left eye (OS) never having improved to more than present levels and with history of wearing glasses since childhood. Cycloplegic refraction was −5 DS/−2.5 DC at 132°. The uncorrected HCVA was 20/800, best corrected HCVA was 20/30 and the best corrected LCVA was 20/50, none improving further with pin hole and/or contact lens. Preoperative slit lamp examination showed a normal anterior segment. Extraocular movements were normal and fundus evaluation showed temporal crescent and a tessellated appearance. Macula was normal.

Orbscan showed astigmatism of 1.7 D at 50° with irregularity coefficient ±1.3 D and ±2 D at 3 mm and 5 mm zones respectively. Central corneal thickness measured was 569 microns. Anterior segment OCT was within normal limits.

The mesopic pupil size of the patient was 4.05 mm and aberrometry was taken at this pupil size. Preoperative total RMS was 1.77 micrometers, HORMS was 0.05 micrometers, third order RMS was 0.08 and fourth order RMS was 0.04 micrometers for 4.05 mm pupil. We then dilated the pupil to 6 mm with topical phenylephrine 1% and again performed aberrometry.

The patient underwent wavefront guided LASIK with Zyoptix work station which includes Zywave (Hartmann Shack aberrometer with Orbscan) and Technolas 217 laser system. Postoperative uncorrected HCVA was 20/10 while the LCVA was 20/20. Orbscan showed astigmatism of 0.6 D at 70° with irregularity coefficient ±1.7 D and ±2.7 D at 3 mm and 5 mm zone respectively. Central corneal thickness measured was 424 microns postoperatively. Postoperative total RMS was 0.47 micrometers, HORMS was 0.020, third order RMS was 0.038 and fourth order RMS was 0.008 microns respectively **(Table 19.1)**. At the three months postoperative follow-up examination, the patient maintained the same distance uncorrected HCVA of 20/10.

Patient 2

The second patient was a 19-year-old male with history of wearing glasses since early childhood. He also gave history of visual acuity in OS never improving beyond present levels with either glasses or contact lenses since early childhood. His distance uncorrected high contrast visual acuity (HCVA) in OS measured by Snellen visual acuity chart was 20/2000 which improved to 20/40 with spectacle correction. His best spectacle corrected low contrast visual acuity (LCVA) detected by CSO digital contrast sensitivity projector was 20/60. There was no further improvement over these levels with either contact lens and/or pinhole. The cycloplegic refraction in OS was found to be –7.5 DS. Anterior segment by slit lamp evaluation was normal. Corneal topography obtained by Orbscan showed 1.6 D astigmatism at 99 degrees with irregularity coefficient ±0.8 D and ±1.4 D at 3 mm and 5 mm zone respectively. Central corneal thickness measured was 513 microns. Anterior segment OCT was within normal limits. Fundus evaluation was within normal limits.

The mesopic pupil size of the patient was 4.18 mm. Preoperatively, total RMS was 2.34 micrometers, HORMS was 0.019 micrometers, third order RMS was 0.038 and fourth order RMS was 0.005 micrometers before surgery.

The patient underwent wavefront guided LASIK in OS with the Zyoptix work station. On the first postoperative day, the patient's uncorrected HCVA and LCVA was 20/15 which improved to 20/10 with –0.5 DS. After 2 months follow-up, the patient still has best corrected HCVA of 20/10. Postoperatively, the total RMS was 0.47 and HORMS was 0.017. Third order RMS and fourth order RMS were 0.022 and 0.022 microns respectively **(Table 19.2)**. Postoperatively, a change from positive spherical aberration (+ 0.010) to negative spherical aberration (–0.048) was observed. Orbscan showed 0.9 D at 87° with irregularity coefficient ±1.1 D and ±2.8 D at 3 mm and 5 mm zone respectively. Central corneal thickness measured was 402 microns.

DISCUSSION

Wave front guided LASIK is a relatively new technology which takes the patient's subjective refraction, ocular optical aberrations and corneal topography into consideration not only for diagnosis, but also for therapeutic treatment, in order to design a personalized treatment based on the total structure of the eye. The wavefront technology in Zyoptix uses the Hartmann-Shack aberrometer based on the Hartmann-Shack principle[1] demonstrated by Liang et al[2,3] to measure the ocular aberrations. The Bausch and Lomb Technolas 217 Z laser into which the topography and aberrometry data is fed provides individualized treatments set to correct lower and higher order aberrations. The treatment is mainly aberrometry based,

Table 19.1 RMS, equivalent defocus and Strehl's ratio for patient 1

Patient 1	Root Mean Square (RMS)		Equivalent Defocus	
Pupil diameter: 4.05 mm	Micrometers		Diopters	
	Preoperative	Postoperative	Preoperative	Postoperative
Total RMS	1.77	0.470	2.988	0.795
HORMS	0.05	0.020	0.091	0.034
3rd order	0.08	0.038	0.145	0.064
4th order	0.04	0.008	0.075	0.064
5th order	0.009	0.002	0.016	0.037
Strehl's ratio	0.66	1.2		

Table 19.2 RMS, equivalent defocus and Strehl's ratio for patient 2

Patient 2	Root Mean Square (RMS)		Equivalent Defocus	
Pupil diameter: 4.18 mm	Micrometers		Diopters	
	Preoperative	Postoperative	Preoperative	Postoperative
Total RMS	2.343	0.47	3.716	0.744
HORMS	0.019	0.017	0.0311	0.0275
3rd order	0.038	0.022	0.059	0.035
4th order	0.005	0.022	0.007	0.035
5th order	0.001	0.002	0.002	0.003
Strehl's ratio	1.2	1.22		

though it also takes certain parameters such as pachymetry from the Orbscan data into account. Zernike polynomials are used to describe ocular aberrations.[4-6]

Considering our two patients, both had subnormal visual acuity but after refractive surgery, they were able to read up to 20/10. These patients had been diagnosed preoperatively as being amblyopic and therefore, it was surprising to see this improvement in their BCVA as refractive surgery in adulthood should not correct amblyopia since amblyopia functions at the cortical and not the optical level. So, was it the alteration brought about in their higher order aberrations that made possible a visual acuity that was never before experienced by the patients by any means?

We hypothesize that amongst the large sub-group of so called "amblyopia" patients, there will be a sub-set of patients who are not actually amblyopic but only aberropic but since ordinary testing methods do not reveal HOA and hence aberropia, the patient would have all along been mistakenly labeled as having amblyopia.

The role of higher order aberrations (HOA) in defining visual acuity has not yet been fully understood. There have been studies which state that as aberrations increase, the visual performance decreases but this study included patients with gross abnormalities such as keratoconus, penetrating keratoplasty, corneal trauma etc.[7], and this inverse correlation between aberrations and acuity was found to much lesser in eyes over a lower aberration range.[8,9] Recently, Applegate and associates[10] found that for low levels of aberration, the root-mean-square (RMS) wavefront error is not a good predictor of visual acuity. Levy Y et al[11] also stated that that the amount of ocular HOAs in eyes with natural supernormal vision (UCVA) ≥ 20/15) is not negligible, and is comparable to the reported amount of HOAs in myopic eyes.

It is important to know the effectiveness of correcting HOA in improving the visual acuity over this lower aberration range that compose the majority of normal and refractive surgery patients. Two important points should be kept in mind while considering this.[12] One is that because the magnitude of the Zernicke coefficient reflects its relative contribution to the total wavefront RMS error, it does not indicate that the largest Zernike coefficient will affect vision the most. This is because different Zernicke modes affect vision to different extents. Secondly, we also need to consider the effect of aberrations when they interact with each other. Combinations of Zernike polynomials have been known to improve or worsen visual performance.[12] Thus some beneficial aberrations overcome the detrimental effects of other aberrations and help in reducing the point spread function from a large blur to a smaller spot of light. This interaction for the better or worse occurs independently of the increase or decrease in the total wavefront error, i.e. they may interact for the better, leading to better visual performance, despite an overall increase in the wavefront error. Analysis of the first patient's wavefront map showed an overall flattening in the central area overlying both 4 and 6 mm pupil as compared to the preoperative map which might have been responsible for the improvement in vision **(Figure 19.1)**. Previous studies[10] have contended that the greater the area in the center of the pupil over which the wavefront error is reasonably flat, the better the visual acuity. Patient 1 had an overall decrease in HORMS, 3rd, 4th and 5th order RMS postoperatively **(Figure 19.4)**.

Analysis of Patient 2 showed that though the HORMS and 3rd order RMS decreased slightly postoperatively, the 4th and 5th order RMS increased **(Figure 19.5)**. These changes in the HOA along with interaction must have been responsible for his increase in vision, both HCVA and LCVA. This interaction can especially be beautifully demonstrated by the fact that his BCVA further improved from 20/15 to 20/10 on addition of –0.5 DS. Analysis of his postoperative wavefront map **(Figures 19.6A and B)** shows a predominant negative spherical aberration at both 4.18 and 6 mm pupils. Applegate et al have stated that Zernike modes with like signed coefficients 2 radial orders apart (e.g. radial orders 2 and 4) and having the same angular frequency (e.g. angular frequencies 0, –2, or 2) can interact positively[12] and this is seen well in our case.

Logically, in the perfect scenario, a zero higher order aberration would provide the best visual performance. A zero higher order aberration system is a pure diffraction limited system. In a pure diffraction limited system, Fraunhofer diffraction produces an Airy disc, the diameter of which varies inversely with the diameter of the pupil, hence the best possible vision would be obtained with a larger pupil size. Considering

Chapter 19: Ocular Higher Order Aberration Induced Decrease in Vision... 205

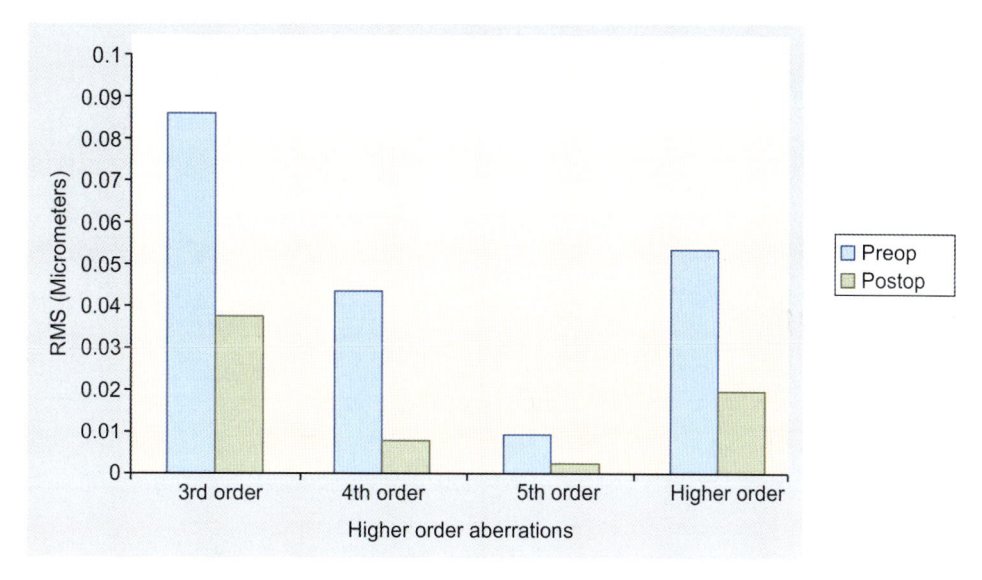

Figure 19.4 Comparison of pre- and postoperative HOA for patient 1

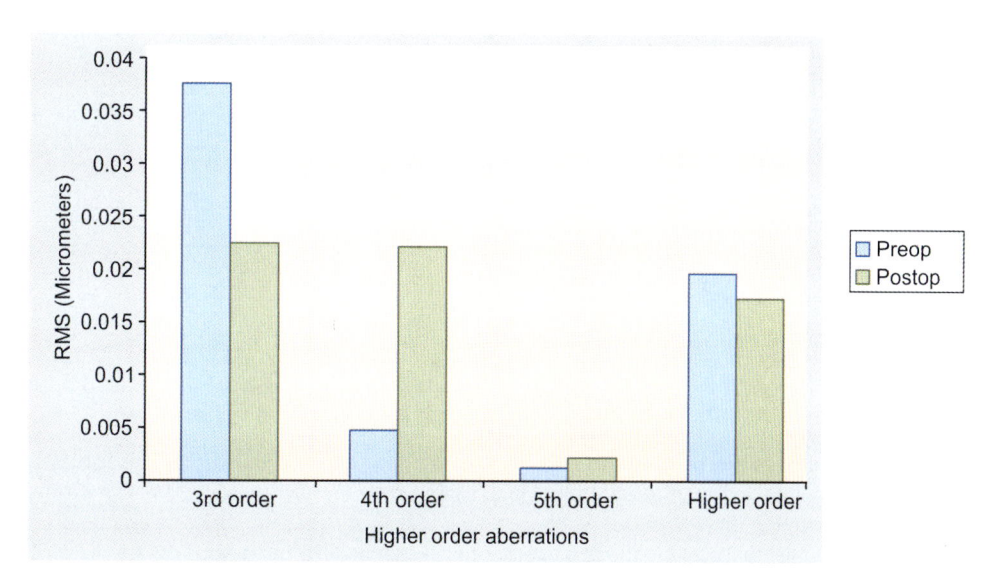

Figure 19.5 Comparison of pre- and postoperative HOA for patient 2

a similar scenario, with a zero order aberration system in the eye extending over the entire scotopic pupil size, i.e. in an aberration free, diffraction limited system, an increase in the size of the pupil would result in better visual acuity. Pupil size smaller than 3 mm would of course lead to deteriorating vision (in a pure diffraction limited aberration free system) due to Fraunhofer diffraction which leads to a larger Airy disc diameter with a smaller pupil size.

In the less than perfect but more common situation, it is an advantage to have positively interacting wavefront aberrations to cancel or neutralize the wavefront aberrations that deteriorate visual quality. In our case report, the patients had an improvement in their BCVA to never before experienced levels which could not be explained by any other reason. The patients did not postoperatively have an aberration free optics and therefore, the improved visual acuity in these patients must have been due to obtaining a set of aberrations which interacted positively to improve visual performance. The question of magnification factor improving visual acuity does not arise as these patients preoperatively did not improve with contact lenses. Further the refractive error in these patients was not very large.

Our case report included two patients with an improvement in best corrected HCVA and LCVA postrefractive surgery.

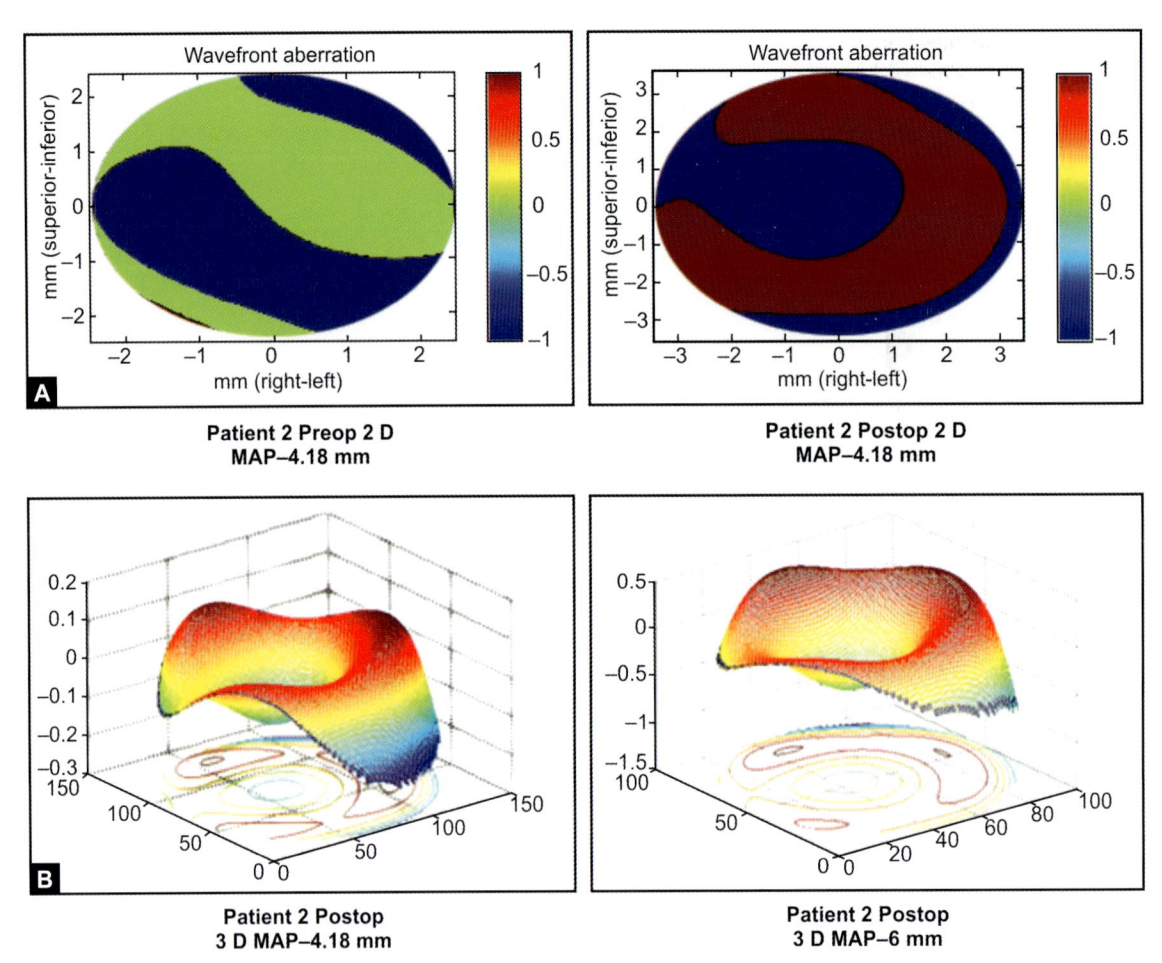

Figures 19.6A and B Comparison of pre- and postop 2 D map at 4.18 mm (mesopic pupil) (A); Postop 3 D wavefront map at mesopic and 6 mm pupil size showing negative spherical aberration (B)

Aberropia need not be limited to this but would refer to any significant improvement in the visual acuity or quality which is brought about by altering/removing the wavefront error.

Considering the reverse of these two cases, there would also be post-LASIK patients who have a decrease in their best corrected visual acuity or visual quality which is not correctable by spherocylindrical combinations and which cannot be explained as being due to media opacities, such as epithelial ingrowth, etc. These could be due to decentered aberrations, central islands, etc. which are conditions that operate in the higher ranges of aberrations. There is also a group of post-LASIK patients whose total wavefront error is not too large but who still do not improve with spherocylinders. These patients despite being in the lower aberration range may be having net detrimental aberrations. It might at least theoretically, be possible to treat them either by inducing aberrations which interact positively with these detrimental aberrations or more ideally, by bringing the total wavefront error to zero, i.e. making it an aberration free optics.

In healthy eyes with pupil_size more than 3.0 mm and having clear media, the wavefront error is the main contributor to image degradation. These aberrations present in the eye can be anywhere in the optical media and can be corrected at the corneal plane. Thus correction of any significant wavefront error in patients with unexplained decreased visual performance might give them the benefit of improved visual acuity or quality. Identification of this subgroup of patients, possibly with preoperative testing with customized wavefront glasses, adaptive optics or some other such modality might allow one to perform customized wavefront guided LASIK and if the treatment is applied over at least the scotopic pupil size, it should neutralize their optical aberrations and allow them improved visual performance. It would be necessary to develop ways of testing these patients in the clinical set-up.

Of course, it is true that getting the best possible optical system and consecutively the best possible retinal image is only the first step in the entire process of visual perception. Limitations are still imposed by the neural transfer function and the sensory system which exists right from the photoreceptors to the cortical level. Also, it has been proposed that each person is adapted to his/her own aberrations (neuroadaptation) and so, the visual acuity with the person's original, less than perfect wavefront may still be better than the visual acuity obtained with a changed but better wavefront.[13]

But would this mean that presenting a better optical sytem would degrade visual quality in every patient? In our two patients, neuroadaptation as well as limits imposed by the neural transfer function would have been expected to bring about an increase in vision to preoperative best corrected visual acuity and not any better than that. The fact that these patients gained significantly in their lines of vision to levels never before experienced by the patient shows that this must have been due to the alteration brought about in their wavefront.

In the present day scenario, with the current limitations in wavefront guided treatment platforms as well as techniques, one may not be totally successful in trying to correct or alter the higher-order aberrations during refractive surgery. But in the future, with greater technological advances, if one can precisely determine preoperatively using either adaptive optics or any other newer modalities which may become available in the future as to what type of correction if applied would lead to an improved or enhanced visual outcome and if the technology for extremely precise application of this wavefront correction to the patients cornea can be developed, then it would definitely be worthwhile to try and do a wavefront "correcting" refractive surgery for every patient. Further research is required to make this kind of wavefront correction a reality and this would be possible only by further improvements in diagnostic modalities as well as refinements in the present wavefront guided LASIK systems available.

We have proposed two systems of classification for this newly defined refractive error based on the etiology and also on the magnitude of aberropia. These are shown in **Tables 19.3 and 19.4**.

Keeping all these facts in mind, we venture forwards to propose a new refractive error—aberropia which was first published by us in 2002.[14-17] We define this as a refractive error which results in a decrease in the visual quality that can be attributable to higher order aberrations.[18] This is either due to the helpful aberrations being inadequate in overcoming the detrimental aberrations or due to a situation where, there are only detrimental aberrations present in the eye. Thus we have coined this term for a refractive error which is due to a net detrimental HOA, postinteraction between different types of aberrations. Correction of this refractive error could be by changing the different aberrations so that they interact differently, thus having a net effect of clear visual performance despite the fact that the total wavefront error is not zero. Correction could also be achieved by bringing down the total wavefront error to zero. Both these situations would yield improved visual performance. Extremely asymmetric HOA between the two eyes during the period of plasticity of the visual

Table 19.3 Classification of aberropia based on etiology

I. Congenital Aberropia
Here, the person is born with these aberrations. If unilateral and large enough to interfere with normal binocular interaction between the two eyes, these could possibly lead to amblyopia in that eye.[16,17]

II. Acquired Aberropia
A. Post Surgical
   a. Corneal:
      - Postpenetrating keratoplasty
      - Postrefractive surgery
   b. Lenticular:
      - IOL induced aberrations: either inherent in the IOL or due to malpositioned IOL
      - Aberrations due to capsular abnormalities
B. Others
   a. Corneal:
      - Keratoconus and other ectatic disorders
      - Corneal trauma, scars, etc.
      - Other causes of irregular astigmatism
   b. Lenticular:
      - Incipient cataract
      - Lenticonus
      - Subluxated lens, coloboma lens
   c. Vitreous: Vitreous opacities and floaters
   d. Retinal:
      - Thickened posterior hyaloid
      - Very fine ERMs not causing traction on the retina.

Table 19.4 Classification of aberropia based on magnitude

> **Higher range aberropia:** Keratoconus, postpenetrating keratoplasty, corneal trauma, lenticonus, etc. Here the visual performance has a good correlation with the amount of higher order aberrations.
>
> **Lower range aberropia:** Majority of normal and refractive surgery patients, where the correlation between the range of aberrations and the visual performance is no longer present. This loss of correlation is due also to interaction between the different aberrations besides other factors such as neural transfer function, etc.

system could similarly lead to aberropia induced amblyopia (Table 19.3).[18-20]

All this does cause one to think what happens when a person with aberropia who is treated presents with age related changes in his wavefront aberrations, either due to loss of accommodaton or due to lens changes or any other cause. This would be similar to the present day problem of calculating IOL power for post-LASIK patients. One may have to treat the patient further for his/her wavefronts or use customized wavefront glasses, contact lenses or even IOLs. There may also develop in the future, some newer modality of optical correction utilizing adaptive optics as done in astrophysics at present.

CONCLUSION

We know that not all wavefront aberrations may be bad for the eye and that these aberrations may sometimes interact positively or negatively to increase or decrease visual performance. We propose a new refractive entity – aberropia- where there is a net negative interaction between the higher order aberrations so that there is deterioration in the visual performance of the patients. We hypothesize that selected cases of unexplained poor vision and so called "amblyopia" maybe actually be due to aberropia and that these are treatable and these patients can obtain an improvement in the BCVA/ visual quality. Thus, similar to the conventional "hyperopia", "myopia" and "astigmatism" which are corrected with spherocylinders, it is only logical that this HOA induced loss of vision would be a new refractive entity — aberropia, which could be correctable by removing or altering these aberrations.

This new field definitely needs a lot of research before attaining its full potential but as research has always been stimulated by what has not been fully understood, and as identification is the first step towards understanding, it is essential that we first recognize and identify aberropia as a new refractive error and try to understand it fully so that all venues are opened for obtaining, not super vision in terms of 20/10 or better, but the best possible vision that is optically possible for a particular person. It will be interesting to see what the future holds.

REFERENCES

1. Platt B and Shack RV. "Lenticular Hartmann screen" Opt Sci Center News (University of Arizona). 1971;5:15-6.
2. Liang J, Grimm B, Goelz S, Bille J. "Objective measurement of the wave aberrations of the human eye with the use of a Hartmann-Shack wavefront sensor". J Opt Soc Am. 1994;11:1949-57.
3. Liang J, Williams DR, et al. Aberrations and retinal image quality of the normal human eye. J Opt Soc Am A. 1997;14(11):2873-83.
4. Thibos LN, Applegate RA, Schwiegerling JT, Webb R. Standards for reporting the optical aberrations of eyes; VSIA Standards Taskforce Members. OSA Trends in Optics Photonics. 2000;35:232-44.
5. MacRae SM, Krueger RR, Applegate RA. Customized Corneal Ablation: the Quest for SuperVision. Thorofare, NJ, Slack, 2001; appendix 1:347-61.
6. Thibos LN, Applegate RA, Schwiegerling JT, Webb R. Standards for reporting the optical aberrations of eyes. J Refract Surg. 2002;18:S652-61.
7. Applegate RA, Hilmantel G, Howland HC, et al. Corneal first surface optical aberrations and visual performance. J Refract Surg. 2000;16:507-14.
8. Hong X, Thibos LN, Bradley A, et al. Impact of monochromatic aberrations on polychromatic image quality and vision. Invest Ophthalmol Vis Sci. 2001;42(suppl):S162.
9. Cheng X, Bradley A, Hong X, Thibos LN. Relationship between refractive error and monochromatic aberrations of the eye. Optom Vis Sci. 2003;80:43-9.
10. Applegate RA, Marsack JD, Ramos R, Sarver EJ. Interaction between aberrations to improve or reduce visual performance. J Cataract Refract Surg. 2003;29:1487-95.
11. Levy Y, Segal O, Avni I. Ocular higher order aberrations in eyes with supernormal vision. AJO. 2005:139;225-28.
12. Applegate RA, Sarver EJ, Khemsara V. Are all aberrations equal?. J Refract Surg. 2002;18:S556-62.
13. Artal P, Chen Li, Fernandez EJ et al. Neural compensation for the eye's optical aberrations. Journal of Vision (2004) 4, 281-87.
14. Amar Agarwal, Soosan Jacob, Athiya Agarwal, et al. Aberropia: a new refractive entity. Ocular Surgery News, U.S. Edition, No.19, October 1, 2002;20:14-19.
15. Amar Agarwal, Soosan Jacob, Nilesh Kanjani, et al. Aberropia: A New Refractive Entity. In: Boyd BF, Agarwal A (eds). Wavefront Analysis, Aberrometers and Corneal Topography. Panama, Republic of Panama: Highlights of Ophthalmology International; 2003.pp.333-42.
16. Aberropia: A new Refractive Entity. Highlights of Ophthalmology. Indian Edition, 2003:31;1:29-35.
17. Chalita MR, Krueger RR. Refractive Surgery In: Agarwal A (Ed) Handbook of Ophthalmology. Thorofare, NJ: Slack Incorporated; 2006.pp.630-32.
18. Agarwal A, Jacob S, Agarwal A. Aberropia: A new refractive entity. JCRS (In Press).
19. Prakash G, Sharma N, Chowdhary V, et al. Association between amblyopia and higher-order aberrations. J Cataract Refract Surg. 2007;33:901-04.
20. de Faber. Higher-order aberrations: Explanation of idiopathic amblyopia? J Cataract Refract Surg. 2007;33:753.

Chapter 20

Topographic and Aberrometer Guided Laser

Amar Agarwal (India), Athiya Agarwal (India)

INTRODUCTION

Since as early as middle of 19th century it has been known that the optical quality of human eye suffers from ocular errors (aberrations) besides the commonly known image errors such as myopia, hyperopia and asigmatism.[1] In early 1970's Fyodorov introduced the anterior radial incisions to flatten the central cornea to correct myopia.[2] Astigmatic keratotomy,[3] keratomileusis and keratophakia, epikeratophakia[4] and currently excimer laser[5] have been used to manage the various refractive errors. These refractive procedures correct lower order aberrations such as spherical and cylindrical refractive errors however higher order aberrations persist, which affect the quality of vision but may not significantly affect the Snellen visual acuity. Refractive corrective procedures are known to induce aberrations.[6] It is the subtle deviations from the ideal optical system, which can be corrected by wavefront and topography guided (customized ablation) LASIK procedures.[7]

ABERRATIONS

Optical aberration customization can be corneal topography guided which measures the ocular aberrations detected by corneal topography and treats the irregularities as an integrated part of the laser treatment plan. The second method of optical aberration customization measures the wavefront errors of the entire eye and treats based on these measurements.[7] Wavefront analysis can be done either using Howland's aberroscope[8] or a Hartmann-Shack wavefront sensor.[9] These techniques measure all the eye's aberrations including second-order (sphere and cylindrical), third-order (coma–like), fourth-order (spherical), and higher order wavefront aberrations. Based on this information an ideal ablation plan can be formulated which treats lower order as well as higher order aberrations.

ZYOPTIX LASER

Zyoptix™ (Bausch and Lomb) is a system for Personalized Vision Solutions, which incorporates Zywave™ Hartmann-Shack aberrometer coupled with Orbscan™ IIz multi-dimensional device, which generates the individual ablation profiles to be used with the Technolas® 217 excimer laser system. Thus, this system utilizes combination of wavefront analysis and corneal topography for optical aberration customization.

ORBSCAN

The orbscan uses a slit scanning system wherein the slits are projected on to the anterior segment of the eye: the anterior cornea, the posterior cornea, the anterior iris and anterior lens. The data collected from these four surfaces are used to create a topographic map. This technique provides more information about anterior segment of the eye, such as anterior and posterior corneal curvature and corneal thickness.[10] It improves the diagnostic accuracy and it has passive eye-tracker from frame to frame, 43 frames are taken to ensure accuracy. It is easy to interpret and has good repeatability. Three different maps are taken, and the one featuring the least eye movements is used. The maximum movements considered acceptable are 200 µ.

ABERROMETER

Zywave™ is based on Hartmann-Shack aberrometry (**Figure 20.1**) in which a laser diode (780 nm) generates a laser beam that is focused on the retina of the patient's eye (**Figure 20.2**). An adjustable collimation system compensates for the spherical portion of the refractive error of the eye. Laser diode is turned on for approximately 100 milliseconds. The light reflected from the focal point on the retina (source of wavefront) is directed through an array of small lenses (lenslet) generating a grid-like pattern (array) of focal points

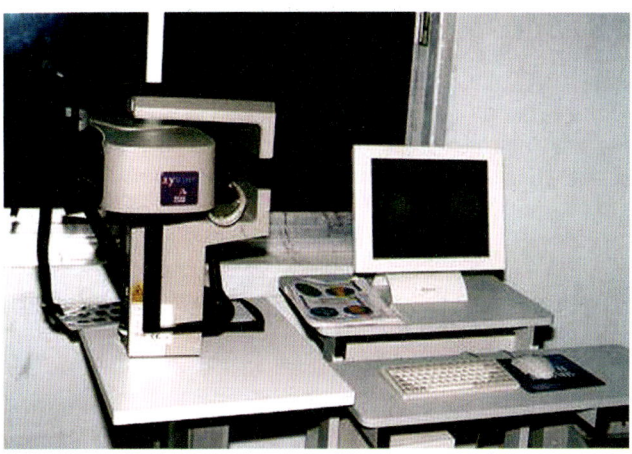

Figure 20.1 Hartmann-Shack aberrometer

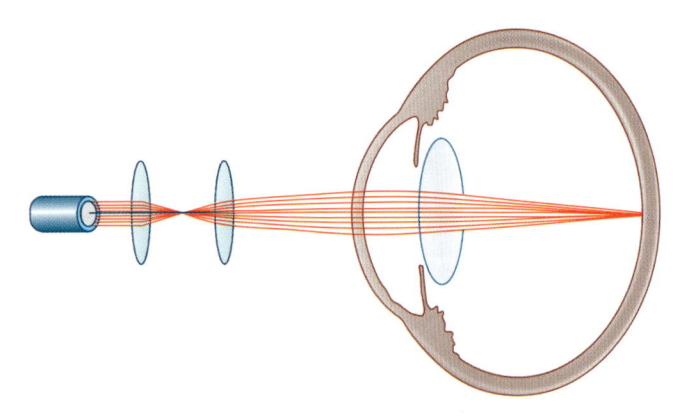

Figure 20.2 Zywave projects low-intensity HeNe infrared light into the eye and use the diffuse reflection from the retina

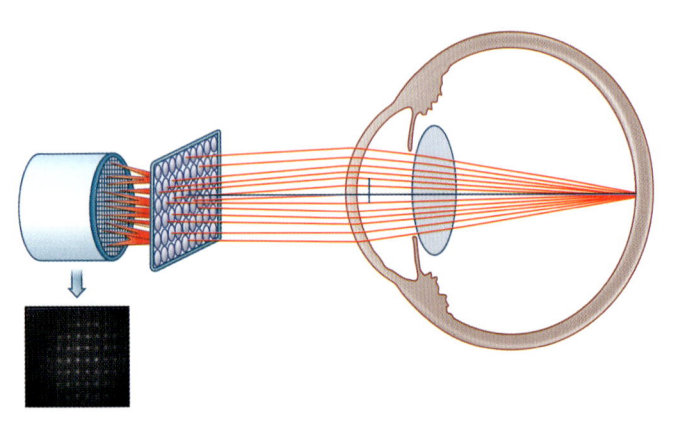

Figure 20.3 Bausch and Lomb Zywave aberrometer. A low-intensity HeNe infrared light is shone into the eye; the reflected light is focused by a number of small lenses (lenslet-array), and pictured by a CCD-camera. The capture image is shown on the bottom left

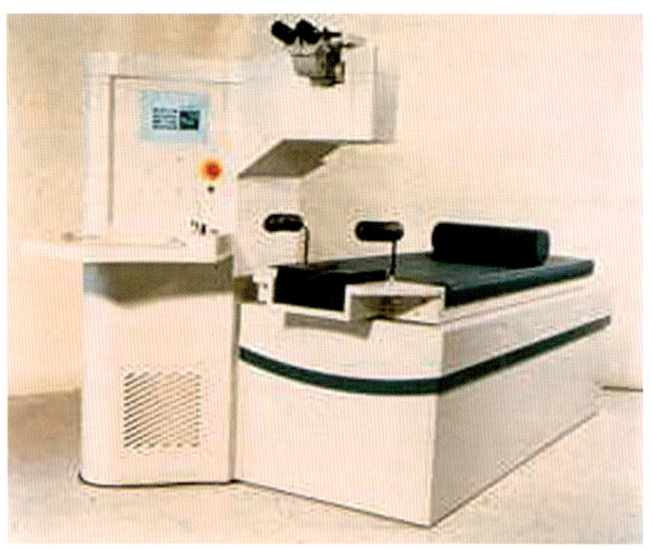

Figure 20.4 Technolas 217 z excimer laser system

(**Figure 20.3**). The position of the focal points are detected by Zywave™. Due to deviation of the points from their ideal position, the wavefront can be reconstructed. Wavefront display shows (a) higher order aberrations, (b) predicted phoropter refraction (PPR) calculated for a back vertex correction of 15 mm. (c) simulated point spread function (PSF). Zywave™ examinations are done with (a) single examination with undilated pupil and (b) five examinations with dilated pupil (mydriasis) noncycloplegic, using 5% phenylephrine drops. One of these five measurements, which matched best with the manifest refraction of the undilated pupil, is chosen for the treatment.

ZYLINK

Information gathered from Orbscan and Zywave are then translated into treatment plan using Zylink™ software and copied to a floppy disk. The floppy disk is then inserted into the Technolas 217 system (**Figure 20.4**), fluence test carried out and a Zyoptix treatment card was inserted. A standard LASIK procedure is then performed with a superiorly hinged flap. A Hansatome™ or Zyoptix XP™ microkeratome is used to create a flap. Flap thickness can be varied from 120–200 μm. A residual stromal bed of 250 μm or more is left in all eyes. Optical zone varied from 6–7 mm depending upon the pupil size and ablation required. Eye tracker is kept on during laser ablation. Postoperatively all patients are followed up for at least 6 months.

RESULTS

We did a study comprising 150 eyes with myopia and compound myopic astigmatism. Preoperatively, the patients underwent corneal topography with Orbscan II z™ and wavefront analysis with Zywave™ in addition to the routine pre-LASIK work-up. The results were assimilated using Zylink™ and a customized treatment plan was formulated. LASIK was then performed with Technolas® 217 system. All the patients were followed up for at least six months.

Mean preoperative best spectacle-corrected visual acuity (BSCVA) (in decimal) was 0.83 ± 0.18 (Range 0.33–1.00). Mean postoperative (6 months) BCVA was 1.00 ± 0.23 (Range 0.33–1.50). Difference was statistically significant ($p = 0.0003$). Out of 150 eyes that underwent customized ablation, 3 eyes (2%) lost two or more lines of best spectacle corrected visual acuity (BSCVA).

Safety index = mean postoperative BSCVA/Mean preoperative BSCVA = 1.20 (**Figure 20.5**). Mean preoperative UCVA was 0.06 ± 0.02 (Range 0.01–0.50). Mean postoperative UCVA was 0.88 ± 0.36 (Range 0.08–1.50). Difference was statistically significant ($p = 0.0001$).

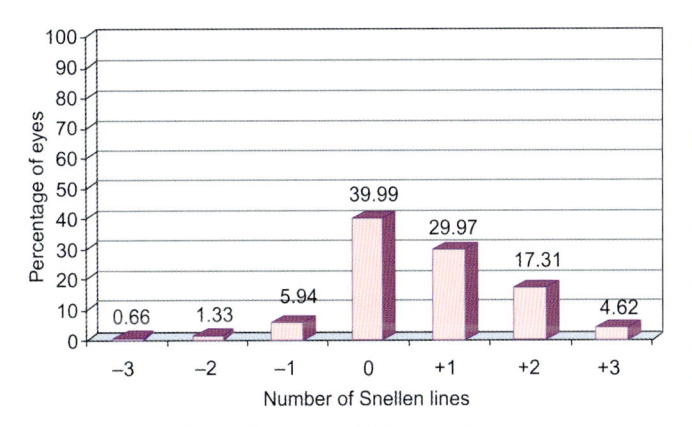

Figure 20.5 Safety-Changes in BSCVA 6 months postoperatively

Efficacy index = mean postoperative UCVA/Mean preoperative UCVA = 14.66 (**Figure 20.6**). Preoperatively, none of the eyes had UCVA of 6/6 or more and one eye (0.66%) had UCVA of 6/12 or more. At 6 months postoperatively, 105 eyes (69.93%) had UCVA of 6\6 or more and 126 eyes (83.91%) had UCVA of 6/12 or more.

Mean preoperative spherical equivalent was −5.25 D ± 1.68 D (Range −0.87 D to −15 D). Mean postoperative spherical equivalent (6 months) was −0.36 D ± 0.931 D (Range −4.25 D to +1.25). Difference between the two was statistically significant ($p < 0.05$) (**Figure 20.7**). 132 eyes (87.91%) were within ±1.00 D of emmetropia while 120 eyes (79.92%) were within ± 0.05 D of emmetropia. One eye (0.66%) was overcorrected by > 0.5 D and 1 eye (0.66%) was overcorrected by >1D. The mean pupil diameter was 5.1 mm ± 0.62 mm. Preoperatively, 95 eyes (63.27%) had third order aberrations. Forty-two eyes (28%) had second order aberration alone, while 13 eyes (8.65%) had fourth and fifth order aberrations. Post-operatively, 60 eyes (40%) had third order aberration. 75 eyes (50%) had second order alone while 15 eyes (10%) had higher order aberrations.

DISCUSSION

Hartmann-Shack wavefront sensor was first used by Liang and colleagues to detect ocular aberrations.[11] They applied an adaptive optics deformable mirror to correct the lower and higher order aberrations of the eye. They reported a 6 times increase in contrast sensitivity to high spatial frequency when the pupil was large. This study demonstrated that correction of higher order aberrations could lead to supernormal vision in normal eyes. **Figures 20.8 to 20.10** are same example of various aberrations.

In our series, using Zyoptix and Technolas 217 system, which is wavefront and corneal topography guided, we yielded results that are comparable to standard LASIK procedure.[12] In a series of 347 eyes, McDonald, et al 12 reported a postoperative refraction of −0.29 ± 0.45 D (−0.36 ± 0.93 D in our series) with standard LASIK. 57% of the eyes in their series had postoperative UCVA of ≥ 6/6. In our study, 70% of the eyes had UCVA of ≥ 6/6, six months postoperatively.

Higher order aberrations were reduced postoperatively in our study. Third-order aberration (coma) was most common in our series, followed by second-order (defocus and astigmatism) and fourth-order (spherical aberration). Postoperatively, after 6 months, there was considerable decrease in third-order and fourth-order aberrations. While most of the eyes had only defocus and astigmatism (i.e. second-order aberration). A slight increase in fourth-order aberration (spherical) was noted. Spherical aberration is known to increase after LASIK.[13-15] Roberts has reported that cornea changes its shape in response to ablation and this change, along with wound healing effects have to be taken into account before customized correction

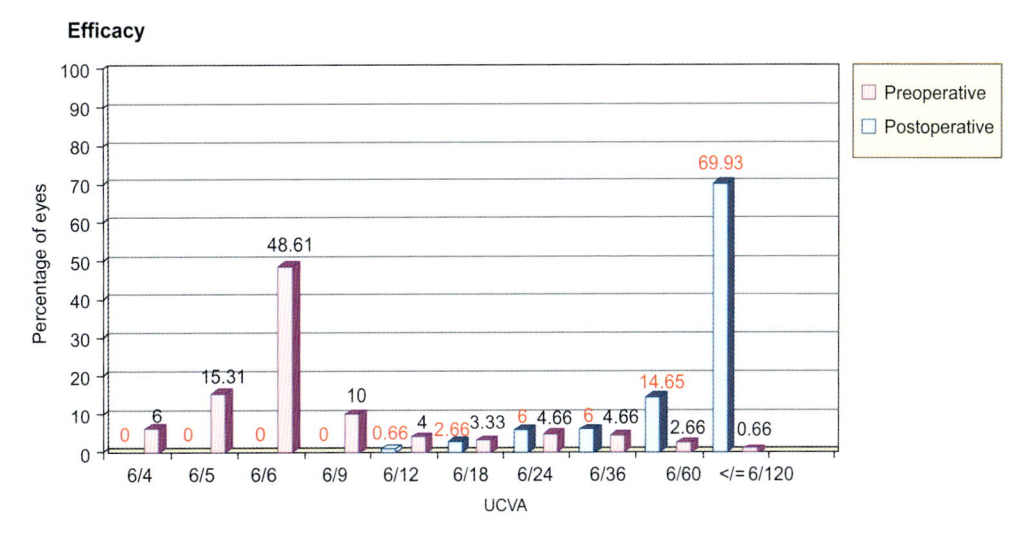

Figure 20.6 Compares preoperative and postoperative UCVA (Efficacy)

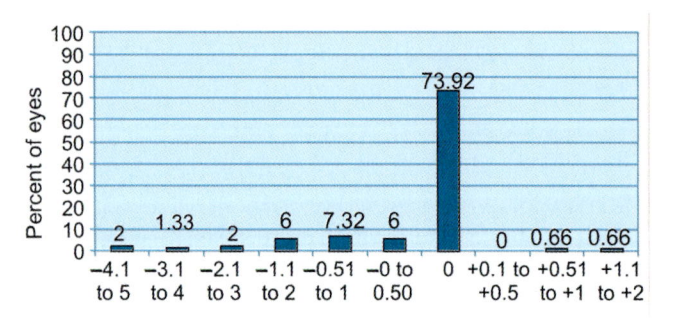

Figure 20.7 Refractive results postoperatively after 6 months

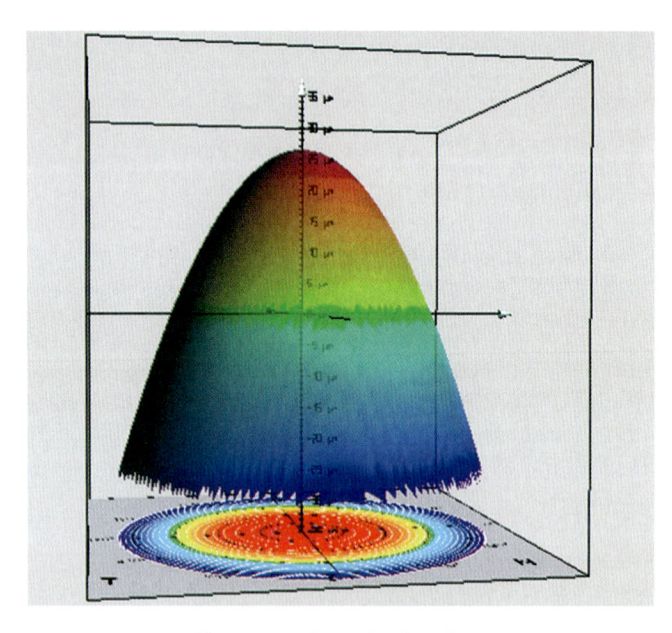

Figure 20.8 Second-order sphere

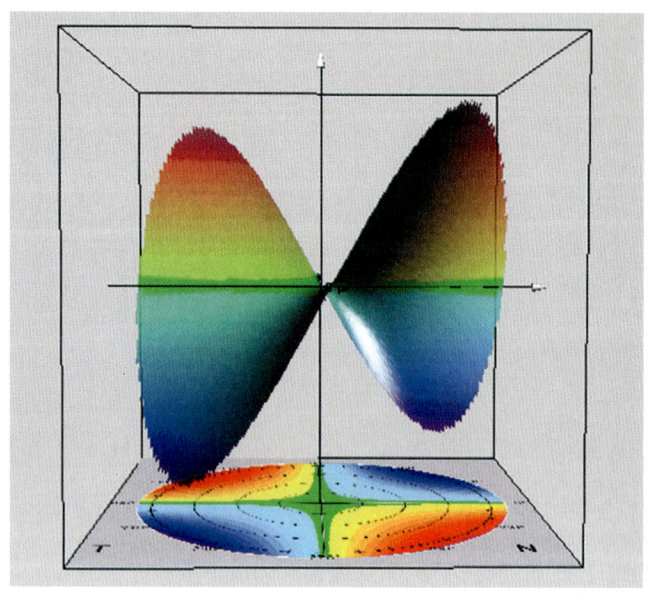

Figure 20.9 Second-order astigmatism

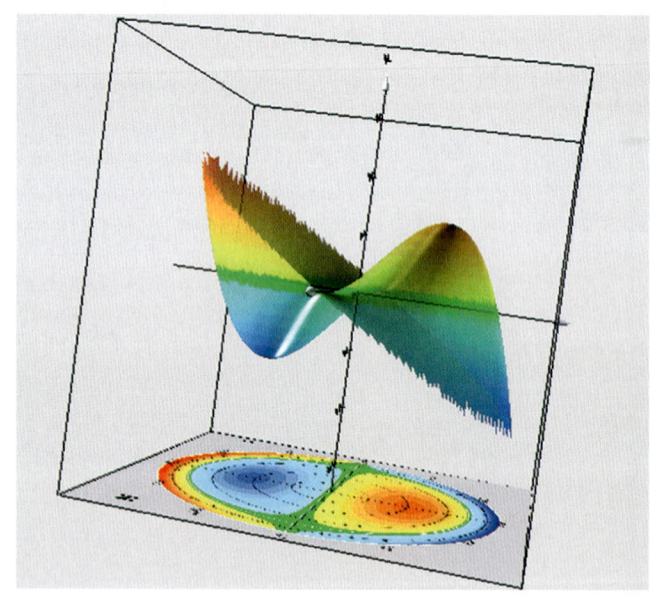

Figure 20.10 Third-order coma

can nullify higher-order aberrations. Roberts and coworkers suggest that increase in spherical aberrations following LASIK may be caused by a biomechanically induced steepening and thickening that may occur in mid-periphery of the cornea.[13] MacRae and coworkers have reported that simply creating a LASIK flap increases higher-order aberrations in unpredictable manner.[14] They suggest that improved results can be obtained using a surface ablation such as PRK or LASEK, or by doing a two-stage LASIK, with the second stage adjusting for the aberration created by the flap and initial ablation.

Scotopic visual complaints have been the bugbear of LASIK procedures, ranging from mild annoyance to severe optical disability.[16,17] Nighttime starbursts, reduced contrast sensitivity and haloes are the most common complaints.[16,17] Spherical aberration that is induced during LASIK may account for this scotopic complaints.[14] Pupil diameter is another factor that is important. When pupil diameter is large, as in young patients, dim light vision is improved after customized correction.[18,19] In our series, 11% of the patients complained of haloes around light at night and difficult night driving. In dim light, the mean pupil diameter in these patients was 4.2 mm while it was 5.9 mm in other patients. Smaller pupil diameter and induced higher-order aberration may account for these scotopic visual complaints.

Twenty-five percent of the patients in our series reported improvement in bright light vision, while 40% showed improvement in dim light vision. A similar improvement was noted by Cox and co-workers (presentation by Cox IG at Zyoptix Alliance meeting, 2002 reported in *Ocular Surgery News*, July 2002 volume 13, number 7). In our series, treatment optical zone ranged from 6 mm to 7 mm. Treatment with larger optical zones and transition zones as compared to conventional LASIK may be possible since entire corneal topography and not just the central cornea overlying pupil along with wavefront ablation in dilated pupil are considered during treatment. This may induce lesser spherical aberration post-LASIK and account for improved scotopic vision.

Though we did not measure contrast sensitivity and glare acuity postoperatively, our results suggest improved quality of vision and fewer glare problems with Zyoptix treatment. A more temporal appraisal of the procedure has to be carried out with comparison to standard LASIK. Short-term results suggest wavefront and topography guided LASIK may be a safe and effective procedure which improves the visual performance.

CONCLUSION

Wavefront and topography guided LASIK procedure leads to better visual performance by decreasing higher order aberration. Scotopic visual complaints may be reduced with this method.

REFERENCES

1. Helmholtz H. Handbuch der physiologischen optik. Leipzig: Leopold Voss; 1867. pp. 137-47.
2. Fyodorov SN, Durnev VV. Operation of dosaged dissection of corneal circular ligament .
3. Binder PS, Waring GO III. Keratotomy for astigmatism. In Waring GO III (Ed). Refractive keratotomy for myopia and astigmatism. Mosby Year Book 1085–1198, 1992. in cases of myopia of mild degree. Ann Ophthalmol II; 1979. pp. 1885-90.
4. Kaufmann HE. Correction of aphakia. Am J Ophthalmol. 1980; 89:1.
5. McGhee CNJ, Taylor HR, Garty DS, et al. Excimer Lasers in Ophthalmology: Principles and Practice. Martin Duntz: London, 1997.
6. MacRae S, Porter J, Cox IG, et al. Higher-order aberrations after conventional LASIK. ISRS: Dallas, Texas, 2000.
7. MacRae SM. Supernormal vision, hypervision, and customized corneal ablation. Guest Editorial J Cat Refract Surg. 2000.
8. Howland HC, Howland B. A subjective method for the measurement of monochromatic aberrations of the eye. J Opt Soc Am. 1977;67:1508-18.
9. Liang J, Williams DR, Miller DT. Supernormal vision and high-resolution retinal imaging through adaptive optics. J Opt Soc Am; 1997. pp. 2884-92.
10. Fedor P, Kaufman S. Corneal topography and imaging. Medicine Journal; 2001.pp. (2)6.
11. Liang J, Williams D. Aberrations and retinal image quality of the normal human eye. J Opt Soc AM A. 1997;14:2884-92.
12. McDonald MB, Carr JD, Frantz JM, et al. Laser in situ keratomileusis for myopia up to –11 diopters with up to –5 diopters of astigmatism with summit autonomous LADARVision excimer laser system. Ophthalmology. 2001;108:309-16.
13. Roberts C. The cornea is not a piece of plastic. J Refract Surg. 2000; 16:407-13.
14. MacRae SM, Roberts C, Porter J, et al. The biomechanics of a LASIK flap. ISRS Mid –Summer Meeting: Orlando, Florida, 2001.
15. Applegate RA, Howland HC, Klyce SD. Corneal aberration and refractive surgery. In MacRae S (Ed). Customized Corneal Ablation. Thorofare NJ: Slack, Inc., 2001.
16. Holladay JT, Dudeja DR, Chang J. Functional vision and corneal changes after laser in situ keratomileusis determined by contrast sensitivity, glare testing, and corneal topography. J Cataract Refract Surg. 1999;25:663-9.
17. Perez-Santonja JJ, Sakla HF, Alio JL. Contrast sensitivity after laser in situ keratomileusis. J Cataract Refract Surg. 1998;24:183-9.
18. Applegate R, Howland H, Sharp R, et al. Corneal aberrations and visual performance after refractive keratectomy. J Refract Surg. 1998;14:397-407.
19. Oshika T, Klyce S, Applegate R, et al. Comparison of corneal wavefront aberrations after photorefractive keratectomy and laser in situ keratomileusis. Am J Ophthal. 1999;127:1-7.

Chapter 21

NAVWave: Nidek Technique for Customized Ablation

Masanao Fujieda (Japan), Mukesh Jain (Australia)

INTRODUCTION

NAV Wave is a coupling of two brilliant technologies, to deliver customized ablation for the correction of refractive error. The OPD-Scan[R] system, combining wavefront analysis with corneal topography to map the aberrations of the entire optical system, is linked with Nidek's unique Final Fit Software to evaluate and convert the data to produce the precise ablation parameters for customized excimer laser ablation of the cornea.

OPD-SCAN

The OPD-Scan (Optical Path Difference Scanning System) is equipped with corneal topography, aberrometry, refractometry, keratometry and pupilometry functions within a single device overcoming the potential problems of inter-device misalignment. The OPD-Scan[R] measures both corneal topography using Placido disk reflection method as well as total ocular aberrations using dynamic skiascopy technology. Dynamic skiascopy currently provides the most direct measurement of any wavefront system without using a lenslet array or the projection of a grid target onto the retina. The technique of skiascopy has been successfully used in auto-refractometers but has now been modified to permit the additional measurement of higher order aberrations. The major difference between the dynamic skiascopy based OPD-Scan[R] and other skiascopy based auto-refractometers is that the OPD-Scan[R] can measure the distribution of refractive error in a wider corneal zone as it provides internally with a photo diode array at a conjugate position with the cornea.

A constant-speed single direction slit shaped infrared ray is projected towards the entrance pupil center as a thin beam and onwards to strike the retina. An aperture and a photo-diode array that is conjugate with the retina for emmetropia collect the reflected light from the retina. There are four photodetectors above and four photodetectors below the optical axis. There are also two photodetectors, one of each side, which detect the center of the photodetector pairs. The basic principle is in many ways similar to confocal microscopy in which only the light reflected from the retina that passes through the aperture would reach the photo-diode array. How the reflected light reaches the photo-diode array, depends on the positional relationship between the retina and aperture. We have just said only the reflected light that passes through the aperture will be collected.

In the case of emmetropic eye, the aperture is positioned on the retina, and the slit shape light goes across the aperture, the reflected light hits all the photodiode cells simultaneously. Therefore, there is no time lag between different detection time and the time difference should be zero. In hyperopia, the aperture is positioned behind the retina and hence there is a time lag between different diodes detection time.

In the myopic eye, the aperture stop is located in front of the retina. The incoming slit-shaped light bundle bounces off the retina and the reflecting slit moves in an opposite direction compared to the incoming slit. This causes some photodetector cells to be stimulated earlier that the others. By correlating the time differences with refractive errors, a refractive error at each position on the cornea (photo-diode position) with respect to the corneal center can be derived. By simple rotation of the measurement system through 180°, the distribution of refractive errors can be obtained through 360-degree meridians.[1-2] The OPD scan also measures corneal topography using a Placido ring method and which has been widely utilized for almost two decades.

TOPOGRAPHY AND WAVEFRONT ANALYZER

The OPD-Scan is a combined corneal topography device and wavefront analyzer. The purpose of laser keratorefractive surgery is to photo ablate the cornea to alter its refracting power, and thereby improve unaided vision. The early systems were effective at reducing primary defocus and astigmatism but often led to increased higher order aberrations. Customized ablation now offers the potential to correct not just the lower order errors but also the majority of significant higher-order aberrations to achieve better vision.[3] Generally, the Transition Zone is also thought to play an important role in improving visual performance under Scotopic conditions as the pupil enlarges, however, it is impossible to design the Transition Zone from Wavefront Analyzer information alone without thought to the cornea overelying areas outside the entrance pupil.

A major functional difference between Dynamic-Skiascopy and Hartmann-Shack type devices lies in the range of measurements capability:

OPD-Scan principle: Sphere: −20 to +22 D
 Cylinder: 0 to ±12 D
Hartmann-Shack principle: Sphere: −15 D to +7 D,
 Cylinder: 0 to ±6 D

OPD POWER MAP

The data generated by the OPD is typically displayed in map form showing the distribution of wavefront errors of the entire eye (D). **Figure 21.1A** illustrates the OPD map of a –4.75 D spherical model eye. In this map, the refractive error at a desired position on the cornea within a 6 mm diameter is displayed. Since the map is of a spherical model eye uncorrected for spherical aberration, the measured errors vary with each concentric zone; the outermost concentric zone being more negative (reddish) than the central zone. In this figure, the terms, sphere, cylinder, and axis have their conventional meaning and are displayed in the middle left for the central zone as: S: –4.75, C: –0.00, A: 0.0. This is repeated for 3 mm and 5 mm annulus zones immediately below the central data and show increasingly negative defocus errors in the periphery. **Figure 21.1B** illustrates the OPD map of a 3D cylindrical model eye. In this map of with-the-rule astigmatism, the steeper meridian (in the 90° to 270° direction) and flatter meridian (in the 0° to 180° direction) are observed as a color-coded butterfly pattern. It is also clear from the map that even in this cylindrical model eye, there is significant spherical aberration.

The OPD-Scan^R also allows the mapping of various individual aberrations described in terms of Zernike coefficients from the wavefront data. The low-order components (up to 5) that can be corrected with spectacle lenses and some high-order components (6 and higher) can be displayed. **Figure 21.2A** illustrates an OPD map of an emmetropic human eye. This map is color-coded in three greenish colors for simple pattern recognition. **Figure 21.2B** shows an eye with myopic astigmatism and **Figure 21.2C** shows a hyperopic astigmatism eye. The OPD-Scan^R produces maps that are easily interpreted, using display techniques familiar to corneal topography maps. Just as computer assisted corneal topography devices raised the standard of keratometry, so too do wavefront devices provide us with a wealth of information over and above sphere, cylinder and axis.

In addition, it is easily perceived whether the map has a butterfly pattern and illustrates symmetric or asymmetric astigmatism from the symmetry of the butterfly pattern. The OPD map provides us with more visual and multifactorial

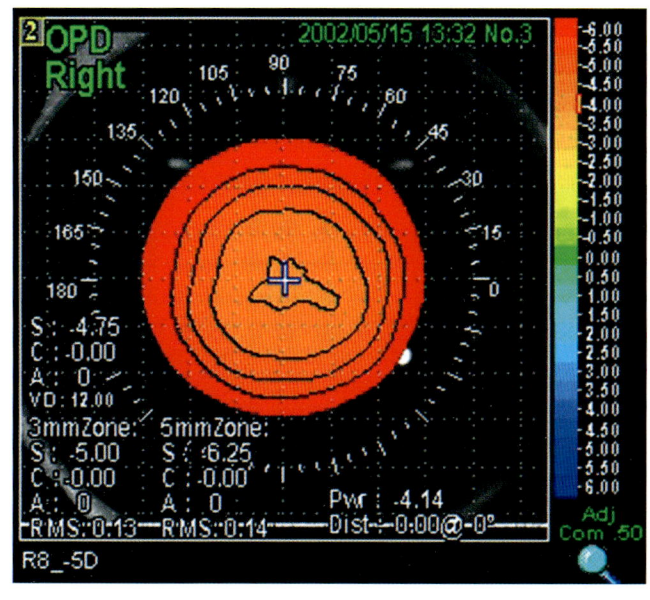

Figure 21.1A OPD map of a –4.75 D spherical model eye

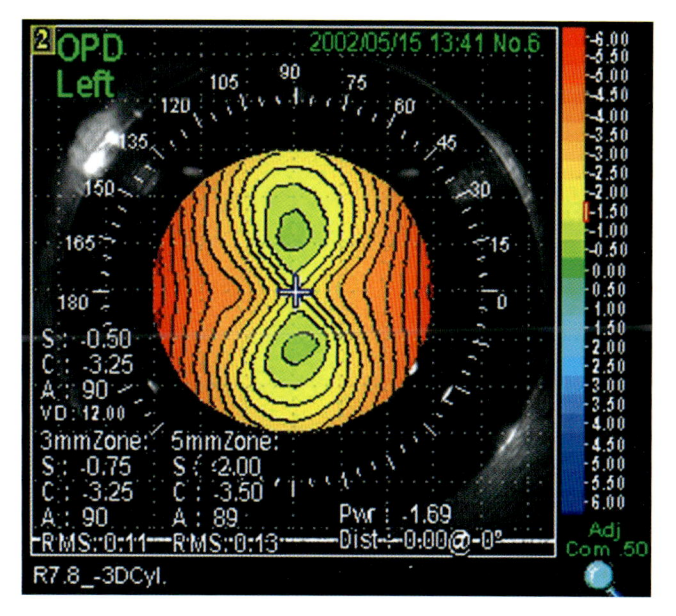

Figure 21.1B OPD map of a 3D cylindrical model eye

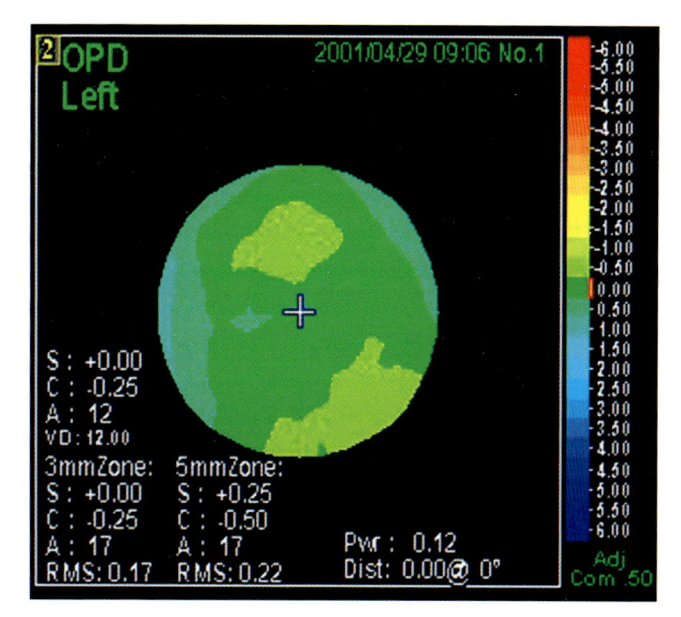

Figure 21.2A OPD map of an emmetropic human eye

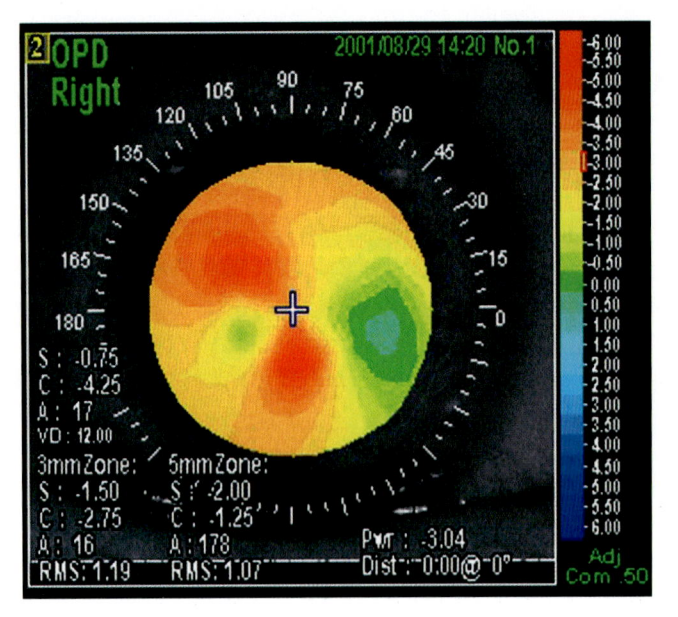

Figure 21.2B OPD map of a myopic astigmatism eye

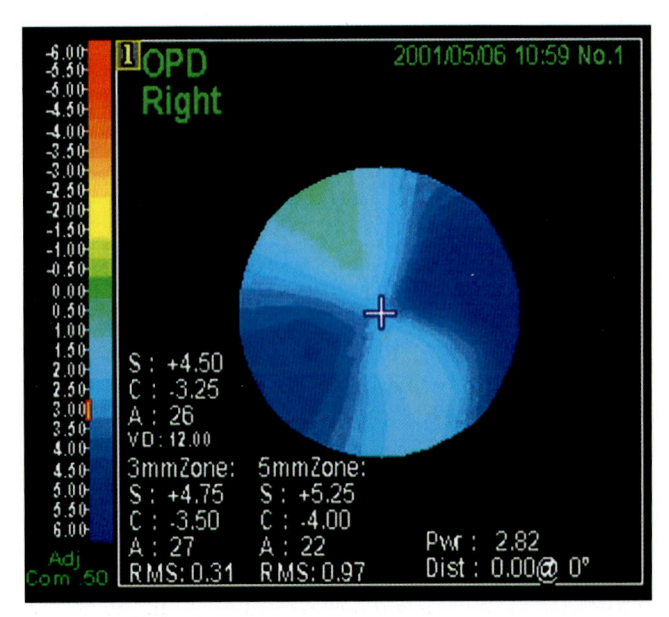

Figure 21.2C OPD map of a hyperopic astigmatism eye

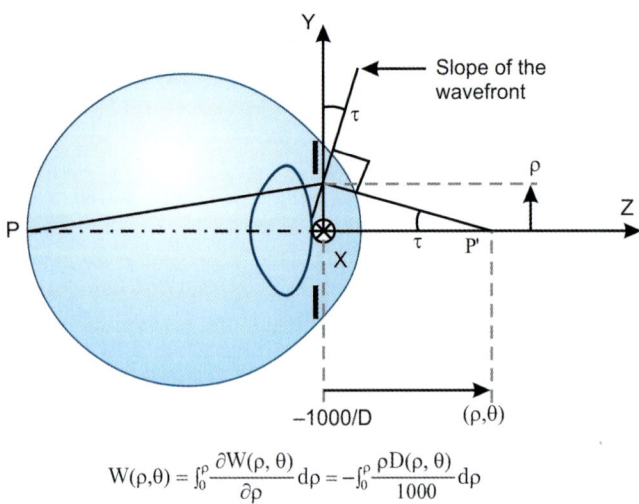

$$W(\rho,\theta) = \int_0^\rho \frac{\partial W(\rho, \theta)}{\partial \rho} d\rho = -\int_0^\rho \frac{\rho D(\rho, \theta)}{1000} d\rho$$

Figure 21.3 Conversion between wavefront aberration and refractive errors

refractive information compared to a conventional auto-refractometer that provides S, C and A data only.

OPD POWER MAP AND WAVEFRONT MAP

To explain how the OPD-Scan^R measures optical aberrations begins with the duality of light, and that light can be thought to propagate in waves. The wavefront is defined as a plane perpendicular to the direction in which light travels and deviations from the ideal wavefront are termed wavefront errors and these errors tell us about the optical properties of the system. To illustrate this point consider the diagram in **Figure 21.3**, which shows a simplified schematic eye with light reflected back out of the eye, from a single point P on the retina. For a perfectly emmetropic eye, the exiting wavefront will be a plane wave perpendicular to the Z-axis. However in this case, the eye is myopic, so the wavefront converges to a point P' where it intersects the reference axis. The difference in slope between the wavefront and the ideal wavefront allows the construction of the wavefront error map for multiple discrete points. The difference is often described using Zernike polynomials with each coefficient relating to a particular type of aberration such as Defocus, Astigmatism, Coma, Trefoil and so on[4]. Thus, one can tell the type and amount of aberrations that the eye produces. This information is useful for comparing preoperative and postoperative changes in ocular aberration quantitatively.

OPD MAP AND CORNEAL TOPOGRAPHY MAP

This section describes one example in which a comparison between corneal topography and OPD map provides new information. **Figure 21.4** illustrates the OPD map of total ocular refraction and the corneal refractive power map among corneal topographic maps for the same eye. The corneal refractive map illustrates the distribution of corneal refractive powers calculated by Snell's law showing corneal astigmatism of about 2 D. The OPD map on the left reveals total refractive astigmatism of 0.5 D at most with the difference being most likely due to crystalline lens astigmatism perpendicular to and therefore canceling the corneal astigmatism of 2 D. Quite clearly the full corneal astigmatism of 2 D should not be corrected whether it be by contact lenses or refractive surgery. To surgically correct refractive error demands an understanding of both the total

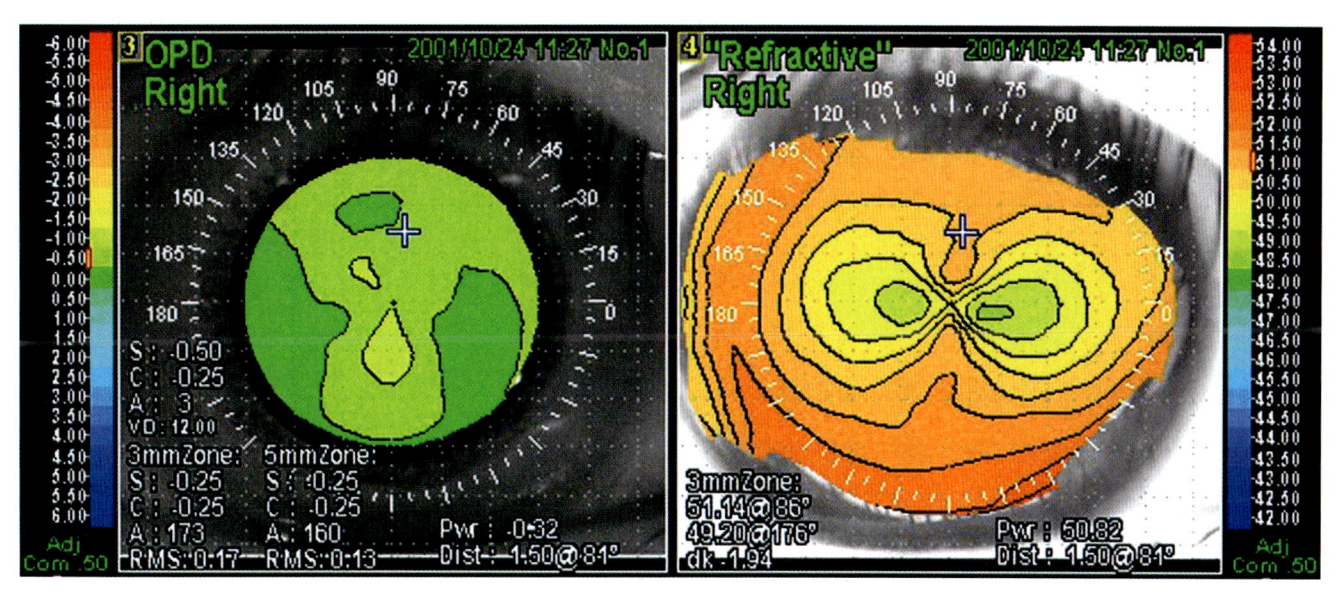

Figure 21.4 OPD map of total ocular refraction and corneal topography map for the same eye

ocular refractive status and the corneal surface ensuring a quick and correct diagnosis. The change in total refraction can be converted into an equivalent change in corneal surface shape and power. The Target Refractive map, method of calculating a shape of ablation, is obtained by adding the ocular refractive error map as measured by the OPD, to the corneal refractive power map. Either of them can be optically calculated from each other, but Axial and Instantaneous maps among topography maps cannot be calculated directly from the OPD map.

Relational expression: Refractive + OPD ≈ Target Refractive

ALIGNING TOPOGRAPHY DATA WITH OPD DATA

The abovementioned Target Refractive maps merge corneal information (Refractive) and total refractive information (OPD). It is important to avoid problems due to any change in eye alignment when moving from one device to another when collecting total ocular refraction data and corneal topography data. This potential problem is overcome with the OPD-scan by incorporating the two devices within the one instrument. The OPD-Scan^R compensates for any positional shift between the Refractive map and OPD map by determining the location of the First Purkinje images its reference point.

MEASUREMENT OF PUPILLARY DIAMETER

The OPD-Scan^R can measure the diameter and center position for both Photopic and Scotopic pupils as shown in **Figure 21.5**. To prevent halos and glare, the ablated area should be outside the nighttime dilated pupil. It would be ideal to compare a pupil image exposed to the laser with Photopic and Scotopic pupil diameters and respective pupil centers, and to align the laser axis with Scotopic pupil center. To avoid halo and glare due to poorly sized optical zones, the ablated area should be larger than the pupil under Scotopic conditions.

FINAL FIT SOFTWARE: OUTLINE AND FEATURES

The Final Fit Software is designed to calculate ablation profile through analysis of both topography and OPD data obtained by the OPD-Scan^R and generation of exact laser pulse shot data that controls the laser delivery system such as the movable apertures with the Nidek EC5000CX II refractive laser. With the Final Fit Software, the ablation profile data is divided into three components, as shown in **Figure 21.6**, so that they correspond to the ablation mechanism of the EC-5000CXII. Radially symmetric components are ablated by scanning and rotating the rectangular laser beam controlled by the opening and closing of a diaphragm, linearly symmetric components are ablated by the laser beam controlled by the opening and closing of a slit mask, and irregular components are divided into small spots of 1 mm in diameter and ablated respectively, Multi Point Ablation.

The Final Fit software also displays preoperative and postoperative topography maps at the upper part of the screen, allowing the operator to optimize the conditions for operation such as the amount of correction, Optical Zone (OZ) and Transition Zone (TZ) for each eye (**Figure 21.6**).

Figure 21.5 By aligning a bright corneal reflex of Photopic pupil image with that of Scotopic pupil image, it is possible to display the each pupil diameter, pupil center, and the distance between both pupil centers

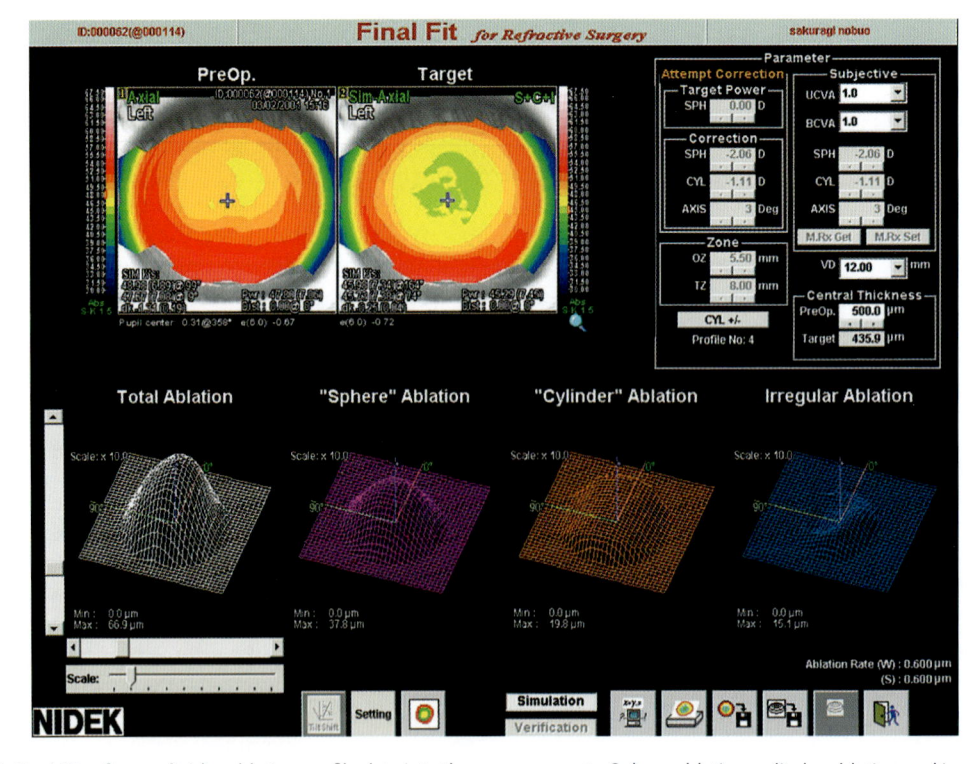

Figure 21.6 Final Fit software divides ablation profile data into three components; Sphere ablation, cylinder ablation and irregular ablation

Customized Ablation

With the Final Fit software, the following ablation modes are available:

OZ
1. Spherical

TZ
OATZ * OATZ (Optimized Aspherical Transition Zone)

2. Topo-guided   OATZ
3. Wavefront-guided OATZ

Spherical with OATZ Ablation

Spherical with OATZ ablation allows for customized ablation surgery in the periphery of the cornea to reduce nighttime halo, glare and the possible resultant decrease in contrast sensitivity. With the customized ablation method, spherical lenses and cylindrical lenses are ablated in accordance with the amount of correction in the optical zone (OZ), and the ablated surface is smoothly connected with the non-ablated periphery of the cornea through the transition zone (TZ), This is to reduce nighttime halo, glare and a decrease in contrast sensitivity thought to be caused by abrupt changes in shape in the TZ.[5] The TZ shape can be determined by selecting the appropriate profile in Final Fit Software.

The Instantaneous corneal topography map is ideal for grasping subtle changes in corneal shape because the map better represents local corneal shape. **Figure 21.7** shows that the position of the red ring representing the area with abrupt change in curvature changes with each power profile. As the profile moves up from a to c, the red ring moves to the periphery of the cornea, increasing the OZ and increasing the depth of ablation.

Topo-guided Customized Ablation

Topo-guided with OATZ ablation allows customized ablation for correcting pathological or postoperative corneal irregularities, such as decentered ablations. With the Topo-guided ablation method, the larger irregularities are removed first. This ablation method allows the operator to ablate corneal irregularities with the minimum ablation depth. In these cases manifest refraction results can be unreliable but by removing much of the irregularities and then re-measuring and re-analyze the eye with the OPD-Scan superior results can be achieved.

Wavefront-guided Customized Ablation

Unlike some other wavefront analyzers, which calculate ablation depth directly from the amount of aberration, the OPD-Scan calculates ablation depth from what is required to change corneal surface power. As mentioned earlier, the preoperative refractive map and OPD map are used to generate the Target Refractive map, as well as corneal elevation data and the difference between the data used to determine the shape of ablation.

Wavefront-guided ablation allows for the display of an aberration-free area (OD) and to optimize the transition zone. The wavefront-guided ablation method is intended to reduce the amount of aberrations in the entire treatment zone (OZ + TZ). Although the above explanation presumes a target refractive endpoint of emmetropia, this can be programmed to achieve various levels of emmetropia as desired for example –1 D of myopia.

Features of the Final Fit Software

The features of the Final Fit are listed below:

Safety

- Preoperative and postoperative simulated topography data allows an estimation of postoperative outcome.
- The three ablation modes, normal (spherical lens)/topo-guided/wavefront-guided ablation are selectable according to the eye to be operated on.

Quality of Vision

- Vision quality can be enhanced by a smooth TZ with an OATZ (Optimized Aspherical Transition Zone).
- The comparison function allows the operator to display preoperative, and postoperative topography map, the OPD map, and differential maps.

Evaluation of Postoperative Outcome

- The topography data of the entire cornea and pupil contour displayed allows the operator to easily check the positional

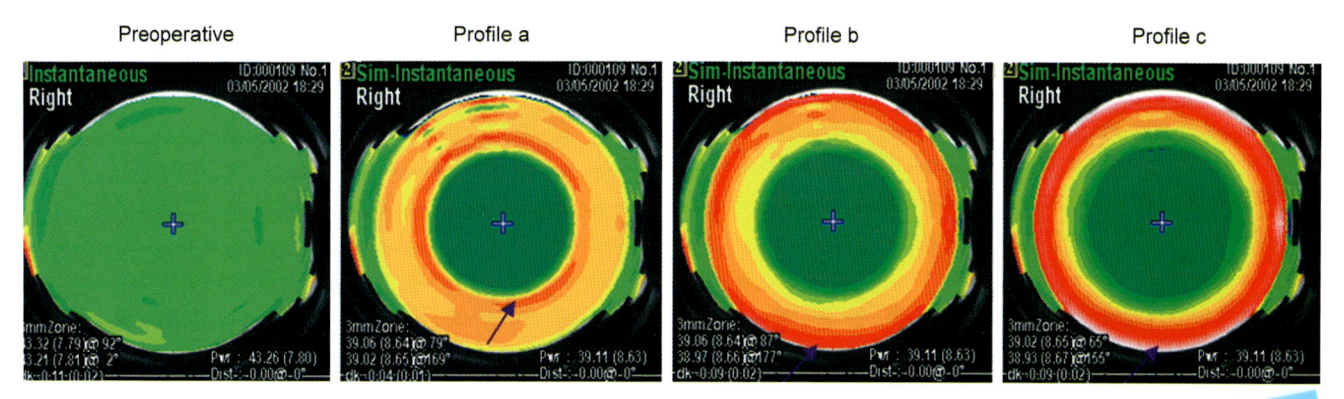

Figure 21.7 As the profile moves up from a to c, the red ring (indicated by "↑") moves outward, the OZ and ablation depth increase. PMMA model eye; Hemisphere, 43.27 D (7.8 mm), Parameter; Sph:-5 D, Cyl:0 D, OZ:5.0 mm, TZ:9.0 mm, Ablation rate: 0.3 um/shot

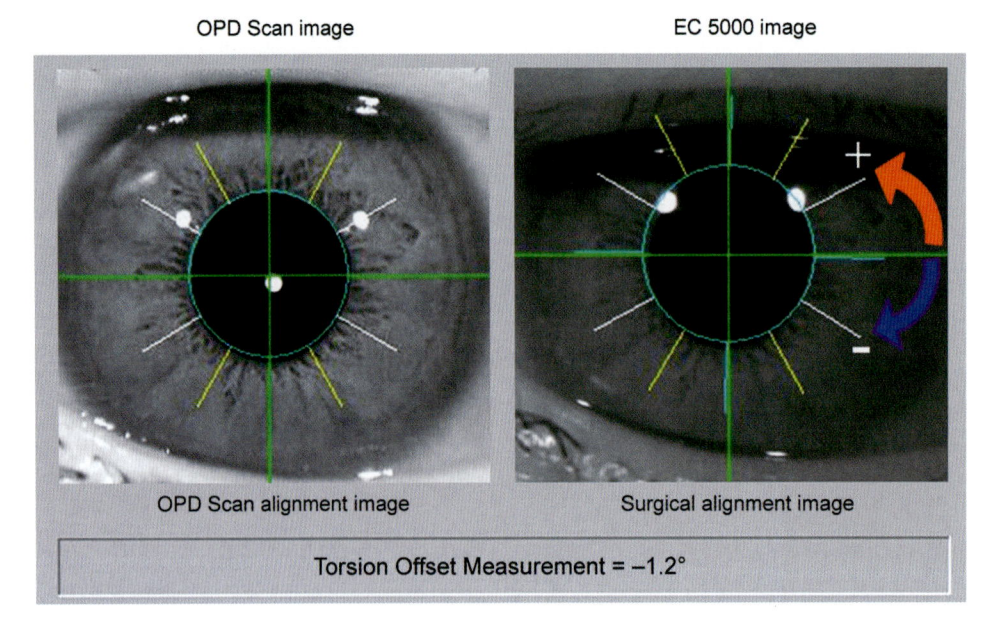

Figure 21.8 Torsion offset measurement calculated from eye images taken by OPD scan and EC-5000CXII

relationship between the treatment area and pupil, and distribution of powers. In addition, the OPD map allows the operator to check the distribution of refractive errors within a pupil (This is also available with the OPD-Scan).

Correction of Cyclo-Torsion

Little attention has been previously given to the possible shift of cylinder axis due to cyclotorsional rotation of the eye and many ophthalmic devices measure patients in the upright sitting position whereas during refractive surgery, the patient is in a recumbent position.[6] For this reason, when using the data obtained by the OPD-Scan in corneal refractive surgery, the eye rotation caused by this counter-rolling of the eyeball must be compensated. The OPD-Scan^R analyzes iris pattern, pupil contour, pupil center and pupil size by capturing anterior eye images just after topography measurement. The pupil position information is then used for image registration and alignment as part of the Final Fit calculations. The Final Fit Software generates ablation profiles and sends this together with the iris image registration data to the excimer laser system.

The iris image of the patient's eye lying on a bed will be captured by CCD camera installed in EC-5000CXII laser system and then pupil center is calculated. Pupil center will also be determined against the iris image obtained by OPD Scan. Similar distinctive iris patterns will be detected from both iris images. The angle for some distinctive iris pattern will be measured from the baseline, which will go through each Pupil center and the angle difference between both images will be torsional angle error as shown in **Figure 21.8**.

REFERENCES

1. MacRae S, Fujieda M. Customized ablation using the NIDEK Laser, customized corneal ablation. Slack. 2001;17:211-17.
2. Campbell CE, Benjamin WJ, Howland HC. Objective refraction: Retinoscopy, autorefraction and photorefraction, In: Benjamin W J, Borlish I M. Borish's Clinical Refraction. Saunders, 1998;18: 594-600.
3. Thibos LN, Applegate RA. Assessment of Optical Quality Customized Corneal Ablation: The Quest for SuperVision. Slack Incorporated, New Jersey, USA, 2001.
4. Thibos LN, Applegate RA, Schwiegerling JT, Webb R, et al. Standards for Reporting the Optical Aberrations of Eyes. Vision Science and Its Applications (OSA Trends in Optics and Photonics, Vol. 35), 232-44, Optical Society of America, Washington, DC, 2000.
5. Wachler BS, Durrie DS, Assil KK, Krueger RR. Role of clearance and treatment zones in contrast sensitivity: significance in refractive surgery. J Cataract Refract Surg. 1999;25 NO.1:16-23.
6. Miller EF, Counter-rolling of the human eyes produced by head tilt with respect to gravity. Acta Otolaryngol. 1962;54:479-501.

Section V

Refractive Procedures and Conditions

CHAPTERS

22. Post-LASIK Iatrogenic Ectasia
23. Decentered Ablations
24. Irregular Astigmatism: LASIK as a Correcting Tool
25. Posterior Chamber ICL and Toric ICL
26. Nidek OPD Scan in Clinical Practice

Chapter 22

Post-LASIK Iatrogenic Ectasia

Melania Cigales (Spain), Jairo Hoyos-Chacón (Spain), Jairo E Hoyos (Spain)

INTRODUCTION

Iatrogenic ectasia may manifest months or years after LASIK surgery in the form of topographic steepening causing progressive myopia together with irregular astigmatism and loss of visual acuity. With an incidence ranging between 0.12 and 0.8 % according to the different series in the literature[1-4] post-LASIK ectasia is an uncommon, but potentially visually disabling complication.

The source of the ectasia may be a subclinical keratoconus that goes undetected during the preoperative examination and is then decompensated as a result of induced corneal thinning. There are cases where there is no prior corneal disorder and ectasia results from excess corneal thinning during surgery. Although ectasia has been described since the early implementation of lamellar techniques for refractive surgery,[5] in recent years, limits to surgical corneal thickness have become more stringent and important advances have been made in preoperative diagnostic tools used for detecting diseased corneas that may lend themselves to this complication. We will analyze risk factors and treatments for post-LASIK iatrogenic corneal ectasia.

SUBCLINICAL KERATOCONUS

Corneal ectatic degenerations **(Figure 22.1)** such as keratoconus and pellucid marginal degeneration are caused by corneal thinning leading to progressive corneal steepening, progressive myopia, irregular astigmatism and, eventually, reduced visual acuity.

In the initial phases, ectatic degenerations usually show a normal biomicroscopic appearance with the only symptom being a visual defect that cannot be properly corrected with spectacles. Topography is usually the examination of choice for detecting early curvature changes **(Figure 22.2)**. Pachymetry may also be used for measuring corneal thinning, long before it can be seen under the slit-lamp; however, because of significant variability among normal subjects, it is an elusive diagnosis. Since the early years of refractive surgery, ectatic degenerations of the cornea have been known to be a counterindication for surgery, but the challenge lies in the ability to arrive at a clear diagnosis. It has been reported[6] that close to 6% of patients coming for refractive surgery are rejected because of a forme fruste keartoconus that might result in post-LASIK corneal ectasia. In 1946, Amsler[7] offered one of the initial descriptions of forme fruste keratoconus (FFKC). Since then, many more diagnostic tools have been developed and much knowledge has been gained for diagnosing this disease.

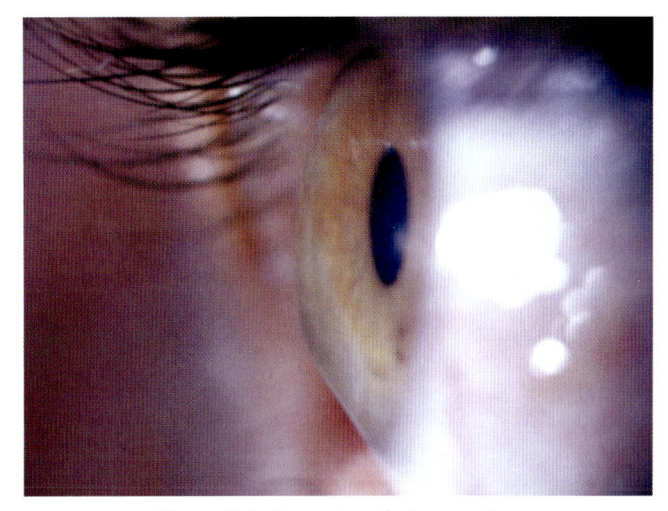

Figure 22.1 Corneal ectatic degeneration

The preoperative examination provides information that may suggest the presence of a forme fruste keratoconus as a risk factor for post-LASIK iatrogenic ectasia.

Clinical History

Etiological factors associated with keratoconus are also predisposing factors for post-LASIK ectasia. Keratoconus is usually idiopathic and is not associated with race or sex, although there is a group of cases that follow an inheritance pattern, and there are descriptions of keratoconus associated with atopia.[8] Even in the absence of atopia, the incidence of keratoconus has been found to be greater in patients with chronic persistent eye-rubbing.[9] Hence, the need to ask patients interested in refractive surgery about potential family history of keratoconus or a personal history of atopia or chronic eye-rubbing, considering the higher risk of postoperative corneal ectasia.

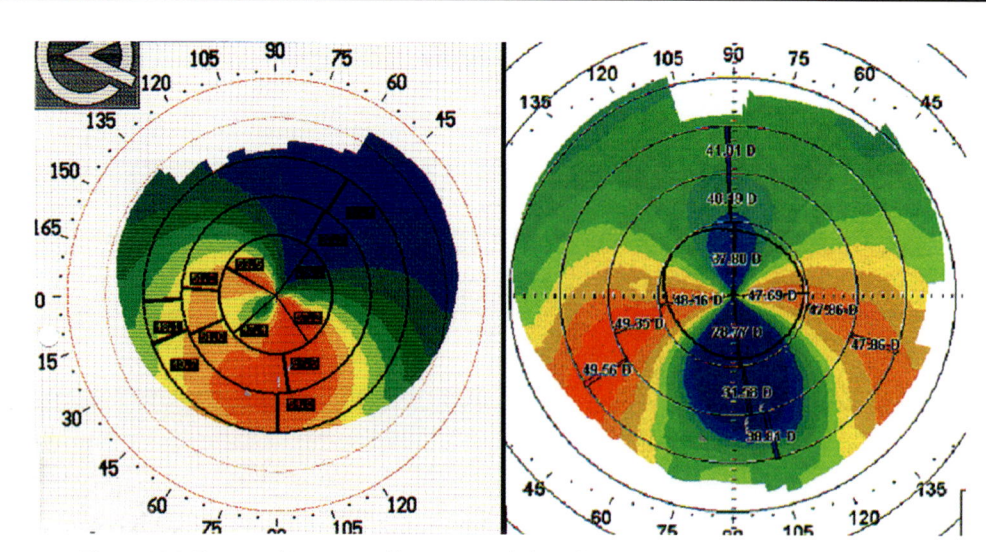

Figure 22.2 Topographic images of keratoconus (left) and pellucid marginal degeneration (right)

Refraction

While current technological breakthroughs have led to sophisticated diagnostic systems for detecting early signs of keratoconus, we must not forget the important information derived from the basic ophthalmological examination. For instance, even in very early stages of keratoconus, it is possible to see the scissor reflex on retinoscopy or the oil droplet sign through a dilated pupil with back-illumination.[10] Moreover, keratoconus must be suspected in those cases where 20/20 vision is not attained with best refraction and there is no logical explanation for this usually mild form of amblyopia.

Anterior Corneal Curvature

The best system to study anterior corneal curvature is computer-assisted topographic analysis of videokeratoscopic images. When there is an established keratoconus, the topographic image provides a clear diagnosis (see **Figure 22.2**). But topography may also reveal subtle signs, not diagnostic of keratoconus by themselves but, when added together in the same patient, especially if associated with other findings, may lead to the diagnosis of FFKC.

The most common suspicious topographic findings on the anterior curvature include:[2,11,12]
1. Corneal curvature greater than 47 D.
2. Asymmetry between inferior and superior curvatures (I-S), where the inferior curvature is 1.4 D greater than the superior curvature **(Figure 22.3)**.
3. Skew of steepest radial axes (SRAX) greater than 20° in corneas with astigmatism greater than 1.5 D **(Figure 22.4)**.
4. Difference in central corneal power between fellow eyes greater than 1 D.
5. Distance between the apex and the center of the cornea greater than 1 mm.

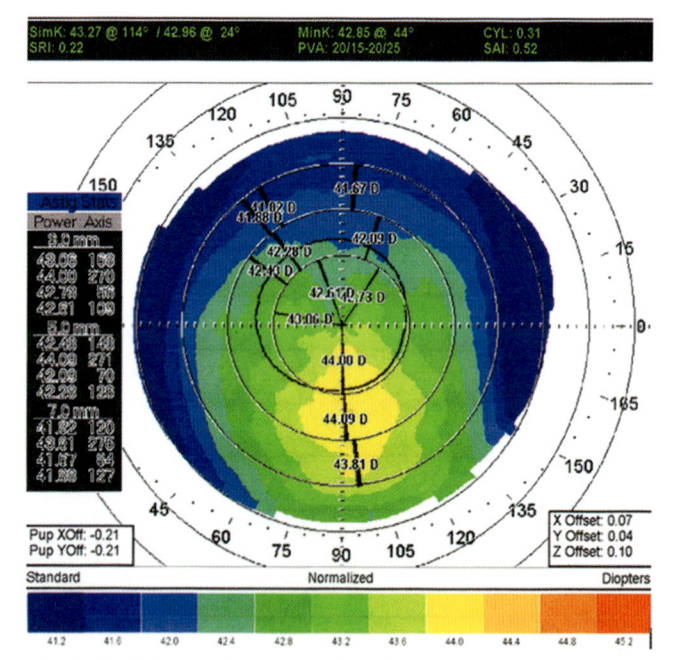

Figure 22.3 Asymmetry between the inferior and superior curvatures, with a difference greater than 1.4 D

The combination of different quantitative topographic indices including central diopter value (central K), simulated keratometry (Sim K), inferosuperior asymmetries (I-S), nasal-temporal asymmetry and skewed radial axis value (SRAX), may help with the early diagnosis of keratoconus.[13] There are new programs for topographic detection of keratoconus using quantitative measurements, including the Rabinowitz, Klyce/Maeda o Smolek/Klyce methods. Using these software packages for analyzing suspicious topographic readings it is possible to recognize early signs or keratoconus and FFKC.

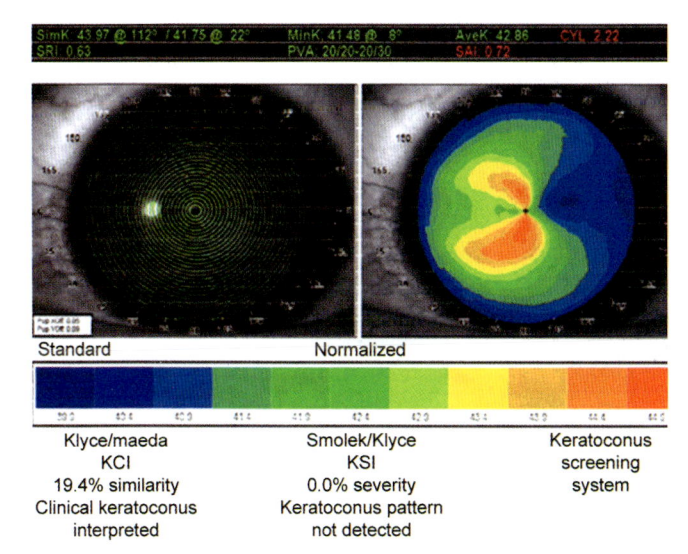

Figure 22.4 Angulation of radial axes (SRAX = skewed radial axis) in a cornea with normal curvature (Sim 43,97/41,75) and 2,22 D cylinder. The keratoconus screening system using clinical keratoconus Interpreted Klyce/Maeda (KCI) shows a 19.4% similarity

Faced with an irregular or suspicious topographic image, it is mandatory to rule out contact lens-induced corneal warpage.[14] Contact lens-induced topographical abnormalities of the cornea include central irregular astigmatism, loss of radial symmetry, reversal of the normal topographic pattern of progressive flattening of corneal contour from the center to the periphery, and keratoconus-like images **(Figure 22.5)**.[15] Contact lens wear should be discontinued before refractive surgery and should any topographic signs of corneal warpage be observed, they must be followed until they normalize.[16] In the event topographic signs do not normalize, a forme fruste keratoconus must be suspected and surgery must be discouraged.

Posterior Corneal Elevation

The topographer has become an indispensable diagnostic system in corneal refractive surgery. At first, Placid ring-based topographers offered the possibility of analyzing the anterior surface of the cornea almost to its full extent. Elevation topographers that measure the height of different points on the cornea in relation to a perfect sphere came about years later. One of the first elevation topographers was the PAR System[17] that analyzed the elevation of the anterior surface of the cornea by means of a grid projection. But the advent of the Orbscan (Bausch and Lomb, Rochester NY)[18] **(Figure 22.6)** based on a slit scan created a whole new concept in corneal analysis—the study of the posterior surface. In keratoconus posterior surface abnormalities may be present, even before significant changes are seen on the anterior surface, and keratoconus is suspected in cases with a posterior surface elevation greater than 40 µm as measured by the Orbscan **(Figure 22.7)**.[19] New technologies have been developed in recent years for the study of the posterior surface of the cornea, including the Pentacam HR (Oculus Inc, Lynnwood WA) **(Figure 22.8)**, that uses a rotating Scheimpflug camera and appears to offer more accurate results.[20] In tests performed with the Pentacam, keratoconus is suspected with posterior surface elevations greater than 25 µm **(Figure 22.9)**.[21] Future studies will determine whether the Pentacam underestimates the posterior vault or if the Orbscan overestimates this height.

Preoperative Pachymetry

Most surgeons advice against corneal refractive surgery when the central corneal thickness is less than 480 microns. Today, even central thicknesses of less than 500 microns may be a risk factor for post-LASIK iatrogrenic ectasia.[22] A thin cornea in a patient seeking refractive surgery poses two problems. First, the

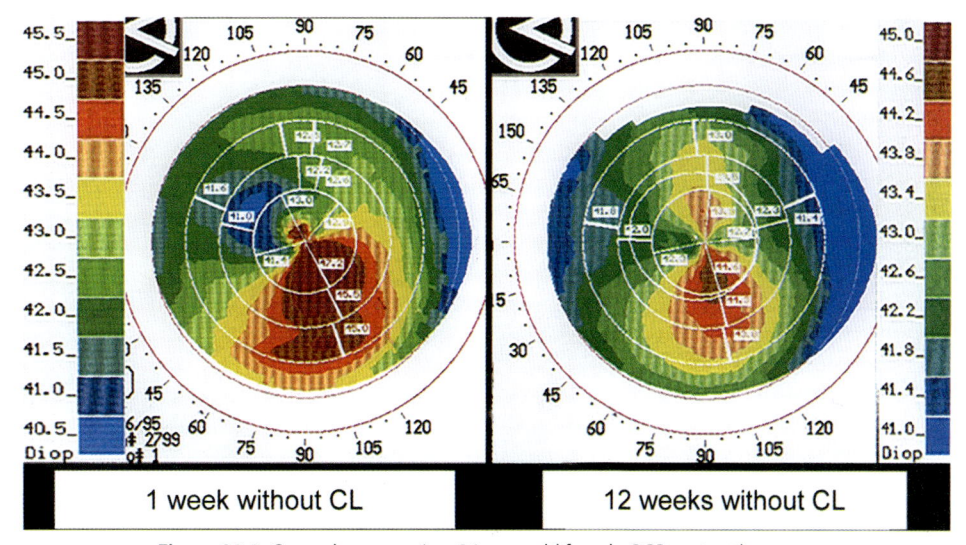

Figure 22.5 Corneal warpage in a 26 years old female, RGP contact lens wear (CL wearer for 10 years, 14 hours/day), with a topographic keratoconus-like image

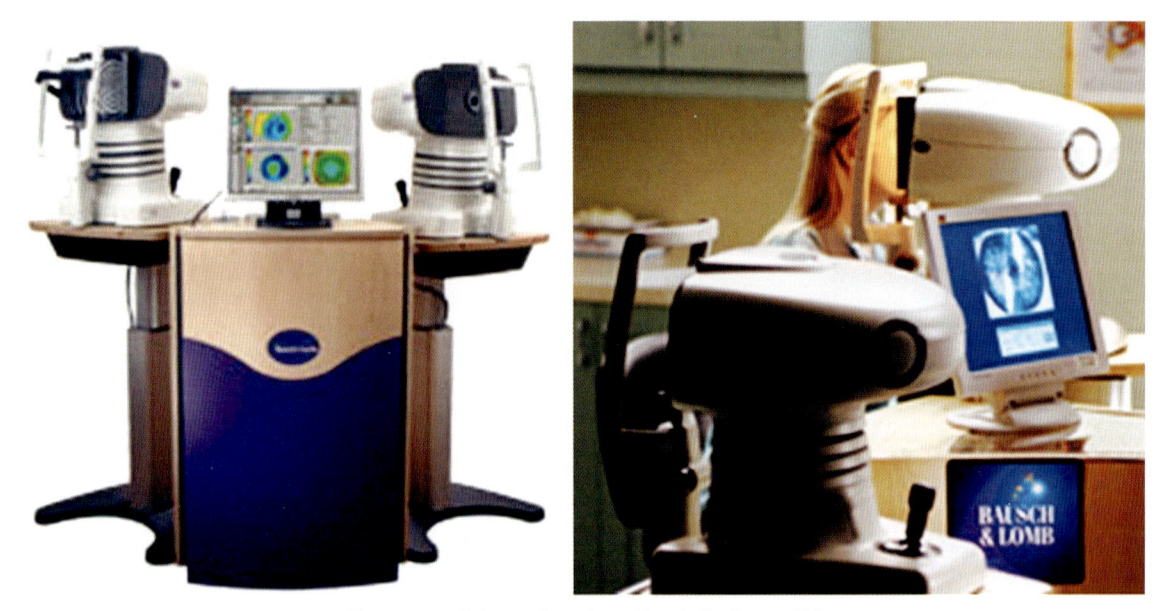

226 Section V: Refractive Procedures and Conditions

Figure 22.6 Orbscan (Bausch and Lomb, Rochester NY)

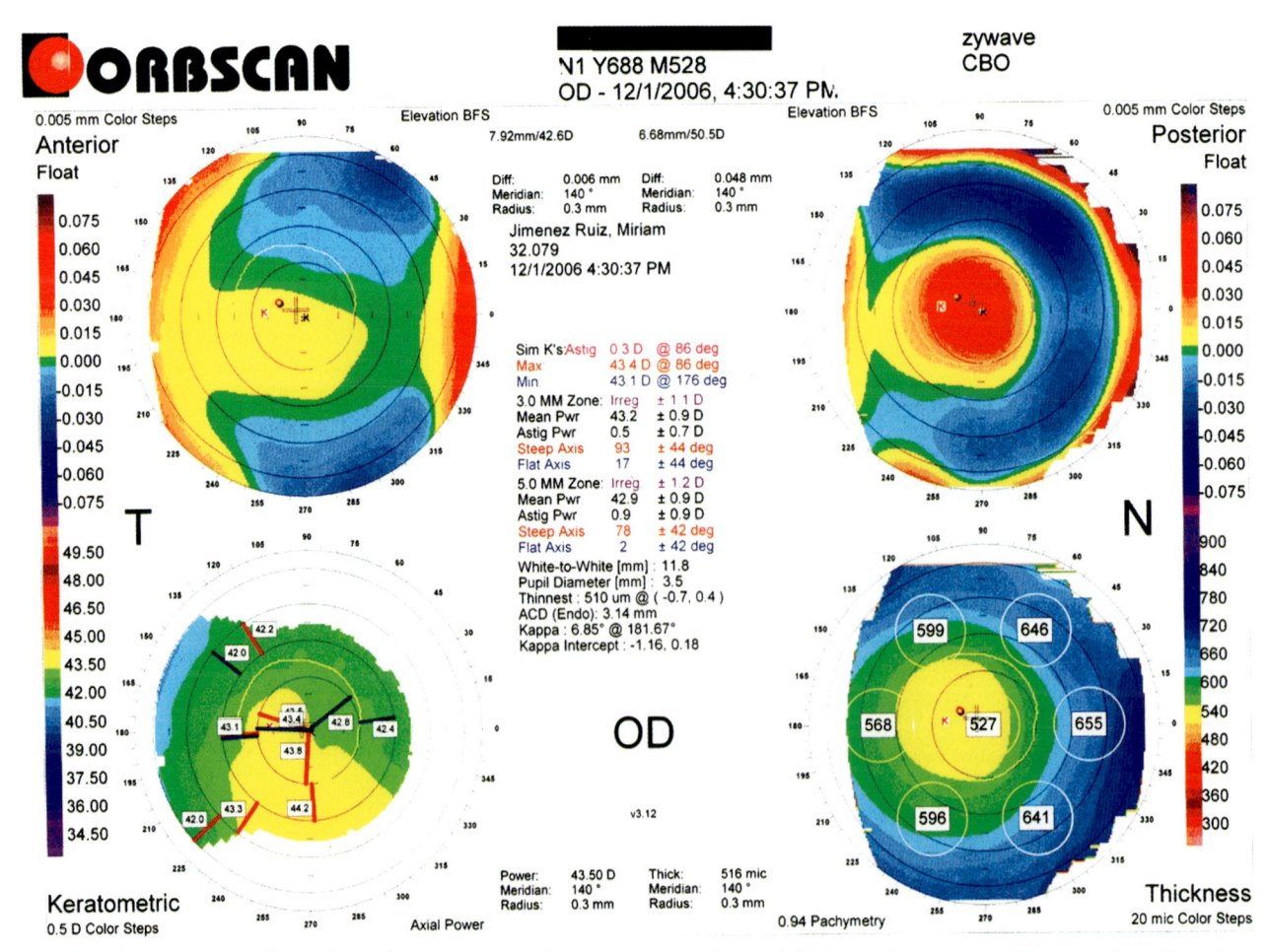

Figure 22.7 Orbscan topography in a forme fruste keratoconus. The curvature map (bottom left) shows I-S asymmetry with a posterior surface elevation (top right) of 48 microns; the pachymetric map (bottom right) shows apical eccentricity. This patient was refused for refractive surgery with a −1,5 D of refraction and 20/15 of BCVA

Chapter 22: Post-LASIK Iatrogenic Ectasia   227

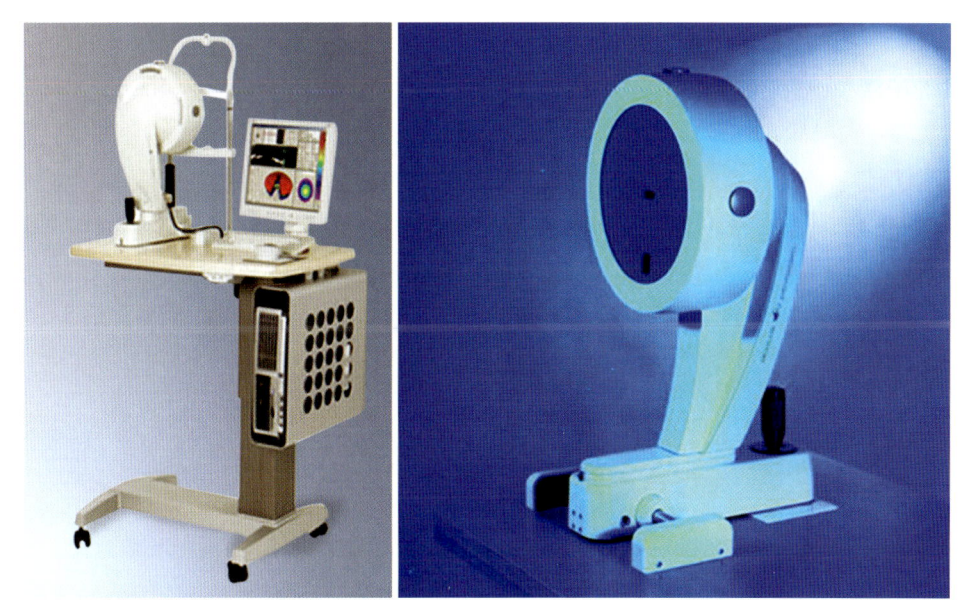

Figure 22.8 Pentacam (Oculus Inc, Lynnwood WA)

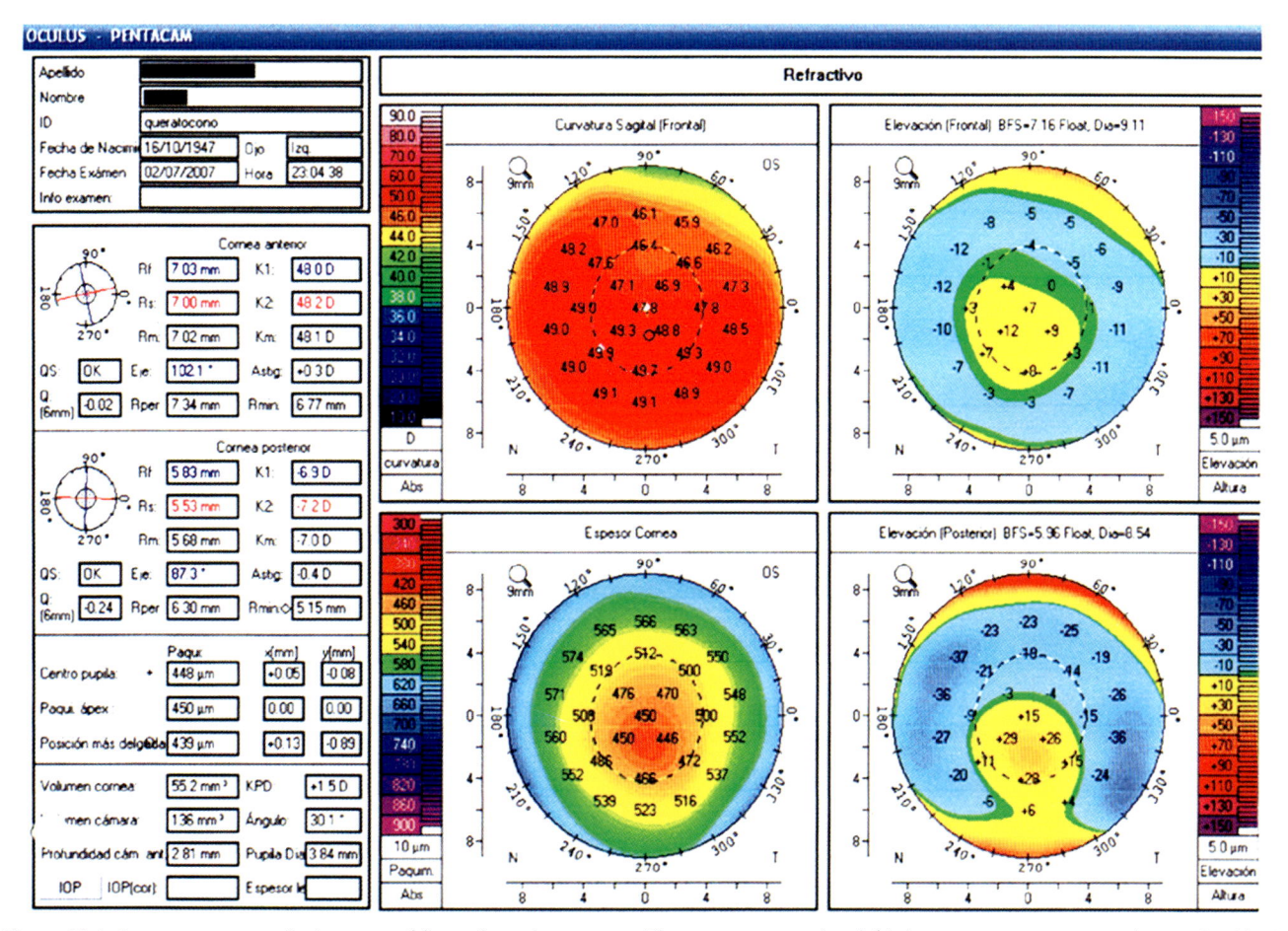

Figure 22.9 Pentacam topography in a case of forme fruste keratoconus. The curvature map (top left) shows a curvature greater than 47 D with I-S asymmetry and a posterior surface elevation (bottom right) of 29 microns; the pachymetric map (bottom left) shows a thin, 450-micron cornea with apical eccentricity. The option of refractive surgery was abandoned in this case with a low refraction (−1,5 −1,25 x 100°) and BCVA of 20/15

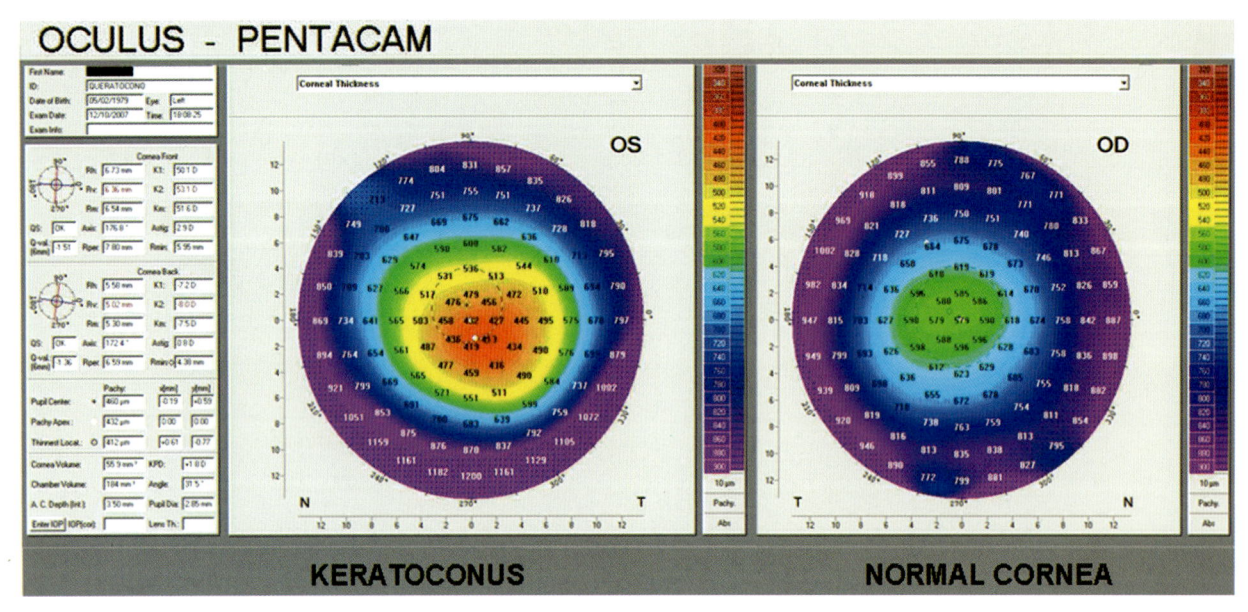

Figure 22.10 Pachymetric map of keratoconus with a thin cornea and a displacement of the thinnest point towards the inferior temporal area. A normal pachymetric map is shown on the right

corneal thickness may be insufficient for correcting ametropia and still respecting the limits of corneal thickness in order to avoid iatrogenic ectasia. Second, a thin cornea may be due to a previous subclinical ectatic disease (keratoconus or pellucid marginal degeneration), and refractive surgery may induce a decompensation. Progressive corneal thinning is common to all ectatic degenerations of the cornea. In keratoconus, corneal thinning is usually central or inferior paracentral, and in pellucid degeneration it is inferiorly located 1 to 2 mm from the limbus.

It is normally assumed that the thinnest portion of the cornea, used as reference for the surgical calculations, is at the center. When the thinnest point of the cornea is not central and, moreover, when it coincides with the steepest anterior curvature and the greatest elevation of the posterior surface, a forme fruste keratoconus must be suspected **(Figure 22.10)**.[19,20] For this reason, aside from determining central corneal thickness during the preoperative examination, a pachymetric map of the entire cornea must be obtained. Ultrasound pachymetry is the most accurate method for measuring corneal thickness, but it is not useful for obtaining a pachymetric map. Although the Orbscan and the Pentacam provide slightly higher corneal thicknesses than those measured by ultrasound, they offer valuable information in the form of a pachymetric map that can help detect FFKC.[23]

Corneal Hysteresis

Corneal hysteresis is a new parameter used to describe the biomechanical strength or elasticity of the cornea. This concept

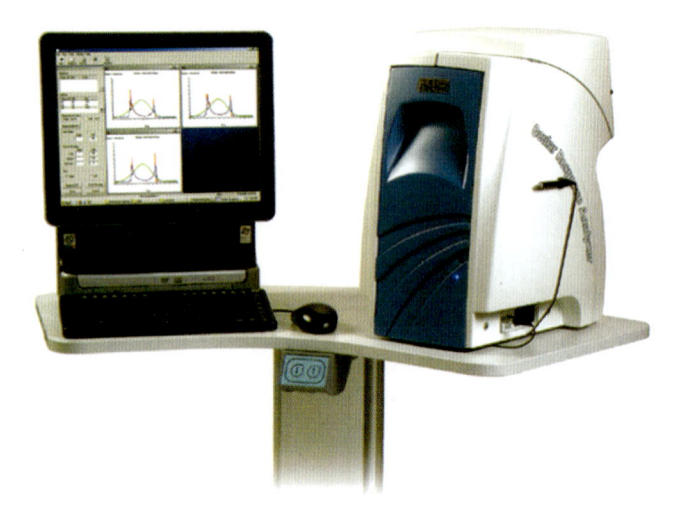

Figure 22.11 Ocular Response Analyzer (ORA; Reichert Ophthalmic Instruments, New York, USA), for measuring corneal hysteresis (CH)

is based on the Ocular Response Analyzer technology (ORA) **(Figure 22.11)**, and uses a rapid air pulse on the cornea. Due to its biomechanical properties, the cornea offers resistance to the air pulse causing a delay in its inward and outward flattening motion and creating two different values. Corneal hysteresis (CH) is the difference between these two pressure values and it measures the properties of the corneal tissues as a result of the cornea's elastic depression. Corneal hysteresis (CH) is low in keratoconus and, theoretically, normal corneas with CH values lower than the mean may be at a higher risk of developing post-LASIK ectasia.[24]

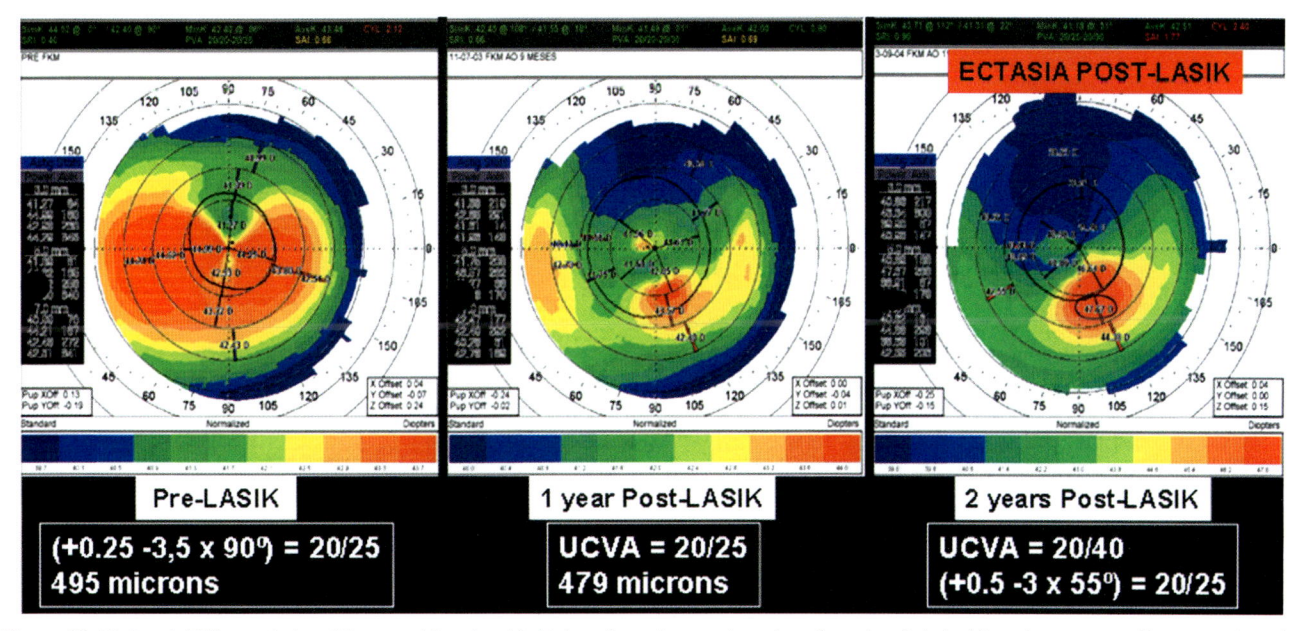

Figure 22.12 Post-LASIK ectasia in a 24 years old male with high astigmatism against the rule and a slightly thinned-out cornea. Two years into the postoperative period, the patient came back complaining of reduced vision, and ectasia was diagnosed. Examining the preoperative topography we can see that the steep astigmatic axis is slightly inferior, there is I-S asymmetry and the cornea is slightly thin in what is a condition consistent with forme fruste keratoconus

Post-LASIK Ectasia in FFKC

Patients who are candidates for LASIK surgery must be worked-up rigorously and carefully in order to avoid iatrogenic ectasia. Most of the reported cases[25,26] had preoperative topographic and/or clinical evidence of forme fruste keratoconus (FFKC), frank keratoconus or pellucid marginal degeneration. There is a growing amount of data on FFKC explaining many post-LASIK ectasias. When faced with an unexplained ectasia, it is important to revisit the preoperative topography in search for any missed signs of subclinical keratoconus **(Figures 22.12 and 22.13)**. **Table 22.1** shows a list of factors that may lead to the suspicion of subclinical keratoconus.

CORNEAL THICKNESS LIMITS

In the absence of prior corneal disease, ectasia may occur when corneal thickness limits are exceeded during surgery. The residual stromal bed **(Figure 22.14)** is considered one of the most important thickness limits ever since JI Barraquer, in his early lamellar techniques, determined that 250 microns must remain behind the ablation in order to avoid iatrogenic ectasia.[5] Several studies report [1,27] that the amount of residual corneal thickness after ablation is critical to the development of post-LASIK ectasia and suggest that the 250 µm limit is safe. In 1996, the US Food and Drug Administration approved a residual stromal bed of 250 µm for LASIK.[28] In the event preoperative surgery planning suggests that the residual stromal bed might be less than 250 µm, PRK or phakic IOL must be recommended. In recent years, and as a result of the growing number of reported ectasias, some authors prefer to increase the limit to 300 microns.[3] Others argue that the residual bed is not a magic number and that what is really important is to leave at least 50 to 55% of the corneal thickness behind the ablation.[22] In any

Table 22.1 Factors for suspected subclinical keratoconus

- Family history of keratoconus
- Personal history of atopia or chronic eye-rubbing
- Retinoscopic scissor reflex and oil droplet sign
- Unexplained mild amblyopia
- Anterior corneal curvature >47 D
- I-S asymmetry with inferior steepening >1.4 D
- Skew of steepest radial axes (SRAX) greater than 20° in astigmatism >1.5 D
- Difference in central corneal power between fellow eyes >1 D
- Apex-to-central corneal distance greater than 1 mm
- Elevation of the posterior corneal surface >40 µm (Orbscan) or >25 µm (Pentacam)
- Thin cornea < 500 µm
- Eccentric location of the thinnest corneal point coinciding with the steepest point and the point of highest posterior surface elevation
- Reduced corneal hysteresis

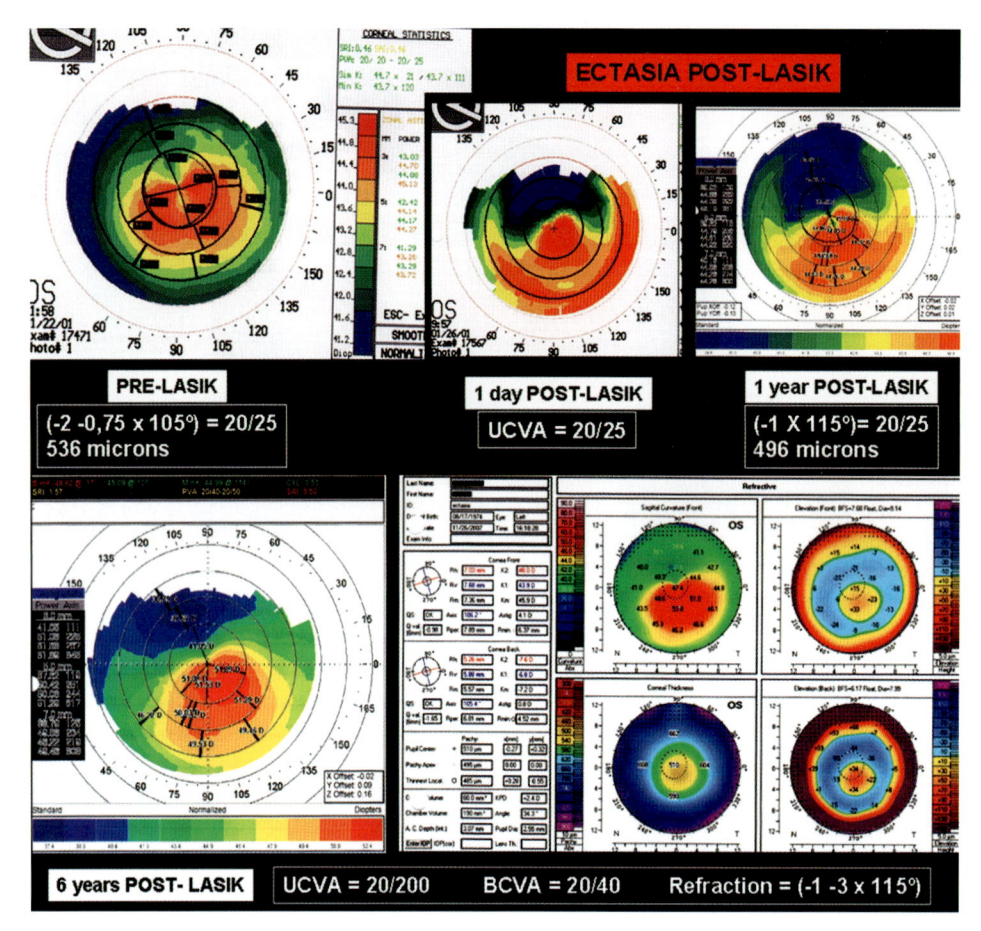

Figure 22.13 Twenty-six years old low myopic male patient with topographic signs of ectasia on the first postoperative day, despite good visual acuity. The patient maintained good visual acuity for 6 years. At that point, he came back complaining of diminished vision, and frank ectasia was diagnosed. The patient had a history of ocular allergy and a mild unexplained amblyopia had been found before surgery (only 20/25 with a refractive error of −2 −0.75 x 105º). Examining the preoperative topography, there is an I-S asymmetry despite a 44 D corneal curvature and a central pachymetry of 536 microns

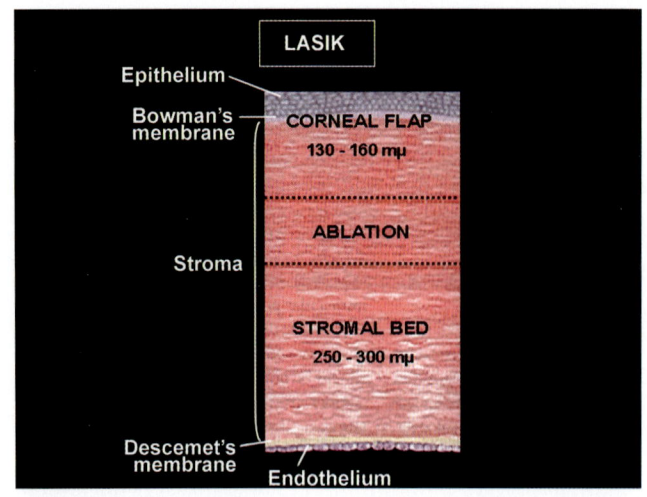

Figure 22.14 The thickness of the LASIK flap is 130–160 microns and includes epithelium, Bowman's membrane and anterior stroma. A stromal bed of at least 250–300 microns must remain under the ablation in order to avoid ectasia

event, a very deep ablation implies a risk factor. The causes for insufficient residual bed are thick flaps or excessive ablations.

Thick Flap

It is widely accepted by LASIK surgeons that the ideal flap thickness is 130 to 160 µm. However, the current trend is towards finer flaps of approximately 100 µm, in order to leave behind a maximum residual bed, thus reducing the risk of keratectasia. Flap thickness is determined by the microkeratome head or plate. However, several pachymetric studies[29] have indicated a high degree of variability in the thicknesses achieved. This variability is associated with corneal K readings, corneal exposure, blade condition and vibration speed, intraocular pressure when cutting, and blade quality.[30] Blade quality varies considerably and that is why it is crucial to check and calibrate the blade in order to set the GAP **(Figure 22.15)**. The GAP is the distance between the blade and plate, and correlates with the thickness of the keratectomy.[31] By calibrating the blades

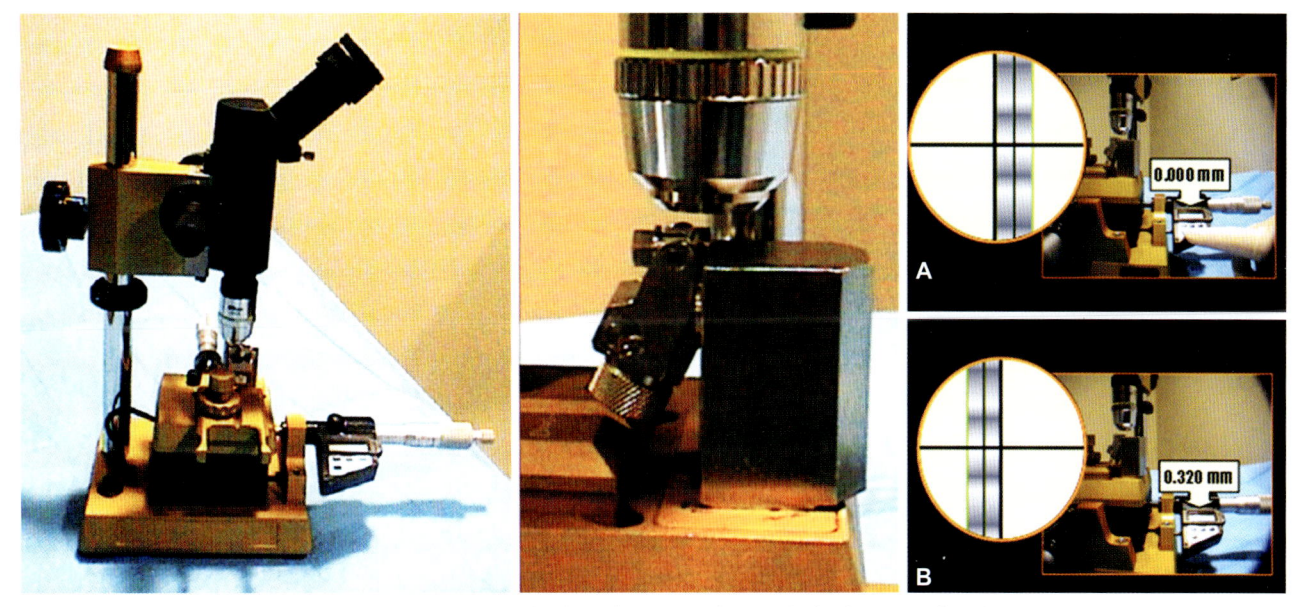

Figure 22.15 GAP measurement (the distance between the blade and plate correlates with the thickness of the keratectomy). The Magnum Diamond Micron-scope, designed to calibrate the RK knife, is useful for checking and calibrating the microkeratome blade. The microkeratome head, set up with the blade and a 160 μm plate, is placed under the microscope in a vertical position using a specially designed metal holder: (A) Using the microscope's controls, the vertical line on the eye piece is aligned with the front end of the blade in the image, and the micrometer's digital marker is set at zero; (B) Next, the same line is aligned with the end of the blade in the image and the digital micrometer indicates the measurement in microns. The image observed through the microscope corresponds to the blade and its mirror image, hence the need to divide it by two in order to obtain the blade GAP. In the picture, the micrometer indicates 320 μm and, therefore, the blade GAP is 160 μm

before using them it is possible to predict flap thickness more accurately in order to select the most appropriate blade for each case.

Some surgeons[26] without checking during surgery, assume that the flap is of the correct thickness, something that may explain some ectasias reported as unexplained. Given the great variability in flap thickness, it is incumbent upon us to perform intraoperative measurements in order to determine the thickness obtained. In the event the flap is found to be too thick, we are required to either to modify the optic zone of the ablation in order to maintain a sufficiently thick residual bed, or to abort the procedure. Subtraction ultrasonic pachymetry can provide quite an accurate estimate of flap thickness. This method measures corneal thickness in the center of the pupil after lifting the flap and subtracting this value from the value of the preoperative pachymetry.

It appears that the newer technologies for creating the flap-like the femtosecond laser—result in greater reproducibility of the flap, thus reducing the risk of iatrogenic ectasias due to exceedingly thick flaps.[32] However, it is fair to say that the femtosecond laser is not free of complications, not to mention its high cost.[33]

obtained in some cases and the rapid development of phakic IOLs led to the narrowing of the range of LASIK corrections. Recent studies have suggested that performing LASIK above –8 D is a risk factor for ectasia.[2,22] It has been speculated that the reason why ectasia develops is because the residual stromal bed is inadequate for sustaining the structural integrity of the cornea.[34] A review of the literature points to a higher incidence of post-LASIK iatrogenic ectasia in high corrections where large ablations are performed. However, there are retrospective studies of large series of LASIK in high myopia showing good stability in time when ablation diameters are decreased so as to ensure maximal preservation of the stromal bed thickness.[2,35] Notwithstanding good results, these studies conclude that high myopia has been considered a risk factor for post-LASIK ectasia, although adherence to proper screening and intraoperative pachymetry data appear to decrease the risk. Cases have been reported of ablations greater than 200 μm that went on to develop progressive ectasia, even after having preserved a 250 μm residual bed.[36] In our practice, we tend to leave a residual bed greater than 250 μm and we try to end with a total corneal thickness greater than 400 μm and not to perform ablations greater than 150 μm.

Large Ablation

Although in the early years of LASIK surgery people undertook to perform high myopic corrections, poor visual results

Retreatments

We must be particularly careful with post-LASIK retreatments and be fully aware of corneal thickness limits in order not to be surprised by the development of ectasia after retreating a small residual defect. Before choosing to retreat after LASIK we must ascertain refractive and topographic stability in order to establish the differential diagnosis between undercorrection and regression. Regression is usually the first symptom of ectasia, and a new ablation may accelerate the process. Moreover, it is important to know the available stromal bed and perform intraoperative pachymetry after lifting the flap, in the event that information is not available as part of the clinical history. There are reports[37] of greater corneal stability and a lower risk of ectasia when retreatment of small post-LASIK undercorrections is performed on the stromal surface of the flap. However, it is important to remember that the goal of refractive surgery, regardless of its modality, is not ametropia but greater independence from optical correction. Right patient selection is paramount in order to avoid the need for retreatments and the associated risk of ectasia.

KERATECTASIA TREATMENTS

The treatment for post-LASIK ectasia depends on the stage of the disease and the patient's needs and attitude. We can often suspect subclinical ectasia or post-LASIK ectatic progression when the patient experiences refractive regression with topographic steepening, while still maintainig best-corrected visual acuity with spectacles. At that stage, we may suspect a mild regression or early ectasia. External pressure applied on a thin cornea may trigger post-LASIK ectasia, as is the case of patients with chronic persistent eye-rubbing.[9] Patients with keratectasia must be made aware of the importance of not rubbing their eyes if they are to avoid rapid progression of the disease. There is even on report on bilateral ectasia resulting from ocular compression by the air-bag in a car accident.[38] Likewise, the effect of the internal intraocular pressure (IOP) on the thin cornea may cause topographic steepening and even transient ectasia when it rises above normal.[39] It has also been shown that when IOP is lowered with medications, even in normotensive patients, there is greater topographic corneal flattening **(Figure 22.16)**. Treatment with ocular pressure-lowering medications is indicated when the first signs of refractive regression and topographic steepening are observed, beside their use as initial treatment for post-LASIK ectasia.[40] Hypotensive drugs stabilize surgically-induced corneal flattening and they even revert small regressions and

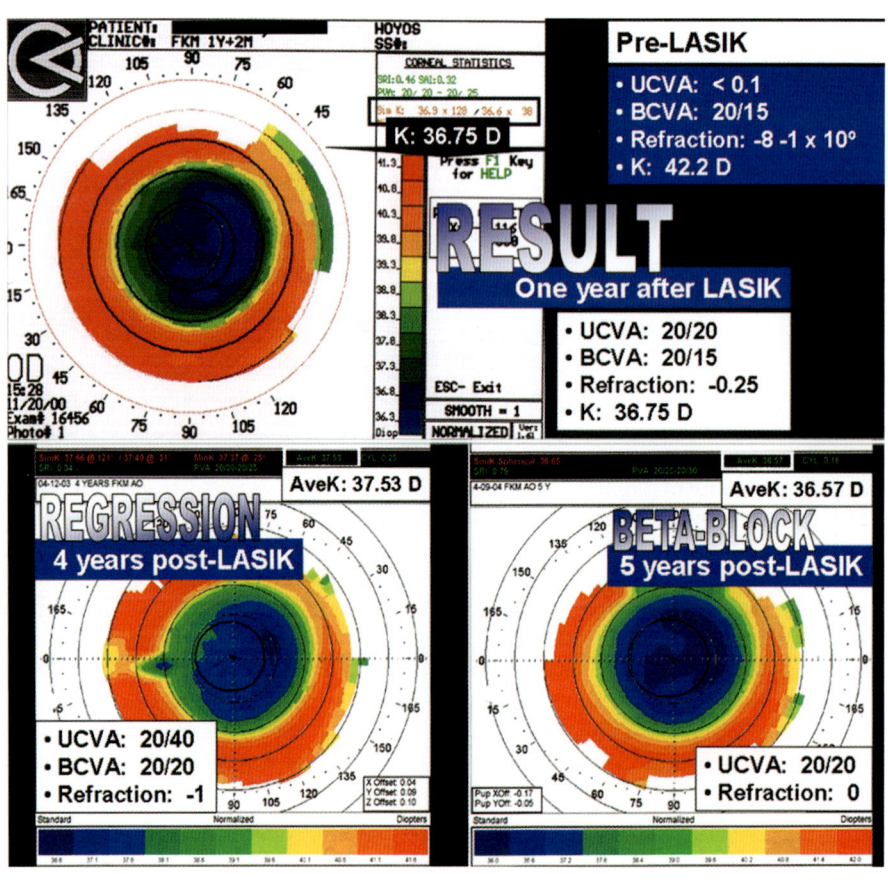

Figure 22.16 Intermediate myopic patient who presented with refractive regression of −1 D and topographic steepening (from 36.75–37.53 D) 4 years after LASIK. The use of topical beta-blockers for lowering intraocular pressure reduced the refractive error and the topographic steepening (from 37.53–36.57 D), stabilizing the cornea

topographic steepenings. The risk of ectasia could be reduced by maintaining a low IOP in LASIK patients, particularly those undergoing high corrections. In our experience, we have found that it is useful to prescribe topical beta-blockers in post-LASIK regressions with topographic steepening, which is not the case with the use of prostaglandin analogues.

On the other hand, visual acuity is compromised in cases of established ectasia. In very early stages, aside from prescribing ocular pressure-lowering agents, we also prescribe contact lenses or spectacles in order to restore visual acuity. Spectacles do not correct irregular astigmatism, a common finding in this complication, which explains why they do not provide good visual rehabilitation. As a result, the treatment of choice is contact lense fitting.[41] Early on, soft contact lenses may be appropriate, in particular in central ectasia. However, in more advanced stages, or in cases of paracentral ectasia, the resilient soft contact lens cannot compensate irregular astigmatism and, therefore, a rigid gas permeable contact (RGP) lens is required. RGP lenses allow for an optically regular surface and good visual acuity.[41] Hard-soft combination lenses (a rigid center with a soft annular ring) or piggy-back (a rigid lens placed onto a soft) may be helpful when a RGP lens cannot be tolerated because of discomfort or staining.[42] But contact lens fitting usually is not a satisfactory treatment for patients who elected to undergo surgery in order not to be dependent on their optical correction. Moreover, contact lenses do not prevent the visual deterioration or the progression of the ectasia. In advanced stages, there is often intolerance to contact lenses and results tend to be poor.

Penetrating keratoplasty, where the ectatic cornea is replaced with a healthy cornea, would constitute definitive treatment **(Figure 22.17)**. However, keratoplasty is not free of complications and visual results are not always as expected. For this reason, it is recommended in very advanced stages when visual results with other forms of treatment are not satisfactory. New treatment options that improve the visual prognosis for these patients have emerged in recent years for not very advanced cases of ectasia. These include crosslinking and intracorneal rings, designed to improve and stabilize the cornea, thus delaying progression and the eventual indication for keratoplasty.[40] On the other hand, the development of lamellar keratoplasty techniques has improved outcomes and prognosis with this procedure when it becomes necessary.[43]

Riboflavin-UVA Crosslinking

Riboflavin and ultraviolet-A (UVA) crosslinking of corneal collagen increases the biomechanical stability of the cornea by inducing additional crosslinking between or within collagen fibers.[44] This treatment produces hardening of the cornea and can arrest, and in some cases partially reverse, the progression of iatrogenic keratectasia after LASIK.[45] The treatment consists of removing the corneal epithelium over the central 8 mm of the cornea and applying riboflavin as photoactivator for approximately 30 minutes (until the aqueous stains yellow from the effect of riboflavin). The cornea is then exposed to a 365 nm UVA light source for 30 minutes while instilling riboflavin at the same time **(Figure 22.18)**. Pachymetry is crucial in selecting patients, given that this procedure is counterindicated in corneas of less than 400 microns in thickness because it may induce endothelial damage.[46]

Intracorneal Rings

Intracorneal rings are semicircular PMMA segments placed in the mid periphery of the ectatic cornea in order to flatten the central cornea and re-center the corneal apex **(Figures 22.19A and B)**. These effects result in refractive improvement because of a lowering of myopia and astigmatism, and also in improvement of visual acuity as a result of the regularization of

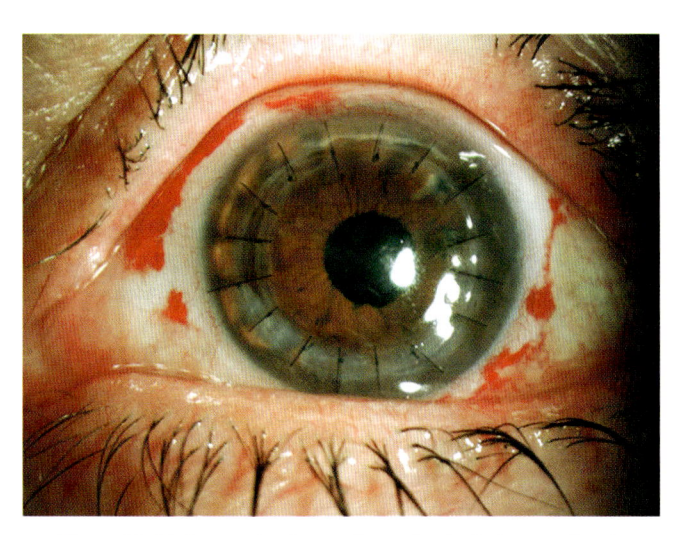

Figure 22.17 Penetrating keratoplasty after *in situ* keratomileusis

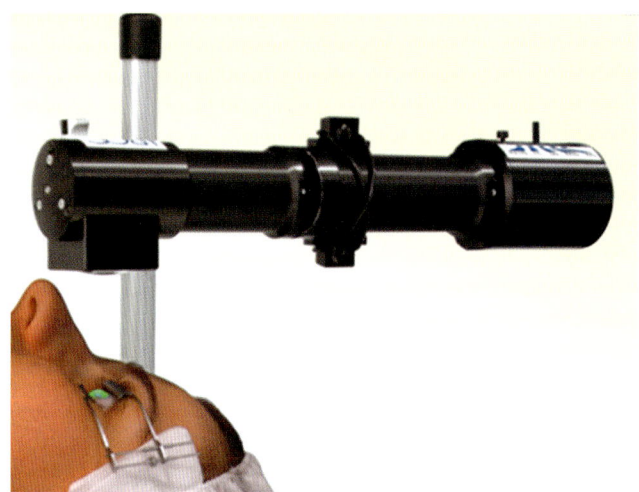

Figure 22.18 Corneal collagen crosslinking in progress
(Courtesy: PESCHKE Meditrade GmbH, Huenenberg -Switzerland)

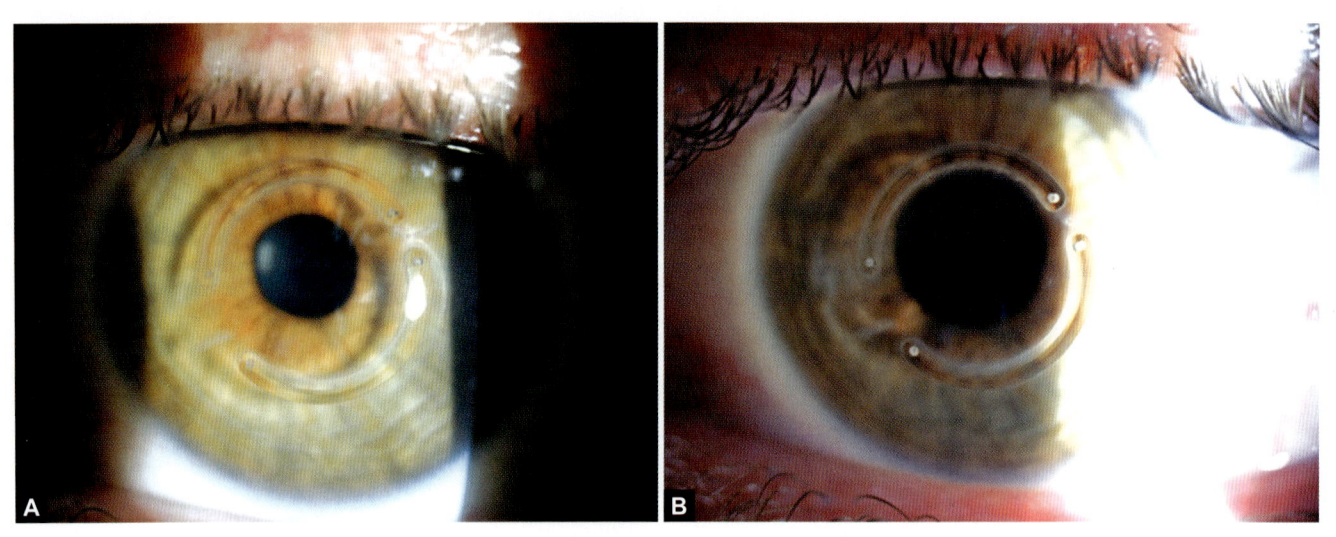

Figures 22.19A and B Intracorneal rings in keratectasia

the corneal surface.[47,48] Considering that ectasia is progressive, the rings are not definitive, but they help improve visual acuity and stabilize the cornea, thus delaying the need for keratoplasty by many years.[49]

There are two types of intracorneal ring segments in the market:
- *Ferrara Ring*[TM] (Ferrara Ophthalmics) and Kerarings (Mediphacos Inc, Belo Horizonte, Brazil) segments: 160° arc length, triangular shape, thicknesses ranging between 150 and 350 microns (50 μm increments); and curvature radius of 4.4 inner and 5.6 mm outer diameters.
- *Intacs*[TM] micro-thin inserts (Addition Technologies LLC, Fremont, CA, USA): 150° arc length, hexagonal cross-section, thicknesses ranging between 250 and 450 microns (50 μm increments) and curvature radius of 6.8 inner and 8.1 mm outer diameters.

Results with both implants are similar, but the higher curvature radius of the Intacs reduce ring show and glare, whereas the smaller radius of the Ferrara Ring appears to increase the applanation effect, since it is closer to the central cornea.[47,48] The ring-induced effect is directly proportional to the thickness of the ring and inversely proportional to its curvature radius. The larger the thickness and the smaller the diameter of the ring, the higher the induced effect. It is also possible to insert 2 rings, one in the steeper hemicornea and a second mirror ring, either of equal thickness or asymmetrical (the thicker in the steeper hemicornea), or to implant a single ring[51] in the steeper hemicornea. The indication depends on the degree and type of ectasia.

The rings may be inserted deep in the corneal stroma through a corneal tunnel. One of the challenges with this technique is the manual shaping of the corneal tunnel, especially in LASIK patients, considering the potential of entering the interphase during dissection and creating a shallow tunnel. Using the femtosecond laser to make the tunnel renders the technique much easier and does not change the results.[52]

Lamellar Keratoplasty

Long-term graft survival rates and endothelial cell counts after penetrating keratoplasty continue to drop for many years after surgery, clearly showing the disadvantage of unnecessary replacement of healthy endothelium in anterior stromal disorders. Recent developments in anterior lamellar keratoplasty enable targeted replacement of corneal stroma without replacement of endothelium, and include procedures such as deep anterior lamellar keratoplasty, and microkeratome or laser-assisted anterior lamellar surgery.[43]

- The *deep anterior lamellar keratoplasty (DALK)* technique is based on surgical manipulation that allows visualization of the lamellar dissection depth using a posterior approach to reach the predescemetic space. Techniques that use air and ophthalmic viscosurgical devices to directly expose Descemet's membrane have dramatically reduced surgery time. The anterior 80% of the central corneal stroma is replaced by a donor button without Descemet's membrane, and sutured in place.[53, 54]
- The development of new artificial chamber models such as automated lamellar therapeutic keratoplasty (ALTK) System®, Moria, have provided simplicity, precision and accuracy to the *microkeratome-assisted anterior lamellar keratoplasty* **(Figures 22.20A and B)**.[55] The ALTK system requires a donor cornea with a scleral rim to guarantee proper vacuum during the microkeratome cut. The microkeratome is used to cut partial-thickness sections through the anterior surface of the donor and host corneas. The donor disk is placed on the recipient bed with interrupted sutures **(Figures 22.21A and B)**.[56]

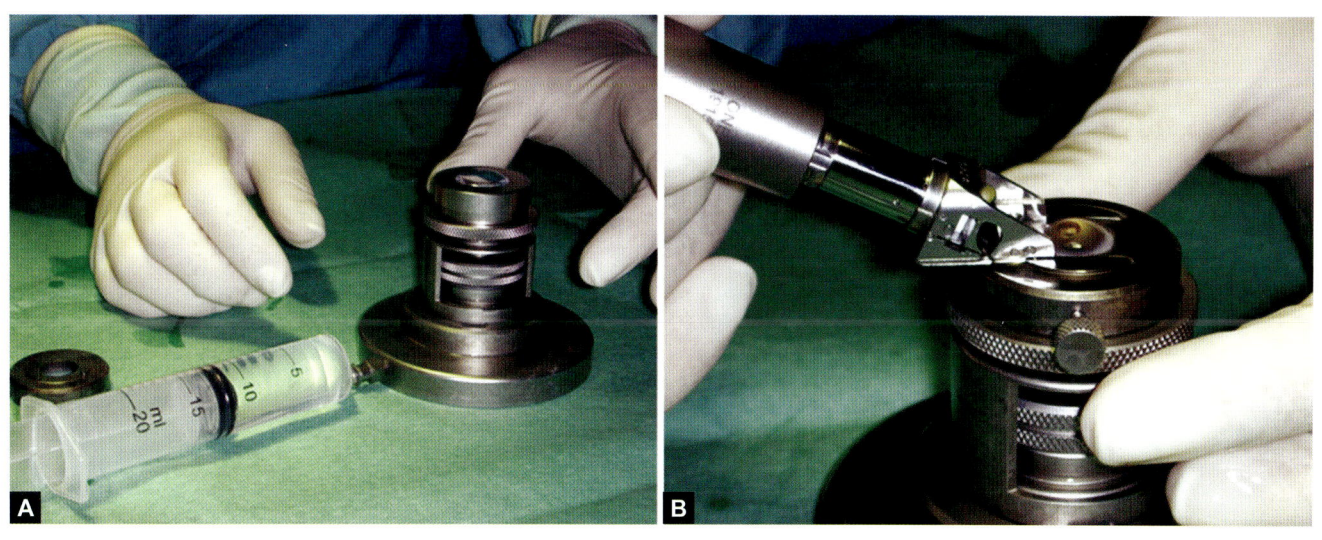

Figures 22.20A and B Cutting the donor cornea with the LSK—One microkeratome and the artificial anterior chamber, AAC, Moria (*Courtesy:* Dr MT Iradier)

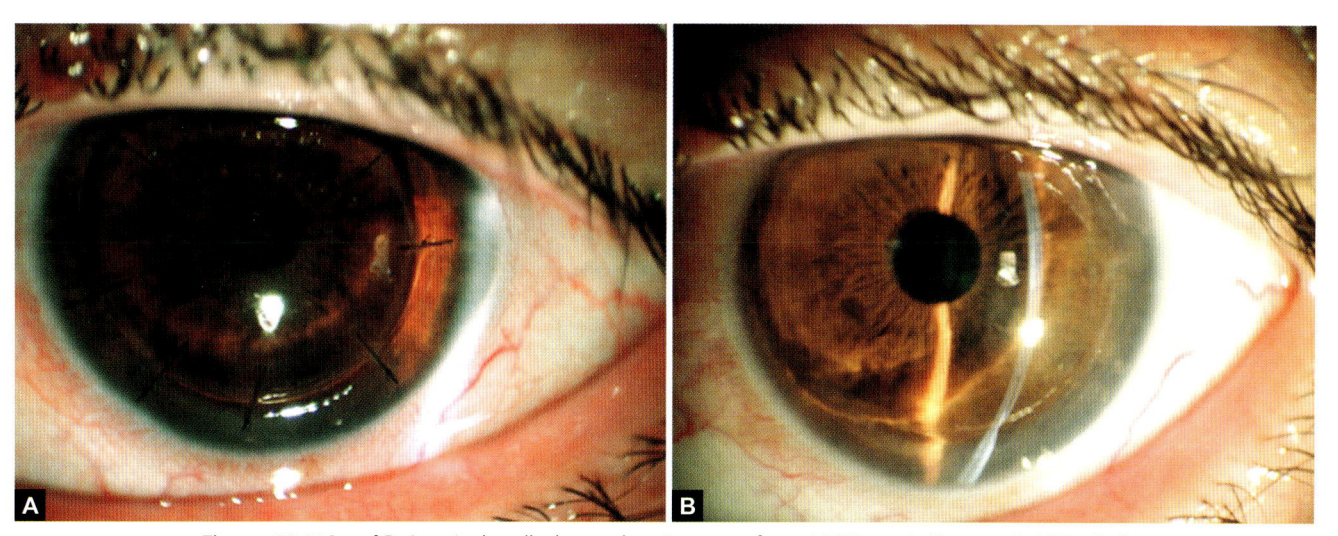

Figures 22.21A and B Anterior lamellar keratoplasty in a case of post-LASIK ectasia (*Courtesy:* Dr MT Iradier)

- *Excimer laser-assisted anterior lamellar keratoplasty* is using to augment thin corneas as corneal ectasia after LASIK. A donor stromal button approximately 350 μm thick received a 100 μm excimer laser ablation on the endothelium. The remaining cornea (epithelium, Bowman's membrane, and stroma) is punched with a 7.5 or 7.7 mm trephine. After transepithelial ablation of the host cornea to 200 μm thickness, the corneal button is sutured with interrupted sutures.[57]

These new forms of surgery are viable alternatives to conventional penetrating keratoplasty and bring added safety profiles for long-term visual rehabilitation and restoration of tectonic integrity in corneal ectasia.

REFERENCES

1. Pallikaris IG, Kymionis GD, Astyrakakis NI. Corneal ectasia induced by laser in situ keratomileusis. J Cataract Refract Surg. 2001;27(11):1796-802.
2. Condon PI, O'Keefe M, Binder PS. Long-term results of laser in situ keratomileusis for high myopia: Risk for ectasia. J Cataract Refract Surg. 2007;33(4):583-90.
3. Reinstein DZ, Srivannaboon S, Archer TJ, Silverman RH, Sutton H, Coleman DJ. Probability model of the inaccuracy of residual stromal thickness prediction to reduce the risk of ectasia after LASIK part II: Quantifying population risk. J Refract Surg. 2006;22(9):861-70.
4. Rad AS, Jabbarvand M, Saifi N. Progressive keratectasia after laser in situ keratomileusis. J Refract Surg. 2004;20(5 Suppl):S718-22.

5. Barraquer JI. Complicaciones postoperatorias profilaxis y tratamiento. In: Cirugía refractiva de la cornea. Instituto Barraquer de America, Bogota (Colombia). 1989; 449-50.
6. Nesburn AB, Bahri S, Salz J, Rabinowitz YS, Maguen E, Hofbauer J, Berlin M, Macy JI. Keratoconus detected by videokeratography in candidates for photorefractive keratectomy. J Refract Surg. 1995;11(3):194-201.
7. Amsler M. Keratocône classique et keratocône fruste, arguments unitaires. Ophthalmologica. 1946;11:96-101.
8. Rabinowitz JS. Keratoconus. Surv Ophthalmol. 1998; 42:297-319.
9. Ioannidis AS, Speedwell L, Nischal KK. Unilateral keratoconus in a child with chronic and persistent eye rubbing. Am J Ophthalmol. 2005;139(2):356-7.
10. Barraquer RI, De Toledo MC, Torres E. Alteraciones corneales ectaticas. In Distrofias y degeneraciones corneales. Espaxs Publicaciones Medicas, Bercelona. 2004;271.
11. Abad JC, Rubinfeld RS, Del Valle M, Belin MW, Kurstin JM. Vertical D: A novel topographic pattern in some keratoconus suspects. Ophthalmology. 2007;114(5):1020-6.
12. Rabinowitz YS. Videokeratographic indices to aid in screening for keratoconus. J Refract Surg. 1995;11:371-9
13. Seiler T, Quurke AW. Iatrogenic keratectasia after LASIK in a case of forme fruste keratoconus. J Cataract Refract Surg. 1998;24(7):1007-9.
14. Lebow KA, Grohe RM. Differentiating contact lens induced warpage from true keratoconus using corneal topography. CLAO J. 1999;25(2):114-22.
15. Wilson SE, Lin DT, Klyce SD, Reidy JJ, Insler MS. Topographic changes in contact lens-induced corneal warpage. Ophthalmology. 1990;97(6):734-44.
16. Wang X, McCulley JP, Bowman RW, Cavanagh HD. Time to resolution of contact lens-induced corneal warpage prior to refractive surgery. CLAO J. 2002;28(4):169-71.
17. Belin MW, Zloty P. Accuracy of the PAR corneal topography system with spatial misalignment. CLAO J. 1993;19(1):64-8.
18. Auffarth GU, Wang L, Volcker HE. Keratoconus evaluation using the Orbscan Topography System. J Cataract Refract Surg. 2000;26(2):222-8.
19. Rao SN, Raviv T, Majmudar PA, Epstein RJ. Role of Orbscan II in screening keratoconus suspects before refractive corneal surgery. Ophthalmology. 2002;109(9):1642-6.
20. Ho JD, Tsai CY, Tsai RJ, Kuo LL, Tsai IL, Liou SW. Validity of the keratometric index: Evaluation by the Pentacam rotating Scheimpflug camera. J Cataract Refract Surg. 2008;34(1):137-45.
21. Quisling S, Sjoberg S, Zimmerman B, Goins K, Sutphin J. Comparison of Pentacam and Orbscan IIz on posterior curvature topography measurements in keratoconus eyes. Ophthalmology. 2006;113(9):1629-32.
22. Binder PS. Analysis of ectasia after laser in situ keratomileusis: Risk factors. J Cataract Refract Surg. 2007;33(9):1530-8.
23. Kim SW, Byun YJ, Kim EK, Kim TI. Central corneal thickness measurements in unoperated eyes and eyes after PRK for myopia using Pentacam, Orbscan II, and ultrasonic pachymetry. J Refract Surg. 2007;23(9):888-94.
24. Shah S, Laiquzzaman M, Bhojwani R, Mantry S, Cunliffe I. Assessment of the biomechanical properties of the cornea with the ocular response analyzer in normal and keratoconic eyes. Invest Ophthalmol Vis Sci. 2007;48(7):3026-31.
25. Rao SN, Epstein RJ. Early onset ectasia following laser in situ keratomileusis: Case report and literature review. J Refract Surg. 2002;18(2):177-84.
26. Amoils SP, Deist MB, Gous P, Amoils PM. Iatrogenic keratectasia after laser in situ keratomileusis for less than −4.0 to −7.0 diopters of myopia. J Cataract Refract Surg. 2000;26(7):967-77.
27. Seiler T, Koufala K, Richter G. Iatrogenic keratectasia after laser in situ keratomileusis. J Refract Surg. 2002;18(2):177-84.
28. Ophthalmic Devices Advisory Panel, Food and Drug Administration. Checklist of information usually submitted in an investigational device exemption (IDE) application for refractive surgery lasers. J Refract Surg. 1997;13:579-88.
29. Giledi O, Daya SM. Unexpected flap thickness in laser in situ keratomileusis. J Cataract Refract Surg. 1998;14(3):312-7.
30. Buratto L, Brint S, Ferrari M. Surgical instrument. In: Buratto L, Brint S (Eds). LASIK: Principles and Techniques. Thorofare, NJ, SLAK Inc. 1998; 35-68.
31. Cigales M, Hoyos JE J. Thin flaps and buttonholes. In: Buratto L, Brint S (Eds). Custom LASIK: Surgical Techniques and Complications. Thorofare, NJ, SLAK Inc.; 2003. pp. 224-5.
32. Kim JH, Lee D, Rhee KI. Flap thickness reproducibility in laser in situ keratomileusis with a femtosecond laser: Optical coherence tomography measurement. J Cataract Refract Surg. 2008;34(1):132-6.
33. Netto MV, Mohan RR, Medeiros FW, Dupps WJ Jr, Sinha S, Krueger RR, Stapleton WM, Rayborn M, Suto C, Wilson SE. Femtosecond laser and microkeratome corneal flaps: Comparison of stromal wound healing and inflammation. J Refract Surg. 2007;23(7):667-76.
34. Spadea L, Palmieri G, Mosca L, Fasciani R, Balestrazzi E. Iatrogenic keratectasia following laser in situ keratomileusis. J Refract Surg. 2002;18(4):475-80.
35. Alio JL, Muftuoglu O, Ortiz D, Perez-Santonja JJ, Artola A, Ayala MJ, Garcia MJ, de Luna GC. Ten-year follow-up of laser in situ keratomileusis for myopia of up to -10 diopters. Am J Ophthalmol. 2008;145(1):46-54.
36. Spadea L, Palmieri G, Mosca L, Fasciani R, Balestrazzi E. Iatrogenic keratectasia following laser in situ keratomileusis. J Refract Surg. 2002;18(4):475-80.
37. Maldonado MJ, Nieto JC, Diez-Cuenca M, Pinero DP. Posterior corneal curvature changes after undersurface ablation of the flap and in-the-bed LASIK retreatment. Ophthalmology. 2006;113(7):1125-33.
38. Mearza AA, Koufaki FN, Aslanides IM. Airbag induced corneal ectasia. Cont Lens Anterior Eye. 2007.
39. Toshino A, Uno T, Ohashi Y, Maeda N, Oshika T. Transient keratectasia caused by intraocular pressure elevation after laser in situ keratomileusis. J Cataract Refract Surg. 2005;31(1):202-4.
40. Randleman JB. Post-laser in situ keratomileusis ectasia: Current understanding and future directions. Curr Opin Ophthalmol. 2006;17(4):406-12.
41. Eggink FA, Beekhuis WH. Contact lens fitting in a patient with keratectasia after laser in situ keratomileusis. J Cataract Refract. Surg. 2001;27(7):1119-23.
42. O'donnell C, Welham L, Doyle S. Contact lens management of keratectasia after laser in situ keratomileusis for myopia. Eye Contact Lens. 2004;30(3):144-6.
43. Tan DT, Por YM. Current treatment options for corneal ectasia. Curr Opin Ophthalmol. 2007;18(4):284-9.
44. Wollensak G, Spoerl E, Seiler T. Riboflavin/ultraviolet-a-induced collagen crosslinking for the treatment of keratoconus. Am J Ophthalmol. 2003;135(5):620-7.
45. Hafezi F, Kanellopoulos J, Wiltfang R, Seiler T. Corneal collagen crosslinking with riboflavin and ultraviolet A to treat induced

keratectasia after laser in situ keratomileusis. J Cataract Refract Surg. 2007;33(12):2035-40.
46. Wollensak G. Crosslinking treatment of progressive keratoconus: New hope. Curr Opin Ophthalmol. 2006;17(4):356-60.
47. Lovisolo CF, Fleming JF. Intracorneal ring segments for iatrogenic keratectasia after laser in situ keratomileusis or photorefractive keratectomy. J Refract Surg. 2002;18(5):535-41.
48. Kymionis GD, Siganos CS, Kounis G, Astyrakakis N, Kalyvianaki MI, Pallikaris IG. Management of post-LASIK corneal ectasia with Intacs inserts: One-year results. Arch Ophthalmol. 2003;121(3):322-6.
49. Kymionis GD, Tsiklis NS, Pallikaris AI, Kounis G, Diakonis VF, Astyrakakis N, Siganos CS. Long-term follow-up of Intacs for post-LASIK corneal ectasia. Ophthalmology. 2006;113(11):1909-17
50. Sharma M, Boxer Wachler BS. Comparison of single-segment and double-segment Intacs for keratoconus and post-LASIK ectasia. Am J Ophthalmol. 2006;141(5):891-5.
51. Pokroy R, Levinger S, Hirsh A. Single Intacs segment for post-laser in situ keratomileusis keratectasia. J Cataract Refract Surg. 2004;30(8):1685-95.
52. Carrasquillo KG, Rand J, Talamo JH. Intacs for keratoconus and post-LASIK ectasia: Mechanical versus femtosecond laser-assisted channel creation. Cornea. 2007;26(8):956-62.
53. Villarrubia A, Perez-Santonja JJ, Palacin E, Rodriguez-Ausin P P, Hidalgo A. Deep anterior lamellar keratoplasty in post-laser in situ keratomileusis keratectasia. J Cataract Refract Surg. 2007;33(5):773-8.
54. Shimmura S, Tsubota K. Deep anterior lamellar keratoplasty. Curr Opin Ophthalmol. 2006;17(4):349-55.
55. Behrens A, Dolorico A, Kara DT, Novick LH, McDonnell PJ, Chao LC, Wellik SR, Chuck RS. Precision and accuracy of an artificial chamber system in obtaining corneal lenticules for lamellar keratoplasty. J Cataract Refract Surg. 2001;27(10):1679-87.
56. Busin M, Zambianchi L, Arffa RC. Microkeratome-assisted lamellar keratoplasty for the surgical treatment of keratoconus. Ophthalmology. 2005;112(6):987-97.
57. Bilgihan K, Ozdek SC, Sari A, Hasanreisoglu B. Excimer laser-assisted anterior lamellar keratoplasty for keratoconus, corneal problems after laser in situ keratomileusis, and corneal stromal opacities. J Cataract Refract Surg. 2006;32(8):1264-9.

Chapter 23

Decentered Ablations

Helen Boerman (USA), Ming Wang (USA), Tracy Schroeder Swartz (USA)

INTRODUCTION

Clinically significant decentered excimer ablations result in symptoms such as glare, shadows, dim lighting disturbances, distortion, and monocular diplopia, as well as loss of best-corrected visual acuity due to irregular astigmatism.[1-31] Decentration can be a corollary of poor fixation due to poor patient instruction, anxiety, over-sedation, or blurry vision due to high refractive error, or the exposed stromal bed causing difficulty seeing the laser's target. It can also result from improper stabilization of the eye with a Thornton ring during excimer ablation.

Centration over the entrance pupil center has been accepted as the standard for many years and still remains the recommendation for many laser systems. However, variations in pupil size can affect the location of the entrance pupil center. Therefore, centration by this technique is not the most reliable estimation of the visual axis. This has led to the use of the coaxially sighted corneal light reflex for more accurate centration during refractive procedures. This reflex represents the corneal intercept of a line from the point of fixation to the center of corneal curvature.

In addition, hyperopic ablations may result in more clinically significant symptoms than myopic ablations following equal magnitude refractive treatments. The functional optical zone in hyperopic treatments is smaller, emphasizing any possible decentration of the ablation zone. This is further accentuated by a greater average angle kappa in hyperopes as compared to myopes.

Proper centration of ablation requires careful preoperative and intraoperative instructions, especially with regard to the fixation target. It is important to keep both eyes open, preparing patients with regards to sounds and smells that may startle them. The head and body must remain still during surgery. The advent of modern laser tracking systems, iris registration software, and wavefront guided excimer laser technology has significantly reduced the incidence of decentration.

CLINICAL DEFINITION

The following clinical signs and symptoms often present in patients with a decentered ablation:
1. Decentration of the ablation zone on corneal topography.
2. Increased higher order aberrations as measured using wavefront aberrometry, predominantly coma.
3. The appearance of a tail on point spread functions.
4. Reduced best spectacle-corrected visual acuity which improves only with gas permeable lenses.
5. A cylinder measurement on autorefraction and wavefront that differs from manifest refraction, and
6. A history of reduced vision immediately following surgery that fails to improve with time.

TOPOGRAPHIC DECENTRATION

To evaluate decentration on corneal topography, both axial curvature and elevation maps are useful. The axial map provides the refractive result of ablation, i.e. the optical zone. A large corneal curvature gradient between treated and untreated cornea, such as that resulting from a highly myopic correction, creates a smaller optical zone, increasing the refractive effect of the decentration. Curvature maps indicate surface shape using the axial radius of curvature, or the distance along the normal from the surface to the optic axis. Once a radius is determined, it is converted to a dioptric value using a paraxial keratometry formula, resulting in error for more peripheral points.

In contrast, elevation maps using an appropriate reference surface describe subtle variations in surface geometry and are valuable when true topography is required. Therefore, elevation maps are far more valuable in both diagnosing and treating corneal decentration, and in monitoring surface changes.

WAVEFRONT ABERRATIONS

The growing application of wavefront aberrometry demonstrates increased higher order aberrations in patients following keratorefractive surgery, specifically those with decentered ablations. Mrochen et al found that subclinical decentrations less than 1 mm significantly increase wavefront aberrations, deteriorating the optical quality of the retinal image. All Zernike coefficients increased postoperatively, with coma being the predominant higher order aberration. Decentrations as small as 0.2 mm increased wavefront aberrations; however, those less than 0.5 mm are considered clinically insignificant.

Wavefront aberrometers offer a variety of displays describing aberrations, including Point Spread Functions (PSF) and Snellen letter appearance simulations. Examples of a wavefront map, simulated Snellen letters, and point spread function with increased coma of a patient with a decentration are illustrated in **Figures 23.1 to 23.3**.

Management of Decentered Ablation

While the diagnosis of decentration is fairly straightforward, reducing or eliminating symptoms associated with decentration can be difficult. The most frequently used nonsurgical method involves gas permeable lenses, which restore visual quality by optically reshaping the anterior cornea surface. Comparing BSCVA to the visual acuity obtained with a gas permeable (GP) lens may provide the prognosis of visual success. Unfortunately, achieving fitting success can be difficult, often requiring novel lens types such as reverse geometry or specialty aspheric designs. An example of such a gas permeable fitting is shown in **Figure 23.4**. Even in cases when the vision significantly improves, failures result due to poor comfort and limited wearing time. Most patients are not receptive to returning to contact lenses after investing time and money in refractive surgery.

We typically address any tear film instability or deficiency by aggressive ocular surface lubrication. Punctal plugs and topical 0.05% cyclosporin (Allergan, Irvine, CA) both work well to smooth the irregular surface and decrease visual symptoms.

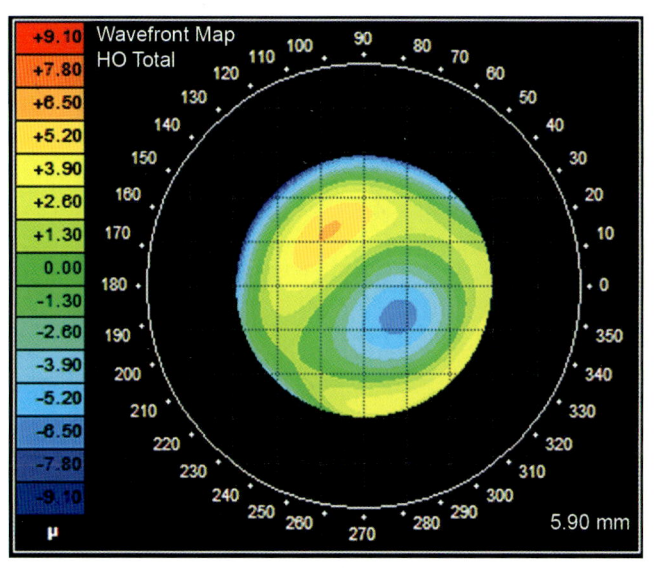

Figure 23.1 Wavefront map in a patient with increased coma

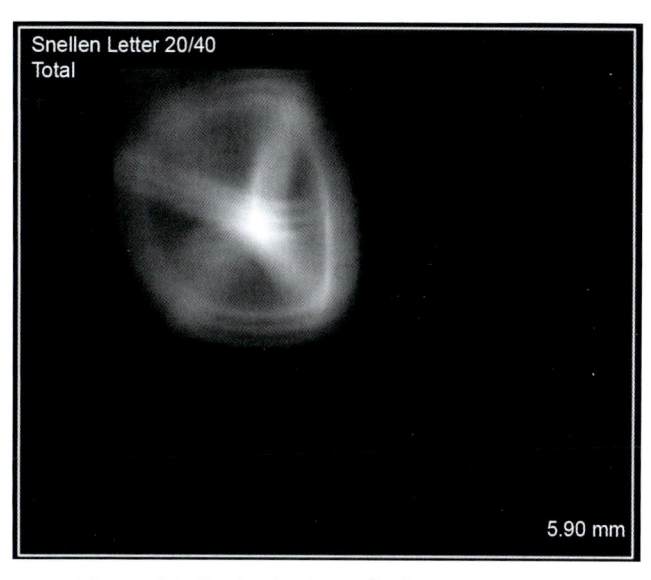

Figure 23.2 Simulated 20/40 Snellen letter "E" in a patient with increased coma

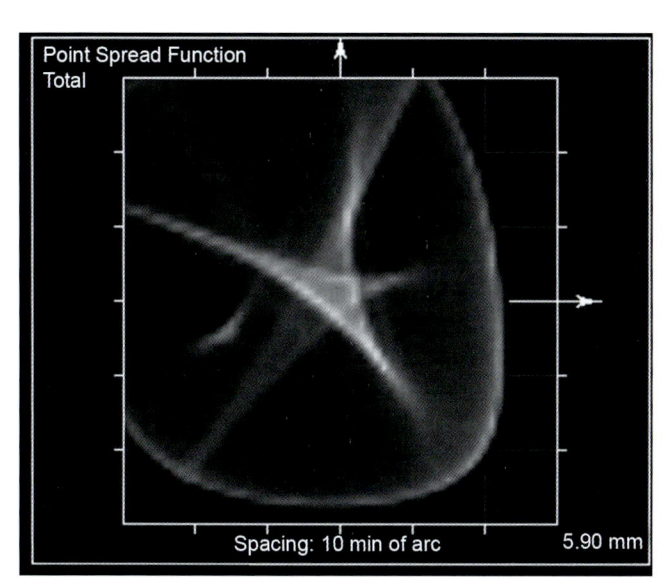

Figure 23.3 Point spread function in a patient with increased coma

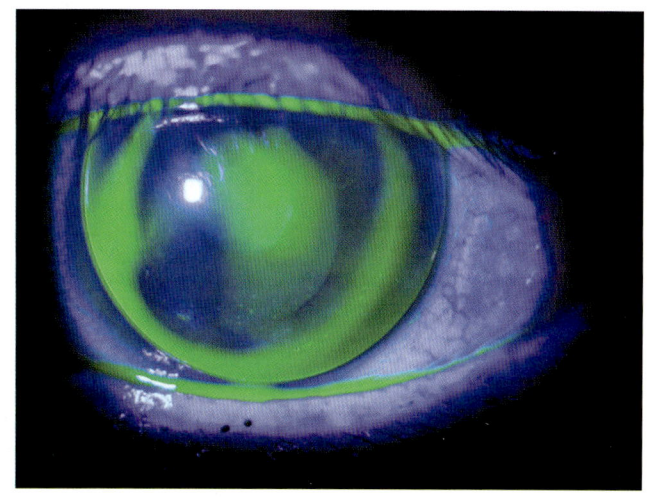

Figure 23.4 Rose K Irregular Corneal (Blanchard Contact Lens Inc, Manchester, New Hampshire) design on a patient with irregular astigmatism resulting from a decentered ablation. Note the asymmetry in the fluorescein pattern. The patient was 20/100 best corrected in spectacles, and 20/20 with this lens

Treatment of meibomian gland disease using oral doxycycline or topical Azacite (Inspire Pharmaceuticals, Durham, NC) may be used to stabilize the tear film, possibly increasing the Snellen acuity and decreasing the aberrations such that the patient appreciates visual improvement without further surgery.

Surgical Correction of Decentered Ablation

Several options for surgical correction of decentered ablations exist with variable results. PTK and purposeful decentered ablation in the opposite direction of the initial treatment[13] have been proposed but such techniques are not widely used. Correction of decentration using wavefront-driven treatment, Custom Corneal Ablation Pattern treatment, and topography-guided treatment are more likely to be used in patients suffering vision loss following keratorefractive surgery.

Wavefront Guided Treatment

Custom wavefront treatments have been used to address the visual effects of a previous refractive surgery, including decentered ablation. Topographical abnormalities translate into wavefront aberrations, which can be addressed with wavefront guided treatment. While severely irregular corneas may not be adequately measured using wavefront aberrometry, when data can be captured, it has been found to improve vision.

In case I, a patient presented after undergoing LASIK followed by an enhancement and epithelial cleaning in her hometown. Uncorrected vision was 20/70, which corrected to 20/20 with a refraction of –1.75 + 0.50 × 128. Topography and aberrometry are shown in **Figures 23.5 and 23.6**. Gas permeable over-refraction yielded 20/20 vision with significant improvement in subjective visual quality. WaveScan-guided (AMO, Santa Ana, CA) PRK using ablation was performed, and the patient reported improved visual quality the following day. Later, she reported although the vision was better than prior to custom treatment, shadows persisted. Postoperative aberrometry is shown in **Figure 23.7**. Note that while the refractive error was greatly reduced, the RMS value did not significantly improve.

Topography Guided Treatment

Topography guided options are limited to Custom-CAP (Carl Zeiss Humphrey, Jeno, Germany) treatments in the United States. Use of Custom-Cap has been shown to be effective in correcting decentered ablation. It enables the surgeon to create a customized excimer laser ablation pattern to reduce areas of topographic irregularity on the anterior corneal surface via computerized simulations. Creation of plans directing the excimer laser beam size, shape, depth, and location to match the corresponding irregularity on the computerized corneal

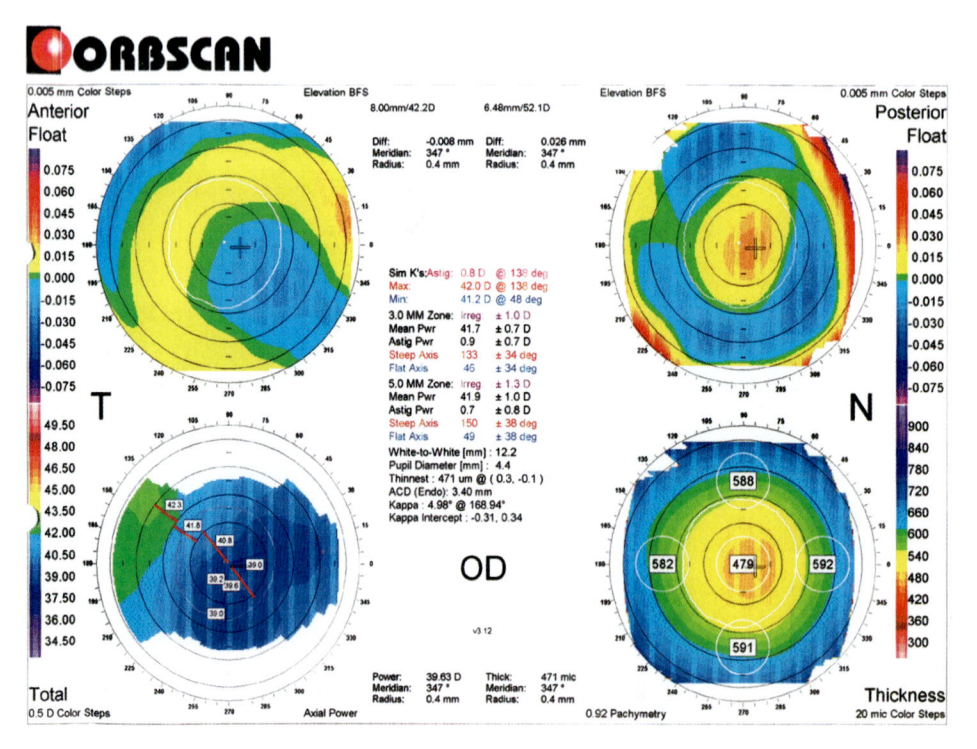

Figure 23.5 Preoperative topographical map showing superior decentration

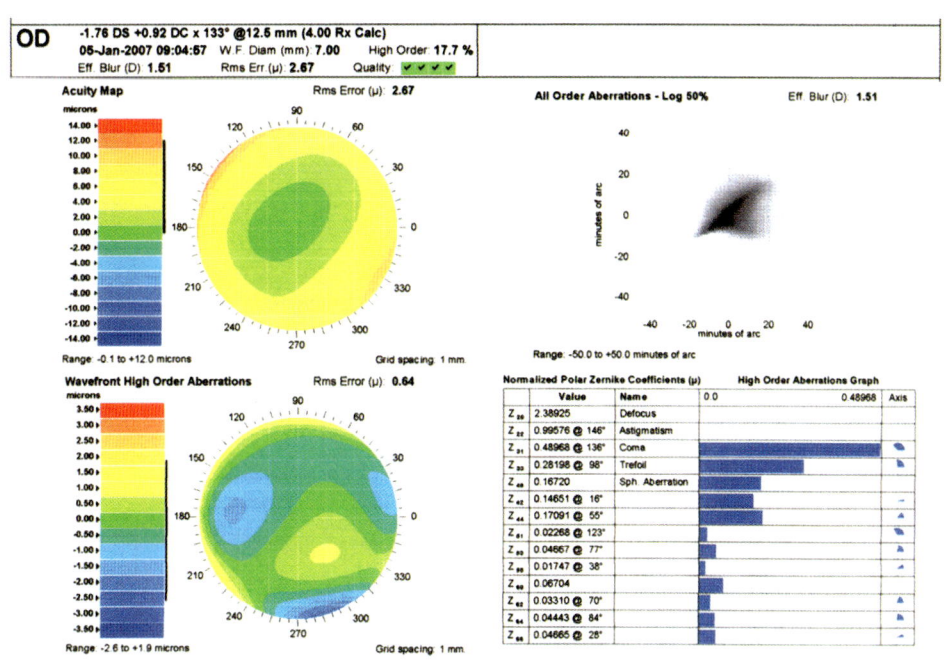

Figure 23.6 Preoperative wavescan aberrometry maps showing coma, as expected with a decentered ablation

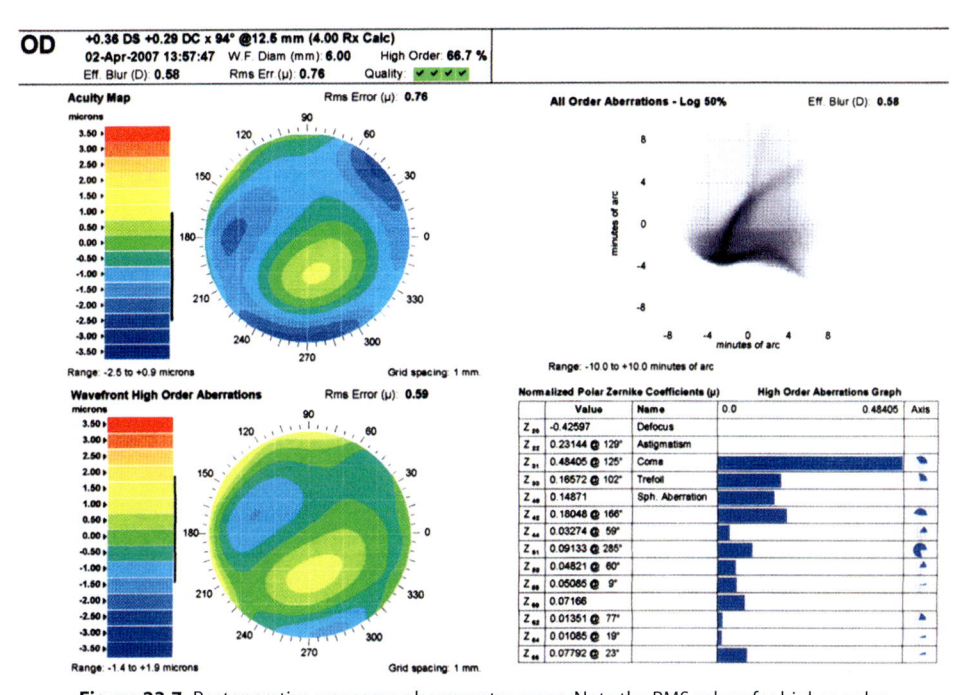

Figure 23.7 Postoperative wavescan aberrometry maps. Note the RMS values for higher order aberrations did not significantly improve

topography elevation map results in a more regular corneal shape. The laser beam varies in diameter from 0.6 to 6.5 mm, and can be centered or offset in any direction from the visual axis. The required VisionPro software (Carl Zeiss Humphrey, Jeno, Germany) allows the programming of up to 20 different sequential ablations.

Case II utilized this technology to correct a decentered ablation in a patient with a history of previous LASIK to correct myopia. She was best corrected to 20/40 and complained of shadows and distorted vision. Her preoperative topography is shown in **Figure 23.8**. The VisionPro software ablation plan is shown in **Figure 23.9**. Following treatment, her best corrected

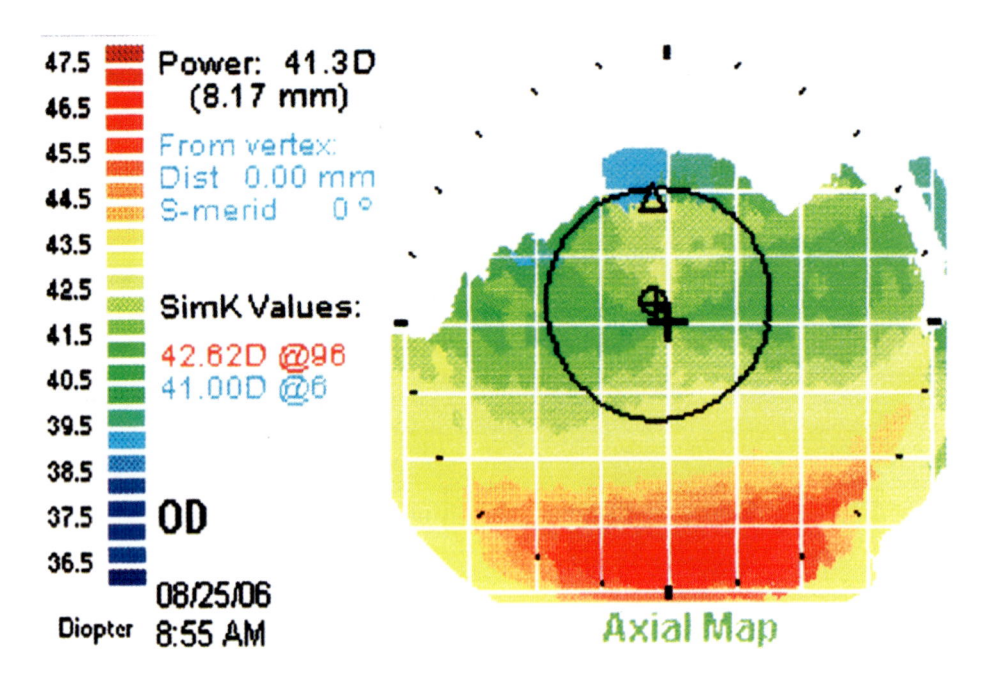

Figure 23.8 Preoperative topographic map in a patient with a decentered ablation

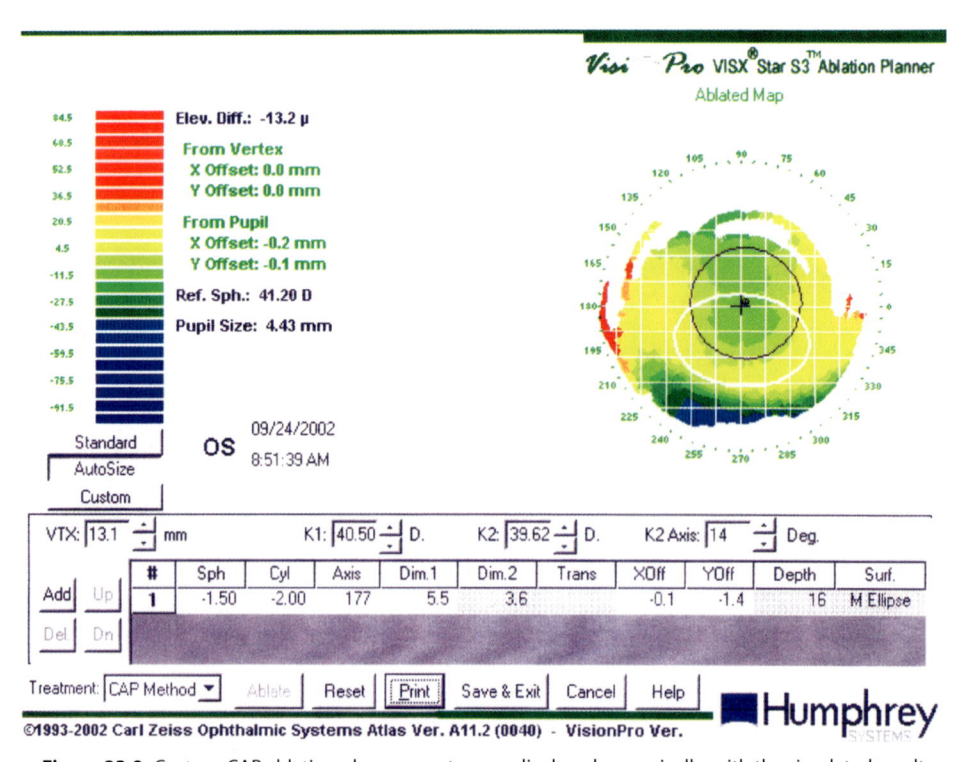

Figure 23.9 Custom-CAP ablation plan parameters are displayed numerically, with the simulated result of the planned ablation pictured in the ablated map, for the patient in Figure 23.8

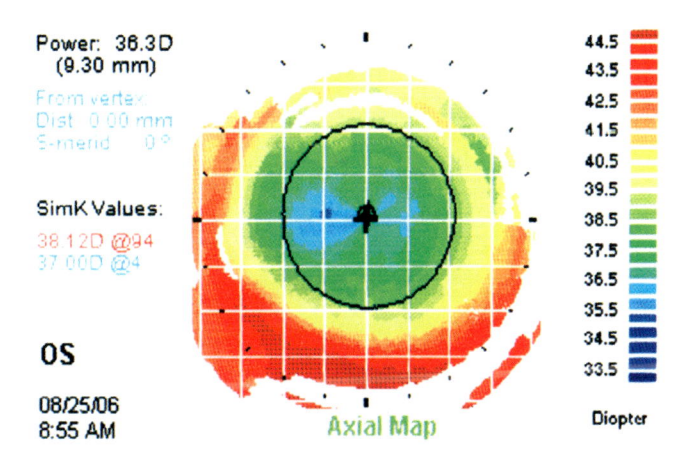

Figure 23.10 The topographical maps following Custom-CAP treatment show a significantly improved topographical regularity

vision improved to 20/25 and the postoperative topography showed improved regularity **(Figure 23.10)**.

Topography guided treatment of decentration may be advantageous compared to wavefront, which addresses topographical irregularities secondarily. Decentration is a topographical phenomenon, which is directly corrected using topographically-driven treatments. Because the ablation is derived from corneal topography data directly, restoration of the natural aspheric shape of the cornea is possible. Topographical treatments may incorporate tissue saving algorithms, important in patients with limited stromal bed thickness. Published reports find topography guided treatment to be effective, improving UCVA, BSCVA and the regularity of the corneal surface. However, residual refractive error, undercorrection of topographic abnormalities and regression have been reported.

Case III illustrates the efficacy of the MEL80 with TOSCA software (Asclepion-Meditec, Jena, Germany) and the CRS-Master (Carl Ziess Meditech, Jena, Germany). This system includes algorithms to correct decentrations and enlarge small optical zones. The CRS-Master features improved control of sphere and cylinder while correcting topographical irregularities. The system incorporates corneal anterior surface wavefront information derived from topography, and whole-eye optical data to determine the refraction of the front surface and the ablation required to remove the irregularities independent of the refractive change. This patient presented with a history of RK rather than LASIK, reporting stable vision for the first 12 years, with progressive hyperopia and reduced visual quality more recently. Her refraction was +3.75–1.00 × 165, which corrected her vision to 20/20. Topography is shown in **Figure 23.11**. Surgery was performed with a target of plano, with the intention of improving the corneal surface regularity. PRK was performed with an optical zone of 7.00 mm. Six months later, the patient was 20/32 uncorrected, and +1.00–0.75 × 85 improved her vision to 20/16. **Figure 23.12** shows the improvement in contrast sensitivity.

Two systems incorporate pupil size, topographic elevation data, and refractive status with surgical recreation of the morphological axis. The morphological axis is defined as the axis of corneal symmetry approximating the best match between the axis of ideal shape and that of the current form of the cornea. Following a decentration, the visual axis shifts in an attempt to correct the induced visual effect of the decentration. Any measurement taken using the patient's fixation, such as autorefraction, wavefront aberrometry, and placido topography, will then measured along the incorrect axis. This is the reason decentration is difficulty to correct using wavefront aberrometry measurements, and why conventional treatments often increase rather than improve the decentration.

Ablation software combines pupil, refractive and corneal elevation information, creating topographically-driven ablations with tissue saving algorithms. The two systems are the Corneal Interactive Programmed Topographic Ablation

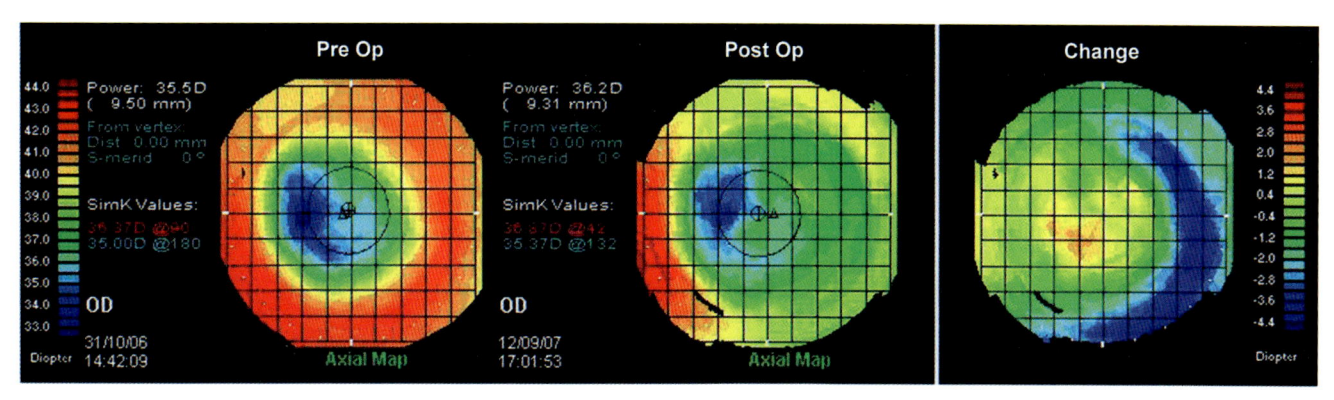

Figure 23.11 Topography maps for Case III, a patient with a decentered optical zone following RK corrected with the Mel80 and CRS-master (Carl Zeiss Meditech, Jena, Germany). (*Courtesy:* Dan Reinstein, MD and Tim Archer)

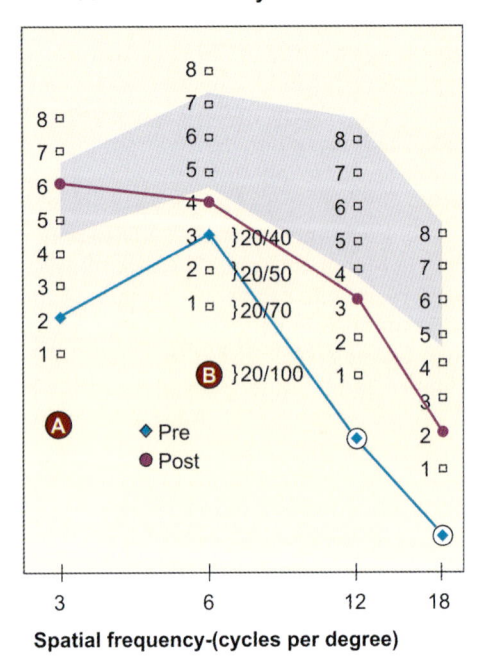

Figure 23.12 Contrast sensitivity testing before (blue) and after (red) PRK custom treatment to correct the decentrated optical zone
(Courtesy: Dan Reinstein, MD and Tim Archer)

(CIPTA) (Ligi, Taranto, Italy) and AstraScan (LaserSight, Orlando, FL). The following two cases illustrate the two systems.

Case IV demonstrates a successful treatment using CIPTA. A patient presented with a decentered ablation following LASIK, which manifested as 2.10 D of astigmatism. Preoperative topography and pachymetry maps are shown in **Figures 23.13 and 23.14**. Incorporation of the pupillometer data, topography, and refraction is illustrated in **Figure 23.15A** which displays the imported topographic map and the idea shape with restoration of the morphological axis. The ablation plan is shown in **Figure 23.15B**, which details the corrective ablation (right) and the predicted elevation topography (left). The actual resulting topography and pachymetry maps are shown in **Figures 23.16 and 23.17**, demonstrating improved centration and decreased pachymetry.

Case V illustrates a case of decentration corrected using AstraScan. **Figure 23.18** shows a superior-temporal decentration on a sagittal curvature map. The axial power map is shown in **Figure 23.19**, where it has been imported into the Astrascan software. The patient's manifest refraction was $-3.75 - 0.25 \times 95$ with a BSCVA of 20/20, and custom LASIK surgery was planned to correct the decentration and address the refractive error. **Figure 23.20** illustrates the planned ablation profile. Note that the pre-enhancement elevation (lower left), when using the optimized postenhancement corneal vertex as the reference axis, shows the same elevated pattern as the enhancement ablation profile (upper right). In this example, the optimized axis is offset of 0.035 mm temporally, and 0.044 mm superiorly from the pre-enhancement corneal vertex axis. **Figure 23.21** shows the postenhancement axial power map showing the decentration has been completely corrected. **Figure 23.22** shows the pre- (left) and postoperative (right) elevation maps. The difference map can be seen in **Figure 23.23**.

CONCLUSION

When a patient with a history of refractive surgery presents with loss of best-corrected visual acuity and expresses symptoms

Figure 23.13 Preoperative topography map for a patient with a decentered ablation following LASIK
(Courtesy: Chuck Stewart, OD and Ligi, Taranto, Italy)

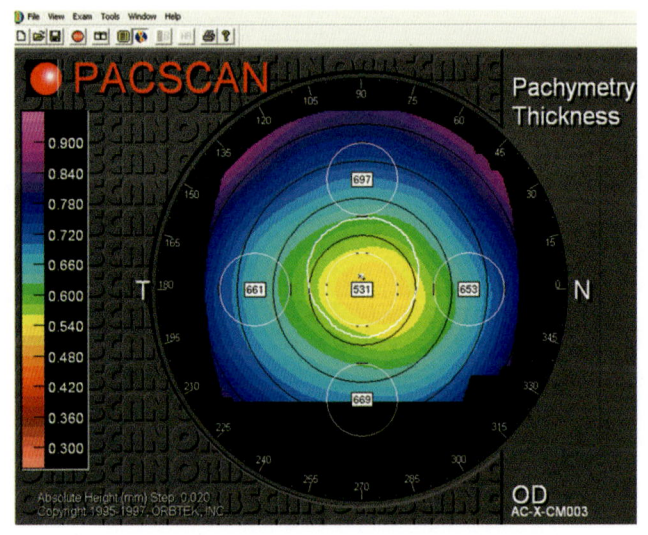

Figure 23.14 Preoperative pachymetry map for the patient in Figure 23.13
(Courtesy: Chuck Stewart, OD and Ligi, Taranto, Italy)

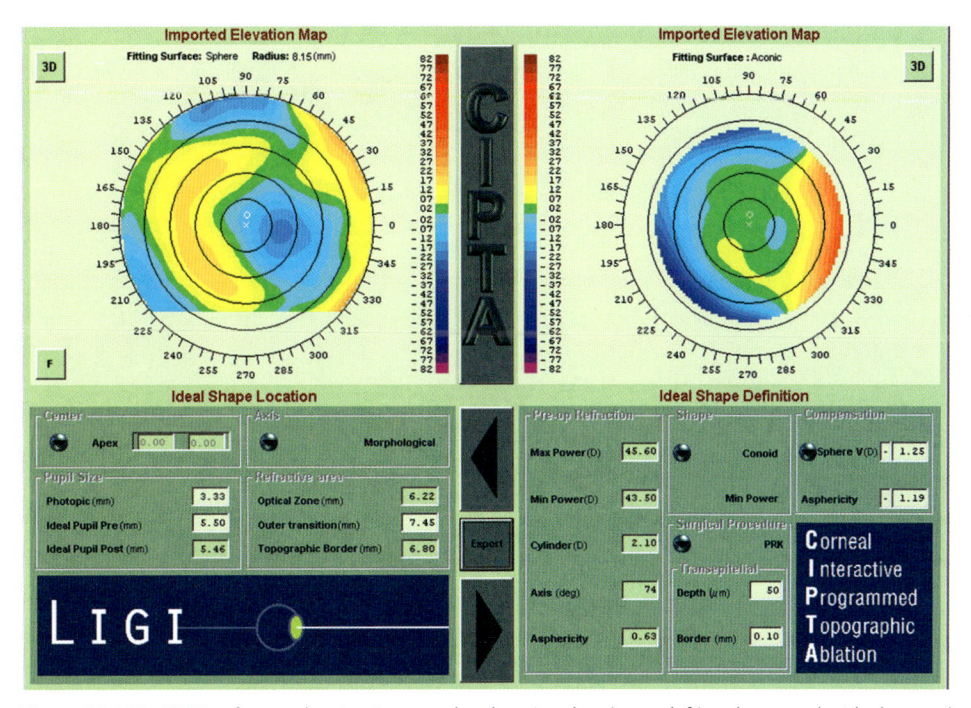

Figure 23.15A CIPTA software planning imports the elevation data (upper left) and creates the ideal corneal surface with reference to the morphological axis (upper right)
(*Courtesy:* Chuck Stewart, OD and Ligi, Taranto, Italy)

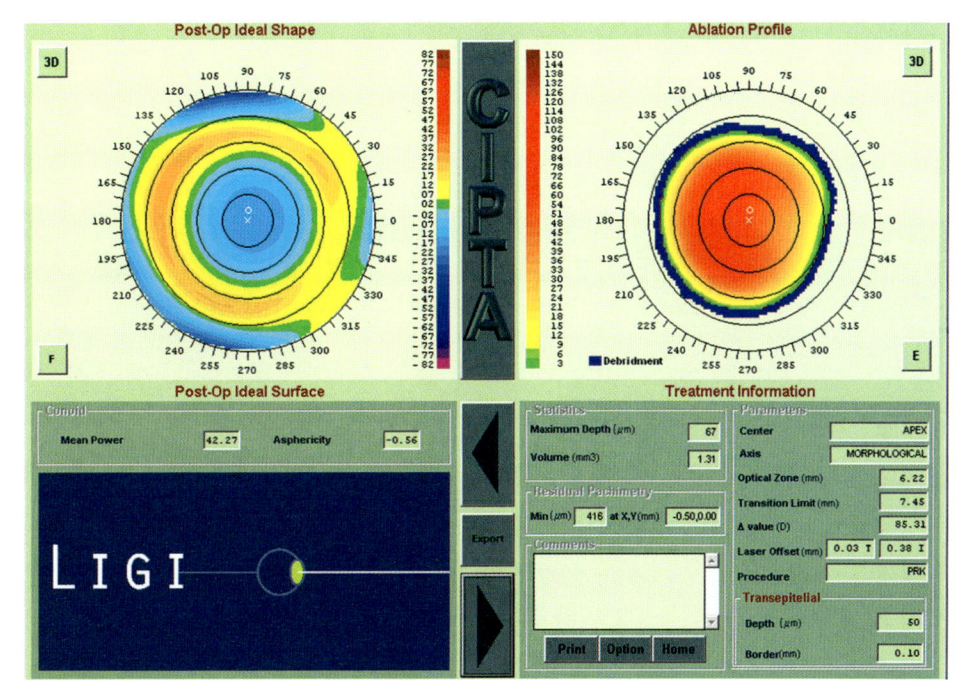

Figure 23.15B CIPTA software creates the ablation profile (upper right) to create the simulated elevation map (upper left)
(*Courtesy:* Chuck Stewart, OD and Ligi, Taranto, Italy)

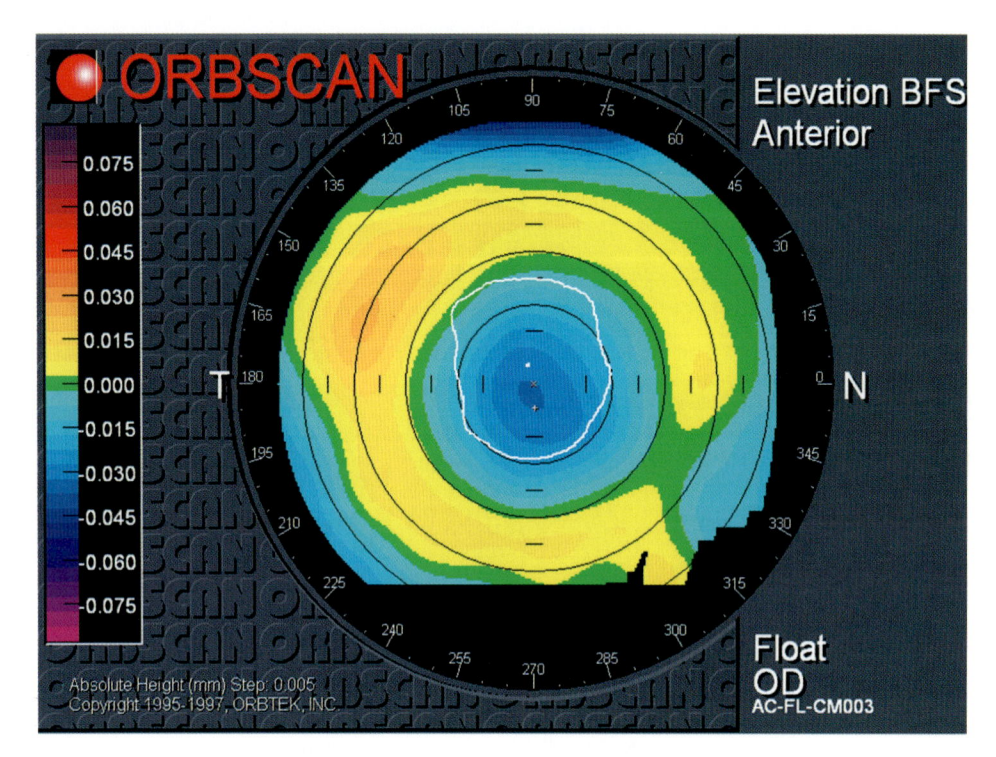

246 Section V: Refractive Procedures and Conditions

Figure 23.16 Actual elevation map following CIPTA treatment
(*Courtesy:* Chuck Stewart, OD and Ligi, Taranto, Italy)

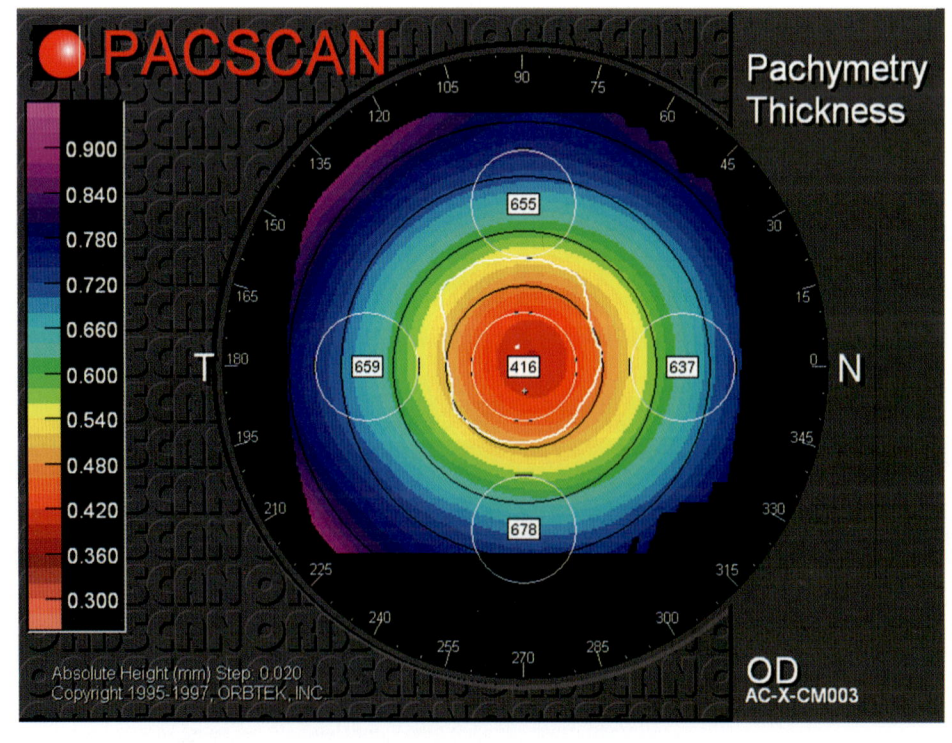

Figure 23.17 Actual postoperative pachymetry map following CIPTA treatment
(*Courtesy:* Chuck Stewart, OD and Ligi, Taranto, Italy)

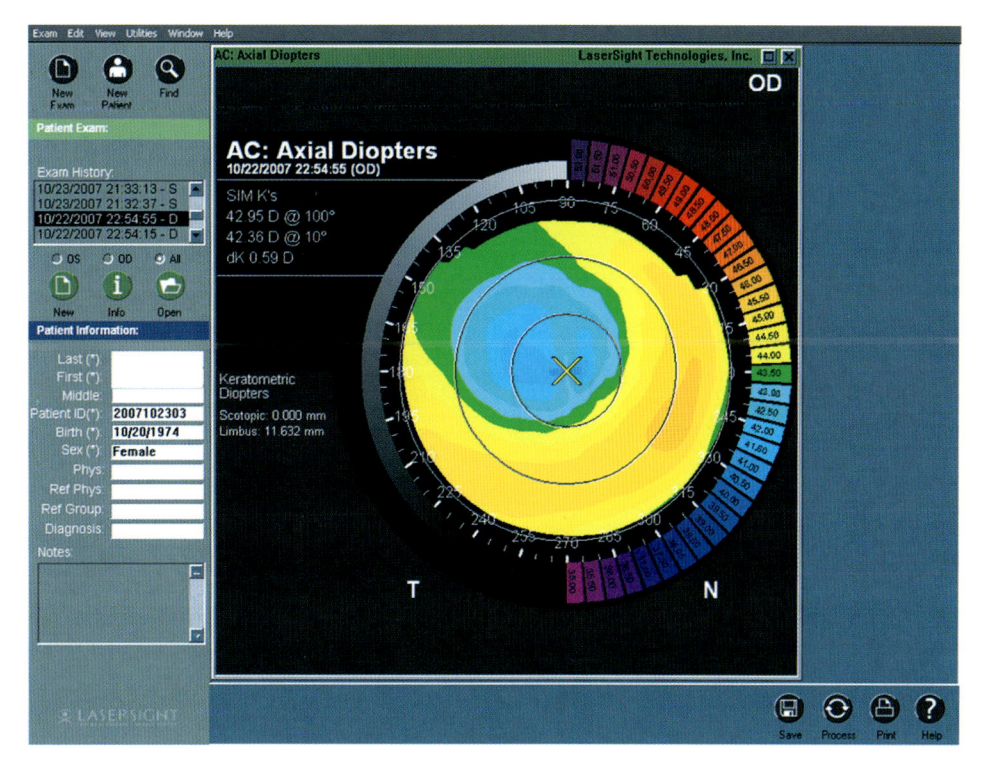

Figure 23.18 Pre-enhancement axial curvature map, showing significant decentration of the ablation superior-temporally
(*Courtesy:* Dr Bing Liu, General Air Force Hospital)

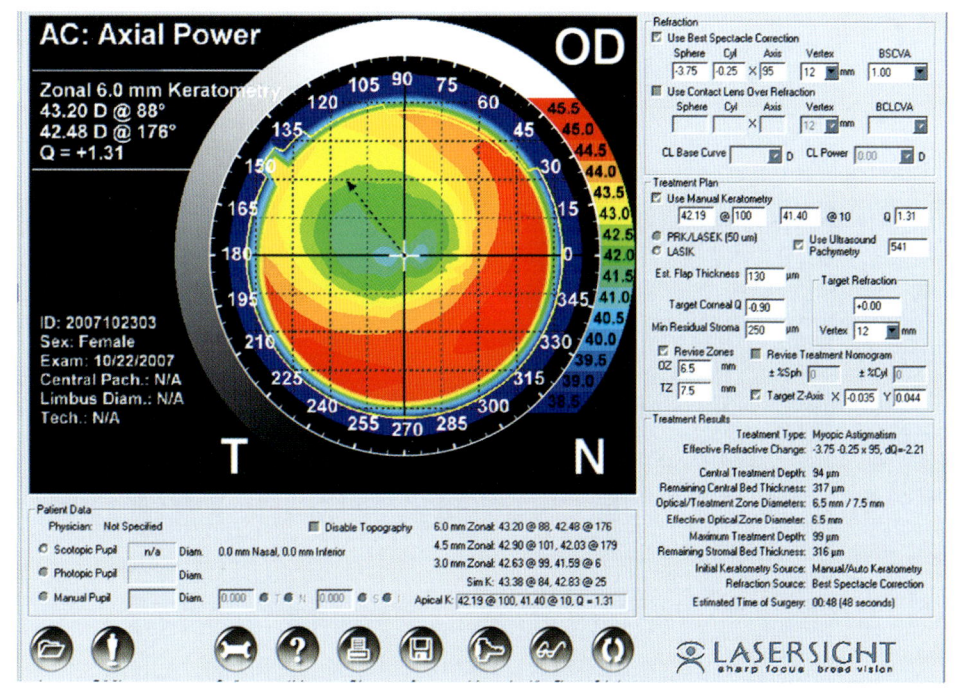

Figure 23.19 AstraPro 2.2Z Custom Planning Software User Interface where the imported power map, pachymetry, keratometry, refractive information, and ablation plan are displayed
(*Courtesy:* Dr Bing Liu, General Air Force Hospital)

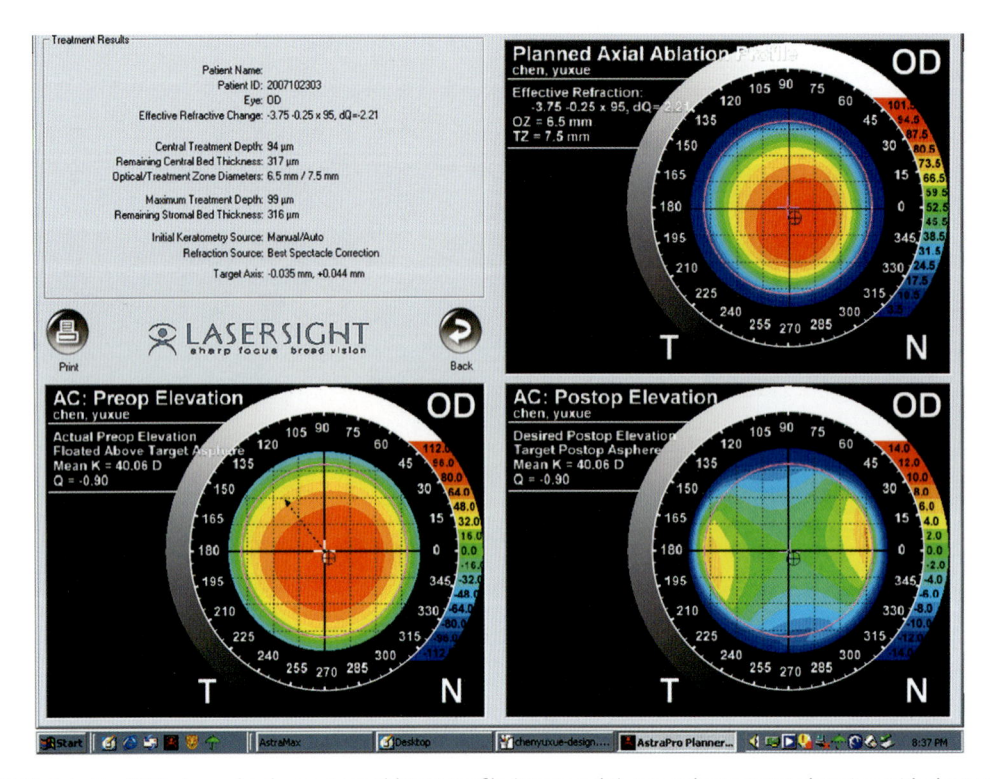

Figure 23.20 AstraPro 2.2Z planned enhancement ablation profile (upper right), pre-enhancement elevation with the target A-axis optimized (lower left) and predicted postoperative elevation map (lower right). Note that the pre-enhancement elevation shows the same elevated pattern as the enhancement ablation profile when using the optimized postenhancement corneal vertex as the reference axis. In this example, the optimized axis is offset 0.035 mm temporally, and 0.044 mm superiorly from the pre-enhancement corneal vertex axis (*Courtesy:* Dr Bing Liu, General Air Force Hospital)

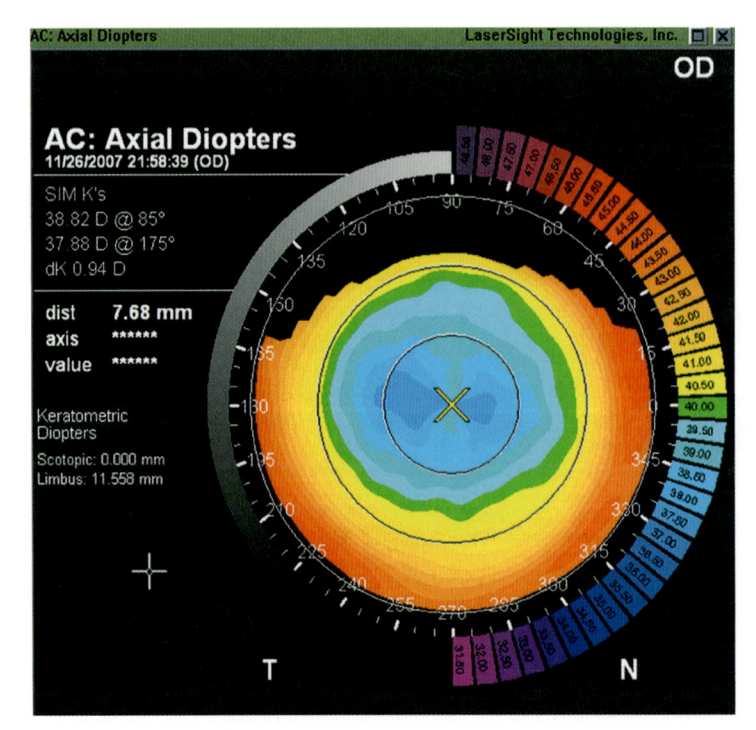

Figure 23.21 Postenhancement axial curvature map showing the decentration has been completely corrected
(*Courtesy:* Dr Bing Liu, General Air Force Hospital)

Chapter 23: Decentered Ablations 249

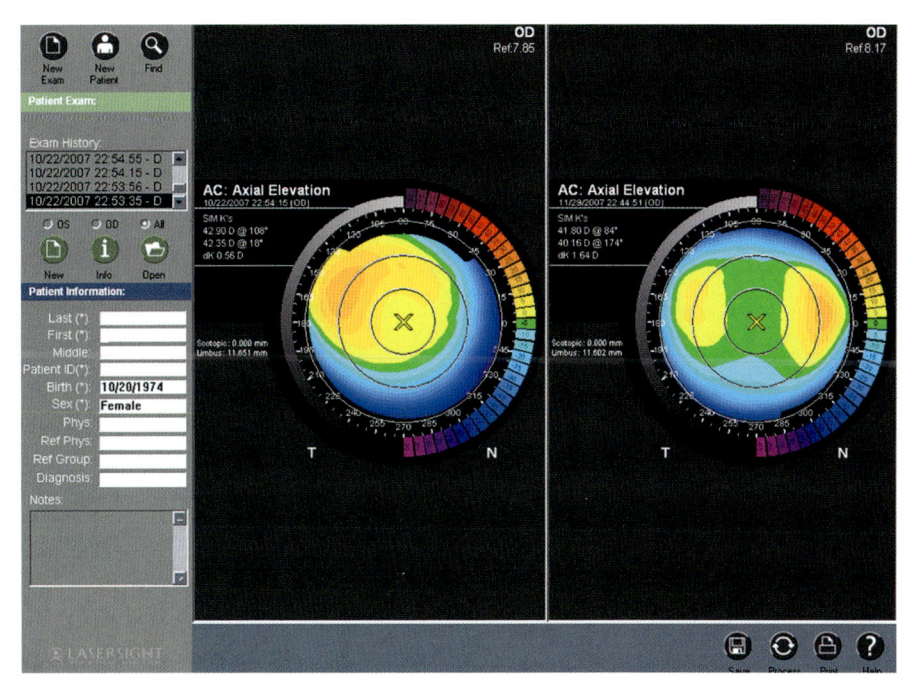

Figure 23.22 Pre-enhancement and postenhancement axial elevation map. Note that when the vertex normal is not changed (as in this Figure), the elevation map of the decentered ablation shows elevation where the cornea was actually ablated for a myopic treatment. This is because the area becomes flatter. Compare this map to the lower left corner of Figure 23.20, where the corneal-vertex normal is optimized (Target Z axis). Using the optimized axis gives an elevated area where no adequate ablation was applied, consistent with the optimized enhancement ablation profile as indicated in Figure 23.20, upper right (*Courtesy:* Dr Bing Liu, General Air Force Hospital)

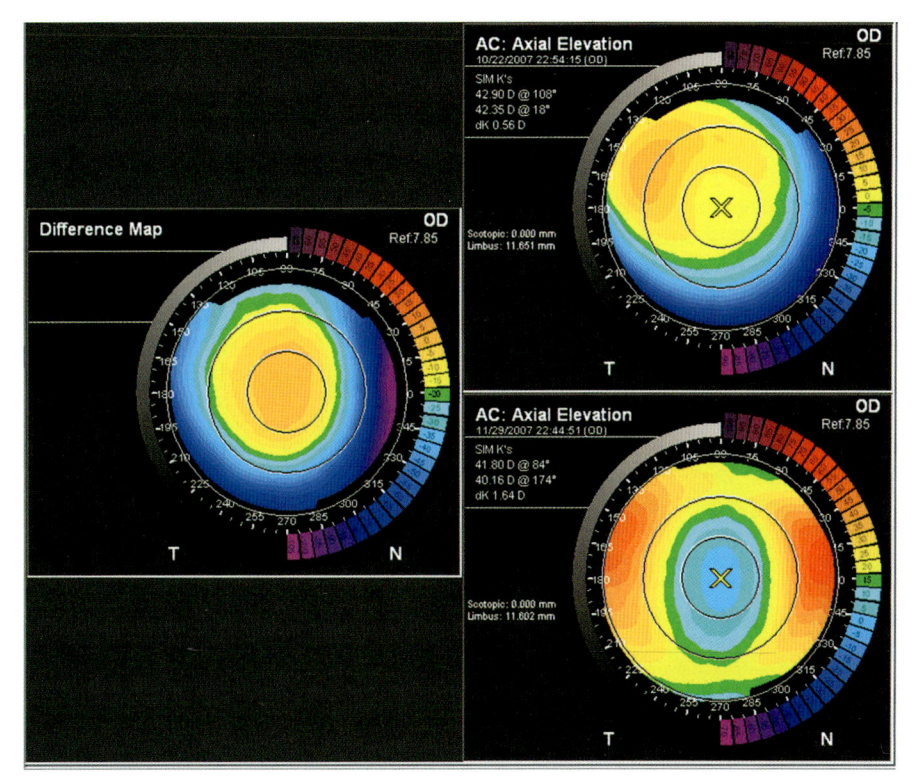

Figure 23.23 Pre-enhancement and postenhancement axial elevation difference map, showing pre-enhancement elevation (upper right), postenhancement elevation (lower right) and elevation difference (left), using a reference sphere of 7.85 mm
(*Courtesy:* Dr Bing Liu, General Air Force Hospital)

of glare, night vision difficulty, and monocular diplopia, decentered ablation needs to be ruled out. Understanding of elevation topography, and aberrometry is crucial for the diagnosis. Modern surgical options are presently evolving and gaining success in addressing this complication to improve visual quality in postrefractive eyes.

REFERENCES

1. Chan CC, Boxer Wachler BS. Centration analysis of ablation over the coaxial corneal light reflex for hyperopic LASIK. J Cataract Refract Surg. 2006;22:467-71.
2. Amano S, Nanba A, Hamada N, et al. Corneal irregular astigmatism after hyperopic laser in situ keratomileusis. Cornea. 2005;24(7):789-92.
3. Gimbel, Howard V. Refractive Surgery: A Manual of Principles and Practice. SLACK Incorporated; 2000. pp. 75-8, 114.
4. Mulhern M, Foley-Nolan A, O'Keefe M, Condon P. Topographic analysis of ablation centration after excimer laser photorefractive keratectomy and laser in situ keratomileusis for high myopia. J Cataract Refract Surg. 1997;23:488-94.
5. Schalhorn SC, Amesbury EC, Tanzer DJ. Avoidance, recognition, and management of LASIK complications. Am J Ophthalmol. 2006;141(4):733-9.
6. Randleman JB. Etiology and clinical presentations of irregular astigmatism after keratorefractive surgery. In: Wang MX (Editor): Irregular Astigmatism: Diagnosis and Treatment. SLACK Incorporated; 2008. pp. 73-5.
7. Ou JI, Manche EE. Topographic centration of ablation after LASIK for myopia using the CustomVue VISX S4 excimer laser. J Cataract Refract Surg. 2007;23:193-7.
8. Vinciguerra P, Camesasca FI. Decentration after refractive surgery. J Refract Surg. 2001;17(2 Suppl):S190-1.
9. Salmon TO, Horner DG. Comparison of elevation, curvature, and power descriptors for corneal topographic mapping. Optom Vis Sci. 1995;72(11):800-8.
10. Rachid MD, Yoo SH, Azar DT. Phototherapeutic keratectomy for decentration and central islands after photorefractive keratectomy. Ophthalmology. 2001;108:545-52.
11. Lafond G, Bonnet S, Solomon L. Treatment of previous decentered excimer laser ablation with combined myopic and hyperopic ablations. J Refract Surg. 2004;20:139-48.
12. Carones F, Vigo L, Scandola E. Wavefront-guided treatment of symptomatic eyes using the LADAR6000 excimer laser. J Refract Surg. 2006;22(9):S983-9.
13. Kanellopoulos AJ, Pe LH. Wavefront-guided enhancements using the wavelight excimer laser in symptomatic eyes previously treated with LASIK. J Refract Surg. 2006;22(4):345-9.
14. Mrochen M, Krueger RR, Bueeler M, Seiler T. Aberration-sensing and wavefront-guided laser in situ keratomileusis: management of decentered ablation. J Refract Surg. 2002;18(4):418-29.
15. Aliã J, Galal A, Montalbán R, Piñero D. Corneal wavefront-guided LASIK retreatments for correction of highly aberrated corneas following refractive surgery. J Refract Surg. 2007;23(8):760-73.
16. Salz JJ. Wavefront-guided treatment for previous laser in situ keratomileusis and photorefractive keratectomy: case reports. J Refract Surg. 2003;19(6):S697-702.
17. Schwartz GS, Park DH, Lane SS. CustomCornea wavefront retreatment after conventional laser in situ keratomileusis. J Cataract Refract Surg. 2005;31(8):1502-5.
18. Montague AA, Manche EE. CustomVue laser in situ keratomileusis treatment after previous keratorefractive surgery. J Cataract Refract Surg. 2006;32(5):795-8.
19. Lin DY, Manche EE. Custom-contoured ablation pattern method for the treatment of decentered laser ablations. J Cataract Refract Surg. 2004;30(8):1675-84.
20. Tamayo Fernandez GE, Serrano MG. Early clinical experience using custom excimer laser ablations to treat irregular astigmatism. J Cataract Refract Surg. 2000;26(10):1442-50.
21. Tamayo F, Serrano MG. Treating Irregular Astigmatism and Keratoconus with the VISX C-CAP Method. Int Ophthalmol Clin. 2003;43(3):103-10.
22. Alessio G, Boscia F, La Tegola MG, Sborgia C. Corneal Interactive Programmed Topographic Ablation Customized Keratectomy for Correction of Postkeratoplasty Astigmatism. Opthalmology. 2001;108:2029-37.
23. Stojanovic A, Suput D. Strategic planning in topography-guided ablation of irregular astigmatism after laser refractive surgery. J Refract Surg. 2005;21(4):369-76.
24. Toda I, Yamamoto T, Ito M, Hori-Komai Y, Tsubota K. Topography-guided ablation for treatment of patients with irregular astigmatism. J Refract Surg. 2007;23(2):118-25.
25. Pedrotti E, Sbabo A, Marchini G. Customized transepithelial photorefractive keratectomy for iatrogenic ametropia after penetrating or deep lamellar keratoplasty. J Cataract Refract Surg. 2006; 32(8):1288-91.
26. Mularoni A, Laffi GL, Bassein L, Tassinari G. Two-step LASIK with topography-guided ablation to correct astigmatism after penetrating keratoplasty. J Refract Surg. 2006;22(1):67-74.
27. Seitz B, Langenbucher A, Kus MED MER, Harrer M. Experimental correction of irregular corneal astigmatism using topography-based flying-spot-mode excimer laser photoablation. Am J Ophthalmol. 1998;125:252-6.
28. Alessio G, Boscia F, La Tegola MG, Sborgia C. Topography-driven Excimer Laser for the Retreatment of Decentralized Myopic Photorefractive Keratectomy. Opthalmology. 2001;108:1695-1703.
29. Kymionis GD, Panagopoulou SI, Aslanides IM, Plainis S, Astyrakakis N, Pallikaris IG. Topographically supported customized ablation for the management of decentered laser in situ keratomileusis. Am J Ophthalmol. 2004;137(5):806-11.
30. Reinstein DZ, Archer TJ, Gobbe M. Topography Guided Ablation with the Carl Zeiss Meditec MEL80 and CRS Master. In: Ming Wang (Ed). Irregular Astigmatism: Diagnosis and Treatment. Slack, Inc, Thoroughfare, NJ. 2007.
31. Stojanoviæ A, Jankov MR. Regularizing the cornea—the concept of an ideal corneal surface (iVIS Suite approach to the treatment of irregular astigmatism). In: Wang MX (Ed). Corneal Topography in the Wavefront Era. Slack, Thoroughfare, NJ, 2007.

Chapter 24

Irregular Astigmatism: LASIK as a Correcting Tool

Jorge L Alió (Spain), José I Belda Sanchis (Spain), Ahmad MM Shalaby (Spain)

INTRODUCTION

Irregular astigmatism represents one of the problems that are very difficult to manage and frustrating in results to refractive surgeons. It is also one of the worst sequelae of corneal injuries. It can also complicate certain corneal diseases as keratoconus. With the recent evolution of refractive surgery techniques and diagnostic tools, new types of irregular astigmatism are being observed.[1,2]

Astigmatism is defined as irregular if the principle meridia are not 90 degrees apart, usually because of an irregularity of the corneal curvature. It cannot be completely corrected with a spherocylindrical lens.[3] Duke-Elder defines irregular astigmatism as a refractive state in which the refraction in different meridians conforms to no geometric plan and the refracted rays have no planes of symmetry.[4]

The alternatives for correction of irregular astigmatism are very scarce and with very limited expectations. Spectacle correction is usually not useful in the correction of corneal irregular astigmatism as it is difficult to define principle meridia. Hard contact lenses represent a good alternative in which the tear fluid layer under the contact lens evens out the irregularity. We should consider that adaptation and stability of contact lenses is limited by irregular corneal surface and the patient's comfort. We also must remember that our patients consented to undergo refractive surgery because they did not want to use contact lens.

Lamellar and full thickness corneal grafting are surgical alternatives. The limited availability of corneal donor as well as the biological and refractive complications of allografic corneal graft limit the clinical applicability of these procedures.

Many surgeons have made great efforts in finding a solution to this problem.[5-7] To this date, we believe there should be safe, efficient and predictable methods to resolve this problem. Accordingly, the approach to new surgical methods for the correction of irregular astigmatism is one of the greatest expectations in today's refractive surgery, especially when the very near future is supposed to bring generalization of corneal refractive surgical techniques.

ETIOLOGY OF IRREGULAR ASTIGMATISM

Primary Idiopathic

There is a general prevalence of low levels of irregular astigmatism of unknown cause within the population. This might explain the mildly reduced best corrected visual acuity (BCVA) in patients presenting for laser vision correction.[1]

Secondary

Dystrophic

In the cornea, keratoconus, which, in optical terms, is primarily an irregularity of the anterior corneal surface, is the best example. Pellucid degeneration and keratoglobus may also be associated with posterior corneal surface irregularity causing irregular astigmatism. In the lens, lenticonus may cause irregular astigmatism; and in the retina, posterior staphyloma.[1]

Traumatic

Corneal irregularity is caused commonly by corneal wounds (incision or excision) or burns (chemical, thermal or electrical).[1]

Postinfective

Postherpetic keratitis is the most common form of postkeratitic healing and scarring that may lead to an irregular surface.[1]

Postsurgical

Irregular corneal astigmatism can complicate any of the following refractive surgical procedures: keratoplasty, photorefractive keratectomy (PRK), laser *in situ* keratomileusis (LASIK), radial keratotomy (RK), arcuate keratotomy (AK), and cataract incisions. Scleral encirclement or external plombage may also contribute.[1]

DIAGNOSIS OF IRREGULAR ASTIGMATISM

Clinically, irregular astigmatism will present with one of those typical *retinoscopy* patterns, the most common being spinning and scissoring of the red reflex. On attempting *keratometry* the mires will appear distorted. *Corneal topography* shows certain patterns for irregular astigmatism that will be discussed in detail later. The most recent and sophisticated technique is the application of *wavefront analysis (aberrometers)*.[8] This emerging method measures the refractive status of the whole internal ocular light path at selected corneal intercepts of incident light pencils. By comparing the wavefront of a pattern of several small beams of coherent light projected through to the retina with the emerging reflected light wavefront, it is possible to measure the refractive path taken by each beam and to infer the specific spatial correction required on each path.

CLINICAL CLASSIFICATION OF IRREGULAR ASTIGMATISM FOLLOWING CORNEAL REFRACTIVE SURGERY

In corneal refractive surgery using laser *in situ* keratomileusis (LASIK) the surgeon uses a microkeratome, whether automated or manual, to fashion a corneal flap and a stromal bed. Once the flap is fashioned and lifted, the excimer laser is used to ablate tissue from the bed for the planned correction, depending on the capabilities of the laser.

In this clinical perspective, irregular astigmatism induced by LASIK can be classified according to its location as:
1. *Superficial:* Due to flap irregularities.
2. *Stromal:* Induced by bed irregularities.
3. *Mixed:* Due to irregularities in both flap and stroma.

CORNEAL TOPOGRAPHY PATTERNS OF IRREGULAR ASTIGMATISM

Topographic classification of irregular astigmatism patterns is very important in the following aspects:
1. To unify terms and concepts when referring corneal topography images.
2. To determine the cause of the subjective symptoms referred by the patient (Haloes, glare, monocular diplopia, etc.).
3. Reaching a topographic basis for retreatment. The topographic approach for treatment patients with a previous unsuccessful excimer laser surgery should allow reshaping the cornea in the pattern appropriate for the specific patient.

Based on the topography, we proposed the following classification for irregular astigmatism:[7]
- Irregular astigmatism with defined pattern, and
- Irregular astigmatism with undefined pattern.

Irregular Astigmatism with Defined Pattern

We define irregular astigmatism with defined pattern when there is a steep or flat area of at least 2 mm of diameter, at any location of the corneal topography, which is the main cause of the irregular astigmatism. It is divided into five groups:
(i) *Decentered ablation:* Shows a corneal topographic pattern with decentered myopic ablation in more than 1.5 mm in relation to the center of the cornea. The flattening area is not centered in the center of the cornea; the optical zone of the cornea has one flat and one steep area **(Figure 24.1A)**.
(ii) *Decentered steep:* Shows a corneal hyperopic treatment decentered in more than 1.5 mm in relation to the center of the cornea **(Figure 24.1B)**.
(iii) *Central Island:* Shows an image with an increase in the central power of the ablation zone for myopic treatment ablation at least 3.00 D and 1.5 mm in diameter, surrounded by areas of lesser curvature **(Figure 24.1C)**.
(iv) *Central irregularity:* Shows an irregular pattern with more than one area not larger than 1.0 mm and no more than 1.50 D in relationship with the flattest radius, located into the area of the myopic ablation treatment **(Figure 24.1D)**.
(v) *Peripheral irregularity:* It is a corneal topographic pattern, similar to Central Island, extending to the periphery. The myopic ablation is not homogeneous, there is a central zone measuring 1.5 mm in diameter and 3.00 D in relation to the flattest radius, connected with the periphery of the ablation zone in one meridian **(Figure 24.1E)**.

Irregular Astigmatism with Undefined Pattern

We consider irregular astigmatism with undefined pattern when the image shows a surface with multiples irregularities; big and small steep and flat areas, defined as more than one area measuring more than 3 mm in diameter in the central 6 mm **(Figure 24.1F)**. The difference between flat and steep areas were not possible to calculate in the Profile Map and Dk showed an irregular line or a plane line. Normally, Dk is the difference between the steep k and the flat k, given in diopters at the cross of the profile map. A plane line is produced when the Dk cannot recognize the difference between the steep k and the flat k in severe corneal surface irregularities.

EVALUATION OF IRREGULAR ASTIGMATISM

In managing irregular astigmatism patients, a meticulous preoperative evaluation is necessary. We perform a complete preoperative ocular examination, including previous medical reports and complete ocular examination: uncorrected and

Chapter 24: Irregular Astigmatism: LASIK as a Correcting Tool   253

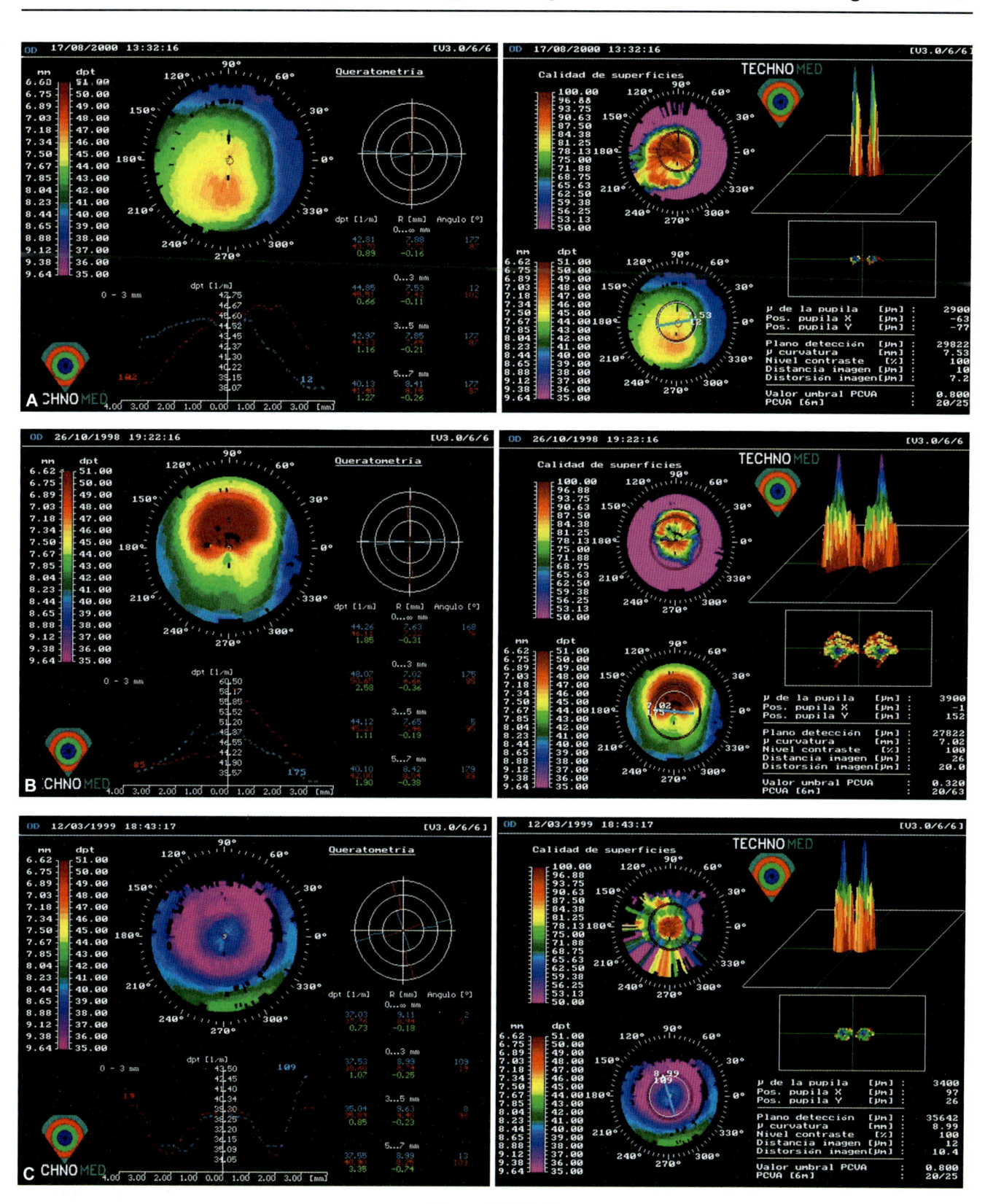

Figures 24.1A to C

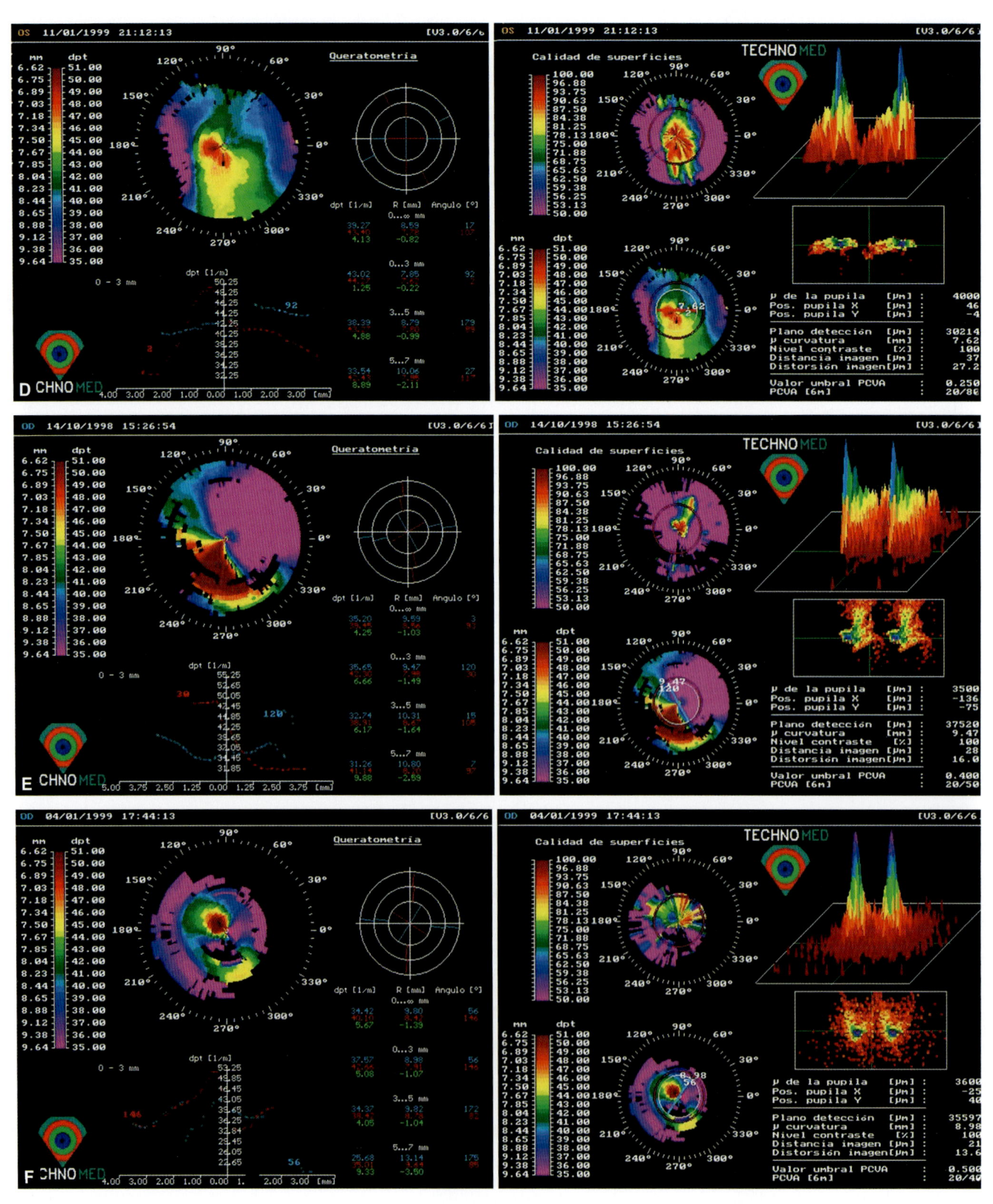

Figures 24.1D to F

Figures 24.1A to F Topographic patterns of irregular astigmatism (with ray-tracing study): (A) Decentered ablation; (B) Decentered steep; (C) Central Island; (D) Central irregularity; (E) Peripheral irregularity; (F) Irregular astigmatism with undefined pattern

best-corrected visual acuity, pinhole visual acuity and cycloplegic refraction, keratometry, contact ultrasonic pachymetry (Ophthasonic Pachymeter Teknar Inc. St. Louis, USA) and computerized corneal topography.

We perform the corneal topography with Eye Sys 2000 Corneal Analysis System (Eye Sys Co., Houston, Texas, USA). We also use the Ray Tracing mode of the C-SCAN Color-Ellipsoid-Topometer (Technomed GmbH, Germany) to determine the Superficial Corneal Surface Quality (SCSQ) and the Predicted Corneal Visual Acuity (PCVA), in addition to the topography. Recently, we have incorporated the elevation topography of the Orbscan system (Orbtek, Bausch & Lomb Surgical, Orbscan II corneal topography, Salt Lake City, Utah, USA) in our evaluation tools.

Follow-up examinations after surgery were performed at 48 hours, and then at one, three and six months. Postoperative follow-up included: uncorrected and best-corrected visual acuity, pinhole visual acuity and cycloplegic refraction, biomicroscopy with slit-lamp and complete corneal topography screening with the previously mentioned instrumentation.

During the preoperative and postoperative period the surface quality of the cornea was studied using the ray tracing module of the C-SCAN 3.0 (Technomed GmbH, Germany). This device determines the Predicted Corneal Visual Acuity from the videokeratography map, by simulating the propagation of rays emanating from 2 light dots, which impinge on the best-fit image plane after projection via the maximum of 10,800 previously determined corneal surface power values. Refraction and reflection of the rays at the optical interfaces, the pupil diameter, and the anterior chamber depth are taken into account according to laws of geometric optics. The ray tracing module calculates the pupil size by the captured image of the pupil during videokeratography. This is measured under the luminance of the videokeratography rings (25.5 cd/m^2) and is automatically integrated into the ray tracing analysis with the videokeratography map. Hence, the projection of objects onto a detection plane can be determined. The ray tracing module calculates the optical function of the eye by means of optical ray tracing, using the cornea as the refractive element of the system. It measured and analyzed the interaction between the corneal shape, the functional optical zone, and the pupil diameter, providing valuable additional information by the resulting diagram. The image points on the detection plane are represented by two intensity peaks that must be spatially resolved to discriminate them separately and individually. The peak distance (distance between the functional maxima) and the distortion index (basic diameter of the point cloud in the detection plane) are parameters defined to help understanding when these two peaks are spatially resolved. They help to objectively quantify the individual retinal image in each subject. We found it very useful to evaluate the corneal surface and corneal healing. It is very useful also to explain visual phenomena referred by the patients, and that cannot be explained by older versions of corneal topographers. We do not consider it a substitution of the Eye Sys 2000 Corneal Analysis System (Houston, Texas, USA), but it showed to be a very useful tool.[9]

Subjective symptoms from the pre- and postoperative periods should be noted in the medical report such as haloes, glare, dazzling, corneal and conjunctival dryness, dark-light adaptation and visual satisfaction reported by the patient.

TREATMENT OF IRREGULAR ASTIGMATISM

Treatment options for irregular astigmatism have expanded greatly during recent years. Excimer laser is gaining priority with the advent of finely controlled corneal ablation. Before that, limited alteration of corneal topography was possible by, for instance, selective incision placement, placement and removal of sutures, or penetrating and lamellar keratoplasty. Other "treatment" options for irregular corneal astigmatism include optical correction with hard contact lenses in which the tear fluid layer under the contact lens "evens out" the irregularity,[1] but the patient's aim to get rid of glasses as well as contact lenses still limits their use. Intracorneal ring segments, originally used for myopia treatment,[10] represent another option that is under investigation.

SURGICAL TECHNIQUES WITH EXCIMER LASER

These represent the main subject of discussion in this chapter. The ultimate goal of excimer laser treatment is to correct the refractive error while reducing corneal astigmatism and topographic disparity but not increasing aberrations within the eye. With the advent of the excimer laser, it may be possible to correct directly some forms of corneal irregularity. Before considering any treatment option, the relationship between the topographical irregularity and the refraction must be considered; a therapeutic balance between refractive and corneal astigmatism must be reached so that overall visual function is optimal. In other word, an optimal treatment should include both topographic and refractive values, rather than excluding one.[1]

We have used different methods for the surgical correction of irregular astigmatism. At this moment we consider three surgical procedures with excimer laser for correction of the irregular astigmatism:

1. Selective Zonal Ablation (SELZA). Designed to improve the irregular astigmatism with defined pattern.[7]
2. Excimer Laser Assisted by Sodium Hyaluronate (ELASHY). Designed mainly to improve the irregular astigmatism with undefined pattern.[11]
3. Topographic linked excimer laser ablation (TOPOLINK). Combines data of the topography and patient refraction in as software to improve the irregular astigmatism with defined pattern and the refractive error, with the same procedure.[12]

The three surgical procedures were performed under topical anesthesia of oxibuprocaine 0.2% (prescaina 0.2%; Laboratorios Llorens, Barcelona, Spain) drops; no patient required sedation. The postoperative treatment consisted of instillation of topical tobramycin 0.3% and dexamethasone 0.1% drops (Tobradex, Alcon-Cusi, Barcelona, Spain) three times daily for the five days of the follow-up and then discontinued. When the ablation was performed onto the cornea (surface ELASHY, some patients of SELZA), a bandage contact lens (Actifresh 400, power +0.5, diameter 14.3 mm, radius of curvature 8.8 mm – Hydron Ltd., Hampshire, UK) was used during the first three days of the postoperative and the patient was examined daily. It was removed when complete re-epithelialization was observed. Then treatment with topical fluorometholone (FML forte, Alcon-Cusi, Barcelona, Spain) was used three times daily for the three months of follow-up and then stopped.[13]

Non-preserved artificial tears (Sodium Hyaluronate 0.18%, Vislube®, CHEMEDICA, Ophthalmic line, München, Germany) were used up to three months in every case. Supplementation with oral pain management medications was also used as necessary.

Statistical analysis. Statistical analysis was performed with the SPSS/Pc+4.0 for Windows (SPSS Inc, Madrid, 1996). Measurements typically are reported as the mean ± 1 standard deviation (using $[n-1]^{1/2}$ in the denominator of the definition for standard deviation, where n is the number of observations for each measurement) and as the range of all measurements at each follow-up visit. Patients' data samples were fitting the normal distribution curves. Statistically significant differences between data sample means were determined by the "t Student's" test; *P* values less than 0.05 were considered significant. Data concerning the standards for reporting the outcome of refractive surgery procedures, as the safety, efficacy and predictability, was analyzed as previously defined.[14]

SELECTIVE ZONAL ABLATION (SELZA)

In this study we report the results of a prospective clinically controlled study performed on 31 eyes of 26 patients with irregular astigmatism induced by refractive surgery. All cases were treated with SELZA using an excimer laser of broad circular beam (Visx Twenty/Twenty, 4.02, Visx, Inc. Sunnyvale, California, USA). The surgical planning was applied using the Munnerlyn formula,[15] modified by Buzard,[16] to calculate the depth of the ablation depending on the amount of correction desired and the ablation zone. In this formula the resection depth is equal to the dioptric correction, divided by 3, and multiplied by the ablation zone (mm) squared. We used a correction factor of 1.5 times, to avoid under-correction:

$$\text{Ablation depth} = \frac{(\text{Dioptric correction}) \times 1.5}{3} \times (\text{ablation zone})^2$$

Methods

In general, we use ablation zone of 2.5 to 3.0 mm, depending on the steep area of the corneal topography to be modified. The ablation zone was determined by observing the color map. The form of videokeratoscope provides additional information about the irregular zones, and the profile map gave the values for performed ablation. In cases of irregular corneal surface, treatment was performed on the center of irregularity, which was located using the color map of the corneal topography. First we located the center of the cornea, then we located the exact center of irregularity. Here we use the dotted boxes in the map (each dot represents 1 mm^2) to detect the exact center of irregularity in relation to the center of the cornea. The amount of ablation is determined using the cross-section of the profile map (vertical line corresponding to diopters and horizontal line corresponding to corneal diameter). When the patient had LASIK previously we lift the flap or do a new LASIK cut and then we perform excimer laser using PTK mode.

The technique is based on subtraction of tissues to eliminate the induced irregular astigmatism and to achieve a uniform corneal surface using excimer laser; we center the effect of laser on zones where the corneal surface is steeper.

Results

In patients with *Irregular Astigmatism with a Defined Pattern*, the visual acuity improved significantly, reaching in many cases near the BCVA before the initial refractive procedure. The difference between the BCVA before the therapeutic procedure was highly statistically significant ($P < 0.001$). The mean BCVA after 3 months of surgery it was 20/25 ± 20/100 (range 20/50 to 20/20), which was as good as the initial BCVA 20/29 ± 20/100 (range 20/50 to 20/20). The BCVA before selective ablation improved from 20/40 ± 20/100 (range 20/100 to 20/25) to 20/25 ± 20/100 (range 20/50 to 20/20). We did not have any patients with one or more lines lost of BCVA. The Corneal Uniformity Index (CUI) before versus after selective zonal ablation with excimer laser improved from 55.65 ± 15.90% (range 20 to 80%) to 87.83 ± 10.43% (range 70 to 100), a change that was also statistically significant ($P < 0.005$). The safety index (the ratio of mean postoperative BCVA over mean preoperative BCVA) was equal to 1.55. The efficacy of the procedure in percent UCVA 20/40 was 85%.

The predictability (astigmatic correction) using CUI was expressed as a percentage. The various relationships between the preoperative CUI and the surgically induced postoperative CUI provided the information about the magnitude of irregular astigmatism correction and the corneal surface uniformity. Correction index, which is the ratio of mean postoperative CUI (87.83 ± 10.43%; range 70 to 100%) over the mean preoperative CUI (55.65 ± 15.90%; range 20 to 80%), was equal to 1.58.

The results observed in all cases of *irregular astigmatism without a defined pattern* were poor. Efficacy in percentage of eyes with UCVA of 20/40 was 6%, and predictability (astigmatic correction) was 0.58. In some cases, visual acuity became worse: the refraction error and corneal topography were considerably modified.

Discussion

The results of the selective zonal ablations technique were satisfactory as regards the correction of irregular astigmatism with a defined topographic pattern. Visual acuity improved in the postoperative period, achieving values near the initial BCVA of the patients (before the initial surgical procedure). The corneal uniformity index was used to evaluate the central 3 mm zone of the cornea. It started to improve in the early postoperative period and stabilized after 3 months, just as the issues of visual acuity ($p < 0.005$). Normally, this refractive procedure requires a stable corneal topography (6 months after the last corneal procedure) and its adequate interpretation.[17] However, our results have proven that it is not suitable for correcting all patterns of irregular astigmatism.

EXCIMER LASER ASSISTED BY SODIUM HYALURONATE (ELASHY)

This can be considered as one of the ablatable masking techniques. We report the results of a prospective clinically controlled study performed on 32 eyes of 32 patients with irregular astigmatism.[11] All the patients had been subjected previously to one or more of the following procedures: LASIK, Incisional Keratotomy, Photorefractive Keratotomy, Phototherapeutic Keratotomy, Laser Thermokeratoplasty, and Corneal Trauma. Irregular astigmatism was induced thereafter.

Six months after the last corneal procedure, for the aim of stability, the cases were selected for ELASHY.

Methods

The correction of irregular astigmatism was made with a Plano Scan Technolas 217 C-LASIK Scanning-spot Excimer laser (Bausch & Lomb, Chiron Technolas GmbH, Doranch, Germany) in PTK mode, assisted by viscous masking sodium hyaluronate 0.25% solution (LASERVIS® CHEMEDICA, Ophthalmic line, München, Germany). The physical characteristics of sodium hyaluronate confer important rheological properties to the product. The photoablation rate is similar to that of corneal tissue, forming a stable and uniform coating on the surface of the eye, filling depressions on the cornea and effectively masking tissues to be protected against ablation by the laser pulses.[18,19]

In cases where the irregular astigmatism was induced by a flap irregularity or superficial corneal scarring, ELASHY ablations were performed onto the corneal surface. The epithelium was removed also using the excimer laser assisted by viscous masking. When the irregularity was inside the stroma, at the previous stromal bed, the previous flap was lifted up whenever possible or a new cut was done. Then ELASHY was performed at the stroma and after the procedure the flap was repositioned.

We centered the ablation area at the corneal center and fixed it with the eye-tracking device in the center of the pupillary area. After this, one drop of the viscous masking and fluorescein was scattered on the cornea that should be ablated and spread out with the 23-G cannula (Alcon laboratories, USA) used for the viscous substance instillation. With fluorescein, it was also possible to observe the spot and the effect of laser. Because fluorescent light is emitted during ablation of corneal tissue, cessation of the fluorescence signifies complete removal of the viscous masking solution, i.e. tissue ablation. The laser was prepared for ablation at 15 microns intervals. After each of the intervals, a new drop of the viscous substance was added at the center of the ablation area and again spread out with the same maneuvers with the 23-G cannula. Total treatment was calculated to ablate the prominent areas to the calculated K value at the 4 to 6 mm optical zone or calculated from the tangential map of the Technomed topographer. Assuming a decrease in the ablative effect of the laser due to the use of the viscous agent, we target at a 50% more ablation than the one that corresponds to the real ablation depth necessary for the smoothing procedure.

Results

Corneal topography corresponded to our established classification of irregular astigmatism: Pattern Irregular Corneal astigmatism was identified in 23 eyes (71.9%) and irregularly irregular corneal astigmatism was identified in the other 9 eyes (28.1%).

The mean preoperative BCVA improved from $20/40 \pm 20/80$ (range 20/200 to 20/20) to $20/32 \pm 20/100$ (range 20/200 to 20/20) ($p = 0.013$, Student T test), six months after surgery. There were only 2 eyes losing 2 lines of BCVA (6.3%) and 3 eyes (9.4%) losing 1 line. The procedure was safe with a safety index equal to 1.1 (**Figure 24.2**).

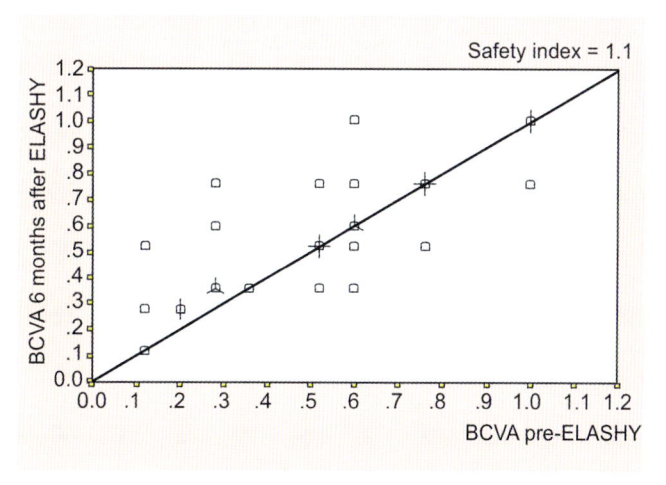

Figure 24.2 Safety of ELASHY procedure

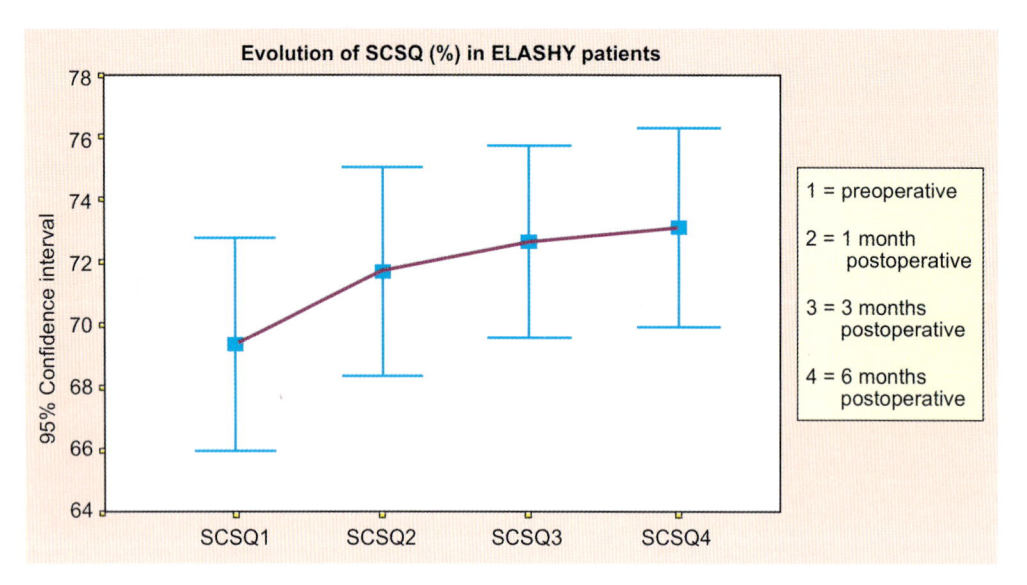

Figure 24.3 Evolution of superficial corneal surface quality (SCSQ)

We had 28.1% of eyes at 6 months with postoperative UCVA of 20/40 or better with 3.1% reaching 20/20. The efficacy index of the procedure (*the ratio [mean postoperative UCVA]/[mean preoperative BCVA]*), was equal to 0.74.

As ELASHY is based on the subtraction of tissues to achieve a smoother corneal surface, we expected improvement in the patients' BCVA and subjective symptoms as glare, haloes, etc. rather than changes in the spherical equivalent. The Astigmatic Correction was evaluated in respect to the improvement of the corneal surface, using the data of the SCSQ provided by the Ray-Tracing study (C-SCAN Color-Ellipsoid-Topometer, Technomed GmbH, Germany). The SCSQ **(Figure 24.3)** pre vs. post therapeutic procedure, evaluated by the Ray-Tracing study, improved from a mean of 69.38% ± 9.48 preoperatively to 73.13% ± 8.87 6 months postoperative ($p = 0.002$, Student T test). Other parameters of the Ray-Tracing study also improved. The PCVA improved from a mean of 20/40 ± 20/80 (range 20/100 to 20/16) preoperatively to 20/32 ± 20/80 (range 20/125 to 20/16) ($p = 0.11$, Student T test) postoperatively. Also the image distortion significantly improved from a mean of 14.39 ± 3.78 (range 8 to 23.2) preoperatively to 13.29 ± 3.87 (range 7.2 to 26) at 6 months ($p = 0.05$, Student T test).

The corneal surface was left smooth. Almost all patients (89.3%) subjectively noted improvement of the visual acuity and disappearance of the visual aberrations that previously impaired their quality of vision. This coincided with the improvement in the peak distortion and the ray tracing **(Figures 24.4A and B)**.

Discussion

The results of this study could add the excimer laser plano Scan surgery assisted by sodium hyaluronate 0.25% (LASERVIS® CHEMEDICA, Ophthalmic line, München, Germany) (ELASHY) to the tools useful for the treatment of irregular astigmatism, both with and without defined pattern. The clinical indications include irregular astigmatism caused by irregularity in flap or irregularity on stromal base induced by laser *in situ* keratomileusis (LASIK).

Excimer laser application in PTK mode may be undertaken to improve various visual symptoms through improving the corneal surface.[20,21] PTK also can help in cases of irregularities and opacities on corneal surface or anterior stroma, induced by LASIK. In 1994, Gibralter and Trokel applied excimer laser in PTK mode to treat a surgically induced irregular astigmatism in two patients. They used the corneal topographic maps to plan focal treatment areas with good results.[5] The correction of irregular astigmatism should be considered one of these therapeutic indications.

The use of a viscous masking agent should increase the efficiency of the procedure, through protection of the valleys between the irregular corneal peaks, leaving these peaks of pathology exposed to laser treatment. In this study, we used the sodium hyaluronate 0.25% (LASERVIS® CHEMEDICA, Ophthalmic line, München, Germany) for this purpose. When the treatment is performed on corneal surface, Bowman's membrane is removed. However, the new epithelium was able to grow and adhere well to the residual stroma. Interestingly, none of our patients developed significant postoperative haze (grade II – III)—normally seen after PRK -, even those subjected to surface treatment. We suggest this effect could be due to the protective properties of the viscoelastic agent, sodium hyaluronate 0.25% (LASERVIS® CHEMEDICA, Ophthalmic line, München, Germany), against the oxidative free radical tissue damage.[22]

Many authors have evaluated different masking agents.[18,19] Methylcellulose is the most commonly used agent and is available in different concentrations. Some properties of the

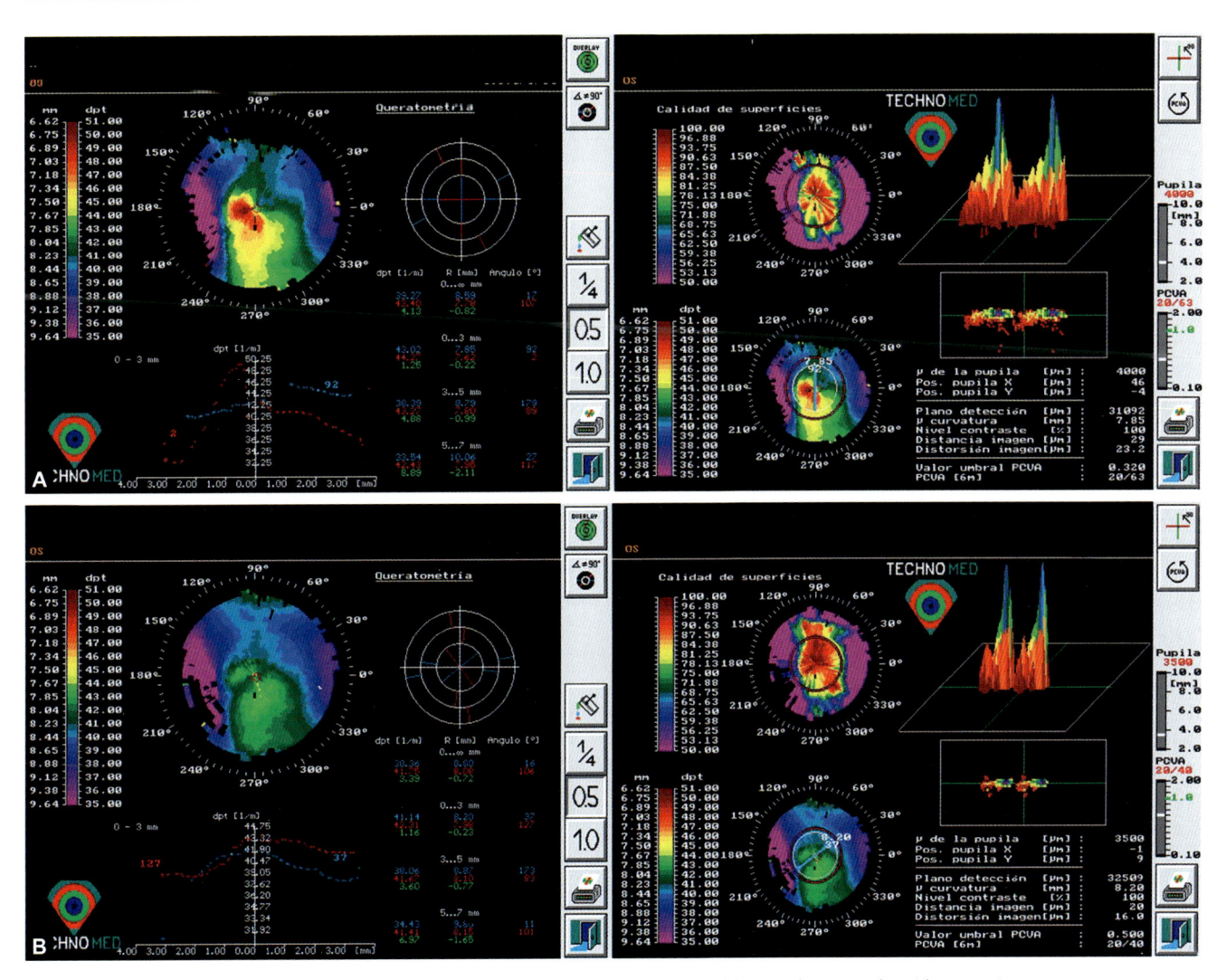

Figures 24.4A and B ELASHY: Preoperative (A) and postoperative (B) corneal topography with ray tracing.
Note the improvement of the ray tracing

methylcellulose, such as to turn white during ablation due to its low boiling point, make this substance not ideal for the purpose of this study.

We found sodium hyaluronate 0.25% (LASERVIS® CHEMEDICA, Ophthalmic line, München, Germany) the most suitable for our purpose. It has a photoablation rate similar to that of the corneal tissue. Its stability on the corneal surface forms a uniform coating that fills the depressions on the cornea, protecting them against ablation by the laser pulses.[18] Adding fluorescein to the viscous masking solution is very useful to observe the excimer laser action during corneal ablation at the corneal surface. With experience, it is very easy to distinguish between the ablated areas (in dark) and the marked areas (in green) while the laser radiation is ablating the cornea during the treatment.

The actual corneal ablation is equal to 63% of the ablation depth programmed in the software of the excimer laser.[23] If the corneal surface has a masking agent, the initial effect of the laser will be ablating the viscous masking.

The viscous masking solution functions to shield the tissues partially. Multiple applications of viscous masking solution often are required, and a familiarity with the ablation characteristics will be learned with experience. When the laser ablation is performed on corneal surface, we increase the ablation by 50 mm, necessary for the epithelium ablation.[24]

ELASHY was originally designed for the correction of those irregular astigmatism cases that did not show a pattern and were not available to SELZA correction, yet it proved to be as effective in cases with pattern irregular astigmatism.

Ray tracing improved considerably, coinciding with the improvement of the visual subjective symptoms. The Superficial Corneal Surface Quality and image distortion were improved, achieving values significantly better than the preoperative values. This demonstrates that a relationship exists between the quality of the corneal surface and the quality of the vision. When the corneal surface is smoothened, the haloes, glare and refractive symptoms improve.[25]

From our results, we can also conclude that the procedure achieves more stability with time, improving from the 3rd to the 6th months. Further follow-up of these cases should be carried on to obtain better judgment of the biomechanical response of these special corneas to the procedure and to decide a proper timing for a re-intervention if necessary.

TOPOGRAPHIC LINKED EXCIMER LASER ABLATION (TOPOLINK)

About 40% of human corneas show some irregularities that cannot be taken into account in a standard basis treatment with excimer laser.[26] For these patients, and for those suffering an irregular astigmatism after trauma or refractive surgery, a custom-tailored, topography-based ablation, which has been adapted to the corneal irregularity, would be the best approach to improve not only their refractive problem but also to improve their quality of vision.

This treatment was the first step in customized ablation depending mainly on the corneal topography as well as the refraction for calculating the treatment. It aimed at obtaining the best corrected visual acuity that can be attained by wearing hard contact lenses. Its requirements were an excimer laser with spot scanning technology, in which a small laser spot delivers a multitude of single shots fired in diverse positions to fashion the desired ablation profile. The laser spot is programmable, thus any profile could be obtained. A videokeratography system that provides an elevation map at high resolution is needed, and specific software is used to create a customized ablation program for the spot scanner laser.

Methods

The aim of this study was to fashion a regular corneal surface in 41 eyes of 41 patients with irregular astigmatism induced by LASIK: 27 eyes (51.9%) had irregular astigmatism with a defined pattern; 14 eyes (48.1%) had irregular astigmatism without a defined pattern.

All cases were treated with a Plano Scan Technolas 217 C-LASIK Scanning-spot Excimer laser (Bausch & Lomb, Chiron Technolas GmbH, Doranch, Germany) assisted by a C-Scan Color-Ellipsoid-Topometer (Technomed GmbH, Germany). We performed several corneal topographies from same eye; the software of the automated corneal topographer selected the four exactly equal. These corneal maps, the refractive error, the pachymetry value and desired k-readings calculated for each patient were sent to Technolas by modem. The information was analyzed and a special software program for each patient was created, including it in the Technolas 217 C-LASIK excimer laser by system modem.

The basis for the topography-assisted procedure was the preoperative topography.[12,27] This data was transferred into true height data and the treatment for correcting the refractive values in sphere and astigmatism, taking into account the corneal irregularities, was calculated. After that, a postoperative topography was simulated. With this technique, real customized treatment should become a reality, not only treating the refractive error but also improving the patient's visual acuity.

Results

After 3 months of the surgery: The mean preoperative UCVA improved from 20/80 ± 0.25 (range 20/400 to 20/60) to 20/40 ± 0.54 (range 20/100–20/32); mean preoperative BCVA improved from 20/60 ± 0.20 (range 20/200 to 20/32) to 20/32 ± 0.15 (range 20/60 to 20/25). This proved to be statistically significant ($p < 0.001$).

Even though emmetropia was our goal, it was considered more important to achieve a regular corneal surface. The spherical equivalent of the individual refraction was taken into account in determining the corneal k-value. Preoperatively, mean sphere was -0.26 ± 4.50 D (range –5.75 to +3.70 D) and mean cylinder was –1.71 ± 3.08 D (range –6.00 to +2.56 D). Three months after surgery, the mean sphere was 0.701. 25 D (range –1.75 to +1.50 D) and the mean cylinder was –0.89 ± 1.00 D (range –1.92 to +1.00).

Corneal topography improved significantly in those cases that presented an irregular astigmatism with a defined pattern. The mean Corneal Surface Quality improved from 45% (range 35–60%) to 76.6% (range 60.06 to 96.43%). The corneal surface is left smooth and the ray tracing improved in the peak distortion, coinciding with the improvement of the visual acuity **(Figures 24.5A and B)**. In 60.29% patients the visual aberrations disappeared.

At 3 months of follow-up, the safety of the procedure was 74.31%, the efficacy **(Figure 24.6)** in %UCVA 20/40 was 63.68% and the predictability for the spherical equivalent within the ± 1HD zone was 68.23%.

Discussion

Using the corneal topographic map as a guide, excimer laser ablation can be used to create a more regular surface with improved visual acuity. In a program consisting of a combination of phototherapeutic and photorefractive ablation patterns, the amount of tissue to be removed is calculated on the basis of the diameter and steepness of the irregular areas of the corneal surface. At present, customized ablation based on topography can improve spectacle-corrected visual acuity.

Limitations for this technique exist. With this procedure some irregular astigmatisms cannot be corrected. Some patients could not be selected as candidates for Topolink because any of the following criteria were present:

1. Differences between steep and flat meridians more than 10 D at the 6.0 mm treatment area.
2. Corneal pachymetry was not thick enough (< 400 mm).

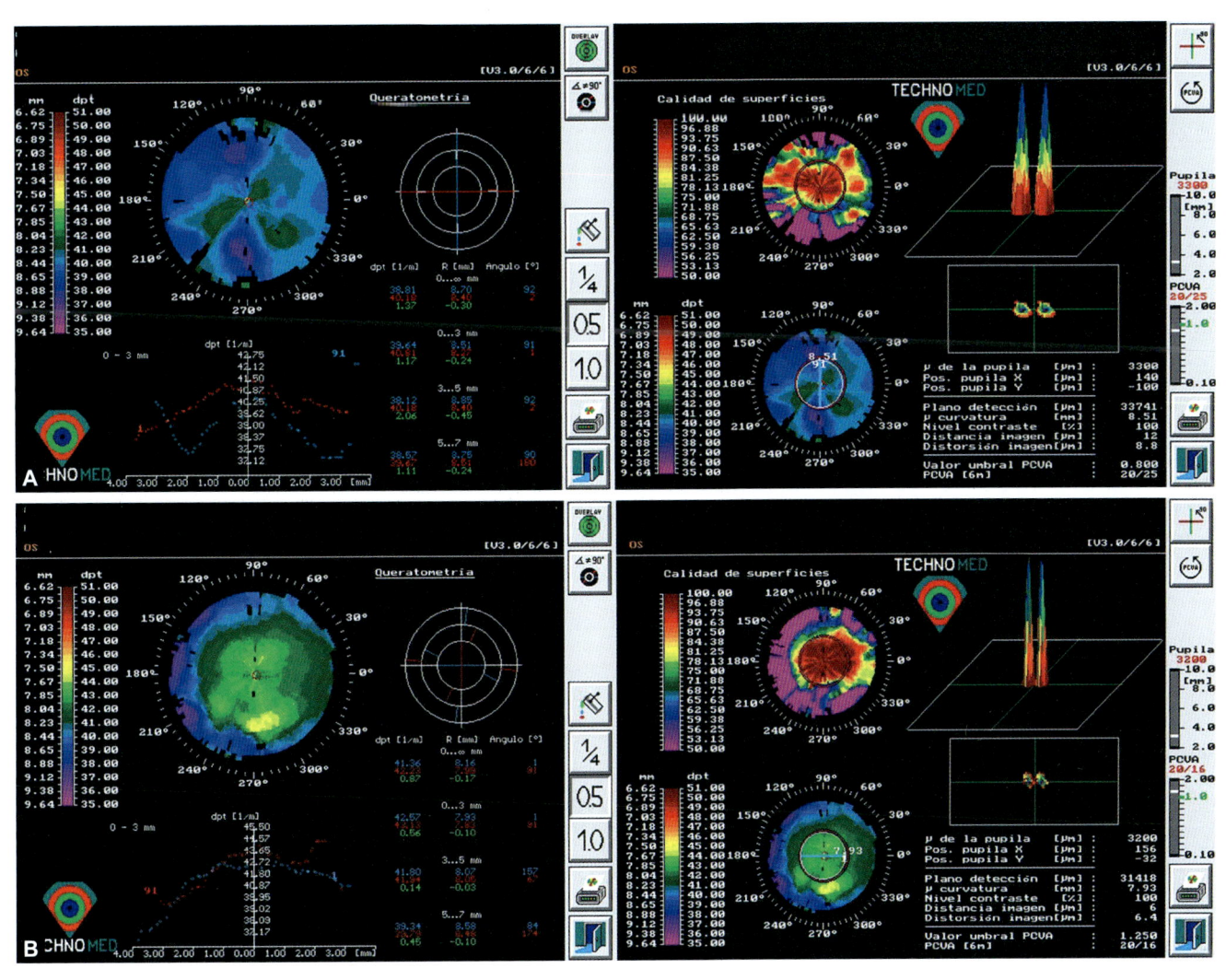

Figures 24.5A and B Topolink: Preoperative (A) and postoperative (B) corneal topography with ray tracing

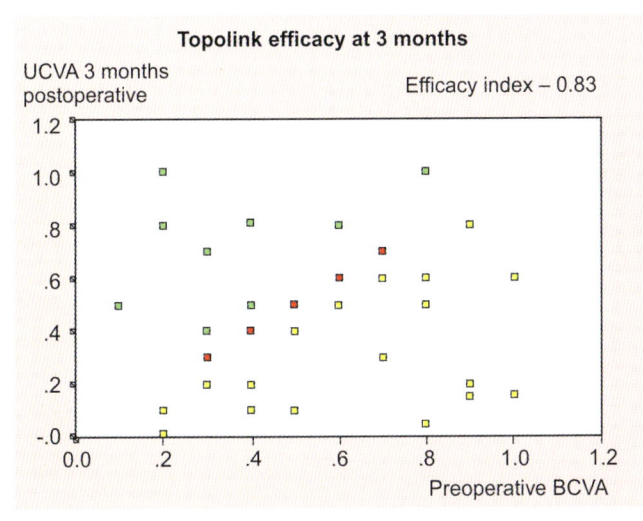

Figure 24.6 Efficacy of the Topolink procedure at 3 months

3. Diameter of the corneal topography more than 5.0 mm.
4. Corneal topography showing an irregular astigmatism with undefined pattern (irregularly irregular).

This preliminary study showed that topographic-assisted LASIK (Topolink) could be a useful tool to treat irregular astigmatism. This technique was, as aforementioned, the early stage of developing customized ablation. The surgeon depends only on the Placido topographic images, their precision and their reproducibility. To the moment, this cannot provide us with the actual customization and we are still left with some patients waiting for a solution.

THE FUTURE

A new view of customization could be achieved with more reliable instruments (elevation topography, aberrometer, etc.). As aforementioned, wavefront analysis (aberrometry,

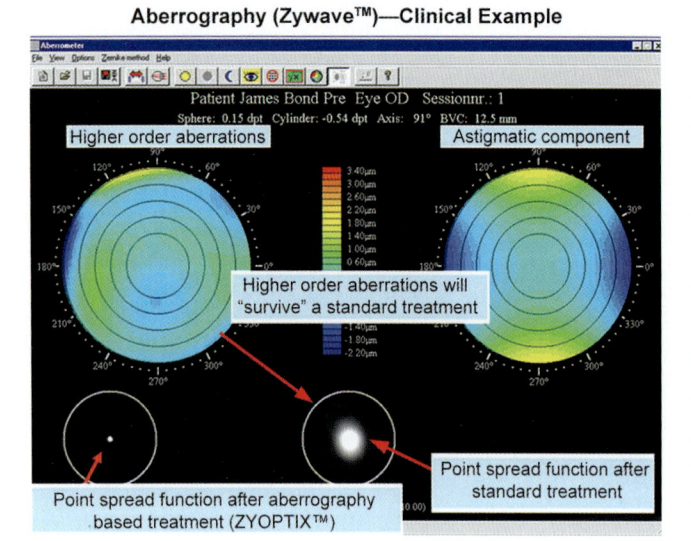

Figure 24.7 Aberrometry, clinical example

Figure 24.7) can measure the refractive state of the entire internal ocular light path.[8] Using this technology, it has been shown that using only the refractive error of the eye to treat the ammetropia can greatly increase optical aberrations within the eye.[28] Increases in wavefront aberrations are evident after both PRK and LASIK,[29] and increased spherical aberration has been shown to occur in cases of increased corneal astigmatism.[30] This increase in spherical aberration and coma will interfere with visual function, particularly in low-light conditions where the pupil size increases, increasing the effect of aberrations within the eye, a condition that is diminished in daylight where the pupil constricts.[31]

We are now conducting the second phase of a study incorporating the data of the wavefront analysis using the Zywave aberrometer (Bausch & Lomb, CHIRON Technolas GmbH, Doranch, Germany) together with the elevation topography of the Orbscan II (Orbtek, Bausch & Lomb Surgical, Orbscan II corneal topography, Salt Lake City, Utah, USA) to correct ammetropia.

To the moment the system is under trial, and is only applicable to regular virgin corneas. With the proper development of the technique, we think that it would provide us with the real customized ablation necessary not only for our desperate irregular astigmatism patients but also for obtaining a super vision for ammetropes who are to be treated for the first time.

OTHER PROCEDURES

Automated Anterior Lamellar Keratoplasty

This technique was originally designed to treat superficial stromal disorders, but it has also been used for the treatment of difficult cases of irregular astigmatism, with very poor results.[32] The surgeon performs phototherapeutic keratectomy or a microkeratome lamellar resection to 250 to 400 mm stromal depth, followed by transplantation of a donor lamella of the same dimension on to the recipient bed.[33] We have limited experience with this subject. We think it is a good option for patients with thin corneas, and with the preservation of the Descemet's membrane, the complications of rejection should be extremely minimized if not eliminated. However, the subject is out of the scope of discussion in this chapter.

Intracorneal Ring Segments (Intacs)

These segments were originally designed to correct low to moderate myopia by inducing flattening of the central cornea through intralamellar insertion of 2 PMMA ring segments in the corneal midperiphery.[34] Studies indicated that the range of corneal asphericity before and after surgery, provided good visual acuity and normal contrast sensitivity.[10, 35] These segments could be used to modify the corneal surface in patients with irregular astigmatism whether natural as in keratoconus or surgically induced.

Contact Lens Management

Contact lenses are sometimes needed in the postoperative management of refractive surgery. This need arises as it has become evident to the refractive surgeon that an undesirable result has occurred. The decision of contact lens fitting has to be based on the impossibility of performing new surgeries, or the willing of the patient.[36]

SUMMARY

It is clear from the previous discussions that the subject of irregular astigmatism is still under investigation. In spite of the availability of various methods attempting to solve this problem, we are left with patients who are not satisfied with their vision and are in need for intervention. Penetrating keratoplasty is an ultimate solution that has to be undertaken only when the patient has no other alternative. More effort should be done to try to help these patients improving their corneal surface quality and BCVA. The evolution of newer techniques and the experience gained by refractive surgeons day after day represent a hope for irregular astigmatism patients.

REFERENCES

1. Goggin M, Alpins N, Schmid LM. Management of irregular astigmatism. Curr Opin Ophthalmol. 2000;11:260-66.
2. Alió JL, Artola A, Claramonte PJ, et al. Complications of photorefractive keratectomy for myopia: Two year follow-up of 3000 cases. J Cataract Refract Surg. 1998;24:619-26.

3. Azar DT, Strauss I. Principles of applied optics. In: Albert DM, Jakobiec FA, (Eds). Principles and Practice of Ophthalmology, Vol 5, Philadelphia, PA, WB Saunders Co; 1994. pp. 3603-21.
4. Duke-Elder S (Ed). Pathological retractive errors. In System of Ophthalmology. London: Publisher. 1970;5:363.
5. Gibralter R, Trokel SL. Correction of irregular astigmatism with the excimer laser. Ophthalmology. 1994;101:1310-15.
6. Alpins NA. Treatment of irregular astigmatism. J Cataract Refract Surg. 1998;24:634-46.
7. Alió JL, Artola A, Rodríguez-Mier FA. Selective Zonal Ablations with excimer laser for correction of irregular astigmatism induced by refractive surgery. Ophthalmology. 2000;107:662-73.
8. Harris WF. Wavefronts and their propagation in astigmatic optical systems. Optom Vis Sci. 1996;73:606-12.
9. Dick HB, Krummenauer F, Schwenn O, et al. Objective and subjective evaluation of photic phenomena after monofocal and multifocal intraocular lens implantation. Ophthalmology. 1999;106:1878-86.
10. Holmes-Higgin DK, Burris TE. The INTACS Study Group. Corneal surface topography and associated visual performance with INTACS for myopia. Phase III clinical trial results. Ophthalmology. 2000;107:2061-71.
11. Alió JL, Belda JI, Shalaby AMM. Excimer Laser Assisted by Sodium Hyaluronate for correction of irregular astigmatism (ELASHY). Accepted for publication to Ophthalmology, September 2000.
12. Wiesinger-Jendritza B, Knorz M, Hugger P, Liermann A. Laser in situ keratomileusis assisted by corneal topography. J Cataract Surg. 1998;24:166-74.
13. Sher NA, Kreuger RR, Teal P, et al. Role of topical corticoids and nonsteroidal anti-inflammatory drugs in the etiology of stromal infiltrates after photorefractive keratectomy. J Refract Corneal Surg. 1994;10:587-8.
14. Koch DD, Kohnen T, Obstbaum SA, Rosen ES. Format for reporting refractive surgical data. [letter]. J Cataract Refract Surg. 1998;24:285-7.
15. Munnerlyn C, Koons S, Marshall J. Photorefractive Keratectomy: A technique for laser refractive surgery. J Cataract Refract Surg. 1988;14:46-52.
16. Buzard K, Fundingsland B. Treatment of irregular astigmatism with a broad beam excimer laser. J Refract Surg. 1997;13:624-36.
17. Seitz B, Behrens A, Langenbucher A. Corneal topography. Curr Opin Ophthalmol. 1997;8:8-24.
18. Kornmehl EW, Steiner RF, Puliafito CA. A comparative study of masking fluids for excimer laser phototherapeutic keratectomy. Arch Ophthalmol. 1991;109:860-63.
19. Kornmehl EW, Steinert RF, Puliafito CA, Reidy W. Morphology of an irregular corneal surface following 193 nm ArF excimer laser large area ablation with 0.3% hydroxypropyl methylcellulose 2910 and 0.1% dextran 70.1% carboxy-methylcellulose sodium or 0.9% saline (ARVO abstracts). Invest Ophthalmol Vis Sci. 1990; 31:245.
20. Trokel SL, Srinivasan R, Braren B. Excimer laser surgery of the cornea. Am J Ophthalmol. 1983;96:705-10.
21. Orndahl M, Fagerholm P, Fitzsimmons T, Tengroth B. Treatment of corneal dystrophies with excimer laser. Acta Ophthalmol. 1994; 72:235-40.
22. Artola A, Alió JL, Bellot JL, Ruiz JM. Protective properties of viscoelastic substances (sodium hyaluronate and 2% hydroxymethyl cellulose) against experimental free radical damage to the corneal endothelium. Cornea. 1993;12:109-14.
23. Kreuger RR, Trokel SL. Quantification of corneal ablation by ultraviolet light. Arch Ophthalmol. 1986;103:1741-2.
24. Seiler T, Bendee T, Wollensak J. Ablation rate of human corneal epithelium and Bowman's layer with the excimer laser (193nm). J Refract Corneal Surg. 1990;6:99-102.
25. Klyce SD, Smolek MK. Corneal topography of excimer laser photorefractive keratectomy. J Cataract Refract Surg. 1993;19:122-30.
26. Bogan SJ, Waring GO III, Ibrahim O, et al. Classification of normal corneal topography based on computer-assisted videokeratography. Arch Ophthalmol. 1990;108:945-9.
27. Dausch D, Schröder E, Dausch S. Topography-controlled excimer laser photorefractive keratectomy. J Refract Surg. 2000;16:13-22.
28. Mierdel P, Kaemmerer M, Krinke H-E, Seiler T. Effects of photorefractive keratectomy and cataract surgery on ocular optical errors of higher order. Graefe's Arch Clin Exp Ophthalmol. 1999;237:725-9.
29. Oshika T, Klyce SD, Applegate RA, et al. Comparison of corneal wavefront aberrations after photorefractive keratectomy and laser in situ keratomileusis. Am J Ophthalmol. 1999;127:1-7.
30. Seiler T, Reckmann W, Maloney RK. Effective spherical aberration of the cornea as a quantitative descriptor in corneal topography. J Cataract Refract Surg. 1993;19(Suppl):155-65.
31. Applegate RA, Howard HC. Refractive surgery, optical aberrations and visual performance. J Refract Surg. 1997;13:295-9.
32. Sugita J, Kondo J. Deep lamellar keratoplasty with complete removal of pathological stroma for vision improvement. Br J Ophthalmol. 1997;81:184-8.
33. Melles GRJ, Remeijer L, Geerards AJM, Beekhuis WH. The future of lamellar keratoplasty. Curr Opin Ophthalmol. 1999;10:253-9.
34. Ruckhofer J, Stoiber J, Alzner E, Grabner G. Intrastromal corneal ring segments (ICRS, KeraVision Ring, Intacs): clinical outcome after 2 years. Klin Monatsbl Augenheilkd. 2000;216:133-42 (abstract).
35. Holmes-Higgin DK, Baker PC, Burris TE, Silvestrini TA. Characterization of the aspheric corneal surface with intrastromal corneal ring segments. J Refract Surg. 1999;15:520-28.
36. Zadnik K. Contact lens management of patients who have had unsuccessful refractive surgery. Curr Opin Ophthalmol. 1999;10:260-3.

Chapter 25

Posterior Chamber ICL and Toric ICL

Mohamed Alaa El-Danasoury (Saudi Arabia)

INTRODUCTION

Since 1983, many phakic intraocular lens (IOLs) have emerged; they can be classified into three major categories; anterior chamber angle fixated lenses, originally introduced by Baikoff and Joly,[1,2] the iris-fixated lens introduced by Fechner and Worst,[3] and the posterior chamber, sulcus-fixated lens introduced by Fyodorov,[4] and modified by Staar company.[5] The penetration of phakic IOLs in the refractive surgery practice was relatively slow during the last 2 decades of the last century due to many factors including the potential complications of intraocular surgery, the poor early designs, the underdeveloped techniques of implantation, the relatively high incidence of complications in the early reports and above all the lack of long-term published results in peer reviewed literature. Also, the introduction of excimer laser refractive surgery and the booming of LASIK in its early years as "the one procedure" that can correct all refractive errors added to the factors that delayed the wide spread use of phakic IOLs.

Over the last decade, phakic IOLs passed through many stages of innovation and development; surgical techniques were made better and more information became available on the long-term results. Refractive surgeons around the world became more interested in phakic IOLs. Also the better understanding of the biomechanical effect of LASIK on the cornea especially in high amounts of myopia, the increasing number of reported corneal ectasia after LASIK and the development of sophisticated wave front analyzers that objectively measured the negative effect of LASIK on the quality of vision especially to surgically induced high order aberrations made many refractive surgeons reconsider the assumption that this alteration of the natural corneal shape is the best way to address myopic and astigmatic refractive errors.[6]

The introduction of the toric phakic IOLs was a great step towards improving the clinical results and widening the range of correction provided by the toric IOLs. To date only 2 toric phakic IOLs are available; the iris fixated toric Artisan lens and the posterior chamber toric implantable collamer lens (ICL).

This chapter summarizes the evolution, indications, patients' selection criteria, surgical techniques, clinical results and possible complications of the posterior chamber implantable collamer lens.

EVOLUTION

The original design of posterior chamber phakic IOL was introduced by Fyodorov in 1986, it had a collar-button optic and a posterior chamber haptic; the lens was made of silicone and was partially implanted in the posterior chamber through fixation wings with the optic at the pupillary plane **(Figures 25.1A and B)**. The prototype of modern ICL was introduced in 1990 in Russia; the fixation wings were replaced with a plate haptic with square edges. In 1993, Pesando implanted the first ICL prototype (IC2020) in Torino, followed by Skorpik in Vienna and Zaldivar in Argentina.[5,7,8]

The ICL is manufactured by Staar Surgical (Nidau, Switzerland). It is a single-piece, plate-haptic lens, designed to vault anteriorly to the crystalline lens and intended to have minimal contact with the natural lens. The lens material is a proprietary hydrophilic collagen polymer (copolymer of 63% hydroxy-ethyl-methyl-acrylate, 0.2% collagen and 3.4% of a benzofenone for UV absorption) known as Collamer, with a water content of 34%, a light transmission of 99%, and a refractive index of 1.45 at 35º C. According to the manufacturer, the Collamer material is biologically quiet, as collagen has an affinity for fibronectin; upon implantation, a monolayer of fibronectin would coat the IOL surface, inhibiting deposition of other proteins. Therefore, the material would not be recognized as a foreign body, and flare, cell deposition, and inflammation would be minimized.

The design of the ICL progressively evolved from the initial prototypes first implanted in 1993 (models IC2020, and IC2020-M) to the currently used model (V4). The optic diameter progressively increased, from 3.5 to 4.5 mm in the myopic IC2020, to 4.65 to 5.50 mm in the myopic V4, and the lens became progressively thinner. Until the second half of 1996, the ICL had no marks to help identify the anterior optic surface. It was therefore difficult to confirm if the lens was in an upside-down position after its injection. The V2 version of the ICL started to be manufactured with orientation marks on the haptics, which lead to an increase in popularity of ICL implantation by injection. Throughout the evolution of the ICL, one of the major changes in the design features was implemented in the lens vaulting; the currently available model (V4) has steeper radius of curvature, this allowed an additional 0.13 to 0.21 mm of anterior vaulting in comparison

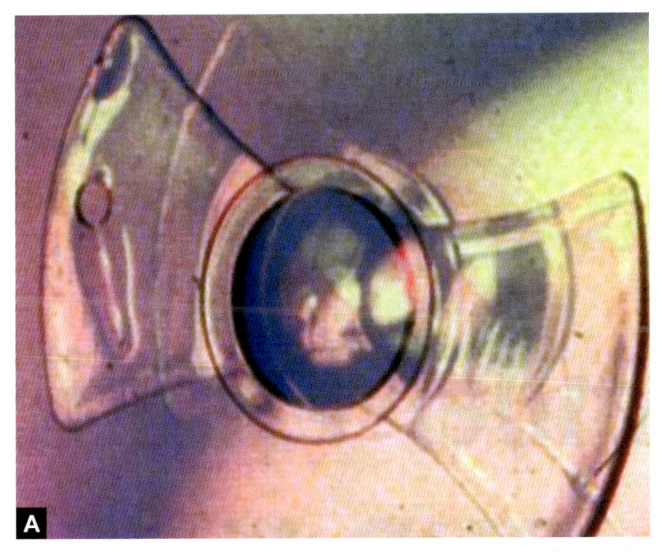

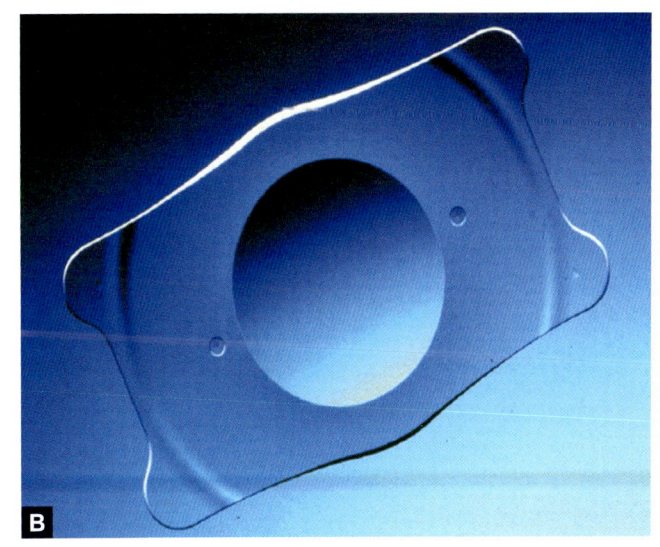

Figures 25.1A and B (A) Original design of phakic posterior chamber lenses (Fyodorov, 1986); fixation wings were implanted in the posterior chamber between the iris and the anterior capsule of the crystalline lens and the collar-button optic was positioned at the pupillary plane; (B) Currently used ICL (model V4). Note the 4 laser marks engraved on the haptic: 2 orientation marks on the leading right and trailing left footplates and 2 alignment marks on either sides of the optic (*Courtesy:* Staar Surgical)

to its predecessor, the V3 depending on the dioptric power of the lens.[9]

Current ICL Models and Powers

Today, three ICL versions are available for use: myopic, hyperopic and toric versions.

Myopic ICL

The myopic version of the ICL (V4) is planoconcave with the anterior surface being plano, the optic diameter ranges from 4.65 to 5.50 mm. The thickness of the lens is less than 50 μm at the center of the optic, and less than 100 μm at the haptic plate. The thickest part of the myopic ICL is the junction between the optic and the haptic and ranges from 300 to 700 μm. The overall length of myopic ICL ranges from 11.50 to 13.00 mm in 0.50 mm increments. Power ranges from –23.00 to –3.00 diopters (D) in half-diopter increments.

Hyperopic ICL

The hyperopic ICL (V3) is concave-convex, with the anterior surface being convex. Optic diameter is fixed at 5.50 mm for all powers; the thickest part is the center of the optic. Overall lengths of hyperopic ICL range from 11.00 to 12.50 mm in 0.50 mm increments. Power ranges from 3.00 to 21.50 D in half-diopter increments.

Toric ICL

The toric ICL (V4) has a toric convex-concave optic that incorporates the desired cylindrical power in a specific axis as required to correct a given patient's astigmatic condition. It is manufactured using the platform of the nontoric design and is similar to the spherical ICL in terms of size, thickness and configuration, with the addition of a toric optic to correct myopia with astigmatism. To minimize rotation required by the surgeon during implantation, the toric ICL is custom made to be implanted on the horizontal axis. The order-delivery time for a toric ICL is between 4 and 6 weeks; to shorten this time, the surgeon has the option to use a readymade toric ICL of the same required power with an axis of the cylinder within 22.5° of the required, in such case the "alternative" toric ICL will have to be rotated inside the eye to compensate for the difference in axis orientation. Each toric ICL is sent to the surgeon with a guide demonstrating the amount and direction of rotation from the horizontal axis required to align the toric ICL cylinder axis to correct the patient's astigmatism. It is recommended that rotation is less than 22.5° from the horizontal.[10] The cylindrical power ranges from 1.0 to 6.0 D with the same range of spherical power as the myopic ICL.

Myopic ICL (V4) was approved by the FDA in 1995 for the full range of powers between –20.00 and –3.00 D. FDA studies for toric and hyperopic ICL are in process. **Table 25.1** summarizes the characteristics and the power ranges for the currently available 3 ICL models. Besides the refractive powers described in **Table 25.1**, which are currently available in international

Table 25.1 Characteristics of the currently available myopic (V4), hyperopic (V3) and toric ICL (V4) models

ICL	Spherical power	Cylindrical power	Optic diameter	Optic/Haptic thickness	Overall height
Myopic model (V4)	−3.0 to −12.0 D	0.0	5.50 mm	0.3 to 0.5 mm	1.15 to 1.77 mm
	−12.5 to −13.5 D	0.0	5.25 mm	0.5 mm	1.08 to 1.78 mm
	−14.0 to −16.5 D	0.0	5.00 mm	0.5 to 0.6 mm	1.12 to 1.89 mm
	−17.0 to −23.0 D	0.0	4.65 mm	0.5 to 0.7 mm	1.19 to 2.05 mm
Hyperopic model (V3)	+3.0 to +12.0 D	0.0	5.50 mm	0.2 mm	1.25 to 2.29 mm
	+12.5 to +13.5 D	0.0	5.50 mm	0.2 mm	1.61 to 2.36 mm
	+14.0 to +16.5 D	0.0	5.50 mm	0.2 mm	1.68 to 2.49 mm
	+17.0 to +21.5 D	0.0	5.50 mm	0.2 mm	1.82 to 2.79 mm
Toric model (V4)	−3.0 to −12.0 D	+1.0 to +6.0 D	5.50 mm	0.3 to 0.5 mm	1.5 mm
	−12.5 to −13.5 D	+1.0 to +6.0 D	5.25 mm	0.5 mm	1.5 mm
	−14.0 to −16.5 D	+1.0 to +6.0 D	5.0 mm	0.5 to 0.6 mm	1.5 to 1.6 mm
	−17.0 to −23.0 D	+1.0 to +6.0 D	4.65 mm	0.5 to 0.7 mm	1.6 to 1.7 mm

markets, Staar can also manufacture customized lenses upon request from surgeons; this includes myopic ICLs from as low as −0.50 D to as high as −23.00 D, hyperopic ICLs from as low as +0.50 D to as high as +21.50 D, as well as toric ICLs with spherical power from −23.00 to +20.00 D, and cylinders from +0.50 to +10.00 D at any axis from 0 to 180º. In addition to these, any combination of the myopic and hyperopic versions with cylinder corrections can be customized.

INDICATIONS OF ICL AND T-ICL

High myopia and high myopic astigmatism remain the most common indications for ICL and toric ICL; LASIK being more commonly performed for low and moderate amounts of myopia. Patients who suffer from high astigmatism and high myopia are usually not suitable candidates for corneal-reshaping procedures because there is an increased risk of corneal ectasia, associated with low visual quality and unpredictability.[11] These cases of high myopia or high compound myopic astigmatism are better candidates for ICL or toric ICL. There is no clear-cut as for the upper limit for safe LASIK, however there is general agreement to be somewhere between 7.00 and 9.00 D of myopia. In a prospective bilateral randomized study we showed that phakic IOLs are more effective, more predictable and safer than LASIK for myopia above 9.00 D; also a subgroup of patients who had LASIK in one eye and phakic IOL in the other eye preferred the phakic IOL eye, better quality of vision was the main reason for their preference,[12] for this reason we routinely perform ICL/toric ICL for correction of myopia of 8.00 D or more, even if there is no contraindication for LASIK.

In lower amounts of myopia we implant ICL/toric ICL for any case that carries any risk of post-LASIK ectasia or flap complications, these include eyes with relatively thin corneas that do not allow leaving 300 μm of stromal bed, corneas steeper than 48.00 D or flat corneas with expected post-LASIK reading flatter than 35.00 D and corneas with suspicious topography including forme fruste keratoconus or keratoconus suspect cases.

Stable keratoconus is another growing indication for ICL and toric ICL, in the last 2 years we performed more than 80 ICL/toric ICL for cases with stable keratoconus with very good results that will be discussed later in the report section.

Other indications of ICL and toric ICL include correction of residual refractive errors after LASIK, corneal grafting, intracorneal ring segments implantation, corneal collagen crosslinking and pseudophakia.

The excellent quality of vision and the high predictability of ICL/toric ICL as compared to excimer laser procedures carry the possibility of reducing the upper limit of keratorefractive procedures in the near future.

Hyperopic ICL are indicated to correct hyperopia up to 10.00 D provided the anterior chamber depth is adequate, since hyperopes usually have shallower anterior chamber and narrower angle compared to myopes, hyperopic ICLs are less commonly used compared to myopic and toric ICLs.

SELECTION CRITERIA AND PREOPERATIVE ASSESSMENT

To be considered a good candidate for ICL implantation a patient should have a stable manifest refraction, an anterior chamber depth of at least 2.7 mm calculated from the endothelium, a central endothelial count of more than 2200 cells/mm^2, and an open angle of the anterior chamber.

Refraction

Manifest refraction is usually sufficient for low and moderately high myopes, however, in extreme myopia contact lens over-refraction is recommended. In hyperopes, a cycloplegic refraction is advisable especially in younger subjects to eliminate the possible effect of accommodation. We perform manifest refraction for myopia less than 15.00 D, contact lens over-refraction for myopia of 15.00 D and above and cycloplegic refraction for all hyperopes. In all cases, the vertex distance of the refraction should be recorded to be used in calculation of the ICL power. A 1.00 mm error in vertex distance was found to correspond to a 1% miscalculation of ICL power.[13]

Stability of Refraction

Simple refractive errors usually stabilize between 18 and 21 years of age. A documented stable refraction for at least one year is advisable if the patient is not to be subjected to a secondary procedure later in his life. There is no published data on ICL implantation in children, however, due to the exchangeability of the ICL it might be a good option for children with anisometropia. A long-term prospective clinical trial is needed to study the efficacy, predictability and safety of ICL implantation in children.

Anterior Chamber Depth

A sufficient anterior chamber depth (ACD) is an important factor to prevent endothelial cell loss after phakic IOLs implantation. ICL is the farthest phakic IOL from the endothelium; it is estimated that an anterior chamber depth of 2.7 mm from the endothelium to the anterior surface of the crystalline lens is the lower limit for safe ICL implantation.

The ACD can be measured using optical devices (IOL Master, Carl Zeiss, Thornwood, NY, USA), anterior segment imaging devices (Pentacam, Oculus, Dutenhofen, Germany and Orbscan; Bausch & Lomb, Rochester, NY, USA) or an A-scan ultrasound. The IOL Master measures the anterior chamber depth via a 0.7 mm wide light section and gives accurate measurements of the ACD. We compared ACD measured with both IOL Master and Orbscan II in 100 consecutive eyes and we found no statistically significant difference between both devices. Reuland et al reported similar results comparing anterior chamber depth values determined by Pentacam and IOLMaster.[14] Contact ultrasound can also be used but it has to be noted that it leads to an impression on the cornea, which influences the true anterior chamber depth. Immersion ultrasound gives accurate measures but it is not widely used because of its being a complicated and time consuming technique.

The Pupil Size

The ICL optic diameter ranges from 4.65 to 5.50 mm depending on the power of the lens. Since the ICL is implanted in the posterior chamber, the effective optic diameter at the corneal plane is larger than the actual diameter; it ranges form 6.17 to 7.30 mm at the corneal plane for the same power range. Patients with scotopic pupil diameter larger than the effective lens optic diameter might experience night glare or haloes around light.

Corneal Topography

Topography is essential for all patients undergoing refractive surgery mainly to help diagnosis early and moderate cases of keratoconus. Abnormal topography is not an absolute contraindication for ICL surgery. Many cases that are not good candidates for excimer laser refractive surgery can safely have ICL; these include steep corneas, flat corneas and keratoconus suspect. Cases with stable keratoconus and good spectacle corrected visual acuity can also benefit from ICL surgery.

Gonioscopy

Gonioscopy is important to exclude patients with narrow or abnormal angle as ICL implantation in such cases may lead to narrowing of the angle of the anterior chamber with secondary glaucoma.

A comprehensive ophthalmic examination has to be performed for all patients before undergoing ICL surgery including but not limited to slit-lamp biomicroscopy, IOP measurement and dilated fundus examination.

ICL Sizing

Estimating the proper size and power for the ICL to be implanted in a given eye is key factor for successful ICL surgery.

Since the ICL was designed so that its haptic plate rests horizontally on the ciliary sulcus, the length of the ICL should ideally be equal to the horizontal sulcus diameter. Nowadays there are two main methods to determine the length of the ICL before implantation; the widely used conventional method based on white-to-white measurement and the relatively new method using high frequency ultrasound imaging devices to measure the actual sulcus diameter.

The conventional method for sizing of myopic ICL is based on adding 0.50 mm to the horizontal white-to-white measurement for anterior chamber depth < 3.5 mm and 1.0 mm to the horizontal white-to-white measurement for anterior chamber depth > 3.5 mm for the myopic ICL model. In Asian eyes and due to some anatomical differences from Caucasian eyes, Chang et al recommended adding 0.5 mm to the horizontal white-to-white measurement for eyes with anterior chamber depth ≤ 3.0 m, and adding 1.0 mm for anterior chamber depth > 3.0 mm.[15]

The white-to-white corneal diameter can be measured manually with calipers, IOL master or Orbscan. The conventional method is more widely used than the high frequency ultrasound method because it is simple and

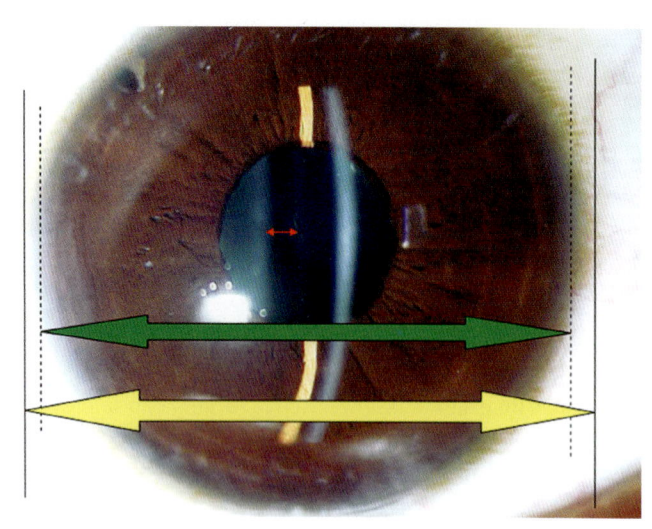

Figure 25.2 An eye with limbal pigmentation and high ICL vault (about 800 μm, red arrow); the ICL was oversized because the actual the white-to-white measurement (green arrow) was overestimated by the Orbscan II as Orbscan measurement included the limbal pigmentation (yellow arrow)

cost effective. In 100 consecutive ICL surgeries, we found no statistically significant difference in the white-to-white measurements using calipers and Orbscan II. The same finding was also reported by Choi and co-workers.[16] In cases with limbal pigmentation it should be noted that Orbscan may overestimate the white-to-white measurement; and in this particular case, calipers measurements are more reliable. **Figure 25.2** shows an eye with limbal pigmentation that received an oversized ICL based on an Orbscan II white-to-white measurement resulting in a high vault.

Choi et al,[16] described a method to calculate the sulcus-to-sulcus horizontal diameter using an ultrasound biomicroscope (UBM) with a 50 MHz probe; they evaluated the vault results of ICL length determined using UBM method and compared the results to those of the conventional method. The UBM used in their study had the limitation of producing only 5 × 5 mm fields per scan making measurement of the direct sulcus-to-sulcus horizontal diameter not possible. In their series, all 13 eyes that had ICL implantation based on the UBM sizing method showed ideal vault, whereas among 17 eyes who received ICL based on the conventional sizing methods; 10 (58.8%) eyes showed ideal vault, 3 (17.6%) eyes showed excessive vault, and 4 (23.6%) eyes showed insufficient vault at 1 month after operation. They concluded that, in their hands, the UBM method, achieved significantly better ICL vaults than the conventional white-to-white method. They also evaluated the ICL footplate locations and found no statistically significant differences between cases where ICL length was determined based on UBM method and the cases where they used the conventional white-to-white measurement.

The introduction of the modern high frequency ultrasound measuring tools was very valuable for understanding the anatomy of the ciliary sulcus and carries a promise to improve the determination of the ICL length. Few of these devices are now commercially available as the Artemis (Ultralink LCC, ST Petersburg, Fla), HiScan (Opticon, Rome, Italy) and the Vumax (Sonomed, NY, USA).

The conventional method for ICL sizing may not be ideal because the correlation between the white-to-white measurement and the sulcus diameter is proven not be accurate,[17] the amount of scleral over-riding on the anterior corneal surface is variable and the point selected for measurement varies among surgeons. However, white-to-white although not ideal is good enough; the rate of ICL replacement for long or short size is extremely low (less than 0.8%).[7] This low rate of incorrect ICL sizing using the conventional white-white method may be at least partly explained by the assumption that the haptic might safely sit in the sulcus, on the zonules or on the ciliary processes with no adverse effects. Vukich and coworkers studied the position of the footplates after ICL implantation and showed that in about 40% of cases the ICL footplates rest on the zonules without causing side effects (Vukich J, personal communication). We believe that the conventional white-to white measurement will remain widely used at least till high frequency ultrasound technology that measures the sulcus diameter reaches maturity and becomes friendly to use and reproducible. A surgeon using the conventional method needs to ensure proper calibration of his instruments, look for scleral over-riding and watch limbal pigmentation in case of using an Orbscan for white-to-white measurement.

ICL Power Calculation

Compared to cataract patients, refractive surgery patients are younger, more demanding and less willing to use spectacles; this entails a very accurate power calculation for ICL. Fortunately, this is made more feasible because the position of ICL in the eye is less variable than that of aphakic IOL after cataract surgery.[7]

Two calculation softwares are provided by the company, one is for spheric and the other for toric ICL power calculation. Calculation softwares provide the surgeon with the ability to calculate the power of the ICL and also the lens size for given preoperative measurements. The software incorporates a formula that derives from a standard IOL power calculation for phakic eyes, described by Holladay in 1993.[18] The only measurements necessary for the calculation are the corneal power, the preoperative refraction, the anterior chamber depth and the vertex distance of the refraction. The power of the lens is calculated based on the desired postoperative refraction. It is not necessary to determine the biometric dimensions of the globe (axial length, crystalline lens thickness, and vitreous chamber), as they remain completely unchanged.

Basically,

$$IOL = \dfrac{1336}{\dfrac{1336}{\dfrac{1000}{\dfrac{1000}{PreRx} - V} + K} - ELP} - \dfrac{1336}{\dfrac{1336}{\dfrac{1000}{\dfrac{1000}{D\,PostRx} - V} + K} - ELP}$$

where ELP is the expected lens position in mm (distance from corneal vertex to principal plane of IOL), IOL is the intraocular lens power in D, K is the net corneal power in D, PreRx is the preoperative refraction in D, D PostRx is the desired postoperative refraction in D, and V is the vertex distance in mm of refractions. The ELP = AA + SF, where AA is the anatomic anterior chamber depth in mm (distance from corneal vertex to plane of iris root), and SF is the surgeon factor in mm (distance from plane of iris root to principal plane of lens, negative in anterior chamber).

The Toric ICL Power Calculation Software incorporates mathematical operations described by Sarver and Sanders in 2004 and used to convert standard toric parameters of sphere, cylinder, and axis to astigmatic decomposition components and vice-versa.[19] These operations can be used to derive equations to calculate the ideal toric IOL power for a phakic or aphakic astigmatic eye, predict the postoperative spectacle correction for a selected toric IOL with power other than the ideal power, and back calculate a parameter to be used to optimize predictability of the calculations based on clinical data. The software also provides a guide for achieving proper alignment of the toric ICL. As described before, a customized lens is manufactured to be implanted on the horizontal meridian while an alternative lens with the same power and different axis can be implanted on a different axis to achieve the desired refractive correction. Example of customized and alternative toric ICL powers is shown in **Figures 25.3A and B**.

SURGICAL TECHNIQUES

Many surgeons prefer to perform two peripheral iridotomies one or two weeks before the surgery using a ND:YAG laser to prevent postoperative pupillary block. Peripheral iridotomies are performed superiorly 90° apart.[7,15,16] Before surgery pupil must be widely dilated; in our practice; 1% cyclopentolate hydrochloride (Cyclogyl; Alcon labs, Inc. Fortworth, TX, USA) and 2.5% phenylephrine hydrochloride (Mydfrin; Alcon labs) instilled every 15 minutes for 1 hour before surgery usually result in efficient pupillary dilation. We routinely perform ICL surgery performed under topical anesthesia (0.5% bupivacaine hydrochloride). It is advisable to double check the white-to-white measurement with calipers before starting the surgery.

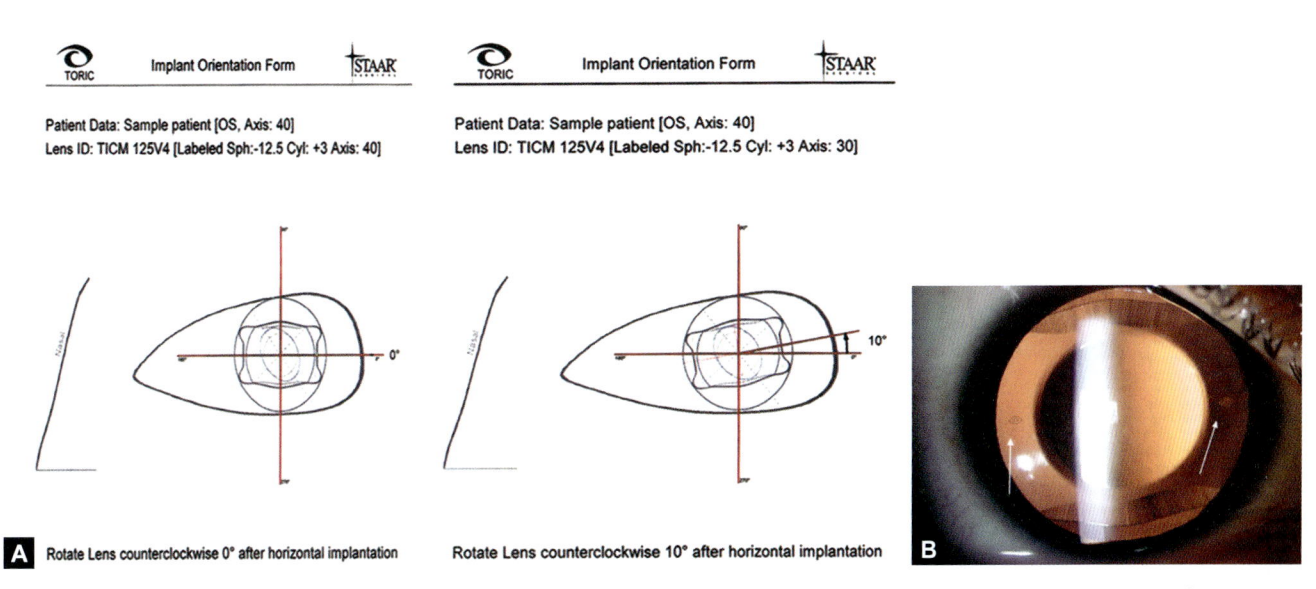

Figures 25.3A and B (A) Examples of a customized lens (Fig. A, left) and an alternative toric ICL (Fig. A, right) for a same preoperative refraction. Note the power calculated for a customized lens is −12.50 +3.00 x 40°, a toric ICL with this power would be implanted at the horizontal meridian (180°); an alternative lens with same power and different axis (−12.50 +3.00 x 30°) can be also used but it will need to be rotated 10° counterclockwise to compensate the difference in axis orientation. The alternative was used in this case and shown after implantation. (B) Note the alignment marks (arrows) are aligned at 10° counterclockwise from the horizontal meridian

ICL Loading

The inside of the insertion cartridge is lubricated with a viscoelastic material (sodium hyaluronate or methyl cellulose). The lens is removed from the sealed glass container and is loaded inside the cartridge preferably under the surgical microscope. For smooth injection of the lens, it is important to load the lens with both longitudinal edges of the haptic symmetrically tucked under the edge of the cartridge with the lens vaulted anteriorly, it is also helpful to align the two holes located on the haptic of the ICL (or the laser engraved axis marks on the toric ICL) with the longitudinal axis of the cartridge. The coaxial forceps designed by Aus Der Au for ICL loading (E. Janach, Como, Italy) is used to pull the lens through the cartridge tunnel. Inspection of the lens inside the tunnel to exclude twisting of the lens helps making the injection inside the anterior chamber symmetrical, smooth and reproducible. If the lens is noticed to be twisted in the cartridge tunnel it is preferable to take it out and reload properly.

ICL Implantation

A clear corneal temporal incision is made with a diamond knife or a metal disposable keratome. The size of the incision can vary from 2.6 to 3.2 mm depending on the surgeon preference; in our first cases we used a 3.2 mm incision; today we are use a 2.8 mm incision; this enables a smooth injection and shown to have negligible effect on postoperative astigmatism.[20]

The anterior chamber is filled with viscoelastic before the lens is slowly injected using the MicroSTAAR injector (Staar, Nidau, Switzerland). It is worth mentioning that the injection should be slow enough to allow the leading footplate to unfold in the anterior chamber before the trailing footplate is injected out of the cartridge, **(Figures 25.4A and B)**. This will prevent the lens from unfolding upside down in the anterior chamber. Once the lens unfolds in the anterior chamber the marks on the distal and proximal footplates are checked for proper orientation. The footplates near the main incision are then tucked under the iris using an ICL manipulator; we use a Battle ICL manipulator (Rhein medical, Inc. Tampa, Fl, USA) that has a small oval tip with a rough lower surface that gives the surgeon good control on the footplate. Keeping the lower surface of the manipulator tip flat on the footplate makes manipulation easier. All manipulations should be as peripheral as possible with no instruments touching the optic or crossing the pupillary zone. The distal footplates are tucked under the iris through a side port. Correct position of the ICL is verified. If laser iridotomies were not done before surgery then a freshly prepared miotic agent (Carbachol 0.01%, Alcon labs, Inc.) is injected to constrict the pupil and surgical iridectomies are performed. We routinely use a vitrector to perform peripheral surgical iridectomy; the tip of the vitrector is inserted, under viscoelastic, through the main incision to touch the peripheral superior iris tissue, vacuum (300 mm Hg) is activated and once the iris tissue is aspirated in the vitrector tip, cutting is activated; one cut is enough to perform a small patent peripheral iridectomy. Alternatively, iridectomy can be performed with forceps and scissors.

In our experience laser iridotomies although effective are sometimes difficult to perform especially on eyes with thick brown irides, we prefer surgical iridectomy with the vitrector over scissors as the size and the site of the iridectomy is more controllable. Once the iridectomy is performed, a thorough irrigation and aspiration of the remaining viscoelastic is

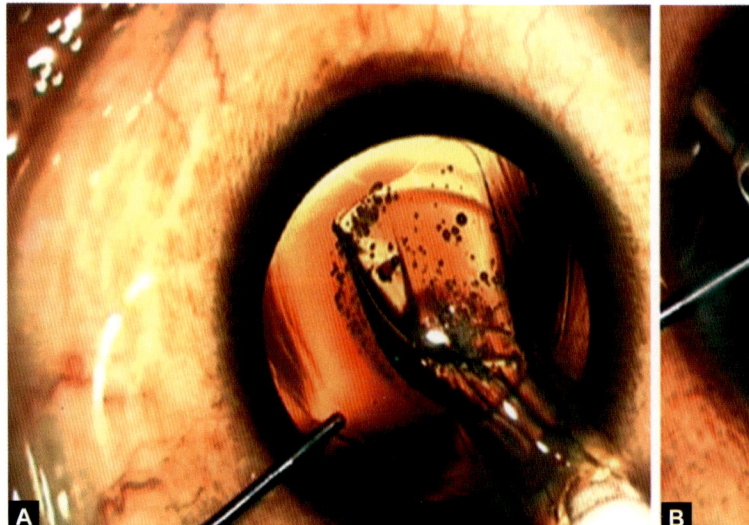

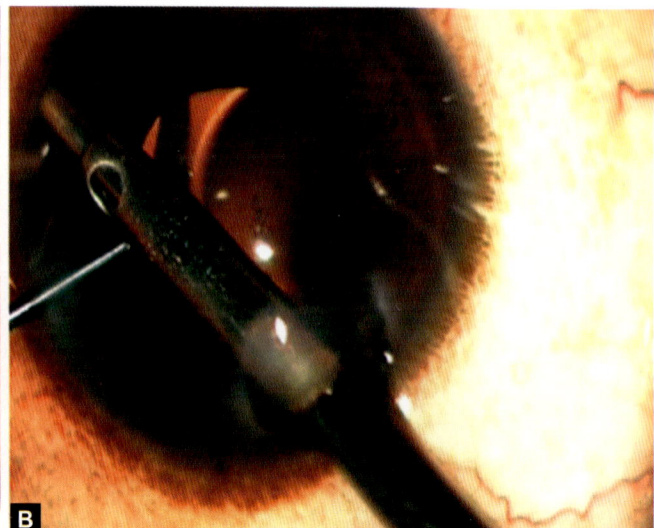

Figures 25.4A and B (A) Allowing the leading footplates to unfold before the trailing footplates are injected prevents the lens from unfolding upside down in the anterior chamber, (B) Using a vitreous cutter helps obtaining a small, patent and reproducible peripheral iridectomy (*Courtesy:* Dr Agarwal's Eye Hospital)

performed meticulously to prevent postoperative high intraocular spikes.

At the completion of the procedure we inject intracameral preservative free antibiotic (vancomycin 1 mg/ml).

Implantation of toric ICL is basically the same as spheric ICL with the exception that the axis of the cylinder of the lens has to be aligned correctly to correct the preoperative astigmatism. If the surgeon is using a custom made lens; the longitudinal axis of toric ICL, marked with laser marks has to be aligned horizontally (0° rotation from the horizontal meridian), in case the surgeon is using an alternative lens that has the same spherocylindrical power and different axis orientation, the lens will need to be rotated to compensate for this axis difference, the manufacturer recommends the rotation to be less than 22.5° from the horizontal axis. In our practice we use alternative lenses with axis difference less than 15° and we center our incision on the axis of implantation to minimize rotation of the toric ICL inside the eye. More than half of toric ICLs we implanted over the last year were alternative lenses to speed the delivery time.

Marking the horizontal axis is best done while the patient is sitting at the slit-lamp biomicroscope prior to surgery. During surgery a Mendez ring (Katena Products, Inc. Denville, New Jersey, USA) can be used to measure the required rotation from horizontal. It is also advisable to recheck the alignment of the laser marks that mark the axis of the cylindrical power on the lens haptic after implantation and before constricting the pupil.

There is a growing interest in performing bilateral surgeries on the same surgical session; we perform bilateral ICL surgery on most of our patients on the same surgical session; each eye is treated as a separate case and separate sets of instruments are used for each procedure.

POSTOPERATIVE CARE

Patients are usually discharged few hours after ICL surgery. Before discharge, it is recommended to measure the intraocular pressure, to ensure patency of the peripheral iridectomy and to assess centration and vaulting of ICL and the depth of the anterior chamber. We prescribe topical antibiotics; moxifloxacin hydrochloride 0.5% (Vigamox; Alcon labs, Inc.) four times a day for 1 week and topical steroids; prednisolone acetate 1% (Predforte; Allergan, Mayo, Ireland) four times a day for 3 weeks.

During subsequent postoperative examinations, a routine ophthalmologic assessment is performed, including corrected and uncorrected visual acuity, refraction, intraocular pressure, etc... ICL vault is important to be assessed on each postoperative examination. Vault is defined as the distance between anterior capsule of the crystalline lens and the posterior surface of the ICL; a vault between 200 and 700 µm is considered safe. There is no clinical evidence as to what

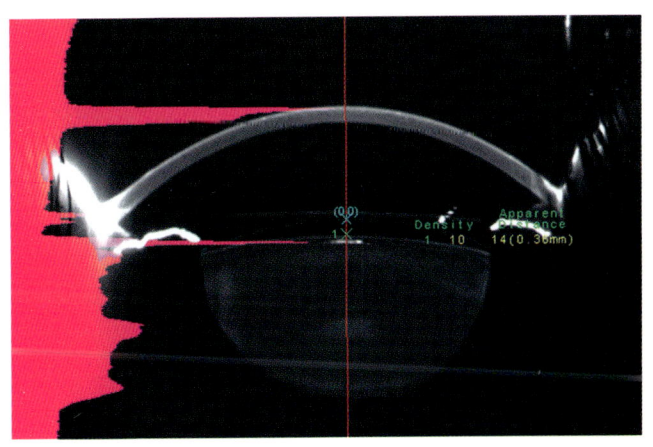

Figure 25.5 Anterior segment image using the Scheimpflug principle (EAS-1000, Nidek, Gamagori, Japan) allows objective measurement of the ICL vault; 360 µm in this case

is the "Ideal vault for an ICL" however, there is a general agreement that it is somewhere between 250 and 500 µm. The ICL length is the major determinant of vault; Choi et al, showed that the ICL power had no statistically significant correlation with the ICL vault if the footplates were located in the ciliary sulcus.[16] The ICL vault can be clinically assessed on the slit-lamp biomicroscope by comparing the vault with the cornea thickness; usually a vault equal to ½-1 ½ corneal thickness is considered acceptable.[7] We recently used the anterior segment analysis system (EAS-1000, Nidek, Gamagori, Japan) to objectively measure the vault of the ICL inside the eye. **Figure 25.5** shows a postoperative image captured from the EAS-1000 allowing objective measurement of the vault.

CLINICAL RESULTS

Clinical results published in literature,[5,8,13,20-27] as well as reports from FDA studies,[7,28] demonstrated impressive results, including a high predictability, efficacy, safety, stability as well as very high level of patients' satisfaction after ICL and toric ICL implantation. Long-term follow-up on a large series already established the safety of spherical ICL.[19] In this section we shall report our results with ICL and toric ICL for different indications over the last 2 years and review some of the results published in the literature.

Over the last 2 years we performed more than 270 cases of spheric ICL and more than 230 cases of toric ICL. ICL is our procedure of choice for all eyes with myopia higher than 8.00 D. We use toric ICL in cases with compound myopic astigmatism when the cylindrical component of the refraction is above 1.00 D. In myopia of 8.00 D or less we perform LASIK provided the corneal topography carries no suspicion and the corneal thickness allows leaving at least 300 microns after an ablation of at least 6.0 mm diameter.

ICL in Myopia above 8.00 D

A series of 42 consecutive eyes of 25 patients received spherical ICL for correction of myopia above 8.00 D; the mean age of this group was 27 yrs (range; 18 to 40 yrs) and the follow-up rate at 12 months was 81% (34 eyes).

Refractive Outcome

At baseline; the mean MRSE was -10.50 ± 2.19 (range; -17.25 to -8.38 D) and the mean refractive cylinder was 0.73 ± 0.29 D (range; 0.00 to 1.00 D). Emmetropia was the refractive target in all eyes. At one year, the mean MRSE was -0.07 ± 0.34 D (range; -0.63 to 0.38 D), the mean manifest refractive cylinder was 0.65 ± 0.43 D (range, 0.00 to 1.25 D). Of the 34 eyes examined at 1 year, 27 eyes (79%) were between ± 0.50 D, 4 eyes (12%) between -0.51 and -1.00 D, 1 eye (3%) between -1.01 and -2.00 D and 2 eyes (6%) between 0.51 and 1.00 D. **Figure 25.6A**, shows the attempted versus achieved spherical equivalent correction 12 months after operation in this group.

Visual Outcome

At baseline, 2 eyes (4.8%) could see 20/16, 31 eyes (73.8%) saw 20/20 or better and 41 eyes (97.6%) saw 20/40 or better. One eye had a spectacle corrected visual acuity (SCVA) worse than 20/50. Twelve months after the operation; 4 eyes (11.8%) saw 20/16 or better, 29 eyes (85.3%) saw 20/20 or better and all eyes could see 20/40 or better without correction. **Figure 25.7A**, shows a comparison between preoperative SCVA and postoperative UCVA in the 34 eyes who completed the 1 year examination. Three eyes (8.8%) lost 1 line of SCVA, 9 eyes (26.5%) did not loose or gain lines, 16 eyes (47.1%) gained 1 line and 6 eyes (17.6%) gained 2 lines or more lines of spectacle corrected visual acuity. After the 1 month examination, the mean change of MRSE was less than 0.50 D at each examination interval.

ICL in Myopia between -2.00 and -8.00 D

As we described earlier, we use ICL as our procedure of choice for correction of myopia less than 8.00 D in cases that are risks for LASIK. In a series of 35 consecutive eyes that received ICL for myopia between -2.00 and -8.00 D; the mean age was 28 yrs, the mean baseline MRSE was -4.69 ± 1.59 D (range; -8.00 to -2.13 D), the mean refractive cylinder was 0.42 ± 0.26 D (range; 0.00 to 1.00 D). Emmetropia was the target in all eyes.

Refractive Outcome

One year after operation; 29 eyes (82.9%) were examined, the mean baseline MRSE was -0.14 ± 0.27 D (range; -0.75 to 0.25 D); 86.2% eyes were between ± 0.50 D and all eyes were between ± 1.00 D of emmetropia. The mean refractive cylinder was 0.43 ± 0.28 D (range; 0.00 to 1.25 D); 25 eyes (86.2%) were between ± 0.50 D and, 4 eyes (13.8%) between -0.51 and -1.00 D. **Figure 25.6B**, shows the predictability of refractive correction in these 29 eyes.

Visual Outcome

Of the 29 eyes that completed the 1 year examination, baseline spectacle-corrected visual acuity was 20/16 or better in 3 eyes (10.3%), 20/20 or better in 24 eyes (82.8%) eyes and 20/32 or better in 28 eyes (96.6%) eyes. One year after operation; 4 eyes (13.8%) saw 20/16 or better, 25 eyes (86%) saw 20/20 or better and all eyes saw 20/32 or better without correction.

Two eyes (6.9%) lost 1 line of SCVA, 14 eyes (48.3%) did not loose or gain any lines, 10 eyes (34.5%) gained 1 line and 3 eyes (10.3%) gained 2 or more lines of SCVA.

Toric ICL

We analyzed the results of toric ICL implantation in a series of 68 consecutive eyes. The mean age was 26 yrs (range; 19 to 45 yrs). The baseline mean MRSE was -7.07 ± 3.35 D (range; -13.38 to -2.25 D), mean refractive cylinder was 2.34 ± 0.81 D (range; 1.25 to 4.75 D).

Refractive Outcome

At 12 months, 58 eyes (85.3%) were examined; mean MRSE was -0.16 ± 0.41 D (range; -1.75 to 1.13 D); 49 eyes (84.5%) were between ± 0.50 D of emmetropia, 5 eyes (8.6%) between -1.00 and -0.51 D, 3 eyes (5.2%) between -2.00 and -1.10 D. One eye (1.7%) was overcorrected by 1.13 D. **Figure 25.6C** shows the attempted versus achieved correction of MRSE for this group of 58 eyes with toric ICL.

Refractive stability was reached at 1 month after operation; mean change in MRSE was less than 0.50 D at all postoperative examination intervals. **Figures 25.7A to C** show a comparison between the baseline SCVA and the one year UCVA in the same three groups.

Mean refractive cylinder at 12 months was 0.38 ± 0.66 D (range; 0.00 to 1.75 D). The stability of the refractive cylinder was documented from the one month examination and afterwards; refractive cylinder changed by less than 1.00 D in all cases and by less than 0.50 D in more than 95.5% of cases. The mean difference was less than 0.05 D at each reporting interval. Sanders and Sarver reported similar stability of the refractive cylinder.[29]

Analysis of the vector stability of cylinder showed that the cylinder is stable from the first month examination and it changed by less than 1.00 D in more than 98.3% of cases and by less than 0.5 D in more than 94.8% of cases at each interval. The mean difference was between 0.20 and 0.28 D at each reporting interval. This shows the stability of the cylindrical correction and supports the data published by Sanders et al who

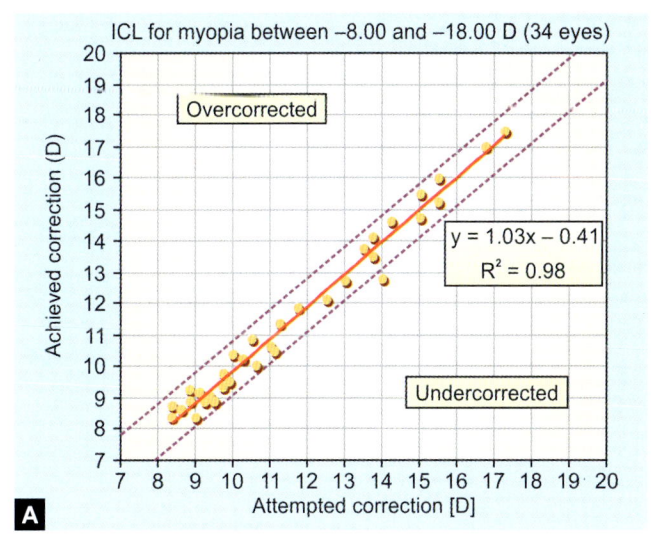

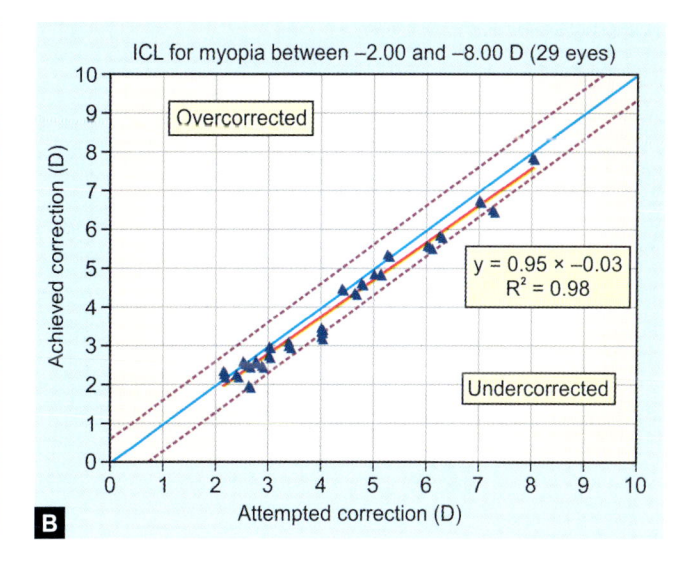

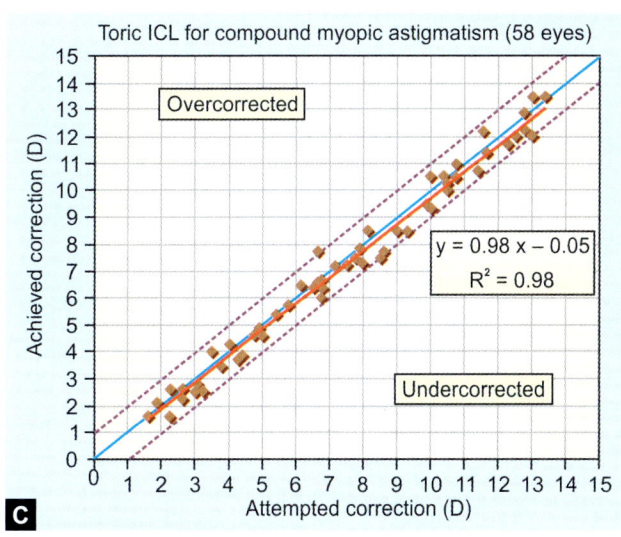

Figures 25.6A to C Scattergrams showing the attempted versus achieved spherical equivalent correction (predictability) 12 months after surgery in 3 different groups. The predictability of ICL for correction of myopia between –8.00 and –18.00 D is shown is graph A and between –2.00 and –8.00 D in graph B. Graph C shows the predictability of toric ICL for correction of compound myopic astigmatism with a spherical equivalent refraction between –2:00 and –14:00 D

reported a change of ≤ 1.00 D in between 96.8% and 97.4% and ≤ 0.50% in between 85.3% and 87.2% of cases.[10] Vector analysis using the double angle minus cylinder method is shown in **Figure 25.8**.

Visual Outcome

At base line, best spectacle-corrected visual acuity was 20/16 or better in 4 eyes (6.9%) eyes, 20/20 or better in 28 eyes (46.6%), 20/32 or better in 52 eyes (89%) eyes, all eyes could see 20/50 or better with spectacles. One year after surgery, uncorrected visual acuity was 20/16 or better in 7 eyes (12.1%), 20/20 or better in 39 eyes (67.2%) and 20/32 or better in 50 eyes (86.2%). All eyes could see 20/40 or better without correction.

21 eyes (36.1%) maintained their baseline spectacle-corrected visual acuity, 1 eye (1.7%) lost 1 line, 29 eyes (43.1%) gained 1 line and 11 eyes (19%) gained 2 or more lines of spectacle-corrected visual acuity.

Stability of Toric ICL Alignment after Implantation

We evaluated the stability of the toric ICL alignment after implantation using the OPD-scan (NIDEK, Gamagori, Japan). The OPD (optical path difference) map measures the objective refraction of the entire eye over a 6 mm pupil while the internal OPD map measures the objective refraction of the entire eye minus the anterior corneal surface over the same pupil diameter. Subtracting the preoperative from the postoperative OPD map of a given eye can reveal the effective power of the implanted ICL at any point within the 6 mm pupil. **Figure 25.9** shows preoperative and postoperative OPD maps of an eye that

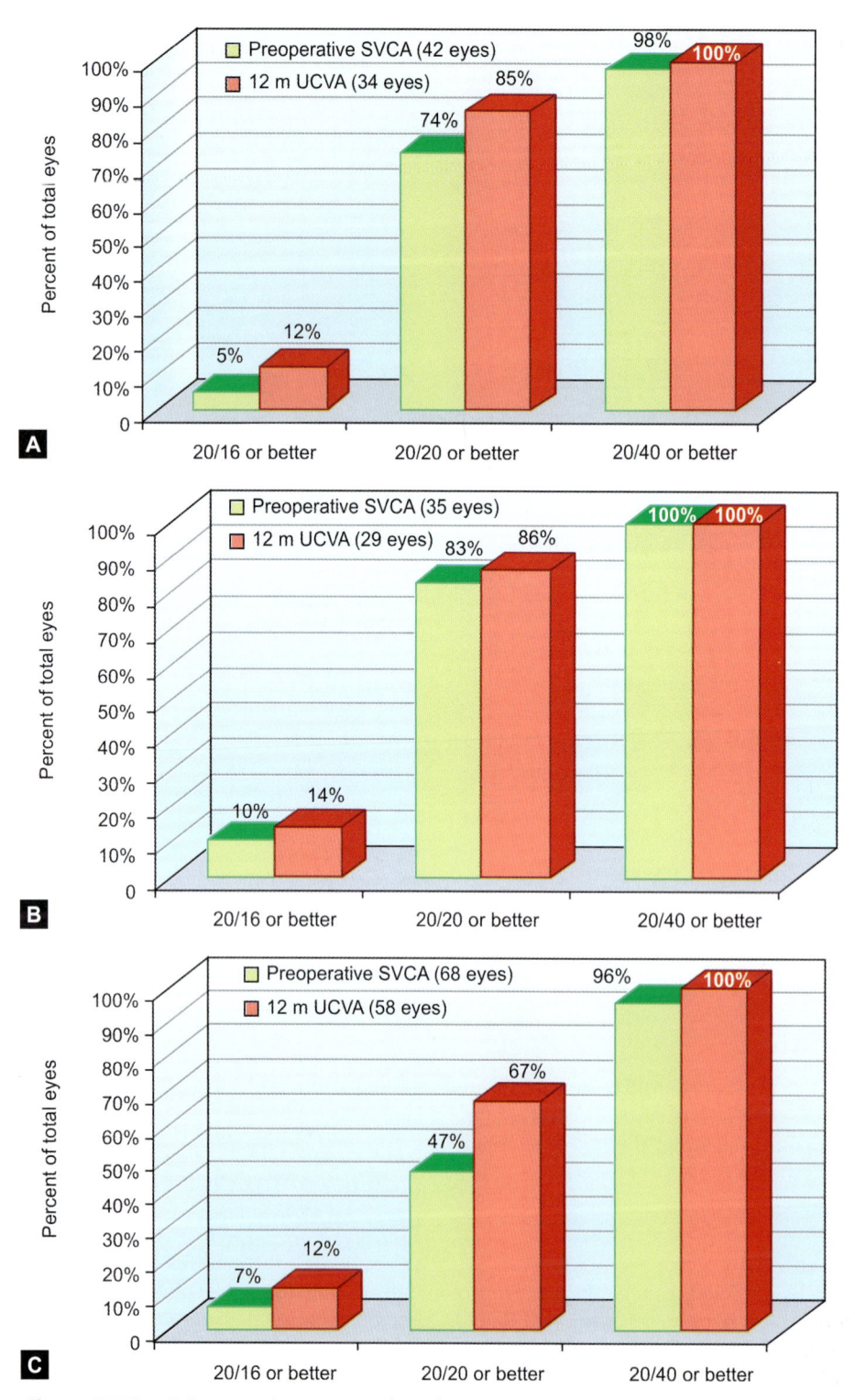

Figures 25.7A to C Postoperative uncorrected visual acuity at 12 months compared to preoperative best spectacle-corrected visual acuity (efficacy) of the same 3 groups shown in Figure 25.6

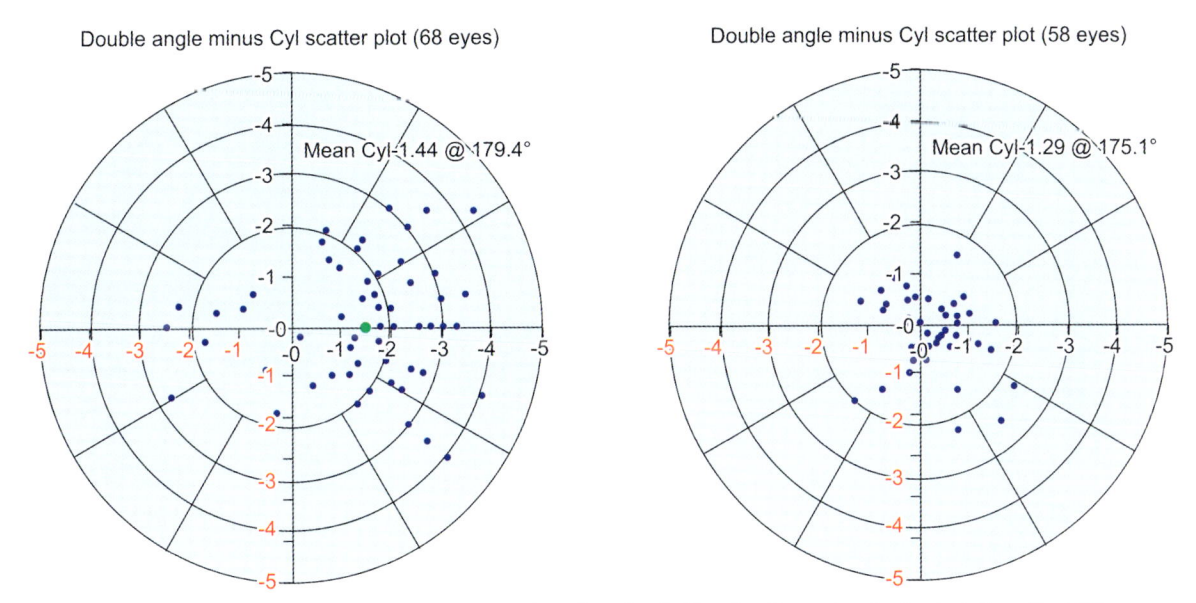

Figure 25.8 Double angle minus cylinder scatter plot at base line (left) and at 12 months after implantation of toric ICL. Mean vector cylinder changed from –1.44 D at 180° to –0.29 at 175.1°

received toric ICL documenting the stability of the refractive correction over 1 year. Also, comparing the axis and power of the cylinder using the internal OPD map at each postoperative examination is a sensitive objective method to detect any late rotation of a toric ICL after implantation. **Figure 25.10** shows baseline and postoperative internal OPD maps of an eye that received toric ICL.

The mean value of rotation of the axis of the cylinder in our series was between 0.06 and 0.9° for all time intervals. Axis misalignment was ≤ 5° at 1 year follow-up in 89.6% of eyes, ≤ 10° in 98.3% and ≤ 20° in all eyes.

One eye had axis misalignment more than 20°, was diagnosed at the end of the first week after operation and was most probably due to misalignment during implantation as the pupil got smaller than the optic diameter during alignment of the axis; realignment was performed on the 8th postoperative day and no rotation was observed afterwards, and at 1 year the axis misalignment of this eye was 2.0°.

Table 25.2 compares our refractive and visual results with similar studies published in the literature.

ICL in Stable Keratoconus

Keratoconus commonly presents during the second decade of life. Many of the cases slowly and gradually progress in severity, but the rate of progression and the length of time that the disease remains actively progressive vary considerably. The ectasia may progress slowly but continuously for years and then stabilizes permanently, or periods of progression man alternate with period during which the ectatic process appears to have arrested. In some cases, the ectasia remains stable after its initial appearance. It is uncommon for the condition to progress after the age of 40 years, but exceptions do occur.[30] ICL and toric ICL can be used to correct myopia and compound myopic astigmatism in eyes with stable keratoconus. Bartels et al used a toric phakic lens to correct high astigmatism in an eye with pellucid marginal degeneration.[31]

We are conducting a prospective randomized clinical trial to assess the efficacy, predictability and safety of toric ICL for correction of compound myopic astigmatism associated with stable keratoconus. We included 23 eyes of 17 patients. All eyes had stable keratoconus documented by videokeratography, clear central cornea, MRSE between –4.00 and –15.00 D, spectacle-corrected visual acuity of 20/40 or better, stable manifest refraction for at least 1 year together with the other previously mentioned selection criteria for ICL implantation including an endothelial cell count above 2200 cell/mm² and anterior chamber depth of 2.7 mm or more calculated from the endothelium. All patients were rigid contact lens intolerant. Each eye received a myopic toric ICL through a temporal clear corneal incision. At baseline; mean MRSE refraction was –9.62 ± 2.89 D (range; –15.00 to –4.38 D), 12 eyes (52%) eyes could see 20/20 or better with correction. At 12 months (follow-up rate, 87%), MRSE was –0.32 ± 0.52 D (range; –1.50 to 0.13 D), uncorrected visual acuity was 20/40 or better in 20 eyes (90%) and 20/20 or better in 11 eyes (55%); 4 eyes (20%) eyes gained 2 or more lines of spectacle-corrected visual acuity. Due to the nature of the disease, longer follow-up and larger series are needed, however based on our 1 year results we believe that toric ICL implantation is effective, predictable and relatively safe for the correction of compound myopic astigmatism associated with stable keratoconus.

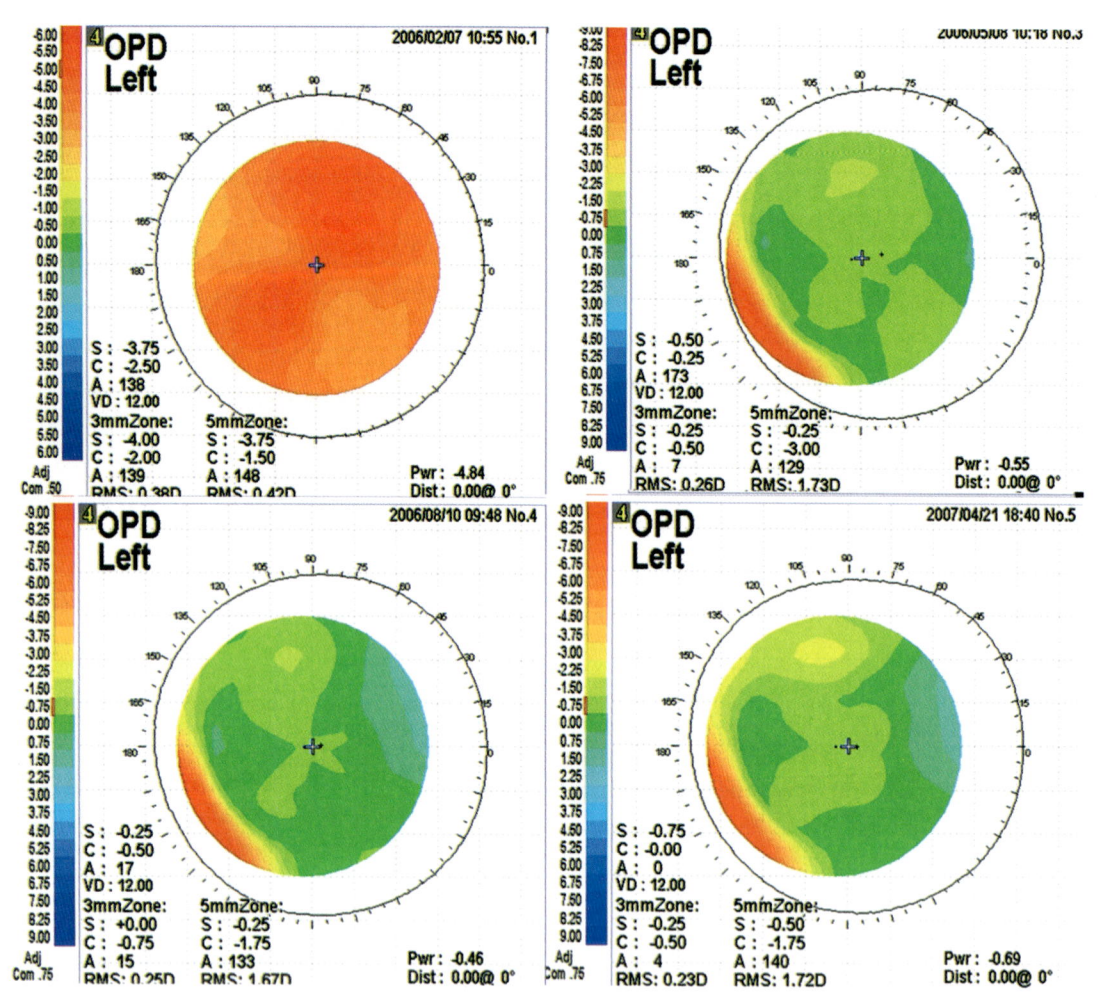

Figure 25.9 The total optical path difference (OPD) of an eye with preoperative refraction of −3.75 −2.50 x 138° (top left), a toric ICL was implanted, the OPD map 3 months after the operation (top right) shows an objective refraction of −0.50 −0.25 x 173. OPD map was stable in the following exams; 6 and 12 months after surgery (bottom)

ICL after Corneal Ring Segments or Collagen Crosslinking in Progressive Keratoconus

Over the last few years many reports showed the possibility of stabilizing a progressive keratoconus using intracorneal ring segments,[32,33] and corneal collagen crosslinking.[34,35] The favorable results published in peer reviewed literature as well as our own unpublished results are encouraging. Implantation of toric ICL after corneal ring segments or crosslinking is possible to correct the residual refractive error. **Figure 25.11** shows an eye with progressive keratoconus that received intracorneal ring segments to stabilize the progression, a toric ICL was implanted one year after the primary procedure to correct residual refractive error.

Toric ICL after Corneal Grafts

Another important indication for toric ICL is the correction of residual refractive errors after corneal grafting in which keratorefractive techniques are not necessarily good or viable option. Tahzib,[36] described the effective reduction of post-keratoplasty astigmatism in 36 eyes from −7.06 ± 2.01 D preoperatively to −2.0±1.53 D at last follow-up. In a prospective study we evaluated the predictability, efficacy and safety of toric ICL implantation in correcting compound myopic astigmatism after deep anterior lamellar keratoplasty (DALKP); 28 eyes of 28 patients with previous DALKP received toric ICL. All eyes had stable refraction for 6 months after removal of corneal sutures, mean MRSE was −9.4 ± 2.6 D

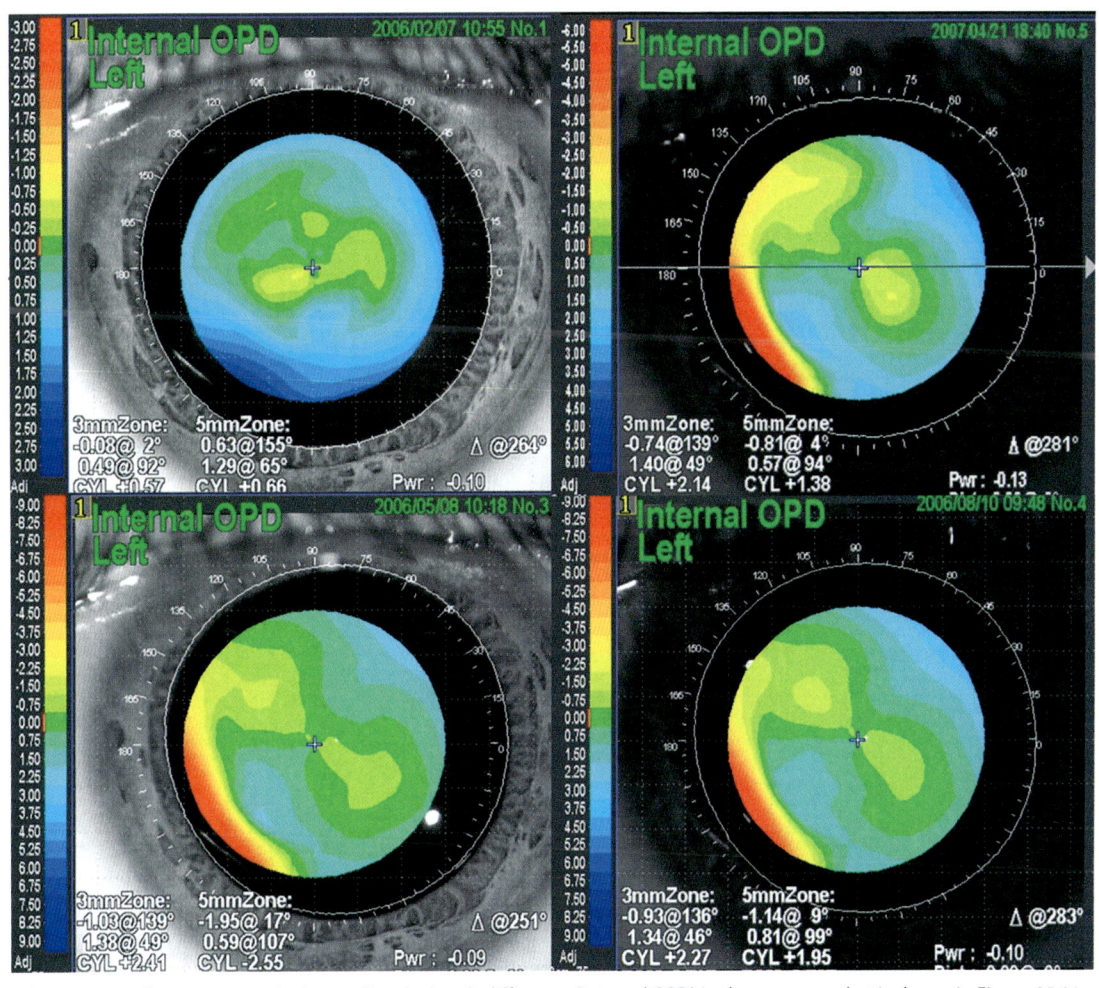

Figure 25.10 Demonstrates the internal optical path difference (internal OPD) in the same eye that is shown in Figure 25.11. Note the stability of the axis of the internal astigmatism (equivalent to the astigmatic axis of the toric ICL) overtime

(range; –16.0 to –5.0 D), SCVA of 20/40 or better in all eyes and 20/20 or better in 14 eyes (50%), endothelial cell count more than 2200 cells/mm^2 and anterior chamber depth 2.7 mm or more calculated from the endothelium. One year after surgery, (follow-up rate, 85.7%); MRSE was –0.3 ± 0.5 D, 14 eyes (58.3%) eyes saw 20/20 uncorrected; 6 eyes (25%) gained 2 or more lines of SCVA. No visual threatening complications were observed. The ICL and toric ICL can also be implanted in eyes with penetrating corneal graft provided the endothelial cell count is at acceptable level (above 2200 cells/mm^2) and the anterior chamber depth is deep enough (more than 2.7 mm from endothelium).

COMPLICATIONS

Long-term follow-up on a large series using the current model of myopic ICL (V4) already established its relative safety,[19] and showed a marked reduction of the rate of complications reported in earlier models.[5,37,38] This dramatic improvement in the safety of ICL shadows our own experience; in our initial series of 100 ICL models V2 and V3 implanted between 1995 and 97, we encountered a relatively high incidence of lens opacities (10%) and sizing issues (6%), this made up stop using ICL till the year 2005 when we restarted implanting ICL and toric ICL using the currently available model (V4) and the newly introduced loading and injecting system. Since then we adopted the ICL and toric ICL as our phakic IOLs of choice. In this section we will review the most important complications that we encountered over the last 2 years or were published in the literature.

Improper Sizing and Poor Vaulting

Proper vaulting is critical in ICL surgery as complications reported after ICL implantation resulted largely from improper sizing. Excessive vault may induce peripheral

Table 25.2 Comparative studies of ICL and Toric ICL for myopia and compound myopic astigmatism

	El-Danasoury et al[‡]	El-Danasoury et al[‡]	El-Danasoury et al[‡]	Sanders et al[10]	FDA clinical trial,[7]	Uusitalo et al[37]	Pienda-Fernandez et al[38]	Zaldivar et al[5]
Dates of surgery	2005–2006	2005–2006	2005–2006	2002–2003	1998–2001	1998–2000	1998	1993–1996
ICL Model	V4	V4	V4 (toric)	V4 (toric)	V4	NA	V3, V4	20202, V1, V2, V3
Population								
Mean age (years)	27	29.5	26	36.4	36.5	39	34.5	34
Eyes operated (eyes)	42	35	68	210	523	38	18	124
Eyes reported (eyes)	34	29	58	186	428	36	18	124
Percent of eyes reported (%)	81	82.9	85.3	88.6	81.8	94.1	100	100
Mean follow-up (months)	12	12	12	12	12	13	26.6	11
Preoperative refraction								
Mean MRSE (D)	−10.50 ± 2.19	−4.69 ± 1.59	−7.07 ± 3.35	−9.36 ± 2.66	−10.05 ± 3.75	−15.1	−15.27 ± 3.47	−13.38 ± 2.23
Range MRSE (D)	−17.25 to −8.38	−8.00 to −2.13	−13.38 to −2.25	−19.50 to −2.38	−20.00 to −3.00	−29.00 to −7.75	−21.25 to −2.75	−18.63 to −8.50
Mean refractive cylinder (D)	0.73 ± 0.29	0.42 ± 2.6	2.34 ± 0.81	1.93 ± 0.84	NA	NA	1.8 ± 1.30	2.13 ± 1.51
Range refractive cylinder (D)	0.00 to 1.00	0.00 to 1.00	1.25 to 4.75	1.25 to 475	NA	NA	0.50 to 4.00	0.00 to 6.00
Postoperative MRSE								
Mean MRSE (D)	−0.07 ± 0.34	−0.14 ± 0.27	−0.16 ± 0.41	0.05 ± 0.46	−0.50 ± 0.98	−2.00 ± 2.48	−0.62 ± n0.81	−0.78 ± 0.87
Range MRSE (D)	−0.63 to 0.38	−0.75 to 0.25	−1.75 to 1.13	−2.25 to 1.00	−8.00 to 1.13*	−13.00 to 0.13**	−2.75 to 0.75	−3.50 to 1.63
Percent within 0.50 D (%)	79	86.2	84.5	76.9	61.6	71.1	22.2	44
Percent within 1.00 D (%)	97	100	93.1	97.3	84.7	81.6	61.1	69
Percent within 2.00 D (%)	100	100	100	100	96.7	NA	NA	NA
Postoperative cylinder								
Mean (D)	0.65 ± 0.43	0.43 ± 0.28	0.38 ± 0.66	0.51 ± 0.48	NA	NA	NA	0.96 ± 0.85
Range (D)	0.00 to 1.25	0.0 to 1.25	0.00 to 1.75	0.00 to 3.00	NA	NA	NA	0.00 to 3.75
Baseline SCVA								
20/16 or better (%)	4.8	10.3	6.9	4.8	NA	NA	NA	NA
20/20 or better (%)	73.8	82.8	46.6	83.1	67.7	23.9	NA	5
20/40 or better (%)	97.6	100	96	NA	96.9	63.2	NA	80

Contd...

Contd...

	El-Danasoury et al[‡]	El-Danasoury et al[‡]	El-Danasoury et al[‡]	Sanders et al[10]	FDA clinical trial,[7]	Uusitalo et al[37]	Pienda-Fernandez et al[38]	Zaldivar et al[5]
Postoperative UCVA								
20/16 or better (%)	11.8	13.8	12.1	NA	NA	NA	NA	NA
20/20 or better (%)	85.3	86	67.2	83.1	60.1	5.3	5.5	2
20/40 or better (%)	100	100	100	NA	92.5	52.6	44.4	68
Postoperative SCVA								
20/16 or better (%)	14.4	20	17	37.6	NA	NA	NA	NA
20/20 or better (%)	94	96	88	96.8	82.4	39.5	NA	19
20/40 or better (%)	100	100	100	NA	98.1	94.7	NA	93
Change in BSCVA								
Loss ≥ 2 or more lines	0	0	0	1.6	0.7	NA	5.6	0.81
Loss 1 line (%)	8.8	6.9	1.7	7.5	5.4	6.2	NA	NA
Unchanged (%)	26.5	48.3	36.1	14.5	44.3	NA	NA	NA
Gain 1 line (%)	47.1	34.5	43.1	57.5	40	31.3	38.8	NA
Gain ≥ 2 or more lines (%)	17.6	10.3	19	18.9	9.6	40.6	NA	36
Complications								
Visually insignificant lens opacities (%)	2.9	0	1.7	2.4	2.1	2.6	5.6	2.42
Visually significant cataract (%)	2.9	0	0	0.5	0.4	2.6	5.6	0
Pupillary block (%)	0	0	0	0	0	7.9***	12.5***	4.8
Percent of secondary interventions (total)	2.9	0	5.3	2.4	2.3	13.2	16.7	
Removal (%)	0	0	0	1.6	0	2	0	3.3
Replacement (%)	0	0	0	0.5	1.7	0	0	1.6
Repositioning (%)	0	3.4	0	0	0.7	0	0	0.8
Axis realignment (%)	0	0	5.3	0.5	0	0	0	0
Removal with cataract extraction (%)	2.9	0	0	0	0.4	5.3	5.6	0
Laser iridotomies enlargement (%)	0	0	0	0	0	7.9	11.1	0

[‡] Ongoing studies
* 9.9 % eyes were not corrected to emmetropia
** 31.6 % eyes were not corrected to emmetropia
*** All eyes that developed pupillary block had laser iridotomies before ICL implantation

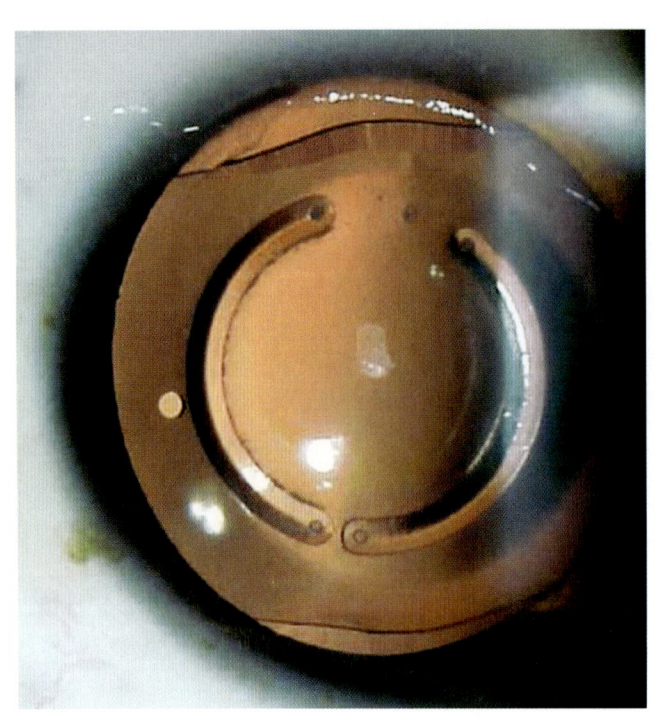

Figure 25.11 An eye with progressive keratoconus; 2 Ferrara ring segments wee implanted to stabilize the ectasia; one year later, a toric ICL was implanted to correct the residual compound myopic astigmatism

anterior synechiae, pigment dispersion and shallowing of the anterior chamber; also a large ICL may distend the pupil with subsequent glare and halos. A low vault may induce cataract formation. Gonvers et al found no anterior subcapsular cataract when vaulting is >90 μm.[39]

Cataract

The relatively high rate of induced cataract after ICL implantation was a main concern with the earlier models,[40] it decreased significantly after the introduction of the latest model (V4) and the introduction of the loading and injection technique described previously in the methods section. In recent reports, where the authors used only the V4 model, the rate of cataract ranges from 0.0 to 2.4%.[7,10,19] A low incidence of late onset cataract was also reported in the US FDA Clinical Trial (0.4%, 2 of 526 eyes).[19] In our hands, we had observed a similar low rate of clinically significant cataract after ICL implantation; 2 of 482 eyes (0.41%). Both patients that developed cataract had ICL implantation for high myopia (above 15.00 D) and were older than 45 years of age. This finding supports Lackner and coauthors suggestion that cataract formation is more likely to occur after ICL implantation in patients who are aged > 45 years.[41] In cases where cataract developed after ICL implantation; removal of the ICL and performing a phacoemulsification with IOL implantation resulted in favorable outcome.[7,37,38]

Pupillary Block

Peripheral iridectomy or iridotomies are mandatory in ICL surgery; otherwise pupillary block will occur during the early postoperative period. Many surgeons prefer to perform laser iridotomies one or two weeks before the ICL implantation. We prefer surgical iridectomy with a vitreous cutter as described earlier; we did not see any case of pupillary block after surgical iridectomy. Pienda-Fernandez and co-workers reported a relatively high incidence of pupillary block after ICL implantation with laser iridotomies (12.5%), they reported no incidence of pupillary block after they shifted to surgical iridectomies.[38]

Other causes of high intraocular pressure during early postoperative period is retained viscoelastic; Chang and Meau noticed that the most common cause for rise of intraocular pressure in early postoperative period in their series was due to retained viscoelastic; they recommended that the surgeon, at the conclusion of the surgery removes the viscoelastic from the region around the peripheral iridotomies before the other parts of the anterior chamber. This led, in their experience, to a significant decrease in the incidence of transient IOP elevation.[15]

Night Glare

Night vision symptoms are less common after ICL implantation compared to anterior chamber lenses. This may be at last partly, due to the relatively larger effective optic diameter of the posterior chamber lenses being closer to the nodal point. Occasionally, night glare can be due to peripheral iridectomy; Chang and Meau reported 3 (4.9%) patients with symptoms of glare after initial surgery due to peripheral iridotomies prior to ICL implantation, symptoms persisted only for a short period. Only 1 (1.6%) patient complained of seeing an extra light 6 months after surgery.[15] In their series of 210 eyes, Sanders et al reported one patient who complained of a line in his vision from the preoperative laser iridotomies; although the patient insisted upon removal of the ICL, it did not correct for the line in his vision.[7]

Residual Refractive Error

The excellent predictability and efficacy of ICL and toric ICL in correcting myopia and compound myopic astigmatism has been proved.[5,7,8,13,20-28] In case of residual refractive errors after ICL implantation, ICL replacement or excimer laser keratorefractive procedure (LASIK or surface ablation) remain valid options. In our practice, we perform LASIK as a secondary procedure to correct residual refractive error after

ICL implantation (Bioptics). LASIK can be performed as soon as the refractive outcome stabilizes and the wound heals. We usually allow 4 weeks before performing LASIK on an eye who received an ICL. Due to the exceptionally high predictability of the calculation software we did not have to perform a secondary refractive procedure after ICL implantation in more than 400 cases performed in the last 2 years.

Endothelial Damage

Compared to other phakic lenses, posterior chamber lenses are the farthest from the endothelium and the least to induce endothelial cell loss. Apart from the endothelial loss directly related to the surgery, little concerns exist over subsequent endothelial loss after ICL implantation.[10] Pienda-Fernandez and coauthors reported an endothelial cell loss of 4.9 and 6.1% at 6 and 36 months respectively after ICL implantation.[38]

Decrease in Accommodation

Chang and Meau reported a case of 39 years old man who complained difficulty in reading 1 month after receiving an ICL for high myopia despite having UCVA of J2 at near and a manifest refraction of 0.13 D and an UCVA of 20/25 at distance. This patient elected to have the ICL removed. After removal, the patient did not lose any lines of SCVA nor did he develop any cataract.[15]

Pigment Dispersion

Pigment dispersion after ICL implantation has been a concern, in an earlier study, Trindade et al found contact between the iris and implanted ICL in all eyes.[40] However, with the better vaulting design of the V4 model, chances of contact between the iris and IOL have been reduced.[7] According to international reports, the ICL is safe for implantation in eyes with a minimum anterior chamber depth of 2.8 mm. However, the United States Food and Drug Administration (FDA) approved lens use for a minimum anterior chamber depth of 2.7 mm. In Chang and Meau series, 23% of eyes had anterior chamber depth between 2.8 and 3.0 mm, but they did not find any significant pigment dispersion in any eye; in another study of 18 eyes with a minimum anterior chamber depth of 3.0 mm, the same authors found no significant pigment changes in any of the eyes.[15]

Retinal Complications

Retinal complications have been reported in high myopic eyes after ICL implantation, these include macular hemorrhage, retinal detachment and progressive dry macular degeneration. The preoperative high myopia and the pre-existing myopic degenerations probably contributed to the eventual hemorrhages and detachment seen in these eyes rather than the ICL surgical procedure.[7,15,19,38] Detailed fundus examination is highly recommended before ICL implantation especially in highly myopic eyes to diagnose and if needed, to treat any pre-existing myopic degenerations prior to ICL implantation.

Future carries promises for improvements including more accurate sizing, more understanding of the ciliary sulcus anatomy, the position of the ICL in relation to ciliary sulcus and zonules, and possible wavefront customized lenses to compensate the pre-existing high order aberrations in highly aberrated eyes.

So far, the excellent predictability and efficacy combined with the very low incidence of postoperative complications and overwhelming patient satisfaction make the ICL and the toric ICL extremely valuable tools for refractive surgeons to address the needs of their patients.

REFERENCES

1. Baikoff GB, Joly P. Comparison of minus power anterior chamber intraocular lenses and myopic epikeratoplasty in phakic eyes. Refract Corneal Surg. 1990;6:252-60.
2. Baïkoff G. Phakic anterior chamber intraocular lenses. Int Ophthalmol Clin. 1991; 31:75-86.
3. Fechner PU, Worst JGF. A new concave intraocular lens for the correction of high myopia. Eur J Implant Refract Surg. 1989;1:41-3.
4. Brauweiler PH, Wehler T, Busin M. High incidence of cataract formation after implantation of a silicone posterior chamber lens in phakic, highly myopic eyes. Ophthalmology. 1999:106:1651-5.
5. Zaldivar R, Davidorf JM, Oscherow S. Posterior chamber phakic intraocular lens for myopia of –8 to –19 diopters. J Refract Surg. 1998;14:294-305.
6. Durrie DS, Lesher MP, Cavanaugh TB. Classification of variable clinical response after photorefractive keratectomy for myopia. J Refract Surg. 1995;11:341-7.
7. The Implantable Contact Lens in Treatment of Myopia (ITM) Study Group. US food and drug administration clinical trial of the implantable contact lens for moderate to high myopia. Ophthalmology. 2003;110:255-66.
8. Pesando PM, Ghiringhello MP, Tagliavacche P. Posterior chamber collamer phakic intraocular lens for myopia and hyperopia. J Refract Surg. 1999;15:415-23.
9. Sanders DR, Vukich JA. ICL in treatment of myopia (ITM) study group. Incidence of lens opacities and clinically significant cataracts with the implantable contact lens; comparison of two lens designs. J Refract Surg. 2002;18:673-82.
10. Sanders DR, Schneider D, Martin R, Brown D, Dulaney D, Vukich J, Slade S, Schallhorn S. Toric implantable collamer lens for moderate high myopic astigmatism. Ophthalmology. 2007; 114:54-61.
11. Marcos S. Aberrations and visual performance following standard laser vision correction. J Refract Surg. 2001;17:S596-601.
12. El Danasoury A, El Maghraby A, Gamali TO. Comparison of iris-fixed Artisan lens implantation with excimer laser in situ keratomileusis in correcting myopia between –9.00 and –19.50 D. Ophthalmology. 2002;109:955-64.
13. Gonvers M, Othenin-Girard P, Bonet C, Sickenberg M. Implantable contact lens for moderate to high myopia; short-term follow-up of 2 models. J Catract Refract Surg. 001;27:380-8.

14. Reuland MS, Reuland AJ, Nishi Y, Auffarth GU. Corneal radii and anterior chamber depth measurements using the IOLMaster Versus the Pentacam. J Refract Surg. 2007;23:368-73.
15. Chang JS, Meau AY. Visian collamer phakic intraocular lens in high myopic Asian eyes. J Refract Surg. 2007;23:17-25.
16. Choi KH, Chung SE, Chung TY, Chung ES. Ultrasound biomicroscopy for determining Visian implantable Contact lens length in Phakic IOL implantation. J Refract Surg. 2007;23:362-7.
17. Pop M, Payette Y, Mansour M. Predicting sulcus size using ocular measurements. J Cataract Refract Surgery. 2001;27:1033-8.
18. Holladay JT. Refractive power calculations for intraocular lenses in the phakic eye. Am J Ophthalmol. 1993; 116:63-6.
19. Sanders DR, Doney K, Poco M. ICL In Treatment of Myopia (ITM) Study Group. United States Food and Drug Administration Clinical Trial of The Implantable Collamer Lens (ICL) for moderate to high myopia; three-year follow-up. Ophthalmology. 2004;111:1683-92.
20. Martin RG, Gills JP. Evaluating outcomes of cataract surgery. In: Sanders DR, Koch DD, (Eds). An Atlas of Corneal Topography. Thorofare, NJ: SLACK Inc. 1993:67-8.
21. Arne JL, Lesueur LC. Phakic posterior chamber lenses for high myopia: Functional and anatomical outcomes. J Cataract Refract Surg. 2000;26:369-74.
22. Menezo JL, Peris-Martinez C, Cisneros A, Martinez-Costa R. Posterior chamber phakic intraocular lenses to correct high myopia: A comparative study between STAAR and Adatormed models. J Refract Surg. 2001;17:32-42
23. Assetto V, Benedetti S, Pesando P. Collamer intraocular contact lens to correct high myopia. J Cataract Refract Surg. 1996;22:551-6.
24. Fink AM, Gore C, Rosen E. Cataract development after implantation of the Staar Collamer posterior chamber phakic lens. J Cataract Refract Surg. 1999;25:278-82.
25. Jimenez-Alfaro I, Benitez del Castillo JM, Garcia-Feijoo J, et al. Safety of posterior chamber phakic intraocular lenses for the correction of high myopia. Anterior segment changes after posterior chamber phakic intraocular lens implantation. Ophthalmology. 2001;108:90-9.
26. Kaya V, Kevser MA, Yilmaz OF. Phakic posterior chamber plate intraocular lenses for high myopia. J Refract Surg. 1999;15:580-5.
27. Rosen E. Gore C. Staar collamer posterior chamber phakic intraocular lens to correct myopia and hyperopia. J Cataract Refract Surg. 1998;24:596-606.
28. Sanders Dr, Brown DC, Martin Rg, et al. Implantable contact lens for moderate to high myopia; phase I FDA clinical study with 6 month follow-up. J Cataract Refract Surg. 1998;24:607-11.
29. Sanders DR, Sarver EJ. Standardized Analyses of correction of astigmatism with the Visian toric phakic implantable collamer lens. J Refract Surg. 2007;23:649-60.
30. Leibowitz HM, Morello S. Keratoconus and noninflammatory thinning disorders in Leibowitz HM, Waring GO: Corneal disorders, clinical diagnosis and management. WB Saunders 1998, chap 12:349-74.
31. Bartels MC, Saxena R, van den Berg TJ, et al. The influence of incision-induced astigmatism and axial lens position on the correction of myopic astigmatism with the Artisan toric phakic intraocular lens, Ophthalmology. 2006;113:1110-7.
32. Kymionis G, C Siganos C, Tsiklis N, Anastasakis A, Yoo S, Pallikaris A, N Astyrakakis N, Pallikaris I. Long-term Follow-up of intacs in keratoconus. Am J Ophthalmol. 2003;143:236-44.
33. Colin J, Cochener B, Savary G, Malet F, Holmes-Higgin D. INTACS Inserts for Treating Keratoconus: One Year Results. Ophthalmology. 2001;108:1409-14.
34. Spoerl E, Wollensak G, Seiler T. Increased resistance of crosslinked cornea against enzymatic digestion. Curr Eye Res. 2004;29(1): 35-40.
35. Chan CCK, Sharma M, Boxer Wachler BS. The effect of inferior segment Intacs with and without corneal collagen crosslinking with riboflavin (C3-R) on keratoconus. J Cataract Refract Surg. 2007;33:75-80.
36. Tahzib Ng, Cheng YY, Nuijts RM. Three-year follow-up analysis of Artisan toric lens implantation for correction of postkeratoplasty ametropia in phakic and pseudophakic eyes. Ophthalmology. 2006;113:976-84.
37. Uusitalo RJ, Aine E, Sen NH, Laatikainen L. Implantable contact lens for high myopia. J Cataract Refract Surg. 2002;28:29-36.
38. Pienda-Fernandez AP, Jaramillo J, Vargas J, Jaramillo M, Jaramilo J, Galindez. Phakic posterior chamber intraocular lens for high myopia. J Cataract Refract Surg. 2004;30:2277-83.
39. Gonvers M. Bornet C, Othenin-Girard P. Implantable contact lens for moderate to high myopia: relationship of vaulting to cataract formation. J Cataract Refract Surg. 2003;29:918-24.
40. Trindade F, Pereira F, Cronemberger S. Ultrasound biomicroscopic imaging of posterior chamber phakic intraocular lens. J Refract Surg. 1998;14:497-503.
41. Lackner B, Pieh S, Schmidinger G, Simader C, Franz C, Dejaco-Ruhswurm I, Skorpik C. Long-terms results of implantation of phakic posterior chamber intraocular lens. J Cataract Refract Surg. 2004;30:2269-76.

Chapter 26

Nidek OPD Scan in Clinical Practice

Gregg Feinerman (USA), N Timothy Peters (USA), Hoo Yeun Kim (USA),
Marcus Solorzano (USA), Shiela Scott (USA)

INTRODUCTION

Corneal topography and wavefront analysis are both essential data that provide useful information to the refractive surgeon. Unlike corneal topography, wavefront analysis provides us with information about the overall refractive status of the eye, including the cornea, lens and retina. It also demonstrates aberrations that occur with pupillary dilation.

Over the past 5 years, wavefront technology has been proven to be useful in both custom ablation planning and in screening patients for refractive surgery. Wavefront analysis helps explain visual aberrations when they are not obvious on corneal topography. Patients with visual aberrations following refractive surgery may have unremarkable corneal topography maps, but their symptoms may be explained on wavefront analysis.[1] In such cases, wavefront analysis will commonly show elevated values for vertical coma and trefoil.

NIDEK OPD SCAN

The Nidek OPD Scan is a scanning slit refractometer using skiascopic technology with simultaneous Placido disc corneal topography **(Figure 26.1)**. It is the first diagnostic instrument to combine corneal topography, autorefraction, and wavefront analysis. The Nidek OPD Scan takes the autorefraction, keratometry, and wavefront measurements simultaneously in 0.4 seconds. Compared to other autorefractors, it measures the largest range of spherocylinder refractive error in the industry. It measures between –20 D and +22 D of sphere and 12 D of cylinder. After performing the autorefraction, the technician performs the corneal topography (also in less than one second). Unlike Hartmann-Shack systems, the Nidek OPD-Scan uses dynamic retinoscopy to measure aberrations through 1,440 data points (highest number among all wavefront machines).[2] These points create refractive power maps with more data than on other systems. Unlike the grid on Hartmann-Shack wavefront systems, there is no mixing of data points with the scanning slit technology.

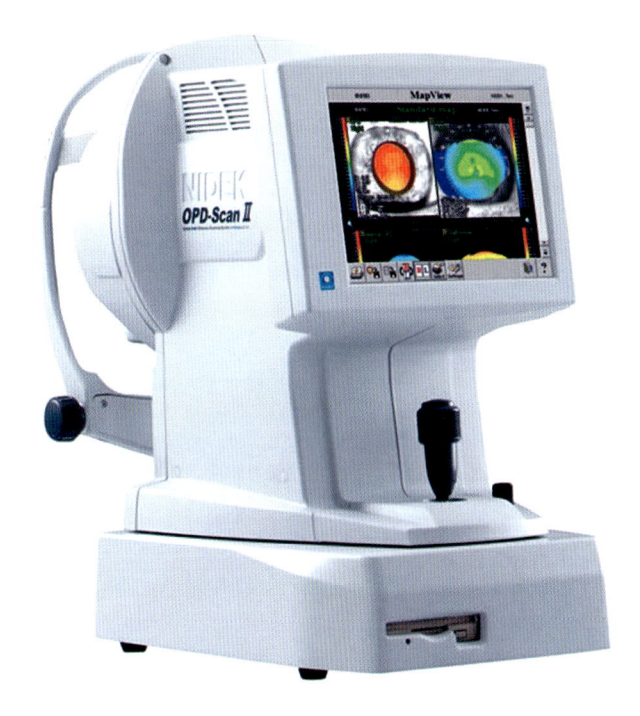

Figure 26.1 Nidek OPD scan

Guide to Clinical Interpretation with the Nidek OPD Scan

Nidek OPD Scan Six Map Display

Refractive (Snell's Law) map: Look at the color and topography patterns, keratometry, and Sim K values, as you would normally do for corneal topography maps. The scale should be set so that green represents 44 diopters in the scale settings section of the software. The dioptric power steps should be set to either 0.5 diopter or 1 diopter steps.

IROC (Tangential) map: Look at peripheral color patterns to look for peripheral changes beyond the 4 mm zone. The scale

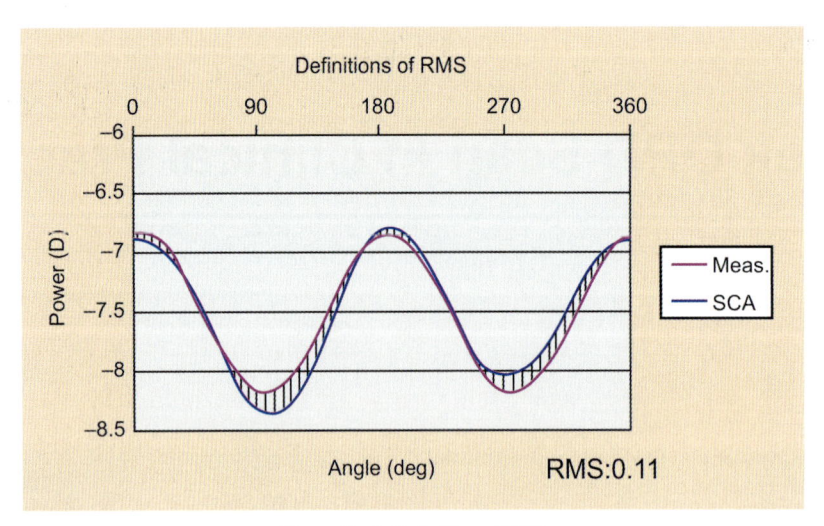

Figure 26.2 Definition of RMS

should be set so that green represents 44 diopters in the scale settings section of the software. The dioptric power steps should be set to either 0.5 diopter or 1 diopter steps.

OPD (Optical Path Difference to Emmetropia) map: Look at color patterns and overall dioptric power error scale for the 6 mm optical zone. ARK (Sphere/Cylinder/Astigmatism) values are displayed at the 2.5 mm, 3 mm and 5 mm zone. The irregular component of S/C/A at the 3 mm and 5 mm ring zone are quantified using RMS values in diopters. RMS diopter values below 0.5 on the OPD map are regular or near normal sphere and cylinder patterns (radially linear and radially symmetric). The components of S/C/A become more irregular at values greater than 0.5 RMS (diopters). Look for irregular patterns associated with double vision (two or three power lobes similar to a three leaf clover pattern) or ghosting (significant variation in central power from nasal to temporal within the 4 mm zone). The scale should be set so that green equals "0" diopters in the scale settings section of the software. The dioptric power steps should be set to either 0.5 diopter or 1 diopter steps.

Total order aberration map: This map displays how an emmetropic wavefront deviates through the entire optical system. Both lower and higher order aberrations are displayed in this map. The scale should be set so that green equals "0" microns in 0.5 μm or 1.0 μm steps in the scale settings section of the software.

Higher order aberration map: Determine the Higher Order (HO) wavefront percent by dividing Higher Order RMS wavefront error by Total Order RMS wavefront error (HO WF RMS error/TO WF RMS error = % of HO aberrations). This map displays only the irregular S/C/A or Higher Order aberrations of the optical system. The scale should be set so that green equals "0" microns in 0.5 μm or 1.0 μm steps in the scale settings section of the software.

The percentage of HO aberrations that is significant will vary for preoperative and postoperative patients. Preoperative HO/TO percent aberrations are abnormal after 20%, and postoperative HO/TO percent aberrations are suspect after 50%. However, this is a subjective observation that does not have clinical meaning until one reviews all of the available corneal topography, ARK, and OPD wavefront data.

Zernike graph: Examine the coefficients 6 through 27th and look for values of 0.5 RMS mm or higher for clinical significance. As for Zernike, the irregular (higher order) components of S/C/A can be measured and described optically as coma, trefoil and pentafoil and irregular (higher order) sphere can be described and measured by spherical aberrations (12th and 24th coefficient). RMS mm values below 0.5 mm are considered low and not clinically significant. RMS values above 0.5 mm generally correlate to subjective visual complaints. This would apply to all higher order Zernike coefficients starting from 6 to 27th as displayed on the Zernike Graph. The Zernike Graph coefficient values are in microns of light (not tissue).

RMS error is the best measure of dispersion around the best-fit sinusoid (**Figure 26.2**). It expresses a degree of irregularity or reliability of S/C/A values. Emmetropic patients will generally have very uniform topography maps, normal keratometry, low RMS values and low Zernike values. The progression of error increases for conditions such as asymmetrical astigmatism and keratoconus.

Summary

Examine the simulated keratometry and patterns on the topography maps, the ARK Data and RMS values and patterns on the OPD map, the ratio of HO/TO WF error from the wavefront maps and the HO Zernike RMS coefficients from 6 to 27th to determine.

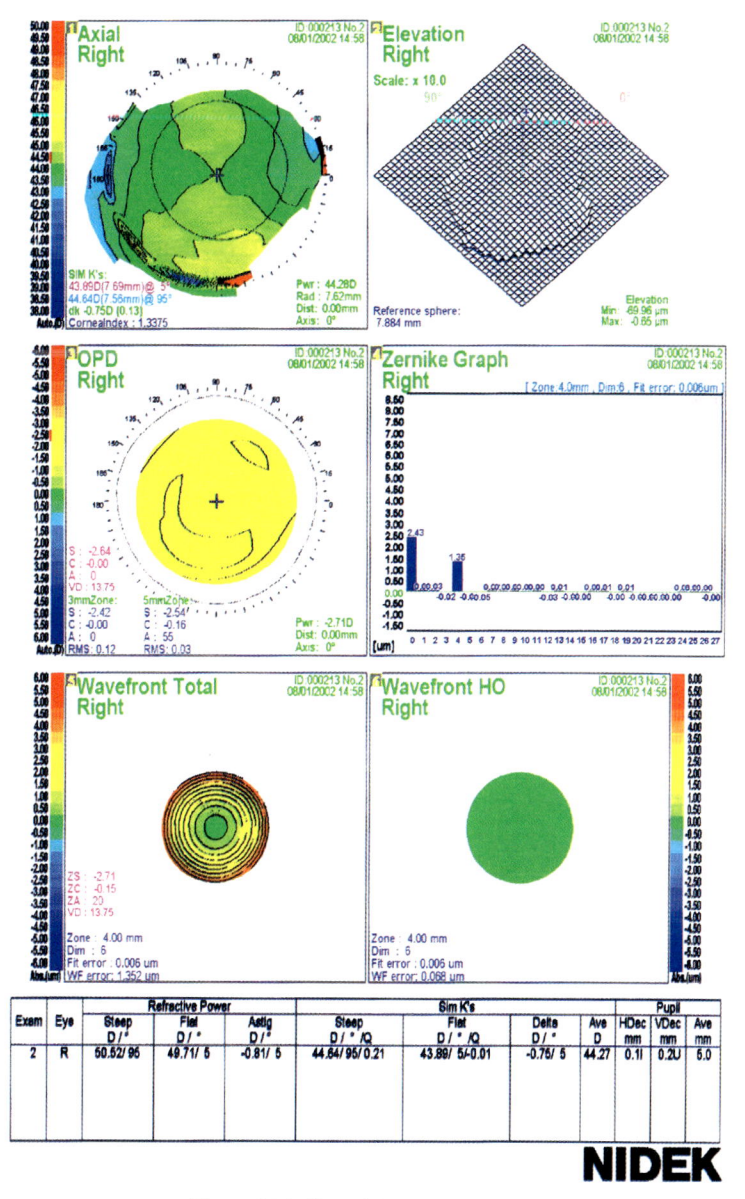

Figure 26.3 Normal Bowtie astigmatism

1. If the visual errors are caused by irregular astigmatism or by irregular spherical error, and to what degree by looking at Zernike coefficients.
2. Compare the RMS OPD values to a known normal range (0.0 to 0.5 diopters) to identify irregular versus regular profiles.
3. Evaluate whether HO/TO WF error percent aberration value is clinically significant by examining the Zernike RMS coefficient values. A value of 0.0 to 0.5 mm is not clinically significant. Values above 0.5 mm are clinically significant. This would apply to all higher order Zernike coefficients starting from 6 to 27th as displayed on the Zernike graph.

CLINICAL EXAMPLES

Normal Bowtie Astigmatism

The following patient demonstrates typical bowtie astigmatism on the axial map **(Figure 26.3)**. The OPD map has RMS values below 0.50 D, which correlates to the clinical picture of regular astigmatism.

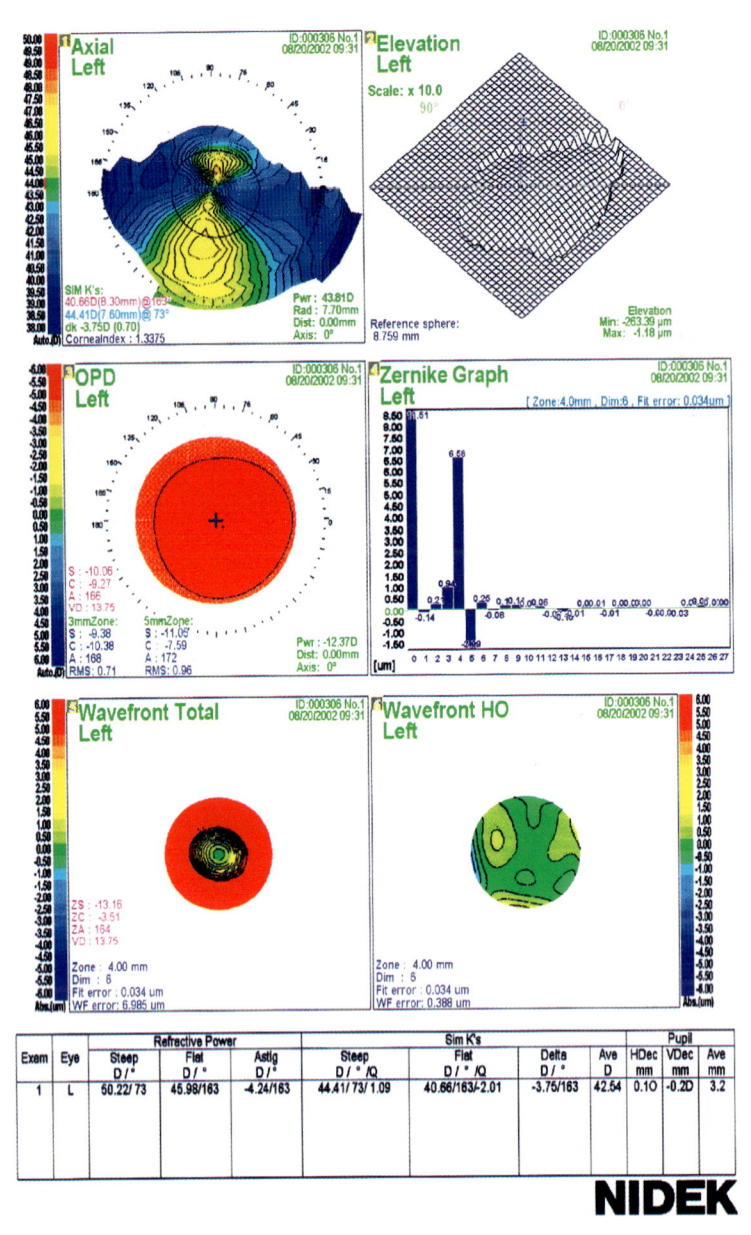

Figure 26.4 Keratoconus

Keratoconus

This 20-year-old male presented for refractive surgery **(Figure 26.4)**. Manifest refraction was −10.00 −8.00 × 165° (20/40). The refractive map revealed high keratometry readings with asymmetric astigmatism. OPD Map readings showed the irregular component of S/C/A at the three and five-millimeter zone using RMS values in diopters. RMS dioptric values measured greater than 0.50 D, which is associated with irregular astigmatism.

Pellucid Marginal Degeneration

This example demonstrates classic loop cylinder on corneal topography which is classic for pellucid marginal degeneration **(Figure 26.5)**. Wavefront RMS values are elevated (2.72 D @ 3 mm and 3.10 @ 5 mm) and consistent with irregular astigmatism.

Decentered LASIK Ablation

This 40-year-old patient was treated at another laser center and presented to the Feinerman Vision Center for correction

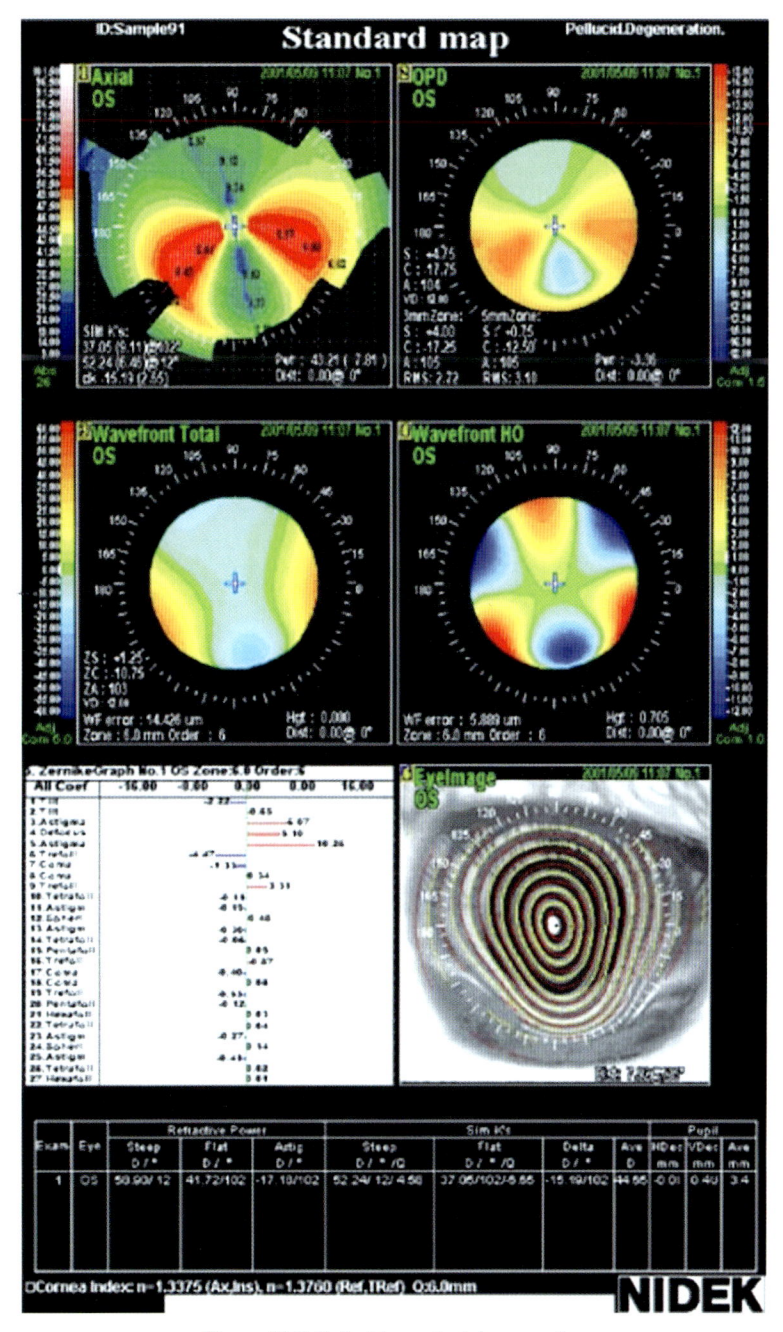

Figure 26.5 Pellucid marginal degeneration

of her LASIK complication. Her main complaint was decreased best-corrected vision and visual aberrations that worsened at night. BCVA was 20/60 in her right eye.

The corneal topography and OPD maps of the right eye demonstrate an inferotemporally decentered ablation **(Figure 26.6)**. RMS diopter values far exceed 0.5 D, which correlate to the patient's visual complaints.

Significant spherical and coma aberrations are present. Individual Zernike RMS values greater than 0.5 D in either direction correlate with the patient's visual problems.

The OPD map is the better indicator of what is wrong in diopters. In this case, I would not place much value in the Zernike coefficients, other than the fact that higher values generally correlate with visual complaints. This patient has an

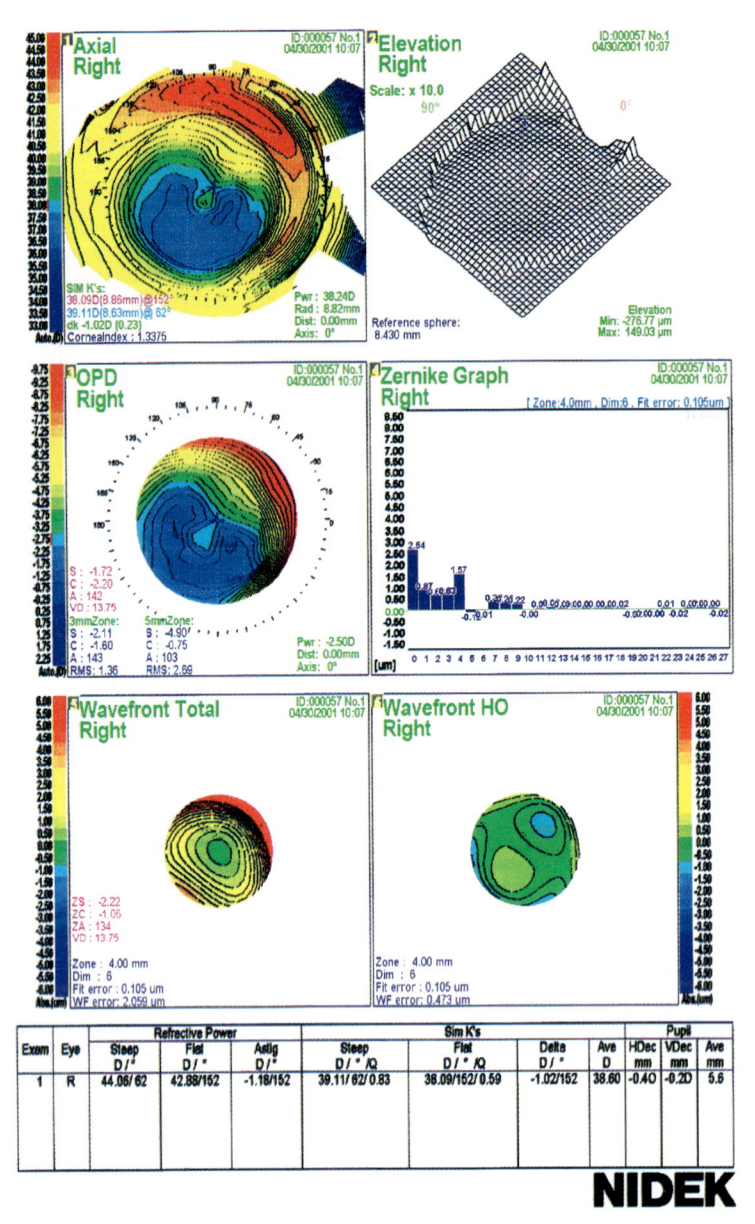

Figure 26.6 Decentered LASIK ablation

off-center power distribution noted on the OPD map. Custom ablation may be an option for cases of decentered ablations.

CONCLUSION

The Nidek OPD Scan is the only diagnostic instrument that incorporates corneal topography, autorefraction, and wavefront analysis in one system. The six map display shows the data in a manner that makes it easy for the surgeon to interpret. In the future, we will be able to utilize Nidek's Final Fit™ software to incorporate this data for custom ablation treatments.

REFERENCES

1. Beyond LASIK - Wavefront Analysis and Customized Ablation. Highlights of Ophthalmology 2001.
2. Nidek OPD Scan Manual, 2002.

Section VI

Cataract

CHAPTERS

27. Corneal Topography in Cataract Surgery
28. Corneal Topography in Phakonit with a 5 mm Optic Rollable Intraocular Lens
29. Glued IOL Position: An OCT Assessment

Chapter 27

Corneal Topography in Cataract Surgery

Athiya Agarwal (India), Amar Agarwal (India)

INTRODUCTION

Topography is defined as the science of describing or representing the features of a particular place in detail. In corneal topography, the place is the cornea, i.e. we describe the features of the cornea in detail.

The word Topography is derived[1,2] from two Greek words:

TOPOS—meaning place
and
GRAPHIEN—meaning to write.

CORNEA

There are basically three refractive elements of the eye, namely; axial length, lens and cornea. The cornea is the most important plane or tissue for refraction. This is because it has the highest refractive power (which is about + 45 D) and it is easily accessible to the surgeon without going inside the eye.

To understand the cornea, one should realize that the cornea is a parabolic curve—its radius of curvature differs from center to periphery. It is steepest in the center and flatter in the periphery. For all practical purposes, the central cornea is the optical zone that is taken into consideration, when you are doing a refractive surgery. A flatter cornea has less refractive power and a steeper cornea has a higher refractive power. If we want to change the refraction we must make the steeper diameter flatter and the flatter diameter steeper.

KERATOMETRY

The keratometer was invented by Hermann Von Helmholtz and modified by Javal, Schiotz, etc. If we place an object in front of a convex mirror we get a virtual, erect and minified image **(Figure 27.1)**. A keratometer in relation to the cornea is just like an object in front of a convex reflecting mirror. Like in a convex reflecting surface, the image is located posterior to the cornea. The cornea behaves as a convex reflecting mirror and the mires of the keratometer are the objects. The radius of curvature of the cornea's anterior surface determines the size of the image.

The keratometer projects a single mire on the cornea and the separation of the two points on the mire is used to determine corneal curvature. The zone measured depends upon corneal curvature—the steeper the cornea, the smaller the zone. For example, for a 36 D cornea, the keratometer measures a 4 mm zone and for a 50 D cornea, the size of the cone is 2.88 mm.

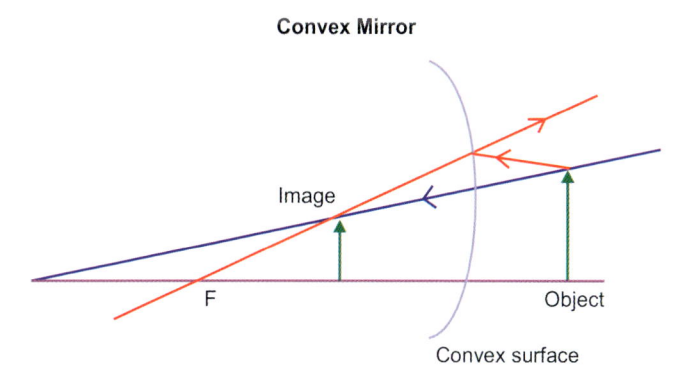

Figure 27.1 Physics of a convex mirror. Note the image is virtual, erect and minified. The cornea acts like the convex mirror and the mire of the keratometer is the object

Keratometers are accurate only when the corneal surface is a sphere or a spherocylinder. Actually, the shape of the anterior surface of the cornea is more than a sphere or a spherocylinder. But keratometers measure the central 3 mm of the cornea, which behaves like a sphere or a spherocylinder. This is the reason why Helmholtz could manage with the keratometer **(Figure 27.2)**. This is also the reason why most ophthalmologists can manage preoperative work-up of cataract surgery with the keratometer. But today, with refractive surgery, the ball game has changed. This is because when the cornea has complex central curves like in keratoconus or after refractive surgery, the keratometer cannot give good results and becomes inaccurate. Thus, the advantages of the keratometer like speed, ease of use, low cost and minimum maintenance are obscured.

The objects used in the keratometer are referred to as mires. Separation of two points on the mire are used to determine corneal curvature. The object in the keratometer can be rotated with respect to the axis. The disadvantages of the keratometer are that they measure only a small region of the cornea. The peripheral regions are ignored. They also lose accuracy when measuring very steep or flat corneas. As the keratometer assumes the cornea to be symmetrical it becomes

292   Section VI: Cataract

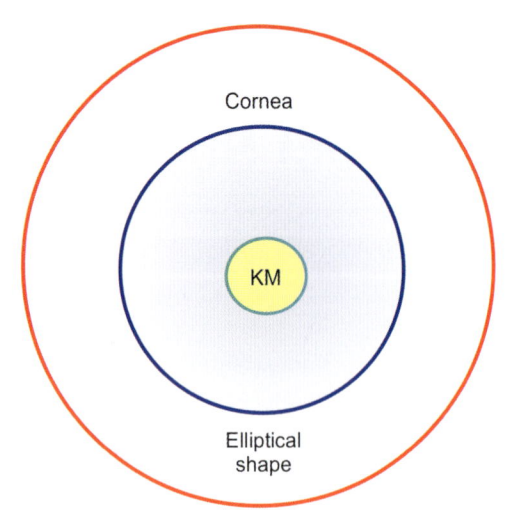

Figure 27.2 Keratometers measure the central 3 mm of the cornea, which generally behaves like a sphere or a spherocylinder. This is the reason why keratometers are generally accurate. But in complex situations like in keratoconus or refractive surgery they become inaccurate

a disadvantage, if the cornea is asymmetrical as after refractive surgery.

KERATOSCOPY

To solve the problem of keratometers, scientists worked on a system called Keratoscopy. In this, they projected a beam of concentric rings and observed them over a wide expanse of the corneal surface. But this was not enough and the next step was to move into computerized videokeratography.

COMPUTERIZED VIDEOKERATOGRAPHY

In this, some form of light like a placido disc is projected onto the cornea. The cornea modifies this light and this modification is captured by a video camera. This information is analyzed by computer software and the data is then displayed in a variety of formats. To simplify the results to an ophthalmologist, Klyce in 1988 started the corneal color maps. The corneal color maps display the estimate of corneal shape in a fashion that is understandable to the ophthalmologist. Each color on the map is assigned a defined range of measurement. The placido type topographic machines **(Figure 27.3)** do not assess the posterior surface of the cornea. The details of the corneal assessment can be done only with the Orbscan (Bausch and Lomb) as both anterior and posterior surface of the cornea are assessed.

ORBSCAN

The Orbscan (Bausch and Lomb) corneal topography system **(Figure 27.4)** uses a scanning optical slit scan that is fundamentally different than the corneal topography that analyzes the reflected images from the anterior corneal surface (Read

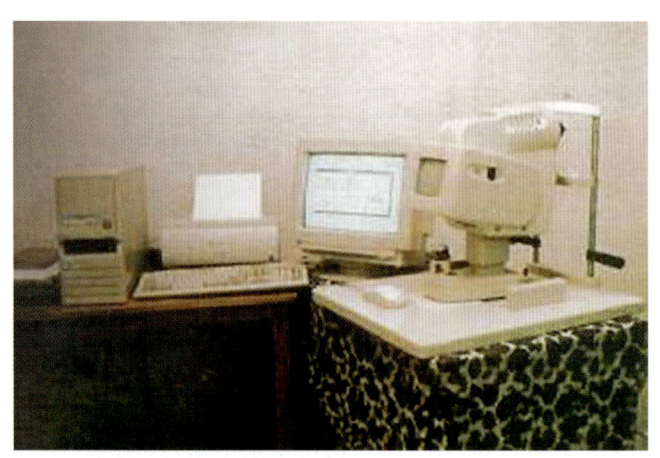

Figure 27.3 Placido type corneal topography machine

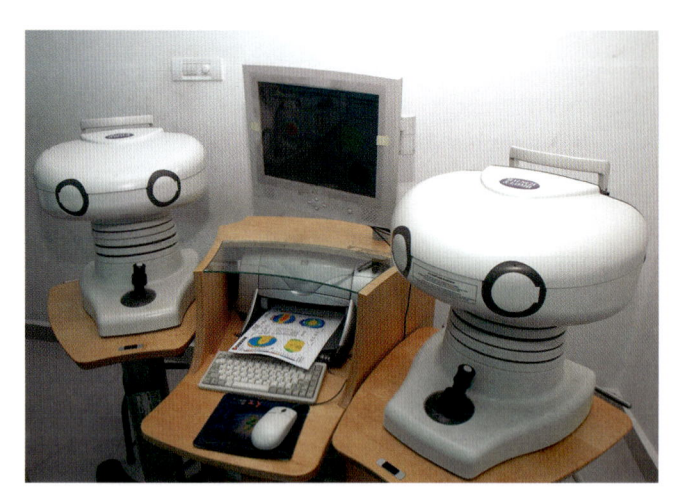

Figure 27.4 Orbscan (*Courtesy:* Dr Agarwal's Eye Hospital)

Orbscan chapter). The high-resolution video camera captures 40 light slits at 45 degrees angle projected through the cornea similarly as seen during slit lamp examination. The slits are projected on to the anterior segment of the eye: the anterior cornea, the posterior cornea, the anterior iris and anterior lens. The data collected from these four surfaces are used to create a topographic map.

NORMAL CORNEA

In a normal cornea **(Figure 27.5)**, the nasal cornea is flatter than the temporal cornea. This is similar to the curvature of the long end of an ellipse. If we see **Figure 27.5** then we will notice the values written on the right end of the pictures. These indicate the astigmatic values. In that is written Max K is 45 @ 84 degrees and Min K is 44 @ 174 degrees. This means the astigmatism is + 1.0 D at 84 degrees. This is with the rule astigmatism as the astigmatism is Plus at 90 degrees axis.

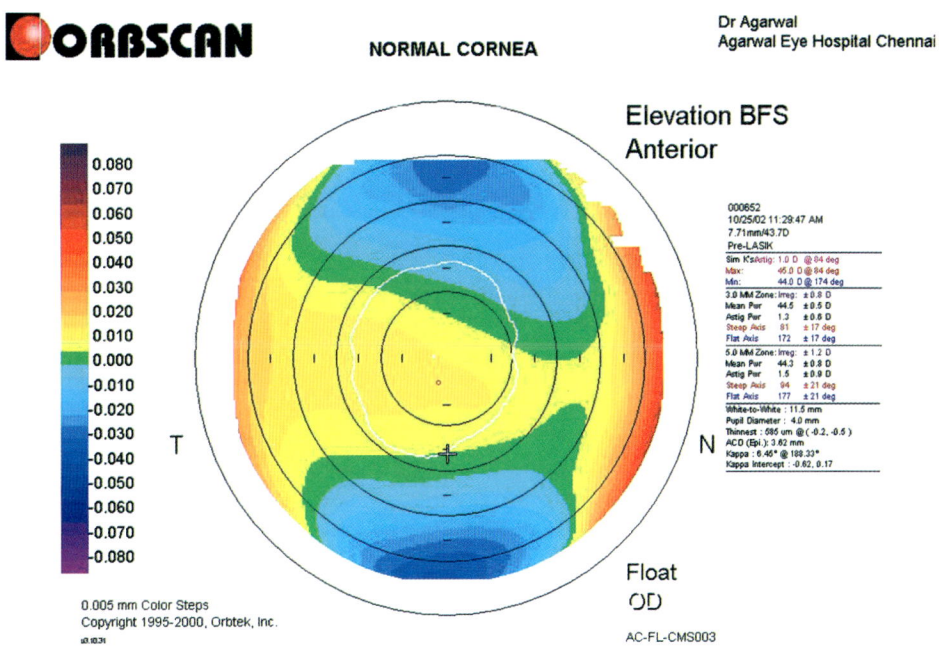

Figure 27.5 Topography of a normal cornea

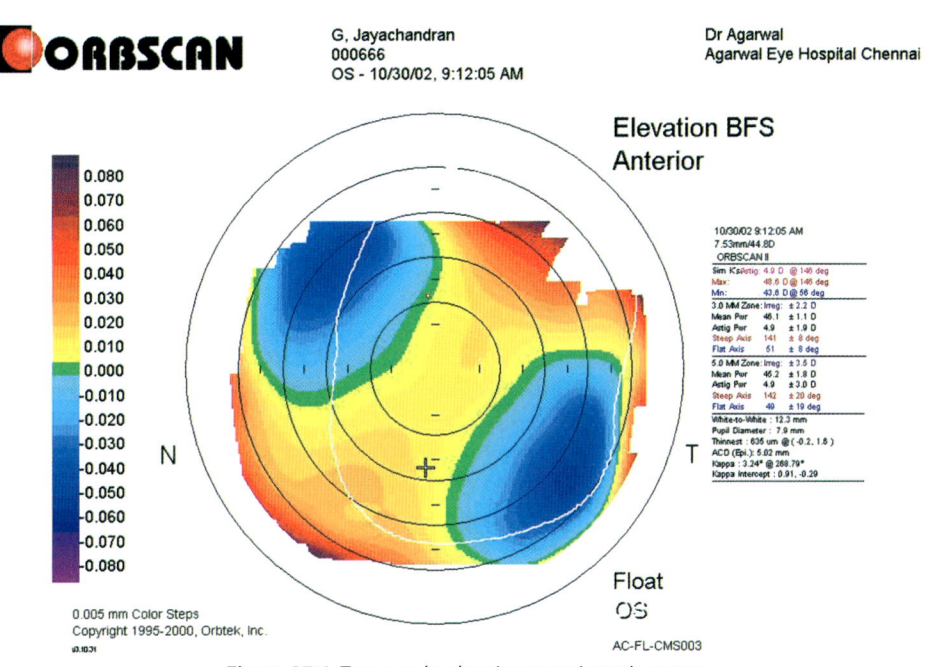

Figure 27.6 Topography showing an astigmatic cornea

If the astigmatism was Plus at 180 degrees then it is against the rule astigmatism. The normal corneal topography can be round, oval, irregular, symmetric bowtie or asymmetric bowtie in appearance. If we see **Figure 27.6**, we will see a case of astigmatism in which the astigmatism is + 4.9 D at 146 degrees. *These figures show the curvature of the anterior surface of the cornea. It is important to remember that these are not the keratometric maps. So the blue/green color denote steepening and the red colors denote flattening.* If we want the red to denote steepening then we can invert the colors.

CATARACT SURGERY

Corneal topography is extremely important in cataract surgery. *The smaller the size of the incision lesser the astigmatism and earlier stability of the astigmatism will occur.* One can reduce

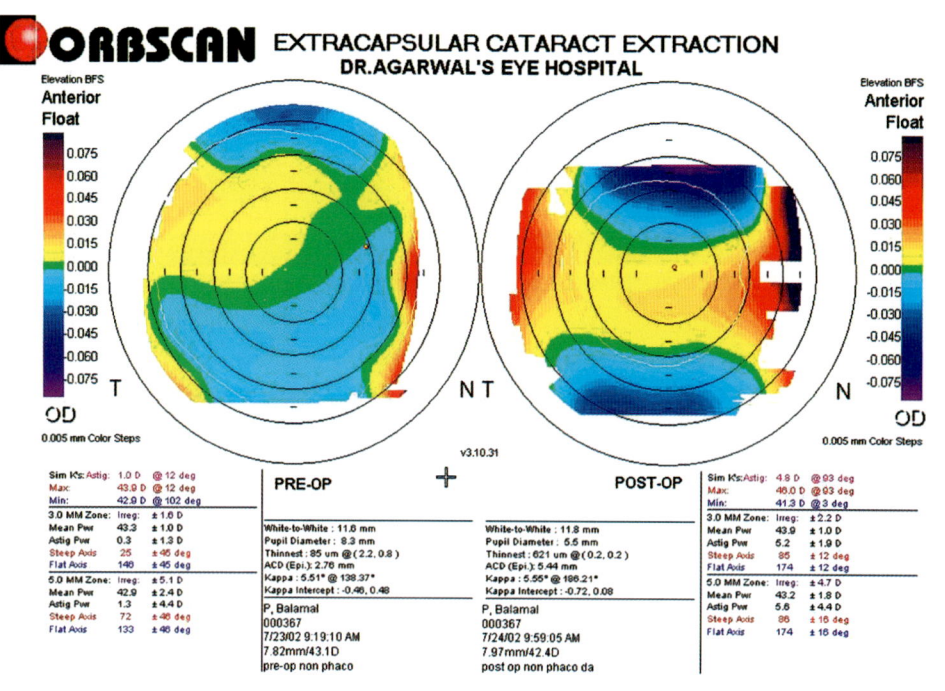

Figure 27.7 Topography after extracapsular cataract extraction (ECCE). The figure on the left shows astigmatism of + 1.1 D at 12 degrees preoperatively. The astigmatism has increased to + 4.8 D as seen in the figure on the right

the astigmatism or increase the astigmatism of a patient after cataract surgery. The simple rule to follow is that—*wherever you make an incision that area will flatten and wherever you apply sutures that area will steepen.*

EXTRACAPSULAR CATARACT EXTRACTION

One of the problems in extracapsular cataract extraction is the astigmatism, which is created as the incision size is about 10 to 12 mm. In **Figure 27.7**, you can see the topographic picture of a patient after extracapsular cataract extraction (ECCE). You can see the picture on the left is the preoperative photo and the picture on the right is a postoperative day 1 photo. Preoperatively one will notice the astigmatism is + 1.0 D at 12 degrees and postoperatively it is + 4.8 D at 93 degrees. This is the problem in ECCE. In the immediate postoperative period the astigmatism is high which would reduce with time. But the predictability of astigmatism is not there which is why smaller incision cataract surgery is more successful.

NONFOLDABLE IOL

Some surgeons perform phaco and implant a nonfoldable IOL in which the incision is increased to 5.5 to 6 mm. In such cases, the astigmatism is better than in an ECCE. In **Figure 27.8**, the pictures are of a patient who has had a nonfoldable IOL. Notice in this the preoperative astigmatism is + 0.8 D @ 166 degrees. This is the left eye of the patient. If we had done a phaco with a foldable IOL the astigmatism would have been nearly the same or reduced as our incision would have come in the area of the astigmatism. But in this case after a phaco a nonfoldable IOL was implanted. The postoperative astigmatism one week postoperative is + 1.8 D @ 115 degrees. You can notice from the two pictures the astigmatism has increased.

FOLDABLE IOL

In phaco with a foldable IOL the amount of astigmatism created is much less than in a nonfoldable IOL. Let us look now at **Figure 27.9**. The patient as you can see has negligible astigmatism in the left eye. The picture on the left shows a preoperative astigmatism of + 0.8 D at 166 degrees axis. Now, we operate generally with a temporal clear corneal approach, so in the left eye, the incision will be generally at the area of the steepend axis. This will reduce the astigmatism. If we see the postoperative photo of day one we will see the astigmatism is only + 0.6 D @ 126 degrees. This means that after a day, the astigmatism has not changed much and this shows a good result. This patient had a foldable IOL implanted under the no anesthesia cataract surgical technique after a phaco cataract surgery with the size of the incision being 2.8 mm.

ASTIGMATISM INCREASED

If we are not careful in selecting the incision depending upon the corneal topography we can burn our hands. **Figure 27.10**,

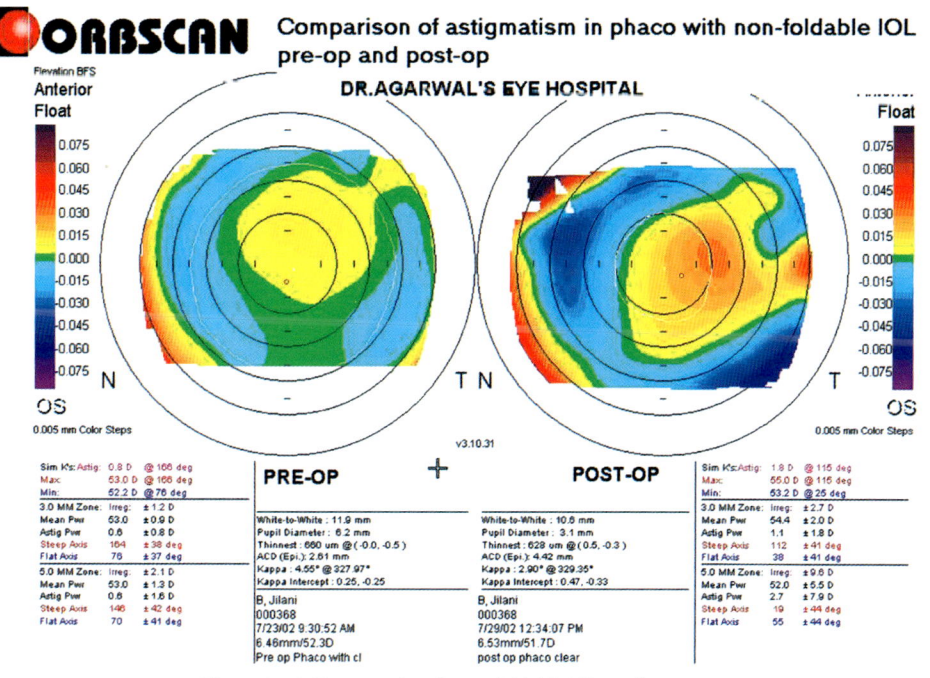

Figure 27.8 Topography of a nonfoldable IOL implantation

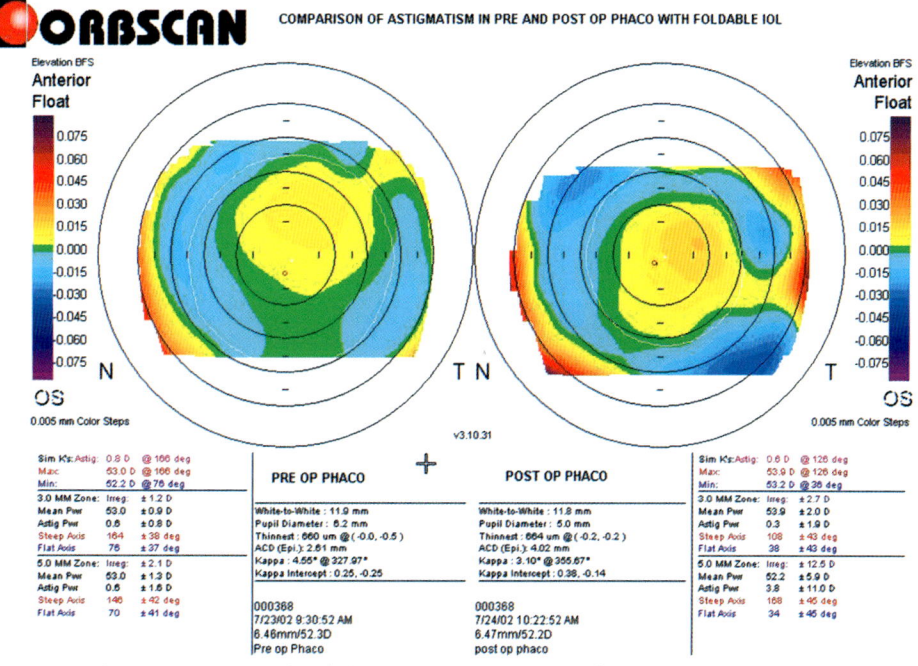

Figure 27.9 Topography of phaco cataract surgery with a foldable IOL implantation

illustrates a case in which astigmatism has increased due to the incision being made in the wrong meridian. The patient had a 2.8 mm incision with a foldable IOL implanted after a phaco cataract surgery under the no anesthesia cataract surgical technique. Both the pictures are of the right eye.

In **Figure 27.10**, look at the picture on the left. In the picture on the left, you can see the patient has an astigmatism of +1.1 D at axis 107 degrees. As this is the right eye with this astigmatism we should have made a superior incision to reduce the preoperative astigmatism. But by mistake we made a temporal

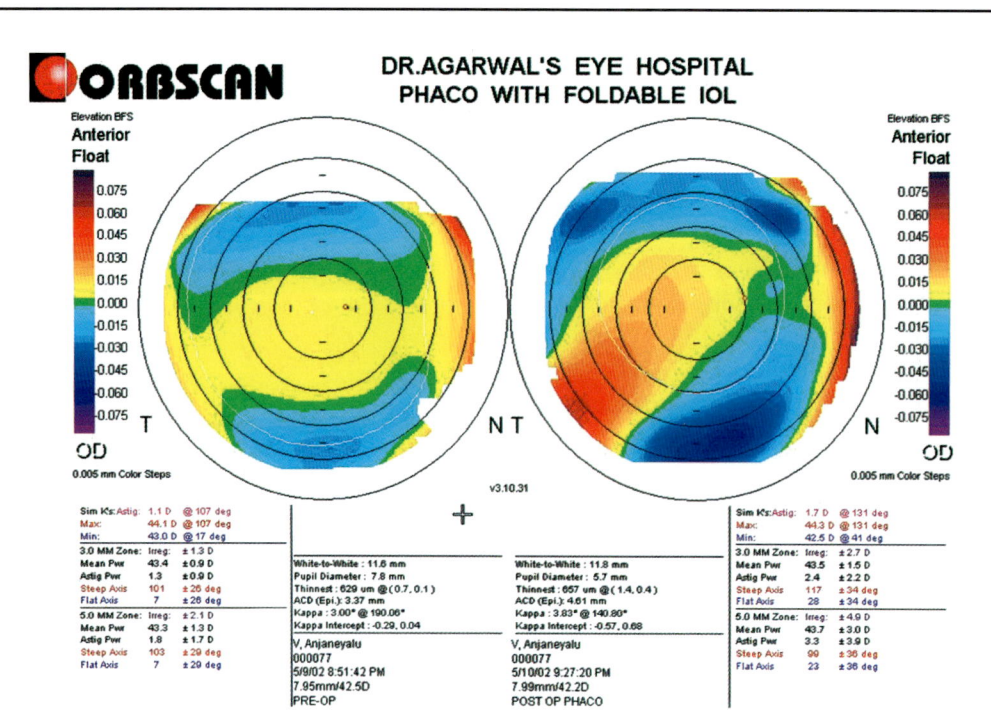

Figure 27.10 Increase in astigmatism after cataract surgery due to incision being made in the wrong meridian. Topography of a phaco with foldable IOL implantation

clear corneal incision. This has increased the astigmatism. Now if we wanted to flatten this case, we should have made the incision where the steeper meridian was. That was at the 105 degrees axis. But because we were doing routinely temporal clear corneal incisions, we made the incision in the opposite axis. Now look at the picture on the right. The astigmatism has increased from + 1.1 D to + 1.7 D. This shows a bad result. If we had made the incision superiorly at the 107 degrees axis, we would have flattened that axis and the astigmatism would have been reduced.

BASIC RULE

The basic rule to follow is to look at the number written in red. The red numbers indicate the plus axis. If the difference in astigmatism is say 3 D at 180 degrees, it means the patient has + 3 D astigmatism at axis 180 degrees. This is against the rule astigmatism. In such cases, make your clear corneal incision at 180 degrees so that you can flatten this steepness. This will reduce the astigmatism.

UNIQUE CASE

In **Figure 27.11**, the patient had a temporal clear corneal incision for phaco cataract surgery under no anesthesia with a nonfoldable IOL. Both the pictures are of the left eye. The figure on the left shows the postoperative topographic picture. The postoperative astigmatism was + 1.8 D at axis 115 degrees.

This patient had three sutures in the site of the incision. These sutures were put as a nonfoldable IOL had been implanted in the eye with a clear corneal incision. When this patient came for a follow-up we removed the sutures. The next day the patient came to us with loss of vision. On examination, we found the astigmatism had increased. We then took another topography. The picture on the right is of the topography after removing the sutures. The astigmatism increased to + 5.7 D. So, one should be very careful in analyzing the corneal topography when one does suture removal also. To solve this problem one can do an astigmatic keratotomy.

PHAKONIT

Phakonit is a technique devised by Dr Amar Agarwal in which the cataract is removed through a 0.9 mm incision. The advantage of this is obvious. The astigmatism created by a 0.9 mm incision is very little compared to a 2.6 mm phaco incision. Today with the rollable IOL and the Acritec IOLs which are ultra-small incision IOLs one can pass IOLs through sub 1.4 mm incisions. This is seen clearly in **Figures 27.12** and **27.13**. **Figure 27.12** shows the comparison after Phakonit with a Rollable IOL and **Figure 27.13** with an Acritec IOL. If you will see the preoperative and the postoperative photographs in comparison you will see there is not much difference between the two. In this case, a rollable IOL was implanted. The point which we will notice in this picture is that the difference between the preoperative photo and the one day postoperative photo is not much.

Chapter 27: Corneal Topography in Cataract Surgery   297

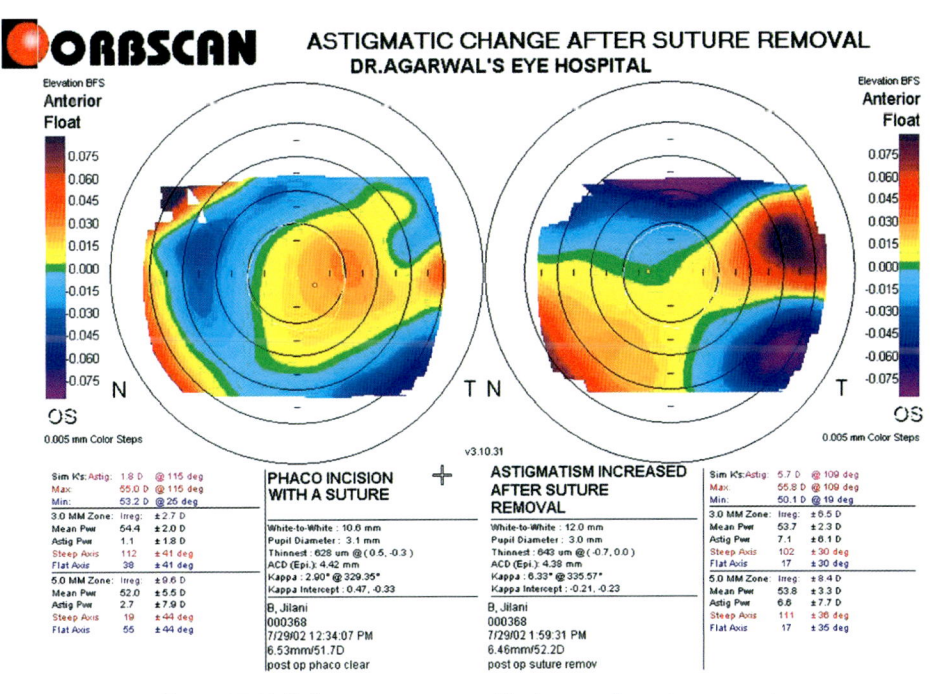

Figure 27.11 Unique case—topographic changes after suture removal

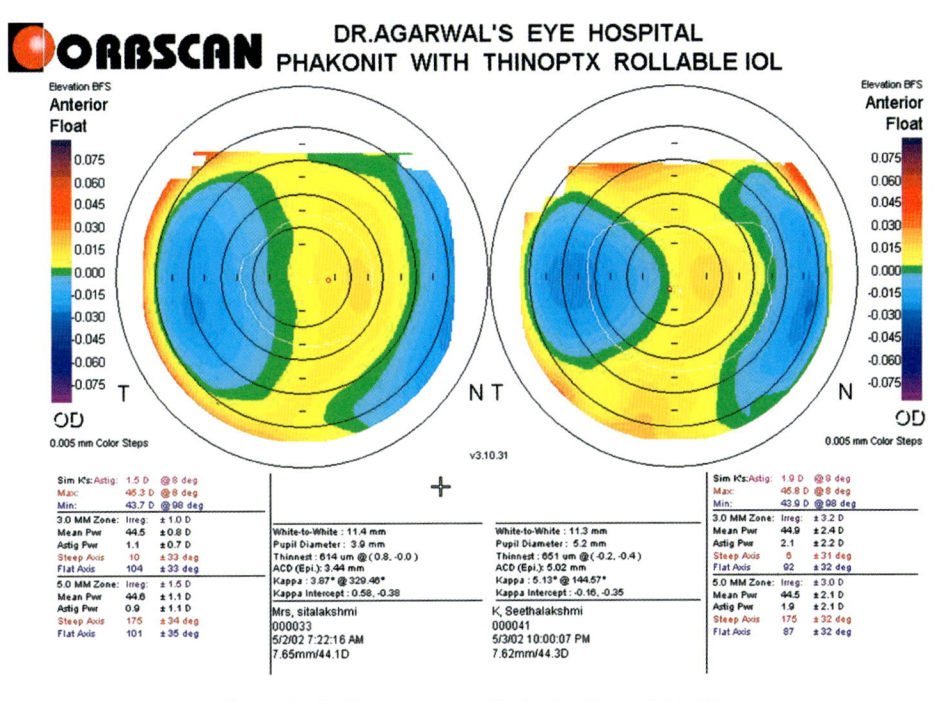

Figure 27.12 Topography of a Phakonit with a rollable IOL

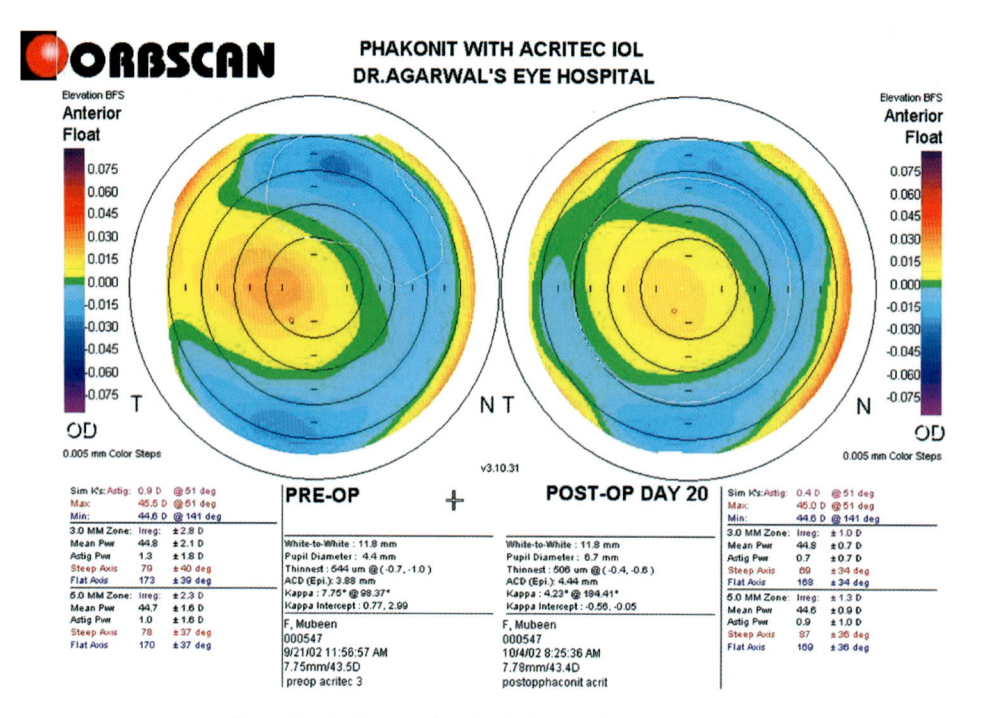

Figure 27.13 Topography of a Phakonit with an Acritec IOL

SUMMARY

Corneal topography is an extremely important tool for the ophthalmologist. It is not only the refractive surgeon who should utilize this instrument but also the cataract surgeon. The most important refractive surgery done in the world is cataract surgery and not LASIK (Laser-in-situ keratomileusis) or PRK (Photorefractive keratectomy). With more advancements in corneal topography, topographic-assisted LASIK will become available to everyone with an excimer laser. One might also have the corneal topographic machine fixed onto the operating microscope so that one can easily reduce the astigmatism of the patient.

REFERENCES

1. Gills JP, et al. Corneal Topography: The State-of-the Art. New Delhi; Jaypee Brothers Medical Publishers (P) Ltd., 1996.
2. Agarwal S, Agarwal A, Sachdev MS, Mehta KR, Fine IH, Agarwal A. Phacoemulsification, Laser Cataract surgery and Foldable IOL's; New Delhi; Second edition; Jaypee Brothers Medical Publishers (P) Ltd., 2000.

Chapter 28

Corneal Topography in Phakonit with a 5 mm Optic Rollable Intraocular Lens

Amar Agarwal (India), Athiya Agarwal (India)

INTRODUCTION

Cataract surgery and intraocular lenses (IOL) have evolved greatly since the time of intracapsular cataract extraction and the first IOL implantation by Sir Harold Ridley.[1] The size of the cataract incision has constantly been decreasing from the extremely large ones used for ICCE to the slightly smaller ones used in ECCE to the present day small incisions used in phacoemulsification. Phacoemulsification and foldable IOLs are a major milestone in the history of cataract surgery. Large postoperative against-the-rule astigmatism were an invariable consequence of ICCE and ECCE. This was minimized to a great extent with the 3.2 mm clear corneal incision used for phacoemulsification but nevertheless some amount of residual postoperative astigmatism was a common outcome. The size of the corneal incision was further decreased by Phakonit[2-4] a technique introduced for the first time by one of us (Am. A), which separates the infusion from the aspiration ports by utilizing a sleeveless phaco probe and an irrigating chopper. The only limitation to thus realizing the goal of astigmatism neutral cataract surgery was the size of the foldable IOL as the wound nevertheless had to be extended for implantation of the conventional foldable IOLs.

ROLLABLE INTRAOCULAR LENS

With the availability of the ThinOptX® rollable IOL (Abingdon, VA, USA), that can be inserted through sub-1.4 mm incision, the full potential of Phakonit could be realized. This lens was created and designed by Wayne Callahan from USA. Subsequently, one of the authors (Am. A) modified the lens by making the optic size 5 mm so that it could go through a smaller incision.

SURGICAL TECHNIQUE

Five eyes of 5 patients underwent Phakonit with implantation of an ultrathin 5 mm optic rollable IOL at Dr Agarwal's Eye Hospital and Eye Research Centre, Chennai, India.

The name PHAKONIT has been given because it shows phacoemulsification (PHAKO) being done with a needle (N) opening via an incision (I) and with the phaco tip (T). A specially designed keratome, an irrigating chopper, a straight blunt rod and a 15° standard phaco tip without an infusion sleeve form the main pre-requisites of the surgery. Viscoelastic is injected with a 26G needle through the presumed site of side port entry. This inflates the chamber and prevents its collapse when the chamber is entered with the keratome. A straight rod is passed through this site to achieve akinesia and a clear corneal temporal valve is made with the keratome **(Figure 28.1A)**. A continuous curvilinear capsulorhexis (CCC) is performed followed by hydrodissection and rotation of the nucleus. After enlarging the side port a 20 Gauge irrigating chopper connected to the infusion line of the phaco machine is introduced with foot pedal on position 1. The phaco probe is connected to the aspiration line and the phaco tip without an infusion sleeve is introduced through the main port **(Figure 28.1B)**. Using the phaco tip with moderate ultrasound power, the center of the nucleus is directly embedded starting from the superior edge of rhexis with the phaco probe directed obliquely downwards towards the vitreous. The settings at this stage are 50% phaco power, flow rate 24 ml/min and 110 mm Hg vacuum. When nearly half of the center of nucleus is embedded, the foot pedal is moved to position 2 as it helps to hold the nucleus due to vacuum rise. To avoid undue pressure on the posterior capsule the nucleus is lifted slightly and with the irrigating chopper in the left hand the nucleus chopped. This is done with a straight downward motion from the inner edge of the rhexis to the center of the nucleus and then to the left in the form of an inverted L shape. Once the crack is created, the nucleus is split till the center. The nucleus is then rotated 180° and cracked again so that the nucleus is completely split into two halves. With the previously described technique, 3 pie-shaped quadrants are created in each half of the nucleus. With a short burst of energy at pulse mode, each pie shaped fragment is lifted and brought at the level of iris where it is further emulsified and aspirated sequentially in pulse mode. Thus, the whole nucleus is removed. Cortical wash-up is then done with the bimanual irrigation aspiration technique.

The lens is taken out from the bottle and placed in a bowl of BSS solution of approximately body temperature to make the lens pliable. It is then rolled with the gloved hand holding it between the index finger and the thumb. The lens is then inserted through the incision carefully **(Figure 28.1C)**. The teardrop on the haptic should be pointing in a clockwise direction so that the smooth optic lenticular surface faces posteriorly. The natural warmth of the eye causes the lens to open gradually. Viscoelastic is then removed with the bimanual

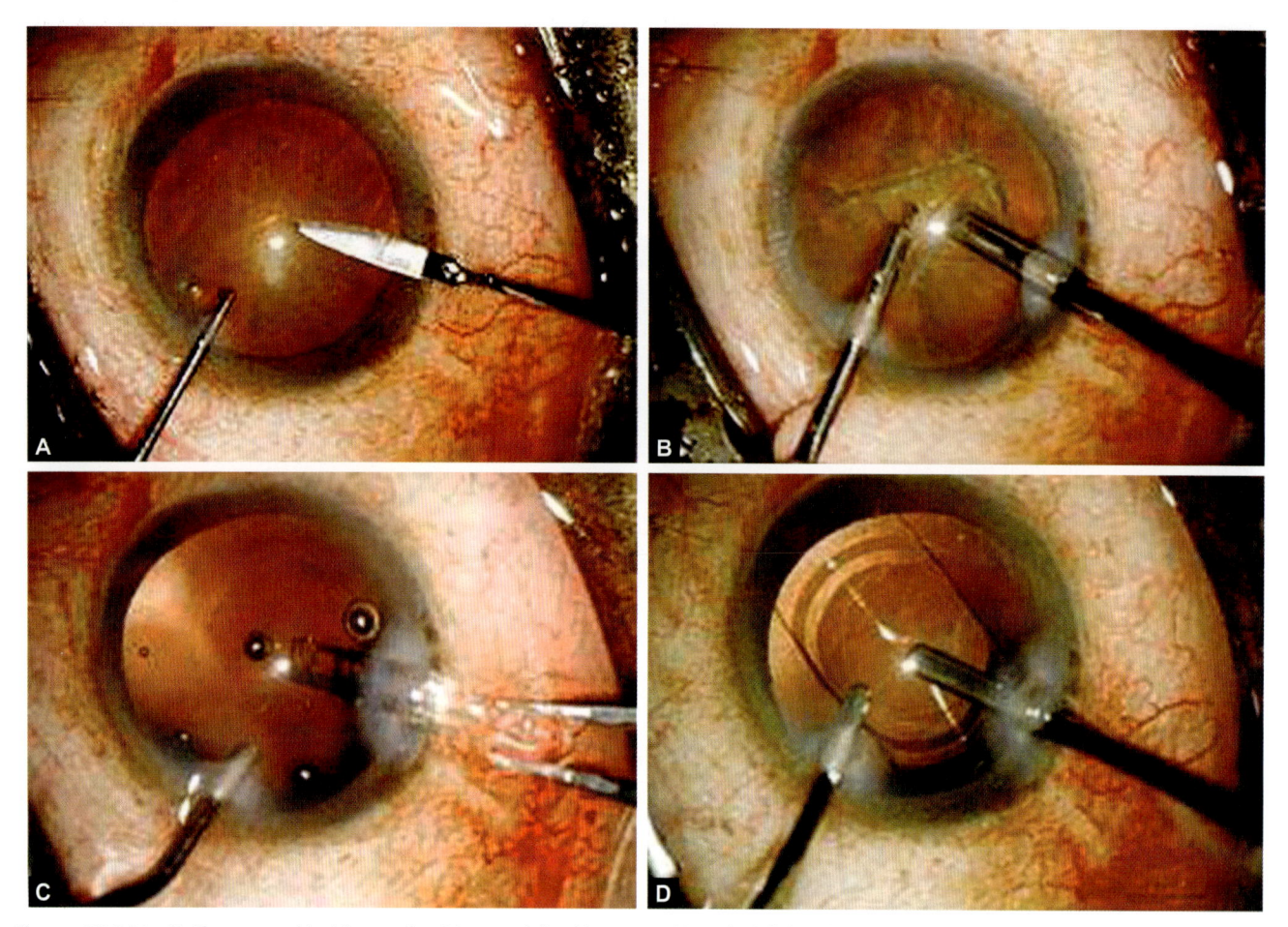

Figures 28.1A to D Clear corneal incision made with a specialized keratome. Note the left hand has a straight rod to stabilize the eye (A); Agarwal's phakonit irrigating chopper and sleeveless phaco probe inside the eye (B); The rollable IOL inserted through the incision (C); Viscoelastic removed using bimanual irrigation aspiration probes (D)

irrigation aspiration probes **(Figure 28.1D)**. **Figure 28.1** shows different steps of the surgery.

TOPOGRAPHIC ANALYSIS AND ASTIGMATISM

The preoperative best corrected visual acuity (BCVA) ranged from 20/60 to 20/200. The mean preoperative astigmatism as detected by topographic analysis was 0.98 D ± 0.62 D (range 0.5 to 1.8 D).

The postoperative course was uneventful in all cases. The IOL was well centered in the capsular bag. There were no corneal burns in any of the cases.

Four eyes had a best-corrected visual acuity of 20/30 or better. One eye that had dry ARMD showed an improvement in BCVA from 20/200 to 20/60. **Figure 28.2** shows a comparison of the pre- and postoperative BCVA. The mean astigmatism on postoperative day 1 on topographic analysis was 1.1 ± 0.61 D (range 0.6 to 1.9 D) as compared to 0.98 D ± 0.62 D (range 0.5 to 1.8 D) preoperatively. The mean astigmatism was 1.02 ± 0.64 D (range 0.3 to 1.7 D) by 3 months postoperatively. **Figures 28.3 and 28.4** show mean astigmatism over time. **Figure 28.5** shows Phakonit being done with an end opening irrigating chopper.

MICROPHAKONIT (CATARACT SURGERY THROUGH A 0.7 MM TIP)

In 1998, Dr Amar Agarwal performed 1 mm cataract surgery by a technique called Phakonit **(Figure 28.5)** (phako being done with a needle incision technology). This used the air pump or gas forced infusion started by Sunita Agarwal to prevent any surge in the eye **(Figure 28.6)**. Dr Jorge Alio coined the term *Microincision Cataract Surgery* (MICS) for all surgeries including laser cataract surgery and phakonit. Dr Randall Olson first used a 0.8 mm phaco needle and a 21-gauge irrigating chopper and called it microphaco. On May 21st 2005, for the first time a 0.7 mm phaco needle tip with a 0.7 mm irrigating chopper was used by Dr Agarwal to

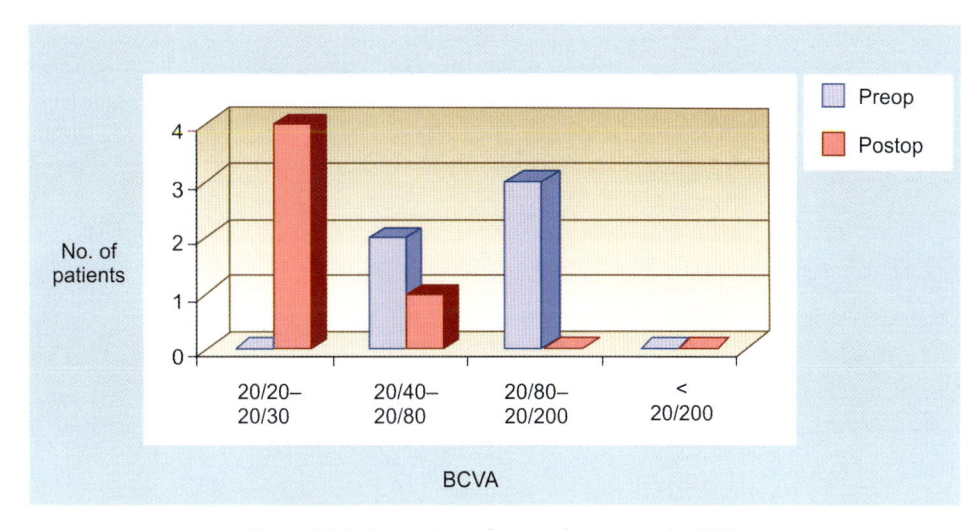

Chapter 28: Corneal Topography in Phakonit with a 5 mm Optic Rollable... 301

Figure 28.2 Comparison of pre- and postoperative BCVA

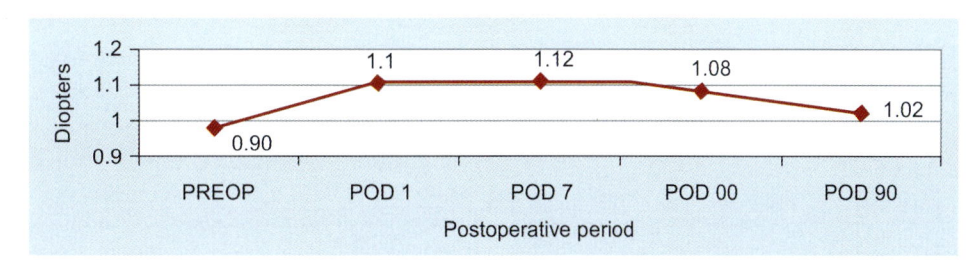

Figure 28.3 Mean astigmatism over time

Time	Eyes	Mean	Std. Dev.	Minimum	Maximum
PREOP	5	0.98	0.62	0.5	1.8
POD 1	5	1.1	0.61	0.6	1.9
POD 7	5	1.12	0.58	0.5	1.7
POD 30	5	1.08	0.62	0.5	1.8
POD 90	5	1.02	0.64	0.3	1.7

Figure 28.4 Showing pre- and postoperative mean astigmatism

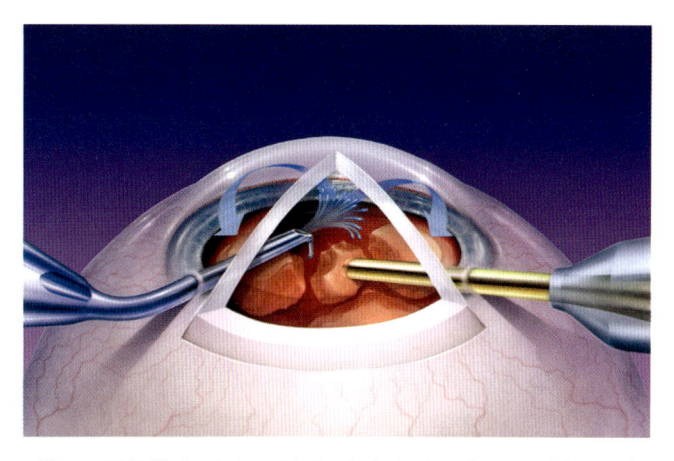

Figure 28.5 Phakonit done. Notice the irrigating chopper with an end opening. (*Courtesy:* Larry Laks, MST, USA)

remove cataracts through the smallest incision possible as of now. This is called microphakonit **(Figure 28.7)**. The 22-gauge (0.7 mm) irrigating chopper is connected to the infusion line with foot pedal on position. The phaco probe is connected to the aspiration line and the 0.7 mm phaco tip without an infusion sleeve is introduced through the clear corneal incision. Using the phaco tip with moderate ultrasound power, the center of the nucleus is directly embedded starting from the superior edge of rhexis with the phaco probe directed obliquely downwards toward the vitreous. The settings at this stage are 50% phaco power, flow rate 24 ml/min, and 110 mm Hg vacuum. Using the karate chop technique, the nucleus is chopped. Thus, the whole nucleus is removed. Cortical washup is then done with the bimanual irrigation aspiration (0.7 mm set) technique. During the micro-phakonit procedure, gas forced infusion is used. The instruments are made by Larry Laks from Microsurgical Technology, USA. At the time of this writing, this is the smallest

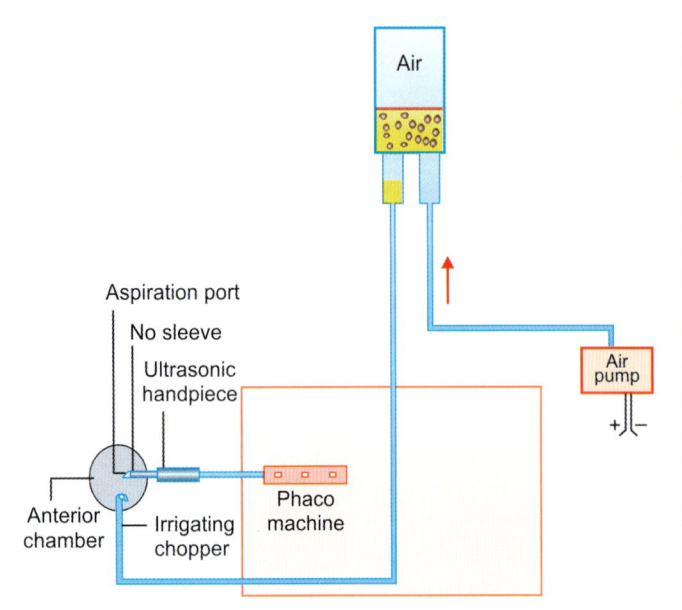

Figure 28.6 Air pump used to prevent surge in phaco and phakonit. In the air pump system, a locally manufactured automated device used in fish tanks (aquariums) to supply oxygen is utilized to forcefully pump air into the irrigation bottle. It has an electromagnetic motor that moves a lever attached to a collapsible rubber cap. There is an inlet with a valve that sucks in atmospheric air as the cap expands. On collapsing, the valve closes and the air is pushed into an intravenous (IV) line connected to the infusion bottle. The lever vibrates at a frequency of approximately 10 oscillations per second. The electromagnetic motor is weak enough to stop once the pressure in the closed system (i.e. the AC) reaches about 50 mm Hg. The rubber cap ceases to expand at this pressure level. A micropore air filter is used between the air pump and the infusion bottle so that the air pumped into the bottle is clean of particulate matter

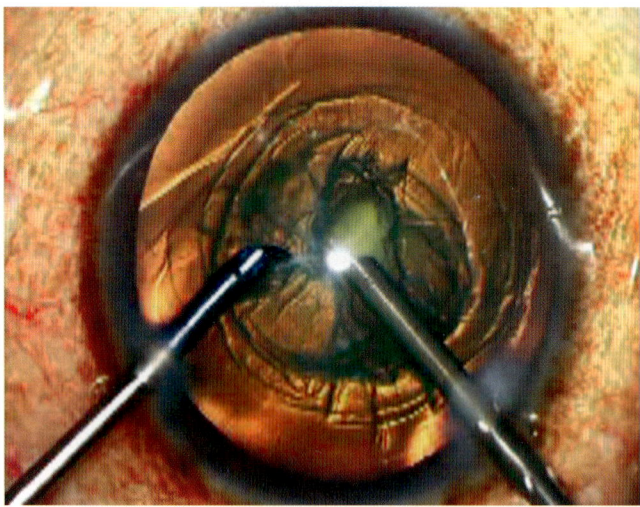

Figure 28.7 Microphakonit being performed with a 0.7 mm irrigating chopper and a 0.7 mm sleeveless phaco needle

one can use for cataract surgery. With time, one would be able to go smaller with better instruments and devices. The problem at present is the IOL. We have to get good quality IOLs going through sub-1 mm cataract surgical incisions so that the real benefit of microphakonit can be given to the patient.

DISCUSSION

Cataract surgery has witnessed great advancements in surgical technique, foldable IOLs and phaco technology. This has made possible easier and safer cataract extraction utilizing smaller incision. With the advent of the latest IOL technology which enables implantation through ultrasmall incisions, it is clear that this will soon replace routine phacoemulsification through the standard 3.2 mm incisions. The ThinOptX® IOL design is based on the Fresnel principle. This was designed by Wayne Callahan (USA). Flexibility and good memory are important characteristics of the lens. It is manufactured from hydrophilic acrylic materials and is available in a range from –25 to +30 with the lens thickness ranging from 30 μm up to 350 μm. One of the authors (Am. A) has modified the lens further by reducing the optic size to 5 mm to go through a smaller incision. The lens is now undergoing clinical-trials in Europe and the USA.

In this study, no intraoperative complications were encountered during CCC, phacoemulsification, cortical aspiration or IOL lens insertion in any of the cases. The mean phacoemulsification time was 0.66 minutes. Previous series by the same authors showed more than 300 eyes where cataract surgery was successfully performed using the sub-1 mm incision.[3] Our experience and that of several other surgeons suggests that with existing phacoemulsification technology, it is possible to perform phacoemulsification through ultra-small incisions without significant complications.[2-6] In a recent study from Japan, Tsuneoka and associates[6] used a sleeveless phaco tip to perform bimanual phacoemulsification in 637 cataractous eyes. All cataracts were safely removed by these authors through an incision of 1.4 mm or smaller that was widened for IOL insertion, without a case of thermal burn and with few intraoperative complications. Furthermore, ongoing research for the development of laser probes[7,8] cold phaco, and microphaco confirms the interest of leading ophthalmologists and manufacturers in the direction of ultra-small incisional cataract surgery (Fine IN, Olson RJ, Osher RH, Steinert RF. Cataract technology makes strides. Ophthalmology Times, December 1, 2001, pp 12-15).

The postoperative course was uneventful in all the cases. The IOL was well centered in the capsular bag. There were no significant corneal burns in any of the cases. Final visual outcome was satisfactory with 4 of the eyes having a BCVA of 20/30 or better. One eye that had dry ARMD showed an improvement in BCVA from 20/200 to 20/60. Thus, the lens was found to have satisfactory optical performance within the eye. In our study, the mean astigmatism on topographical analysis was 0.98 ± 0.62 D (range 0.5 to 1.8 D) preoperatively, 1.1 ± 0.61 D (range 0.6 to 1.9 D) on postoperative day 1 and

1.02 ± 0.64 D (range 0.3 to 1.7 D) by 3 months postoperatively. **Figures 28.8A and B** showing a comparison of the pre- and postoperative astigmatism indicate clearly that Phakonit with an ultrathin 5 mm rollable IOL is virtually astigmatically neutral. **Figure 28.9A and B** depicting the topography comparison in different surgical periods show clearly the virtual astigmatic neutrality of the procedure and stability throughout the postoperative course.

There is an active ongoing attempt to develop newer IOLs that can go through smaller and smaller incisions. Phakonit ThinOptX® modified ultrathin rollable IOL is the first prototype IOL which can go through sub-1.4 mm incisions. Research is also in progress to manufacture this IOL using hydrophobic acrylic biomaterials combined with square-edged optics to minimize posterior capsule opacification.

CONCLUSION

Phakonit with an ultrathin 5 mm optic rollable IOL implantation is a safe and effective technique of cataract extraction, the greatest advantage of this technique being virtual astigmatic neutrality.

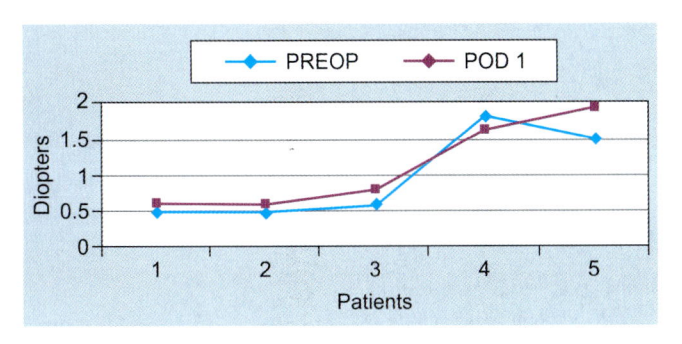

Figure 28.8A Comparison of pre- and postoperative day 1 cylinder

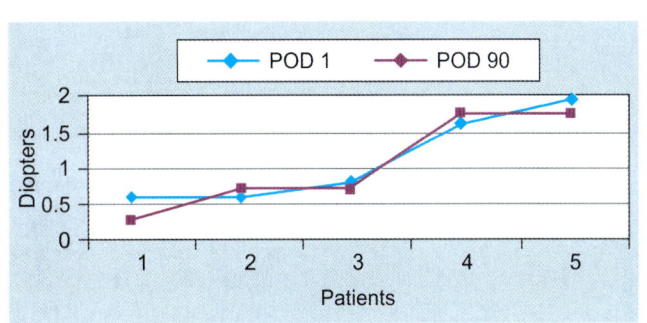

Figure 28.8B Comparison of 1 day postoperative and 3 months postoperative astigmatism

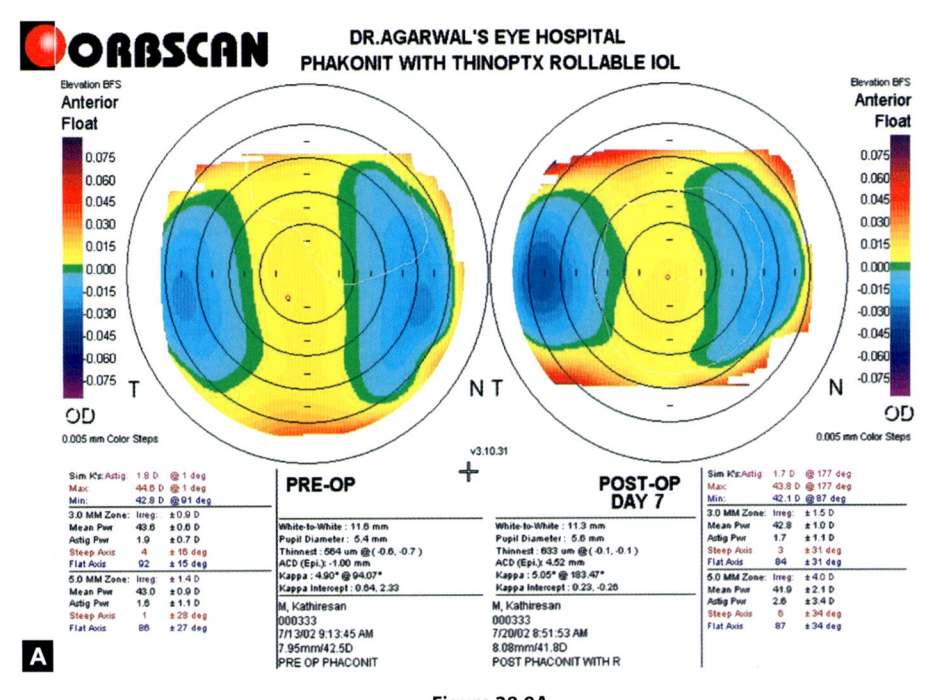

Figure 28.9A

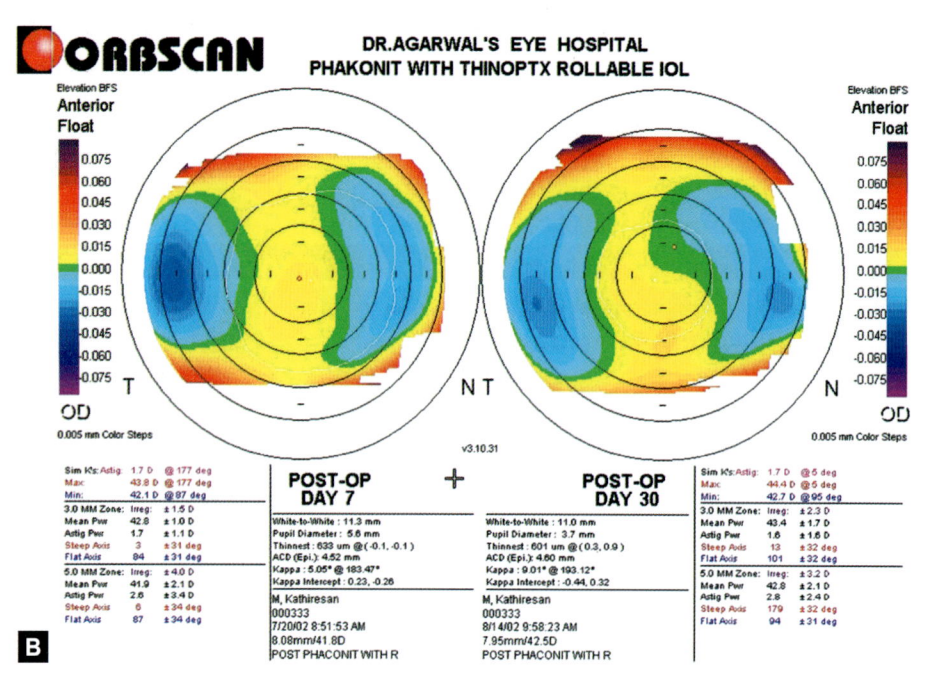

Figures 28.9A and B Topographical comparison during different surgical periods

REFERENCES

1. Apple DJ, Auffarth GU, Peng Q, Visessook N. Foldable Intraocular Lenses. Evolution, Clinicopathologic Correlations, Complications. Thorofare, NJ, Slack , Inc., 2000.
2. Agarwal A, Agarwal A, Agarwal S, et al. Phakonit: Phacoemulsification through a 0.9 mm corneal incision. J Cataract Refract Surg. 2001;27:1548-52.
3. Agarwal A, Agarwal A, Agarwal A, et al. Phakonit: Lens removal through a 0.9 mm incision. (Letter). J Cataract Refract Surg. 2001; 27:1531-2.
4. Agarwal A, Agarwal S, Agarwal A. Phakonit and laser phaconit: Lens removal through a 0.9 mm incision. In: Agarwal S, Agarwal A, Sachdev MS, Fine IH, Agarwal A (Eds) Phacoemulsification, laser cataract surgery and foldable IOLs. New Delhi, India, Jaypee Brothers Medical Publishers (P) Ltd; 2000.pp.204-16.
5. Tsuneoka H, Shiba T, Takahashi Y. Feasibility of ultrasound cataract surgery with a 1.4 mm incision. J Cataract Refract Surg. 2001;27:934-40.
6. Tsuneoka H, Shiba T, Takahashi Y. Ultrasonic phacoemulsification using a 1.4 mm incision: Clinical results. J Cataract Refract Surg. 2002;28:81-6.
7. Kanellpoupolos AJ. A prospective clinical evaluation of 100 consecutive laser cataract procedures using the Dodick photolysis neodymium: Yittrium-aluminum-garnet system. Ophthalmology. 2001;108:1-6.
8. Dodick JM. Laser phacolysis of the human cataractous lens. Dev Ophthalmol. 1991;22:58-64.

Chapter 29

Glued IOL Position: An OCT Assessment

Dhivya Ashok Kumar (India), Amar Agarwal (India)

BACKGROUND

Fibrin glue, which has been used for various indications in ophthalmology, has been known to provide good surgical adhesion.[1-3] Glued IOL technique is one such indication where tissue glue has been used primarily for IOL implantation.[4] Anatomical position similar to a natural lens gives it an additional advantage as compared to the anterior chamber intraocular lenses. Maggi and Maggi pioneered the initial sutureless IOL fixation in eyes with deficient posterior capsule in 1997.[5] In 2006, Gabor Scharioth introduced transscleral needle fixation of IOL in such eyes with deficient capsules.[6] In 2007, Agarwal et al. introduced the glued IOL technique, which was Glued intrascleral haptic fixation of a posterior chamber IOL.[4] In this chapter, we have analyzed the position of glued IOL with high speed anterior segment optical coherence tomography (OCT).

TECHNIQUE

Under peribulbar anesthesia, localized peritomy at the site of exit of the IOL haptics is done. Two partial thickness limbal-based scleral flaps about 2.5 × 2.5 mm are created exactly 180° diagonally (use scleral marker) apart. Infusion cannula or anterior chamber maintainer is inserted. One can use 20 G or 23 G trocar cannula for infusion. Positioning of the infusion cannula should be in the pars plana about 3 mm from the limbus. Anterior segment surgeons can use an anterior chamber maintainer. Two straight sclerotomies with a 20 G needle are made about 1 to 1.5 mm from the limbus under the existing scleral flaps. This is followed by vitrectomy via pars plana or anterior route to remove all vitreous traction. A corneoscleral tunnel incision is then prepared for introducing the IOL in case of a nonfoldable IOL or corneal incision with keratome in case of an injectable three-piece foldable IOL.

The IOL cartridge is passed into the anterior chamber. The glued IOL forceps (Microsurgical Technology, MST, USA) is then passed through the sclerotomy and the tip of the haptic is grasped **(Figures 29.1A to D)**. The IOL is then gradually injected into the eye. Once the optic is unfolded, the glued IOL forceps is used to pull the haptic out and externalize it. The haptic is then held by an assistant or silicone tires. The surgeon now flexes the second haptic into the anterior chamber into the jaws of the glued IOL forceps introduced through the second sclerotomy using the handshake technique **(Figures 29.2A to F)**.[7] This haptic is also thus externalized. A limbus parallel scleral tunnel is made with a 26 G bent needle on either side at the point of haptic externalization. The haptic tips are then tucked into the intralamellar scleral tunnel.

Air is then injected into the anterior chamber and the fluid from the infusion cannula is turned off. This helps to prevent hypotony and also keeps the area of the glue application dry. The reconstituted fibrin glue (Tisseel, Baxter, California, USA) prepared is injected under the scleral flaps. Local pressure is given over the flaps for about 10 to 20s. Corneoscleral wound is closed with 10-0 monofilament nylon in non-foldable three-piece IOL, and in case of foldable IOL, the corneal incision is sealed with fibrin glue. The conjunctiva is closed with the fibrin glue in all eyes irrespective of the type of IOL.

ANTERIOR SEGMENT OPTICAL COHERENCE TOMOGRAPHY

Cross-sectional imaging of the IOL was done with Visante anterior segment OCT (Carl Zeiss Meditec, Dublin, California, USA). Corneal high resolution quad mode was used. Images were taken in 4 axes, namely 180° to 0°, 270° to 90°, 225° to 45° and 315° to 135°. The optics of the IOL were imaged and referred with the position of iris. The images were then analyzed with the caliper tools in the software of AS OCT for iris vault. D1 and D2 were measured as the distances in mm between the iris margin and the anterior surface of IOL optic **(Figure 29.3)**. The mean pupil size was kept as 6 to 7 mm in all the eyes by pharmacological dilatation (0.5% tropicamide). For analysis purpose, OCT images in 180° to 0° (horizontal) and 270° to 90° (vertical) axes has been utilized. All patients underwent refraction (manifest and autorefractometer), retinoscopy, best corrected spectacle vision (BCVA) (Snellen's distant vision acuity charts) and corneal topography (Orbscan, Bausch & Lomb). Slit lamp examination (Topcon slit lamp imaging system, 25X magnification) was performed and the IOL position was clinically examined by experienced ophthalmologist. Ocular residual astigmatism (ORA) using Alpins method[8] was determined and graphical correlation has been performed.

The inclusion criteria were the minimum 5 years follow-up, preoperative indications of surgical aphakia, posterior capsular rupture and subluxated cataract and the patient cooperation

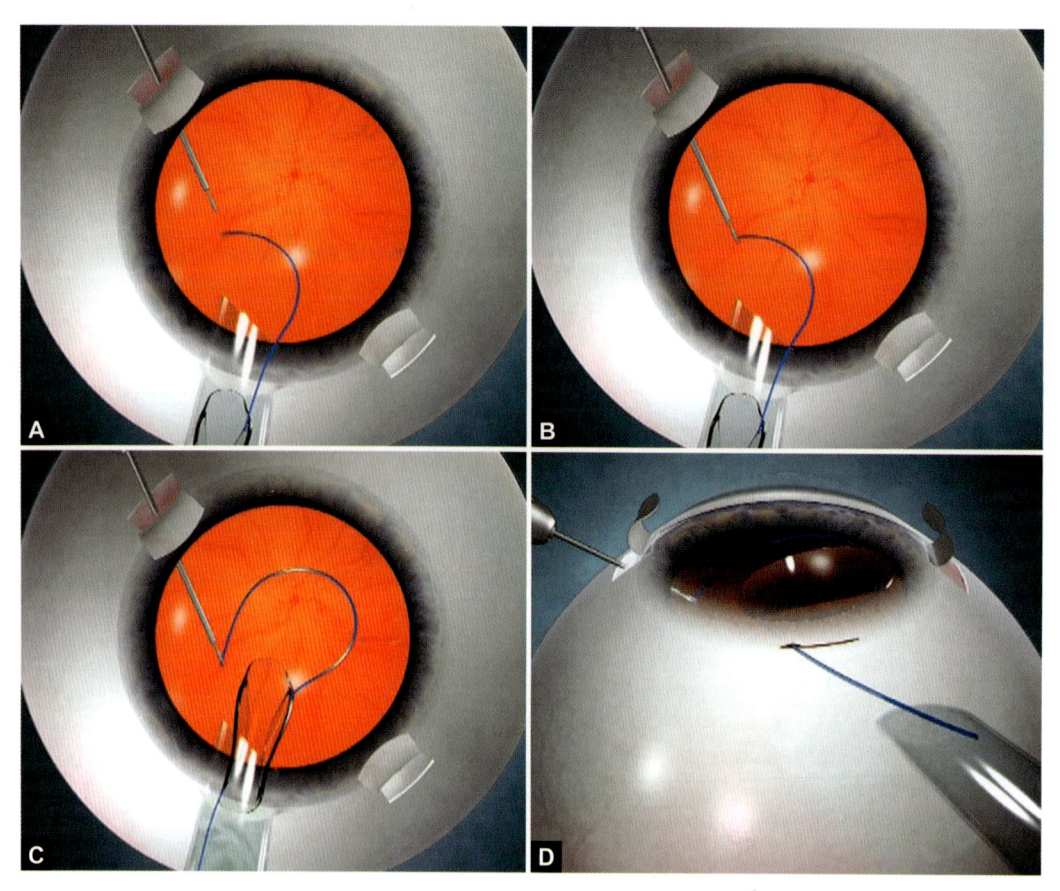

Figures 29.1A to D (A) Haptic outside the cartridge. Glued-IOL forceps ready to grasp the haptic tip; (B) Haptic tip caught with the forceps; (C) Injection of the IOL continued until the optic unfolds inside the anterior chamber; (D) Haptic externalization started

for OCT examination. Patients of pediatric age group and uncooperative for examination were excluded.

IOL TILT ESTIMATION IN OCT

Using MatLab version 7.1, the corneal high resolution images were analyzed.[9] A straight line (L) passing through the iris pigment epithelium on either side of the image was marked as the reference line. A second line (*l*) passing through the horizontal axis of the IOL was marked.[10,11] The slopes were calculated for both the straight lines (**L,** *l*). Slope ratio was obtained by dividing slope of IOL by slope of iris. When the reference line along the iris (L) and the IOL optic (l) were parallel, the optic was not considered to be tilted. A difference of more than 100 microns between the 2 positions (D1 and D2) was considered optic tilt.[11]

IOL OPTIC POSITION IN GLUED IOL

The calculated mean slope of the IOL was 0.009 ± 0.1 and the slope of iris was 0.002 ± 0.1 in 180° to 0° (horizontal) axis. The calculated mean slope of the IOL was 0.008 ± 0.12 and the slope of iris was 0.008 ± 0.10 in 90° to 270° (vertical) axes. There was

significant correlation of slope of the iris with the IOL in both horizontal ($p = 0.000$, $r = 0.854$) and vertical axes ($p = 0.000$, $r = 0.880$) **(Figure 29.4)**. The mean distance D1 and D2 was 0.94 ± 0.36 mm and 0.95 ± 0.36 mm respectively. There was no difference between the D1 ($p = 0.131$) and D2 ($p = -0.181$) between the rigid IOL and foldable IOL groups **(Figure 29.4)**. Both the surfaces of the **(Figure 29.5)** optic were seen in 50 eyes (83.3%). Ten eyes (16.6%) had interrupted reflection from either of the surfaces **(Figure 29.5)**. Ten (16.6%) out of 60 eyes had pigment dispersed on the IOL surface. This was seen hyper-reflective spots on the optic **(Figure 29.6)**. Out of 10 eyes with pigment dispersion, 6 were rigid and 4 were foldable IOL. Iris adhesion to the optic was seen in 4 eyes (6.6%). Out of 60 eyes, 21 eyes (35%) had optic tilt detected on OCT and 39 eyes (65%) had no optic tilt **(Figure 29.7)**. There was no significant association between the IOL tilt and BCVA noted (chi square test, $p = 0.468$).

OCULAR RESIDUAL ASTIGMATISM

The mean ocular residual astigmatism (ORA) was 0.53 ± 0.5 D. There was significant correlation between the ORA and total astigmatism ($r = 0.620$, $p = 0.000$). There was no correlation

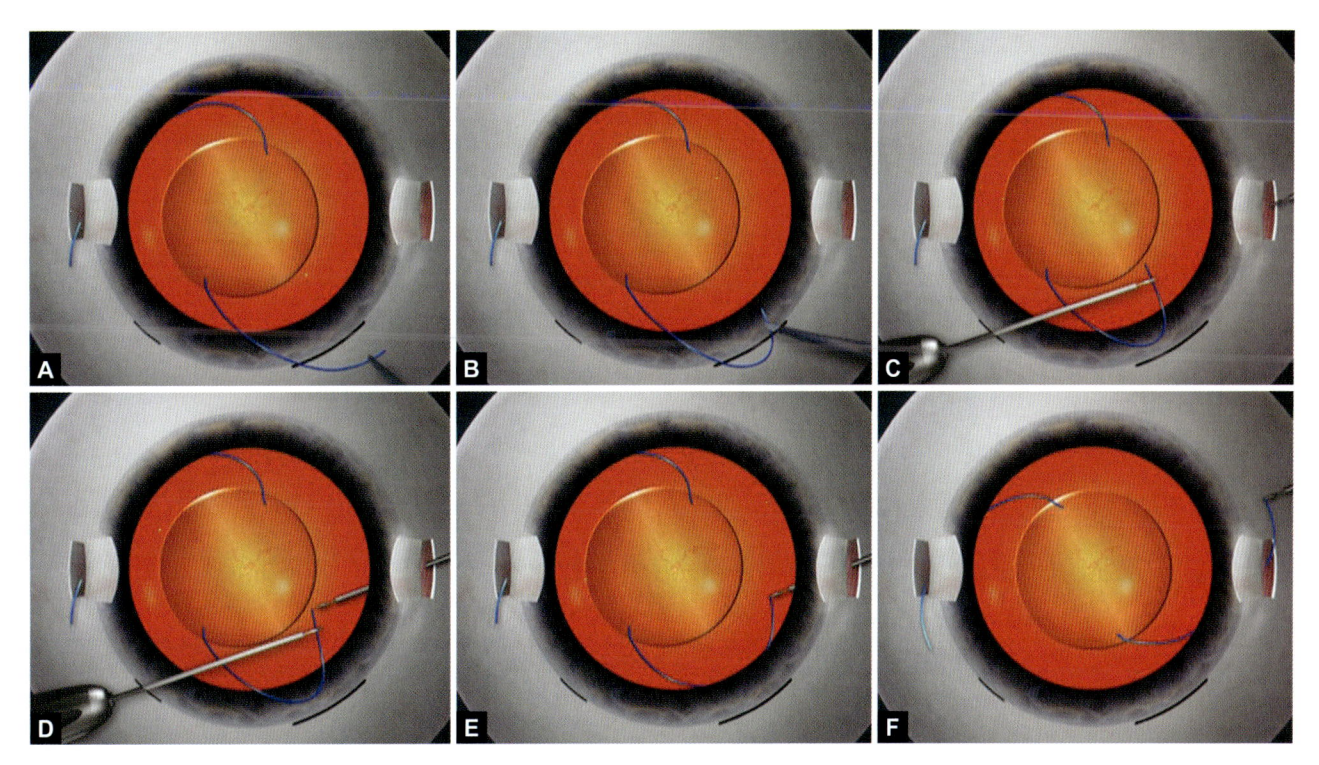

Chapter 29: Glued IOL Position: An OCT Assessment

Figures 29.2A to F (A) Trailing haptic caught with the first glued-IOL forceps; (B) Haptic flexed into the anterior chamber; (C) Haptic transferred from first forceps to the second forceps using the handshake technique. The second forceps is passed through the side port; (D) First forceps is passed through the sclerotomy under the scleral flap. Haptic is transferred from the second forceps back to the first using the handshake technique. Haptic tip is grasped with the first forceps; (E) Haptic is pulled toward the sclerotomy; (F) Haptic externalized

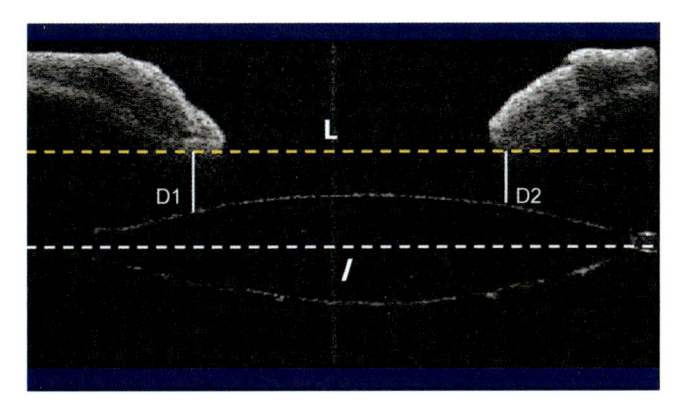

Figure 29.3 Optical coherence tomography image showing the method of intraocular lens (IOL) optic position evaluation. L: Slope of iris, l: Slope of IOL, D1, D2: Distance of IOL from iris

between the IOL slope and the ORA (r = 0.045, p = 0.730). There was also no correlation of ORA with position of IOL at D1 (p = 0.494) and D2 (p = 0.791). There was no association with ORA and optic tilt (p = 0.326). There was no significant difference in the ORA between the eyes with and without optic tilt (p = 0.762). The mean postoperative BCVA was 0.63 ± 0.2. There was a weak correlation (P = 0.013; r = −0.363) between the ORA and BCVA **(Figure 29.8)**. There was no significant correlation of optic position at D1 (p = 0.729) and D2 (p = 0.574) with BCVA. There was no correlation between the slope ratio and BCVA (p = 0.674).

SCLERAL APPOSITION WITH GLUE

Fibrin glue has been shown to provide airtight closure and by the time the fibrin starts degrading, surgical adhesions would have occurred in the scleral bed. This is shown in our follow-up anterior segment optical coherence tomography (OCT) images in which postoperative perfect scleral flap adhesion **(Figure 29.9)** was observed as early as day 1 and was well sealed at 6 weeks.[4]

GLUED IOL IN VARIOUS INDICATIONS

Glued IOL can be performed in eyes with postsurgical or traumatic aphakia. Eyes with subluxated cataract and intraoperative posterior capsular tear or zonular dialysis hindering IOL implantation are ideal candidate for glued intraocular lens.[4,12] Congenital conditions like ectopia lentis and aniridia with lens subluxation are also indications for glued

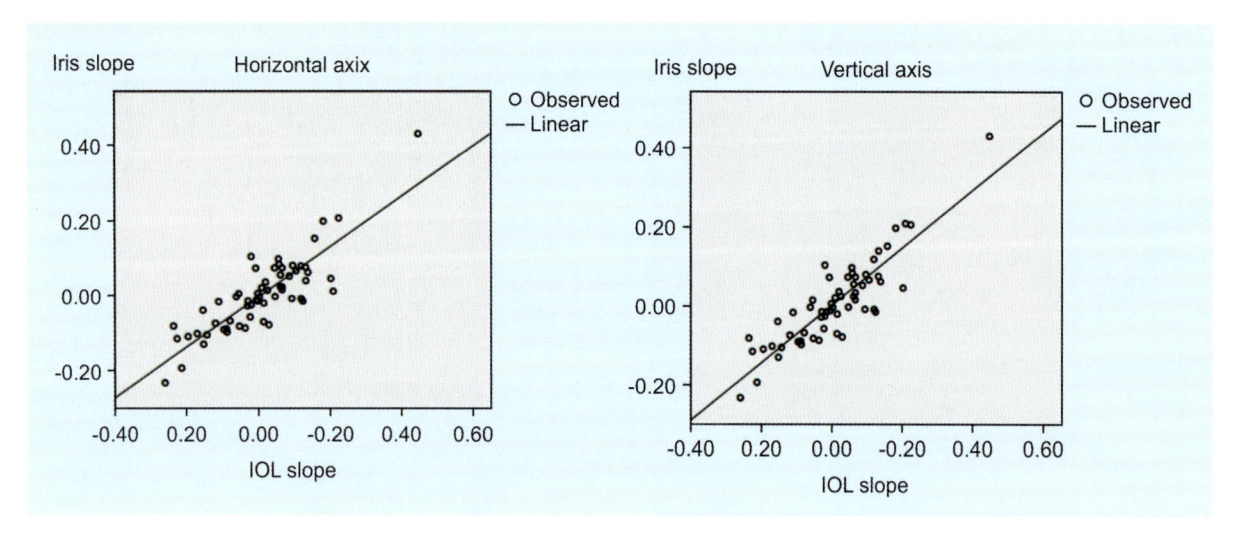

Figure 29.4 Scatter plot showing the correlation of slope of iris and IOL

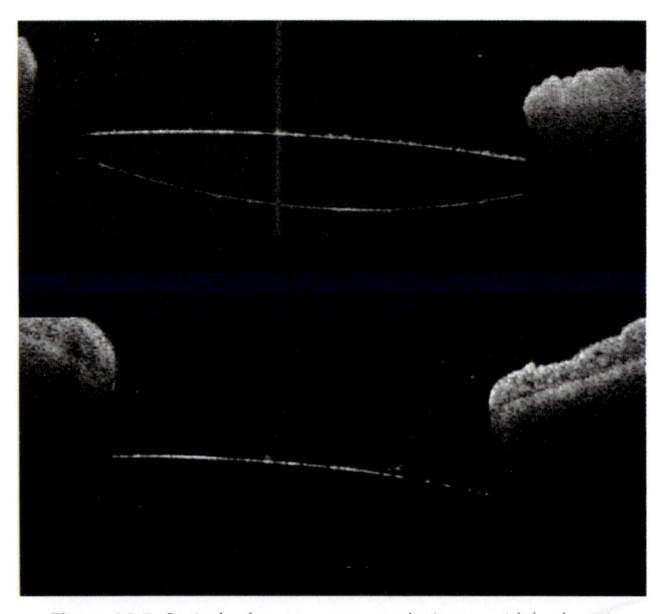

Figure 29.5 Optical coherence tomography image with both optic surfaces clear (above) and only anterior surface clear (below)

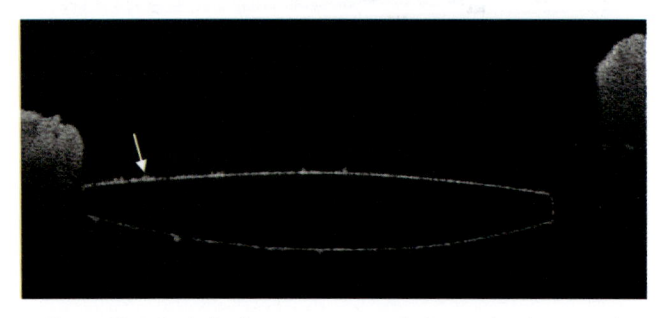

Figure 29.6 Optical coherence tomography image showing an optic surface with pigment dispersion (arrow)

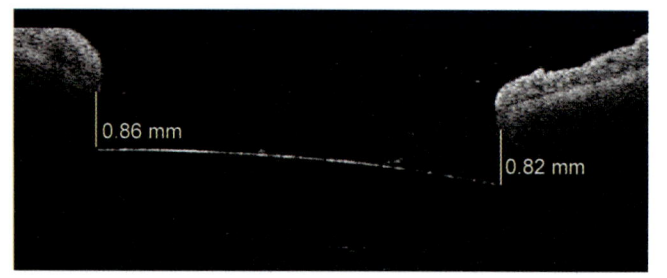

Figure 29.7 Optical coherence tomography image showing a rigid IOL implanted with no tilt

IOL implantation.[13,14] Glued IOL can be performed in eyes with postoperative IOL dislocation either anterior or posterior due to weak zonules **(Figure 29.10 and 11)**.[15]

COMPARISON WITH MICROSCOPIC TILT IN ULTRASOUND BIOMICROSCOPY

In the OCT study, we noted that 65% of the eyes had no microscopic tilt and 35% had microscopic tilt which was not significant to cause vision loss. The incidence of optic tilt seen in this analysis has been noted to be higher than the one with UBM (17.4%) probably due to the greater axial resolution of OCT.[9] The limitation of OCT is that it needs to each time dilate the pupil for IOL visualization as the iris pigment epithelium prevents infrared wavelength transmission. However, OCT offers the noncontact method of evaluating the IOL position with higher resolution **(Figure 29.11)** as compared to UBM. Haptic visualization and pars plicata or plana sclerotomy examination delineation.

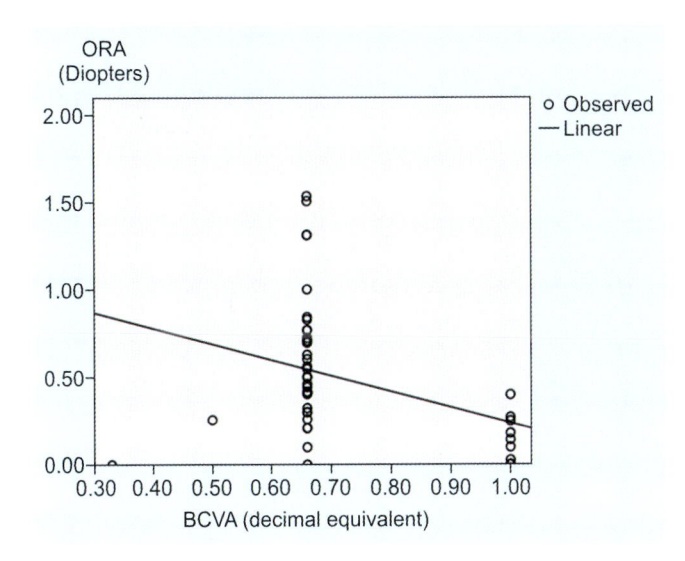

Chapter 29: Glued IOL Position: An OCT Assessment 309

Figure 29.8 Scatter plot showing the correlation of ocular residual astigmatism (ORA) with best corrected visual acuity (BCVA)

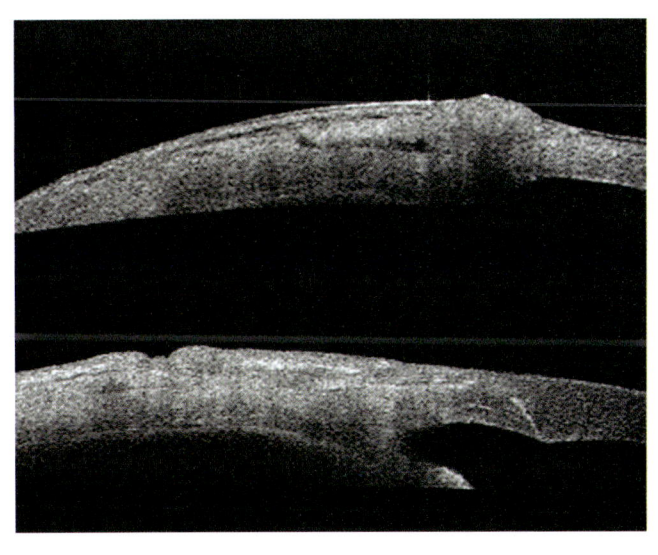

Figure 29.9 OCT section at the scleratomy site showing the flaps. The scleral flap as seen by anterior segment OCT on day 1 (above) and well-sealed scleral flaps at 6 weeks (below)

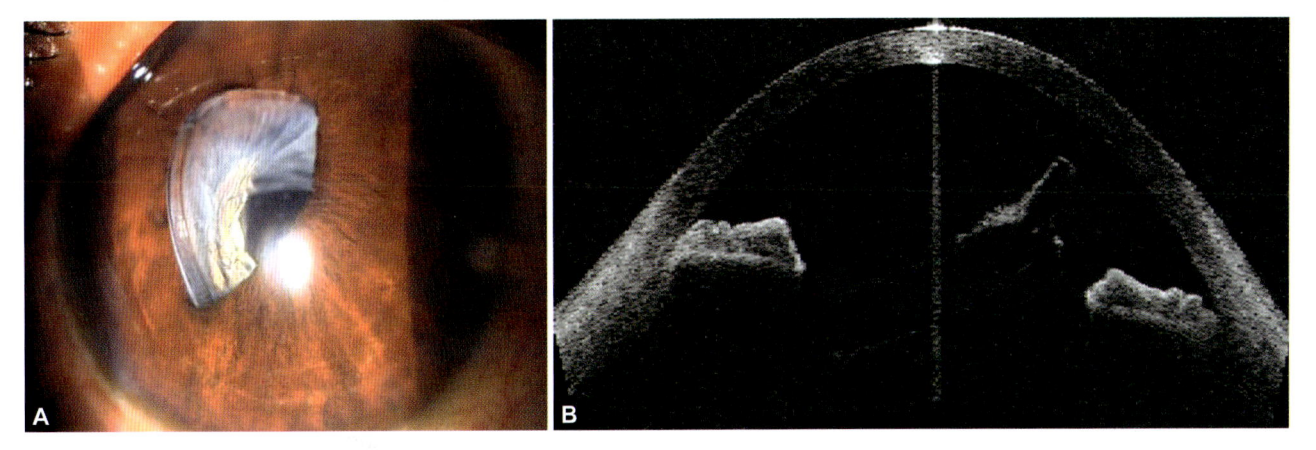

Figures 29.10A and B (A) Partial anterior subluxation of posterior chamber IOL; and (B) The corresponding OCT image

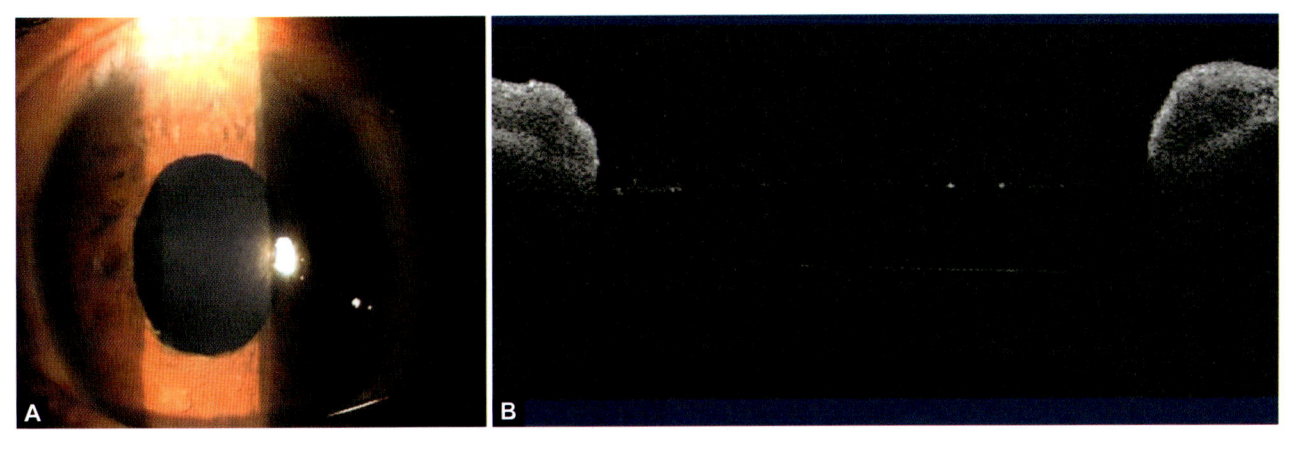

Figures 29.11A and B (A) Same patient postoperatively after luxated IOL removal and transscleral glued IOL fixation performed; and (B) The corresponding OCT image showing the glued IOL

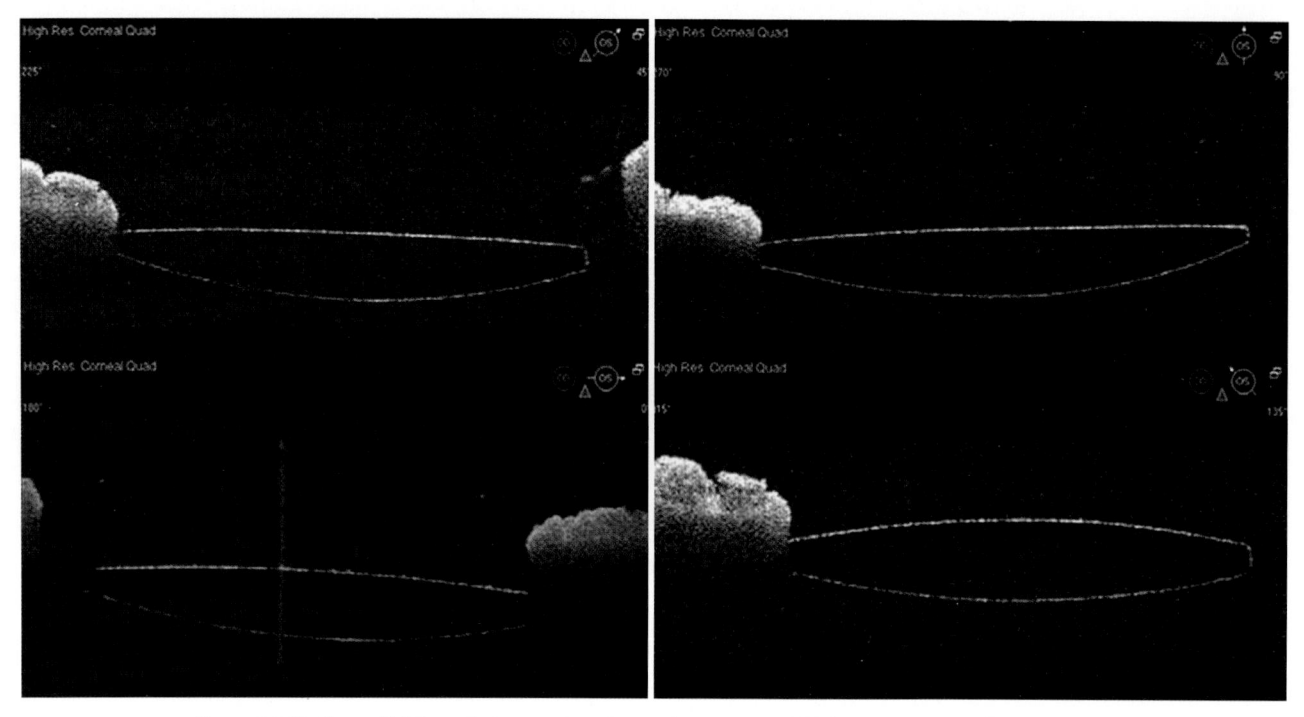

Figure 29.12 Corneal high resolution quad mode anterior segment OCT showing a 360° well-centered IOL

GLUED IOL VERSUS SUTURED SCLERAL FIXATED IOL

In the conventional sutured transscleral-fixated PC IOL technique, IOL tilt occurs because of the torque created by asymmetric suture placement on the IOL. Teichmann and Teichmann studied the combinations of suture configurations and recommended looping the sutures symmetrically through the opposing eyelets.[16] Theoretically, tilt also can be eliminated with radial suture placement. However, this is anatomically undesirable because one suture will exit through the ciliary body in transscleral suture fixation. Asymmetric attachment of the sutures to the haptics; failure to place the needles through the sclera 180° apart; and suture loosening, breakage, or slippage on the haptics can also result in IOL tilt with suture-fixated PC IOLs. However, with glued IOLs, there is no anchoring of haptics with sutures; hence, there are no suture or haptic problems. In the suture-fixated PC IOL technique, the suture needle is blindly passed using the ab externo method. However, in the glued IOL method, the haptics directly come through the sclerotomies made in the measured position on direct visualization. The exact anatomic positioning of the sclerotomy is an important step in the glued IOL method.

Figure 29.12 shows corneal high resolution quad mode anterior segment OCT showing a 360° well-centered IOL.

CONCLUSION

Though there was minimal difference in the axial position of the glued IOL with respect to the normal in-the bag IOL, there was no significant association between the optic position and BCVA noted. We noticed no difference between the foldable and nonfoldable type of IOLs with respect to the iris in axial position. Glued IOL had shown good stability on long-term with no significant IOL tilt.

REFERENCES

1. Hovanesian JA, Karageozian VH. Watertight cataract incision closure using fibrin tissue adhesive. J Cataract Refract Surg. 2007;33:1461-3.
2. Lagoutte FM, Gauthier L, Comte PRM. A fibrin sealant for perforated and preperforated corneal ulcers. Br J Ophthalmol. 1989;73:757-61.
3. Grewing R, Mester U. Fibrin sealant in the management of complicated hypotony after trabeculectomy. Ophthalmic Surg Lasers. 1997;28:124-7.
4. Agarwal A, Kumar DA, Jacob S, et al. Fibrin glue-assisted sutureless posterior chamber intraocular lens implantation in eyes with deficient posterior capsules. J Cataract Refract Surg. 2008;34:1433-8.
5. Maggi R, Maggi C. Sutureless scleral fixation of intraocular lenses. J Cataract Refract Surg. 1997;23:1289-94.

6. Gabor SG, Pavilidis MM. Sutureless intrascleral posterior chamber intraocular lens fixation. J Cataract Refract Surg. 2007; 33:1851-4.
7. Agarwal A, Jacob S, Kumar DA, et al. Handshake technique for glued intrascleral haptic fixation of a posterior chamber intraocular lens. J Cataract Refract Surg. 2013;39:317-22.
8. Alpins NA, Goggin M. Practical astigmatism analysis for refractive outcomes in cataract and refractive surgery. Surv Ophthalmol. 2004;49:109-22.
9. Kumar DA, Agarwal A, Packialakshmi S, Agarwal A. In vivo analysis of glued intraocular lens position with ultrasound biomicroscopy. J Cataract Refract Surg. 2013;39:1017-22.
10. Kumar DA, Agarwal A, Prakash G, et al. Evaluation of intraocular lens tilt with anterior segment optical coherence tomography. Am J Ophthalmol. 2011;151:406-12.
11. Loya N, Lichter H, Barash D, et al. Posterior chamber intraocular lens implantation after capsular tear: ultrasound biomicroscopy evaluation. J Cataract Refract Surg. 2001;27:1423-7.
12. Kumar DA, Agarwal A. Glued intraocular lens: a major review on surgical technique and results. Curr Opin Ophthalmol. 2013;24:21-9.
13. Kumar DA, Agarwal A, Prakash D, et al. Glued intrascleral fixation of posterior chamber intraocular lens in children. Am J Ophthalmol. 2012;153:594-601.
14. Kumar DA, Agarwal A, Jacob S, Lamba M, Packialakshmi S, Meduri A. Combined surgical management of capsular and iris deficiency with glued intraocular lens technique. J Refract Surg. 2013;29(5):342-7.
15. Nair V, Kumar DA, Prakash G, Jacob S, Agarwal A, Agarwal A. Bilateral spontaneous in-the-bag anterior subluxation of PCIOL managed with glued IOL technique: A case report. Eye Contact Lens. 2009;35(4):215-7.
16. Teichmann KD, Teichmann IAM. The torque and tilt gamble. J Cataract Refract Surg. 1997;23:413-8.

INDEX

Page numbers followed by *t* refer to table and *f* refer to figure

A

Aberration 193, 209
  higher order 200, 204, 284
  map, total order 284
  spherical 194, 211
Aberrometer 209
  systems 184
Aberrometry 168, 169, 262*f*
Aberropia 175, 200
  acquired 207
  classification of 207*t*, 208*t*
  congenital 207
  higher range 208
  lower range 208
Ablation
  design 191
  large 231
  management of 239
  surgical correction of 240
  topo-guided customized 219
Agarwal's phakonit irrigating
    chopper 300*f*
Alpins method 169
Angle opening distance 119
Anterior lamellar keratoplasty,
    automated 262
Arcuate keratotomy 251
Astigmatism 172, 294
  irregular 251, 252
  measurement of 168
  second-order 212*f*
Axial diopter displays 10*f*
Axial irregularity map 13*f*
Axial map 10
Axial power map 43*f*
  demonstrating regular astigmatism 43*f*

B

Back-scatter reflection 34*f*
Band scale, normal 36*f*, 90*f*, 91*f*
Bausch and Lomb zywave
    aberrometer 210*f*
Bent cornea 69, 91
Best corrected visual acuity 175, 192, 200,
    251, 300, 309
Best fit sphere 31, 43, 62, 67, 85, 91
Best spectacle corrected visual acuity 194,
    196, 200, 210
Big-bubble technique 139, 140*f*
Bowman's layer 140
Bowman's membrane 65, 121
Bowtie astigmatism, normal 285, 285*f*

C

Cataract 280
  evaluation 105
  incisions 251
  surgery 293, 299
Central cornea, globular
    protrusion of 141*f*
Chamber depth, anterior 126, 267
Chamber evaluation, anterior 107
Chamber phakic lens simulation,
    anterior 109
Collamer lens, implantable 264
Coma 194
Computer assisted videokeratography 168
Confocal microscopy 137*f*
Contact lens 5*f*
  fitting application 14
  management 262
Continuous curvilinear
    capsulorhexis 299
Cornea 291
  astigmatic 293*f*
  curvature of 18*t*
  normal 46*f*, 292
Corneal aberrations 160*f*, 194, 196, 197
  analysis of 192, 194
  higher order 187
Corneal astigmatism 173*f*
Corneal asymmetry, central 87*f*
Corneal central ectasia, bilateral 24*f*
Corneal coma aberration after LASIK 195
Corneal curvature, anterior 224
Corneal ectasia 83
  after LASIK 125*f*
  post-LASIK 83
Corneal ectatic degeneration 223*f*
Corneal ectatic disorders 140
Corneal elevation
  anterior 40, 46*f*, 71
  posterior 40, 43, 71, 225
Corneal herpetic keratopathy, advanced 7*f*
Corneal high resolution quad mode
    anterior segment OCT 310*f*
Corneal hysteresis 228
Corneal inflammation 130
Corneal keratoplasty 139, 140*f*
Corneal maps 9
Corneal pachymetry 260
Corneal power 40
Corneal refractive surgery 252
Corneal scar 120*f*, 121*f*
Corneal spherical aberrations 191
Corneal thickness 40, 71, 130, 229
Corneal topography 3, 113*f*, 120*f*, 145*f*, 155,
    168, 186, 189*f*, 252, 267
  axial map 148*f*
  computerized 190
  in cataract surgery 291
  machine, placido type 292*f*
  map 155
  system 27, 190
Corneal ulcer 131*f*
  healed 133*f*
Corneal wavefront
  analysis 190
  evaluation 109
  guided
    laser surgery for correction of eye
      aberrations 187
    refractive surgery 190
    retreatments for corneas 195
  maps 109*f*
Correction index 169
Crystalens implanted in eye 129*f*
Crystalline lens 126
Cyclo-torsion 220

D

Deep anterior lamellar keratoplasty 139,
    234, 276
Deep corneal infiltration with
    necrosis 131*f*
Descemet and Bowman's layers 137*f*
Descemet's membrane 65, 139
Dry eye syndrome 194

E

Ectasia 62*f*
Ectatic disease, subclinical 228
Efkarpides's orbscan criteria 66*t*
Elevation map 246*f*
Elevation topology 46*f*
Elliptical elevation map 11
Endothelial abscess 133*f*
Endothelial clearance 125
Endothelial damage 281
Endothelial inflammation 131*f*
Epithelial ingrowth after LASIK
    enhancement 123*f*
Equivalent K readings 107
Excimer laser
  assisted anterior lamellar
    keratoplasty 235
  surgical techniques with 255
Extracapsular cataract extraction 294

F
Flap tear, Scheimpflug image of 95*f*
Forme fruste keratoconus 226*f*

G
Global pachymetric map 114*f*, 115*f*
Gonioscopy 267

H
Hartmann-Shack aberrometer 184*f*, 209*f*
Hartmann-Shack principle 214
Height map 10
Higher-order aberrations, impact of 187
Humphrey elevation map 22*f*
Hyperopic ICL 265

I
ICL
    implantation 270
    in myopia 272
    power calculation 69*f*, 268
    sizing 267
Inflammation
    advanced 131
    early stages of 130
International standard scale 9
Intracorneal rings 139*f*, 141, 233
    implantation 138
    in keratectasia 234*f*
    segments 262
Intraocular lens (IOL) 147, 299, 307*f*
    calculation 82, 105
    foldable 294
Intraocular pressure 80
    internal 232
Irregular astigmatism
    evaluation of 252
    treatment of 255

K
K readings 63
Keratectasia
    iatrogenic 80, 81*f*
    treatments 232
Keratoconus 5*f*, 32*f*, 53*f*, 68*f*, 72*f*, 135, 224*f*, 228, 229*t*, 286, 286*f*
    central 13*f*
    detection, subclinical 66*t*
    disease 141*f*
    display 104*f*
    early 74, 77
    pachymetric map of 228*f*
    screening display 104
    subclinical 223
    with normal pachymetry 55*f*
Keratoglobus 141*f*, 142, 155
Keratometric mean power map 87*f*
Keratometry 4, 96, 252, 291
    readings, simulated 10
Keratoplasty 5*f*, 251
    penetrating 139, 233

Keratorefractive surgery, hyperopic 163
Keratoscopic raw image 9
Keratoscopy 4, 292

L
Lamellar keratoplasty 234, 235*f*
Laser *in situ* keratomileusis (LASIK) 161, 251, 252, 258, 298
    ablation, decentered 286, 288*f*
    complication of 140
    flap
        mapping 146
        thickness of 230*f*
Leukoma, adherent 133*f*

M
Marginal pellucid degeneration 140
Mean corneal curvature 66
Mean power map 41*f*
Mean power map demonstrating
    keratoconus 42*f*
    regular astigmatism 42*f*
Microincision cataract surgery 300
Microkeratome assisted anterior lamellar keratoplasty 234
Microphakonit 300
Modern videokeratoscopes 5*f*
Mydriasis 210
Myopia 146*f*, 147
Myopic ICL 265

N
Nidek OPD scan 283, 283*f*
Night glare 280
Night vision symptoms 193
    grading of 192*t*
Nonfoldable IOL implantation, topography of 295*f*
Normal cornea, topography of 14, 293*f*

O
Ocular higher order aberration 200
Ocular residual astigmatism 169, 305, 306
    correlation of 309*f*
OPD
    map and corneal topography map 216
    power map 215, 216
    scan 214
        principle 214
Optical coherence tomography (OCT) 111, 130, 135, 136*f*, 138*f*, 143, 305, 307, 307*f*, 308*f*
    anterior segment 130*f*, 131*f*, 305, 307
    in corneal infiltration 132
    in keratitis, role of 130
    in keratoconus
        evaluation 135
        screening 135
    visante anterior segment 111
Optical path difference scanning system 214

Orbscan 35, 40, 71, 76, 209, 226, 292, 292*f*
    corneal mapping in refractive surgery 61
    normal 54*f*
    slit scanning technology in 63*f*
    topography 226*f*

P
Pachymetry 65, 66, 69, 100
    map 42, 44*f*, 45*f*, 225, 246*f*
Pellucid marginal degeneration 56*f*, 140, 141*f*, 224*f*, 228, 286, 287*f*
Pentacam 95
    topography 227*f*
Phacoemulsification 299
Phakic intraocular lens 124, 264
    model, preoperative 126
Phakic posterior chamber lenses, original design of 265*f*
Phakonit 296
    with acritec IOL, topography of 298*f*
    with rollable IOL, topography of 297*f*
Photokeratoscopy 4
Photorefractive keratectomy 168, 251, 298
Pigment dispersion syndrome 126
Placido's disk 4, 27, 33, 40
Placido's method 5
Posterior elevation map 66, 85, 86*f*, 140*f*
Postfemtosecond laser-assisted *in situ* keratomileusis 146*f*, 147*f*
Post-LASIK
    corneal ectasia 140, 140*f*, 223, 235*f*
    iatrogenic ectasia 223
Postoperative wavescan aberrometry maps 241*f*
Postpenetrating keratoplasty stromal keratitis 131*f*
Power maps 42, 66, 85
Pre-enhancement axial curvature map 247*f*, 248*f*
Pre-existing posterior corneal abnormalities 76
Pre-LASIK topography 125*f*
Ptosis 7*f*
Pupillary diameter, measurement of 217

Q
Quad map 40, 40*f*, 45*f*, 62, 63*f*, 84*t*
Quadruple display map 24*f*

R
Radial axes, angulation of 225*f*
Radial keratotomy 251
Reduced corneal hysteresis 229
Refraction 224, 266
    stability of 267
Refractive laser surgery 168
Refractive map 11, 283
Refractive surgery 130, 143, 192
    wavefront guided 189
Reichert keratometer 155
Retinoscopy 252

Riboflavin-UVA crosslinking 233
Rigid gas permeable contact 233
Ring verification display 5*f*
Rollable intraocular lens 299
Rousch's orbscan criteria 66*t*

S

Scheimpflug image 157*f*
Scheimpflug line 95
Schwind eye-tech solutions 195, 197
Sclerokeratitis 132*f*
Skewed radial axis 225*f*
Snell's law 283
Spectral-domain optical coherence tomography 143, 144*f*, 145*f*, 146, 148, 148*f*, 149*f*
Sphere, second-order 212*f*
Spherical aberration 206*f*
Spherical equivalent refraction 194
Sub-Bowman's region 146
Superficial corneal surface quality, evolution of 258*f*

T

Three step rule 44, 46

Three-dimensional normal band scale map 78*f*
Three-dimensional posterior corneal elevation measured in microns 80*f*
Topographic and aberrometer guided laser 209
Topographic axial power map 140*f*
Topographic indices 99*t*
Topographic linked excimer laser ablation 255, 260
Topographic machines 22
Topographic scales 9
Topography 76, 96
 guided treatment 240
Topolink 261*f*
Toric ICL 265, 272
Total higher-order aberrations 194

U

Uncorrected visual acuity 192, 194, 196

V

Videokeratography, computerized 192, 292
Videokeratoscopy, computerized 5
Vision, quality of 219

Visual acuity 180*f*
 best spectacle-corrected decimal 195
 high contrast 200
 low contrast 200
 uncorrected decimal 195
Vogt's striae 137*f*

W

Wavefront 156
Wavefront aberration 192, 216*f*, 238
Wavefront analysis
 benefits of 185
 display, typical 170*f*
Wavefront
 devices, mechanisms of 184
 guided treatment 240
 irregular 185*f*
 map 216
 spherical 185*f*

Z

Zeiss humphrey systems 22*f*
Zernicke polynomial pyramid 158*f*
Zyoptix laser 209
Zywave raw data 56*f*